CULTURES COVERED IN THE TEXT

People of African American Heritage
The Amish
People of Appalachian Heritage
People of Arab Heritage
People of Chinese Heritage
People of Guatemalan Heritage
People of Egyptian Heritage
People of Filipino Heritage
People of French Canadian Heritage
People of German Heritage
People of Haitian Heritage
People of Iranian Heritage
People of Japanese Heritage
People of Jewish Heritage
People of Korean Heritage
People of Mexican Heritage
People of Russian Heritage
People of Polish Heritage
People of Thai Heritage

CULTURES COVERED ON THE DavisPlus WEB SITE (http://davisplus.fadavis.com)

People of Baltic Heritage: Estonians, Latvians, and Lithuanians
People of Brazilian Heritage
People of Greek Heritage
People of Cuban Heritage
People of Hindu Heritage
People of Irish Heritage
People of Italian Heritage
People of Puerto Rican Heritage
Navajo Indians
People of Turkish Heritage
People of Vietnamese Heritage

Transcultural Health Care

A Culturally Competent Approach
Third Edition

Larry D. Purnell, PhD, RN, FAAN
Professor
College of Health Sciences
University of Delaware
Newark, Delaware

Betty J. Paulanka, EdD, RN
Professor and Dean
College of Health Sciences
University of Delaware
Newark, Delaware

F. A. DAVIS COMPANY • Philadelphia

F. A. Davis Company
1915 Arch Street
Philadelphia, PA 19103
www.fadavis.com

Printed in the United States of America

Last digit indicates print number: 10 9 8 7 6 5 4 3 2 1

Acquisitions Editor: Jonathan D. Joyce
Associate Acquisitions Editor: Thomas A. Ciavarella
Director of Content Development: Darlene D. Pedersen
Art and Design Manager: Carolyn O'Brien

As new scientific information becomes available through basic and clinical research, recommended treatments and drug therapies undergo changes. The author(s) and publisher have done everything possible to make this book accurate, up to date, and in accord with accepted standards at the time of publication. The author(s), editors, and publisher are not responsible for errors or omissions or for consequences from application of the book, and make no warranty, expressed or implied, in regard to the contents of the book. Any practice described in this book should be applied by the reader in accordance with professional standards of care used in regard to the unique circumstances that may apply in each situation. The reader is advised always to check product information (package inserts) for changes and new information regarding dose and contraindications before administering any drug. Caution is especially urged when using new or infrequently ordered drugs.

Library of Congress Cataloging-in-Publication Data

Transcultural health care : a culturally competent approach / [edited by] Larry D. Purnell, Betty J. Paulanka. — 3rd ed.
       p. ; cm.
   Includes bibliographical references and index.
   ISBN-13: 978-0-8036-1865-7
   ISBN-10: 0-8036-1865-4
   1. Transcultural medical care—United States. 2. Transcultural medical care—Canada. I. Purnell, Larry D. II. Paulanka, Betty J.
   [DNLM: 1. Delivery of Health Care—North America. 2. Cross-Cultural Comparison—North America. 3. Ethnic Groups—North America. W 84 DA2 T7 2008]
   RA418.5.T73T73 2008
   362.1089--dc22   2007043727

Preface

The rise in concern for cultural competence has become one of the most important developments in American health care over the past decade. Medicine and health more generally have moved beyond their traditional equanimous approach of application of scientific rationality to clinical problems to one that promotes an easier integration of clinical science with empathy. This development has occurred with a rising tide of the diversity of the population of the United States. Some of this is driven by actual numbers of immigrants, but other dimensions of this awareness come from the visibility of the "new" ethnics and the waning of the social ideology of the melting pot. Beyond all of this is a younger generation that is much more attuned to diversity as part of their cultural landscape and their comfort with the globalization of perspectives resulting from technological and economic change.

From within health care, the advocacy for culturally competent approaches is driven in part by the dawning recognition of the danger to patient safety and overall inadequacy in the quality of outcomes in what we do. The literature around the disparities of outcomes across ethnic, social, and economic groups provides a compelling case to ensure that health care is attentive to these differences. But there is also attention to the costs that are driven up by health care that is not culturally competent and discourages compliance. The excess expenditures are associated with poor communication, the failure to use culturally responsive methods, and ineffective attempts to transfer treatment modalities to make the system cost efficient. Finally, as the health system makes its glacial move to more consumer and individual responsiveness, the system is recognizing that a cultural perspective is essential to provide services that earn high levels of consumer satisfaction.

Much of the activity aimed at advancing cultural competence has been centered on regulations and mandates. However, a generational change that begins with the education of each new practitioner is needed to bring about a culturally informed and competent professional community.

This edition of *Transcultural Health Care* provides the critical lessons to introduce students and practitioners to how different cultures construct the social world and the dramatic impact that culture has on how health care, medicine, community, and family interact. These insights into the rich variety of human culture are only small steps toward developing real wisdom regarding culture competence.

The first step in such a transformation is *awareness* of the other. Most young students and many seasoned practitioners simply do not have an appreciation of the variety of backgrounds and perspectives that people bring to an encounter with the health-care system. They have the expectation that the patient or consumer will "fit" into their clinic or admission process. Moreover, much of what is done in health care follows a "procedure," which implies that there are predetermined steps by which any one receiving the care or service must fit. For an increasingly large part of the population, nothing could be further from the truth. The care-seeking behavior, the attitude toward authority, the comfort with middle-class America culture that makes up so much of the health-care social world, and the relationship between genders are just a few of the literally hundreds of places at which a disconnect between the individual and the system can occur. When disconnects occur, the efforts by the system to maintain or return health may fail.

The second step after awareness is *knowledge*. What is it that we must know as practitioners in a system of care to reach the other person and overcome the cultural barriers? And it is essential that this knowledge pass both ways. What do they need to know about us in order to be an equal part of a team-focused plan to address a problem? Knowledge also speaks to the need for every practitioner to be aware of his/her own attitudes, bias, and prejudices. Everyone has such prejudices; they are not the issue. Awareness of them and the wisdom and insight to adjust care to provide nonjudgmental and supportive interventions is the challenge.

A culturally competent practitioner must also have a sense of comfort with the *experiential* process of engaging others from different cultures. This is perhaps the most difficult of all skills to teach and may only be learned through the practice of engaging others and being able to reflect critically on the experience and its impact on the patient as well as on the provider. This process is a familiar one, of course, as it is the core of clinical education. But students must come to value the variety of life and learn how to adapt their clinical expertise to different cultures and the individual unique development in a multicultural context.

As we focus on cultural competence, one fear is that we will make the knowledge more transactional than *transformational*. It needs to be the latter. For the patient or consumer, health care presented in a culturally competent way must blend the traditions of the older culture with the promise and resources of modern health care. For the practitioner or health-care institution, new patterns of service and organization of care must be transformed using the experience with the new culture. Such a critical perspective of cultural humility is essential for all practitioners in all dimensions of health care and is a vital part of developing into a truly culturally competent provider.

This will be greatly assisted as care delivery moves from profession-specific models of care to more *interprofessional* and team-based approaches. This has long been a hope of many involved in efforts to reform health care. If one is truly committed in becoming culturally competent, then one important lesson to learn is how to expand competence and the facility from the culture of nursing to an interdisciplinary culture that includes pharmacy, medicine, and the allied health professions. This seems obvious, but without these skills of closer adaptation and accommodation among all health professions, how can you imagine practitioners adapting to cultures that are more alien than those we encounter on a routine basis?

Synthesizing cultural adaptations within the health professional perspectives and offering adapted care to patients may not be sufficient to guarantee individual cultural competence. Practitioners who achieve such skill will need to change their orientation from one that is focused on the profession and its clinical world to one that is *patient-centric*. This is easy to affirm but very difficult to deliver because of the power and cultural hegemony of the clinical world. This cultural blindness serves neither the patient nor the practitioner. It is also a source of much of the dysfunction of the current system of care, both in terms of costs and quality.

The final stage in cultural competency is the ability to balance self-awareness with *other-awareness*. Such a balance is the hallmark of an outstanding clinician and is also the basis of all true cultural competence. This value allows for a response ability that transcends the simple knowledge of all practitioners knowing every detail about particular cultures and allows a different relationship to emerge between the provider of service and the recipient. In this way, the work toward developing the skills of a culturally competent practitioner assists in the broader goal of becoming an outstanding clinician in any setting. This edition of *Transcultural Health Care* provides an outstanding guide to the journey of becoming just such a practitioner.

EDWARD O'NEIL, MPA, PHD, FAAN
Professor
Departments of Family and Community Medicine,
Preventive and Restorative Dental Sciences and
Social and Behavioral Sciences, and
Director of the Center for the Health Professions
University of California, San Francisco
San Francisco, California

Acknowledgments

The editors would like to thank all those who helped in the preparation of the third edition of this book. We especially thank acquisitions editor, Jonathan D. Joyce, and associate acquisitions editor, Thomas A. Ciavarella, at F. A. Davis for their support and enthusiasm for the project; and Julie Catagnus, developmental editor, for her attention to detail, timeliness, and patience during the editing process. We thank the copyeditors at F. A. Davis for their assistance in bringing the book to completion. Most importantly, we want to thank the many multicultural populations and health professionals who are the impetus for this book. Finally, we thank our families, friends, and colleagues for their patience and support during the preparation of the book.

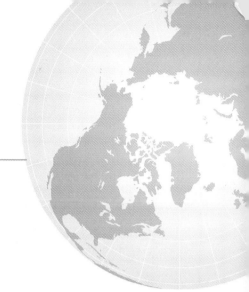

Contributors

Diane Alain, Med, RN
Teacher
La Cité Collégiale
University of Ottawa
Ottawa, Ontario, Canada

Josepha Campinha-Bacote, PhD, MAR, APRN, BC, CNS, CTN, FAAN
Clinical Assistant Professor
Case Western Reserve University
Cleveland, Ohio
President, Transcultural C.A.R.E. Associates
Cincinnati, Ohio

Marga Simon Coler, EdD, APRN-C, FAAN
Professor Emeritus
University of Connecticut
Storrs, Connecticut
Adjunct Professor
University of Massachusetts
Amherst, Massachusetts
Collaborating Professor
Federal University of Paraíba
Paraíba, Brazil

Jessie M. Colin, PhD, RN
Professor
Barry University School of Nursing
Miami Shores, Florida

Ginette Coutu-Wakulczyk, RN, MSc, PhD
Associate Professor
School of Nursing
Faculty of Health Sciences
University of Ottawa
Ottawa, Ontario, Canada

Tina A. Ellis, RN, MSN, CTN
Nursing Instructor
Florida Gulf Coast University
Fort Myers, Florida

Rauda Gelazis, RN, PhD, CS, CTN
Associate Professor
Ursuline College
Pepper Pike, Ohio

Divina Grossman, PhD, RN, FAAN
Dean
College of Nursing and Health Sciences
Florida International University
Miami, Florida

Homeyra Hafizi, RN, MS, LHRM
Occupational Health
Dynamac Corporation
Kennedy Space Center, Florida

Sandra M. Hillman, PhD, MS, BSN
Professor
Nelson Mandela Metropolitan University
Port Elizabeth, South Africa

David Hodgins, MSN, RN, CEN
Indian Health Service
Shiprock, New Mexico

Olivia Hodgins, RN, PhD, MSA, BSN
Map Instructor and Nurse Executive
Indian Health Service
San Fidel, New Mexico

Kathleen W. Huttlinger, PhD, RN
Associate Director for Research and
Interim Director of Graduate Programs
School of Nursing
New Mexico State University
Las Cruces, New Mexico

Eun-Ok Im, PhD, MPH, FAAN
Professor
The University of Texas at Austin
Austin, Texas

Misae Ito, MSN, RN, NMW
Associate Professor, Fundamental Nursing
Department of Nursing, Faculty of Health Sciences
Yamaguchi University School of Medicine
Yamaguchi-Ken, Japan

Anahid Dervartanian Kulwicki, RN, DNS, FAAN
Deputy Director
Wayne County Health and Human Services
Detroit, Michigan
Professor
Oakland University
Rochester, Michigan

Juliene G. Lipson, RN, PhD, FAAN
Professor Emerita
University of California, San Francisco School of
    Nursing
Mill Valley, California

Afaf Ibrahim Meleis, PhD, DrPS(hon), FAAN
Margaret Bond Simon Dean of Nursing
Professor of Nursing and Sociology
University of Pennsylvania School of Nursing
Philadelphia, Pennsylvania

Mahmoud Hanafi Meleis, PhD, PE
Retired Nuclear Engineer
Philadelphia, Pennsylvania

Denise Moreau, PhD, MSc, RN
Assistant Professor and Lecturer
University of Ottawa
Ottawa, Ontario, Canada

Dula F. Pacquiao, EdD, RN, CTN
Associate Professor and Director
Bergen Center for Multicultural Education,
    Research and Practice
School of Nursing
University of Medicine and Dentistry of New Jersey
Newark, New Jersey

**Irena Papadopoulos, PhD, MA, RN, RM, DipNEd,
    NDN Cert**
Professor of Transcultural Health and Nursing
Middlesex University, United Kingdom
Highgate Hill, London

Ghislaine Paperwalla, BSN, RN
Research Nurse in Immunology
Veterans Administration Medical Center
Miami, Florida

Henry M. Plawecki, RN, PhD
Professor of Nursing
Purdue University Calumet School of Nursing
Hammond, Indiana

Judith A. Plawecki, RN, PhD
Professor
University of South Florida
Tampa, Florida

Lawrence H. Plawecki, RN, JD, LLM
Health Law Consultant
Plawecki Consultants, LLC
Highland, Indiana

Martin H. Plawecki, PhD, MD
Faculty
Indiana University School of Medicine
Indianapolis, Indiana

Jeffrey Ross, BFA, MA, MAT
Graphic Designer and Language Arts Teacher
Archbishop Hoban High School
Akron, Ohio

**Ratchneewan Ross, PhD, MSc, RN, Certificate in
    Midwifery**
Assistant Professor
College of Nursing
Kent State University
Kent, Ohio

Maryam Sayyedi, PhD
Adjunct Professor
Department of Counseling
California State University, Fullerton
Fullerton, California

Janice Selekman, DNSc, RN
Professor
University of Delaware
Newark, Delaware

Linda S. Smith, MS, DSN, RN, CLNC
Associate Professor and Director
Idaho State University
Pocatello, Idaho

Jessica A. Steckler, MS, RNBC
National Program Manager
Employee Education System, VHA
Erie, Pennsylvania

Gulbu Tortumluoglu, PhD
Assistant Professor
Nursing Department Chief
Yuksekokulu, Canakkale, Turkey

**Susan Turale, DEd, MNStud, BN,
    DApSci(AdvPsychNurs), RN, RPN, FRCNA,
    FANZCMHN**
Professor of International Nursing
Department of Nursing, Faculty of Health Sciences
Yamaguchi University School of Medicine
Yamaguchi-Ken, Japan

Yan Wang, MSN, RN-BC
Nursing Informatics System Specialist III
Duke University Health System
Duke Health Technology Solutions
Durham, North Carolina

Anna Frances Z. Wenger, PhD, RN, CTN, FAAN
Professor and Director of Nursing Emerita
Goshen College
Goshen, Indiana
Senior Scholar
Interfaith Health Program
School of Public Health
Emory University
Program Consultant
Ethiopia Public Health Training Initiative
The Carter Center
Atlanta, Georgia

Marion R. Wenger, PhD
Retired Professor of Foreign Languages and Linguistics
Emory University
Atlanta, Georgia

Sarah A. Wilson, PhD, RN
Associate Professor
Director, Institute for End of Life Care Education
Marquette University College of Nursing
Milwaukee, Wisconsin

Cecilia A. Zamarripa, RN, CWON
Wound, Ostomy, and Continence Nurse
University of Pittsburgh Medical Center
Pittsburgh, Pennsylvania

Rick Zoucha, APRN, BC, DNSc, CTN
Associate Professor
Duquesne University School of Nursing
Pittsburgh, Pennsylvania

Contents

Contents –
DavisPlus

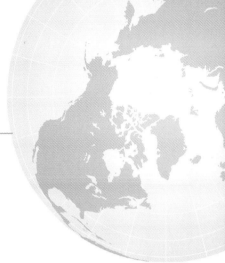

Introduction

The Purnell Model for Cultural Competence and its accompanying organizing framework has been used in education, clinical practice, administration, and research, giving credence to its usefulness for healthcare providers. They have been translated into Spanish, French, Flemish, Portuguese, Turkish, and Korean. Healthcare organizations have adapted the organizing framework as a cultural assessment tool and numerous students have used the Model to guide research for theses and dissertations in the United States and overseas. The Model's usefulness has been established in the global arena, recognizing and including the client's culture in assessment, healthcare planning, interventions, and evaluation. The Model is now being used more with organizational cultural competence as well.

The third edition of *Transcultural Health Care: A Culturally Competent Approach* has been revised based upon response from students and practicing healthcare professionals such as nurses, physicians, physical therapists, emergency medical technicians, and nutritionists to name a few as well as educators from associate degree, baccalaureate, masters, and doctoral programs in nursing. We appreciate their review and suggestions.

Chapter 1 has three important changes: (a) a more extensive section on health disparities, (b) a more extensive section on organizational cultural competence, and (c) a section on evidence-based practice as it relates to culture care. We have made a concerted effort to use nonstereotypical language when describing cultural attributes of specific cultures, recognizing that there are exceptions to every description provided and that the differences within a cultural group may be greater than the diversity between and among different cultural groups. We have also tried to include both the sociological and anthropological perspectives of culture.

Chapter 2 expands the description of the Purnell Model for Cultural Competence to include application of the domains and concepts of culture to the dominant American Culture in a cross-cultural fashion. Chapters 1 and 2 have critical thinking questions dispersed throughout each chapter. The glossary remains as it did in the second edition because users have noted its importance. Cultural specific chapters have changes based on users' suggestions. Instead of one large case study at the end of each chapter, shorter vignettes covering several domains with study questions are dispersed throughout each chapter.

Given the world diversity and the diversity within cultural groups, it is impossible to cover each group more extensively. Space and cost concerns limit the number of chapters that are included in the book; therefore, additional cultural groups, PowerPoint slides, test banks, useful web sites, and additional case studies are include on DavisPlus.

Specific criteria were used for identifying the groups represented in the book and those included in electronic format. Groups included in the book were selected based on any of the six criteria that follow.

- The group has a large population in North America, such as people of Appalachian, Mexican, German, and African American heritage.

- The group is relatively new in its migration status, such as people of Haitian, Cuban, and Arab heritage.

- The group is widely dispersed throughout North America, such as people of Iranian, Korean, and Filipino heritage.

- The group has little written about it in the healthcare literature, such as people of Guatemalan, Russian, and Thai heritage.

- The group holds significant disenfranchised status, such as people of Navajo heritage, a large American Indian group.

- The group was of particular interest to readers in the second edition, such as people from Amish heritage.

Again, we have strived to portray each culture positively and without stereotyping. We hope you enjoy our book and are as excited about the content as we are.

Larry D. Purnell
Betty J. Paulanka

Chapter 1

Transcultural Diversity and Health Care

LARRY D. PURNELL

The Need for Culturally Competent Health Care

Cultural competence in multicultural societies continues as a major initiative for business, health-care, and educational organizations in the United States and throughout most of the world. The mass media, health-care policy makers, the Office of Minority Health, and other Governmental organizations, professional organizations, the workplace, and health insurance payers are addressing the need for individuals to understand and become culturally competent as one strategy to improve quality and eliminate racial, ethnic, and gender disparities in health care. Educational institutions from elementary schools to colleges and universities also address cultural diversity and cultural competency as they relate to disparities and health promotion and wellness.

Many countries are now recognizing the need for addressing the diversity of their society, including the client base, the provider base, and the organization. Societies that used to be rather homogeneous, such as Portugal, Norway, Sweden, Korea, and selected areas in the United States and the United Kingdom, are now facing significant internal and external migration, resulting in ethnocultural diversity that did not previously exist, at least not to the degree it does now. As commissioned by the U.K. Presidency of the European Union, several European countries—such as Denmark, Italy, Poland, the Czech Republic, Latvia, the United Kingdom, Sweden, Norway, Finland, Italy, Spain, Portugal, Hungary, Belgium, Greece, Germany, the Netherlands, and France—either have in place or are developing national programs to address the value of cultural competence in reducing health disparities (Health Inequities: A Challenge for Europe, 2005).

Whether people are internal migrants, immigrants, or vacationers, they have the right to expect the health-care system to respect their personal beliefs, values, and health-care practices. Culturally competent health care from providers and the system, regardless of the setting in which care is delivered, is becoming a concern and expectation among consumers. Diversity also includes having a diverse workforce that more closely represents the population the organization serves.

Health-care personnel provide care to people of diverse cultures in long-term-care facilities, acute-care facilities, clinics, communities, and clients' homes. All health-care providers—physicians, nurses, nutritionists, therapists, technicians, home health aides, and other caregivers—need similar culturally specific information. For example, all health-care providers engage in verbal and nonverbal communication; therefore, all health-care professionals and ancillary staff need to have similar information and skill development to communicate appropriately with diverse populations. The manner in which the information is used may differ significantly based on the discipline, individual experiences, and specific circumstances of the client and provider.

Culturally competent staff and organizations are essential ingredients in increasing clients' satisfaction with health care and reducing multifactor reasons for gender, racial, and ethnic disparities and complications in health care. If providers and the system are competent, most clients will access the health-care system when problems are first recognized, thereby reducing the length of stay, decreasing complications, and reducing overall costs.

A lack of knowledge of clients' language abilities and cultural beliefs and values can result in serious threats to life and quality of care for all individuals. Organizations

1

and individuals who understand their clients' cultural values, beliefs, and practices are in a better position to be coparticipants with their clients in providing culturally acceptable care. Having ethnocultural specific knowledge, understanding, and assessment skills to work with culturally diverse clients assures that the health-care provider knows what questions to ask. Providers who know ethnoculturally specific knowledge are less likely to demonstrate negative attitudes, behaviors, ethnocentrism, stereotyping, and racism. Accordingly, there will be improved opportunities for health promotion and wellness; illness, disease, and injury prevention; and health maintenance and restoration. The onus for cultural competence is on the health-care provider and the delivery system in which care is provided. To this end, health-care providers need both general and specific cultural knowledge to help reduce gender and ethnic and racial disparities in health care.

World Diversity and Migration

The world's population reached 6.5 billion people in the year 2005 and is expected to approach 7.6 billion by 2020 and 9.3 billion by 2050. The estimated population growth rate is 1.14 percent, with 20.05 births per 1000 population, 8.6 deaths per 1000 population, and an infant mortality rate of 48.87 per 1000 population. Worldwide, life expectancy at birth is currently 64.77 years, with males at 63.17 years and females at 66.47 years (CIA, 2007).

As a first language, Mandarin Chinese is the most popular, spoken by 13.59 percent of the world's population, followed by Spanish at 5.05 percent, English at 4.8 percent, Hindi at 2.82 percent, Portuguese at 2.77 percent, Bengali at 2.68 percent, Russian at 2.27 percent, Japanese at 1.99 percent, German at 1.49 percent, and Wu Chinese at 1.21 percent. Only 82 percent of the world population is literate. When technology is examined, more people now have a cell phone than a landline: 1.72 billion versus 1.2 billion. Slightly over 1 billion people are Internet users (CIA, 2007).

We currently live in a global society, a trend that is expected to continue into the future. According to the United Nations High Commissioner for Refugees, there is a global population of 9.2 million refugees, the lowest number in 25 years, and as many as 25 million internally displaced persons. Migrants represent 2.9 percent or approximately 190 million people of the world population, up from 175 million in the year 2000. Moreover, international migration is decreasing while internal migration is increasing, especially in Asian countries. Only two countries in the world are seeing an increase in their migrant stock—North America and the former USSR (CIA, 2007).

The International Organization for Migration completed the first-ever comprehensive study looking at the costs and benefits of international migration. According to the report, ample evidence exists that migration brings both costs and benefits for sending and receiving countries, although these are not shared equally. Trends suggest a greater movement toward circular migration with substantial benefits to both home and host countries. The perception that migrants are more of a burden on, than a benefit to, the host country is not substantiated by research. For example, in the Home Office Study (2002) in the United Kingdom, migrants contributed U.S. $4 billion more in taxes than they received in benefits. In the United States, the National Research Council (1998) estimated that national income had expanded by U.S. $8 billion because of immigration. Thus, because migrants pay taxes, they are not likely to put a greater burden on health and welfare services than the host population. However, undocumented migrants run the highest health risks because they are less likely to seek health care. This not only poses risks for migrants but also fuels sentiments of xenophobia and discrimination against all migrants.

> **What evidence do you see in your community that migrants have added to the economic base of the community? Who would be doing their work if they were not available?**

UNITED STATES POPULATION AND CENSUS DATA

As of 2006, the U.S. population was over 300 million, an increase of 16 million since the 2000 census. The most recent census data estimates that 74.7 percent are white, 14.5 percent are Hispanic/Latino (of any race), 12.1 percent are black or African American, 0.8 percent are American Indian or Alaskan Native, 4.3 percent are Asian, 0.1 percent are Native Hawaiian or other Pacific Islander, 6 percent are some other race, and only 1.9 percent are of two or more races. Please note: These figures total more than 100 percent because the federal government considers race and Hispanic origin to be two separate and distinct categories. The categories as used in Census 2000 are

1. *White* refers to people having origins in any of the original peoples of Europe, the Near East, and the Middle East, and North Africa. This category includes Irish, German, Italian, Lebanese, Turkish, Arab, and Polish.

2. *Black* or *African American* refers to people having origins in any of the black racial groups of Africa, and includes Nigerians and Haitians or any person who self-designates this category regardless of origin.

3. *American Indian* and *Alaskan Native* refer to people having origins in any of the original peoples of North, South, or Central America and who maintain tribal affiliation or community attachment.

4. *Asian* refers to people having origins in any of the original peoples of the Far East, Southeast Asia, or the Indian subcontinent. This category includes the terms *Asian Indian, Chinese, Filipino, Korean, Japanese, Vietnamese, Burmese, Hmong, Pakistani,* and *Thai.*

5. *Native Hawaiian* and *other Pacific Islander* refer to people having origins in any of the original peoples of Hawaii, Guam, Samoa, Tahiti, the Mariana Islands, and Chuuk.

6. *Some other race* was included for people who are unable to identify with the other categories.

7. In addition, the respondent could identify, as a write-in, with two races (U.S. Bureau of the Census, 2006).

The Hispanic/Latino and Asian populations continue to rise in numbers and in percentage of the overall population; although the black/African American, Native Hawaiian and Pacific Islanders, Native American and Alaskan Natives groups continue to increase in overall numbers, their percentage of the population has decreased. Of the Hispanic/Latino population, most are Mexicans, followed by Puerto Ricans, Cubans, Central Americans, South Americans, and lastly, Dominicans. Salvadorans are the largest group from Central America. Three-quarters of Hispanics live in the West or South, with 50 percent of the Hispanics living in just two states, California and Texas. The median age for the entire U.S. population is 35.3 years, and the median age for Hispanics is 25.9 years (U.S. Bureau of the Census, 2006). The young age of Hispanics in the United States makes them ideal candidates for recruitment into the health professions, an area with crisis-level shortages of personnel, especially of minority representation.

Before 1940, most immigrants to the United States came from Europe, especially Germany, the United Kingdom, Ireland, the former Union of Soviet Socialist Republics, Latvia, Austria, and Hungary. Since 1940, immigration patterns to the United States have changed: Most are from Mexico, the Philippines, China, India, Brazil, Russia, Pakistan, Japan, Turkey, Egypt, and Thailand. People from each of these countries bring their own culture with them and increase the cultural mosaic of the United States. Many of these groups have strong ethnic identities and maintain their values, beliefs, practices, and languages long after their arrival. Individuals who speak only their indigenous language are more likely to adhere to traditional practices and live in ethnic enclaves and are less likely to assimilate into their new society. The inability of immigrants to speak the language of their new country creates additional challenges for health-care providers working with these populations. Other countries in the world face similar immigration challenges and opportunities for diversity enrichment. However, space does not permit a comprehensive analysis of migration patterns.

What changes in ethnic and cultural diversity have you seen in your community over the last 5 years? Over the last 10 years? Have you had the opportunity to interact with newer groups?

Racial and Ethnic Disparities in Health Care

A number of organizations have developed documents addressing the need for cultural competence as one strategy for eliminating racial and ethnic disparities. In 1985, the Department of Health and Human Services released

the Secretary's Task Force's report on Black and Minority Health (Perspectives on Disease Prevention and Health Promotion, 1985). Two goals from *Healthy People 2010* are to increase quality and years of healthy life and eliminate health disparities (Healthy People 2010, 2005). In 2005, the Agency for Healthcare Research and Quality (AHRQ) released the Third National Healthcare Disparities Report (Agency for Healthcare Research and Quality [AHRQ], 2005) that provides a comprehensive overview of health disparities in ethnic, racial, and socioeconomic groups in the United States. This report is a companion document to the National Healthcare Quality Report (NHQR) that is an overview of quality health care in the United States. These two documents highlight four themes: (1) Disparities still exist, (2) some disparities are diminishing, (3) opportunities for improvement still exist, and (4) information about disparities is improving. These documents address the importance of clinicians, administrators, educators, and policymakers in cultural competence. Disparities are observed in almost all aspects of healthcare, including

1. Effectiveness, patient safety, timeliness, and patient centeredness.

2. Facilitators and barriers to care and health-care utilization.

3. Preventive care, treatment of acute conditions, and management of chronic disease.

4. Clinical conditions such as cancer, diabetes, end-stage renal disease, heart disease, HIV disease, mental health and substance abuse, and respiratory diseases.

5. Women, children, elderly, rural residency, and individuals with disabilities and other special health-care needs.

6. Minorities and the financially poor receive a lower quality of care (AHRQ, 2005).

When ethnocultural specific populations are examined, although some disparities have shown improvement, many have not improved and some have worsened. With whites as the comparison group, the report shows:

1. Blacks were 10 times more likely to be diagnosed with AIDS, 59 percent less likely to be given antibiotics for the common cold, 9 percent more likely to receive poorer quality care, 17 percent more likely to lack health insurance, 7 percent less likely to report difficulties in getting care, and 10 percent more likely to have worse access to care.

2. Non-white Hispanics/Latinos were 3.7 times more likely to be diagnosed with AIDS, 16 percent more likely to receive poorer quality care, 2.9 times for under age 65 to lack health insurance, 18 percent less likely to report difficulties or delays getting care, and 87 percent more likely to have worse access. However, they were 40 percent less likely to die of breast cancer.

3. Asians were 57 percent more likely to report communication problems with the child's provider,

40 percent less likely to report difficulties or delays in getting care, and 20 percent more likely to have worse access to care.

4. American Indians and Alaskan Natives were twice as likely to lack early prenatal care, 67 percent less likely to develop late-stage breast cancer, 8 percent more likely to receive poorer quality care, twice as likely for the under-age-65 group to not have health insurance, 23 percent more likely to lack a primary-care provider, and 4 percent more likely to have worse access to care.

5. Data for Native Hawaiians and other Pacific Islanders were not available for this report but will be in future reports (AHRQ, 2005).

The health of the lesbian, gay, bisexual, and transgender populations has not been addressed in the *Healthy People 2010* document or in other government publications. However, the Gay and Lesbian Medical Association (www.glma.org) in 2001 developed *Healthy People 2010 Companion Document for Lesbian, Gay, Bisexual, and Transgender Health*. Salient disparities are noted in this publication. Gays and lesbians are more likely than their heterosexual cohort groups to have higher rates of tobacco, alcohol, and recreational drug use. Sexually transmitted infections, HIV (especially for men), suicide and suicide ideation, depression, being a victim of street violence (especially for men) and home violence (especially for women), sexual abuse among men, hate crimes, and psychological and emotional disorders are higher among these groups. They are also more likely to be discriminated against by health-care providers owing to homophobia. Because of the stigma that alternative identity gender discrimination brings, especially among racially and ethnically diverse populations (Purnell, 2003), these populations were less likely to disclose their sexual orientations. They are also less likely to have health insurance, have a primary-care provider, or take part in prevention programs; in fact, 57 percent of transgender people do not have health insurance (*Healthy People 2010 Companion Document for Lesbian, Gay, Bisexual, Transgender Health*, 2001; Purnell, 2003). To help combat violence and crimes against lesbians, gays, and transgender people, several cities such as Washington, D.C.; Fargo, North Dakota; and Missoula, Montana, in the United States have initiated Gay and Lesbian Crime Units (Police Unit Reaches Out to Gay Community, Inspires Others, 2006).

> What health disparities have you observed in your community? To what do you attribute these disparities? What can you do as a professional to help decrease these disparities?

Only broad categories of health disparities are addressed in this chapter. More specific data are included in individual chapters on cultural groups. As can be seen by the overwhelming data, much more work needs to be accomplished to improve the health of the nation. Space does not permit an extensive discourse on racial and ethnic disparities in other countries. However, documents that include other countries, conditions, and policies are listed as a resource herein. Additional information on the role of cultural competence on eliminating racial and ethnic disparities includes:

1. Transcultural Nursing Society, International (www.tcns.org)

2. U.S. Department of Health and Human Services Office of Minority Health: Physician's Toolkit and Curriculum (http://www.omhrc.gov/assets/pdf/checked/toolkit.pdf)

3. Institute of Medicine's Unequal Treatment study (http://www.iom.edu/?id=4475)

4. The Commonwealth Fund Report on Health Care Quality (http://www.cmwf.org/)

5. Delivering Race Equality: A Framework for Action (http://www.londondevelopmentcentre.org/silo/files/577.pdf)

6. Protecting Vulnerable Populations (www.wcc-assembly.info/en/news-media/news/english)

7. Canadian Institutes of Health Research: Reducing Health Disparities and Promoting Equity for Vulnerable Populations (www.cihr-irsc.gc.ca/e/19739.html)

8. American Physical Therapy Association's document and monographs on cultural competence (www.apta.org)

9. Health Inequalities: A Challenge for Europe that includes health policies for the Czech Republic, England, Denmark, Finland, Greece, Germany, Hungary, Ireland, Latvia, the Netherlands, Northern Ireland, Poland Portugal, Scotland, Spain, Sweden, and Wales (www.fco.gov.uk/Files/kfile/HI_EU_Challenge,0.pdf)

10. American Academy of Family Physicians documents on health disparities and cultural competence (http://www.aafp.org)

11. American Academy of Physician Assistants document The Four Layers of Diversity (http://www.aapa.org/)

12. Health Resources and Services Administration publication "Indicators of Cultural Competence in Health Care Delivery Organizations" and Cultural Competence Works (www.hrsa.gov)

13. American Student Medical Association Culture and Diversity Curriculum (http://www.amsa.org/programs/diversitycurriculum.cfm)

14. American Academy of Nursing Standards of Cultural Competence (in press).

15. Diversity Rx (www.diversityRx.org)

Self-Awareness and Health Professionals

Culture has a powerful unconscious impact on health professionals. Each health-care provider adds a new and unique dimension to the complexity of providing culturally competent care. The way health-care providers perceive themselves as competent providers is often reflected in the way they communicate with clients. Thus, it is essential for health professionals to think about their cultures, their behaviors, and their communication styles in relation to their perceptions of cultural differences. They should also examine the impact their beliefs have on others, including clients and coworkers, who are culturally diverse. Before addressing the multicultural backgrounds and unique individual perspectives of each client, health-care professionals must first address their own personal and professional knowledge, values, beliefs, ethics, and life experiences in a manner that optimizes interactions and assessment of culturally diverse individuals.

Self-knowledge and understanding promote strong professional perceptions that free health-care professionals from prejudice and allow them to interact with others in a manner that preserves personal integrity and respects uniqueness and differences among individual clients. The process of professional development and diversity competence begins with self-awareness, sometimes referred to as *self-exploration*. Although the literature provides numerous definitions of self-awareness, discussion of research integrating the concept of self-awareness with multicultural competence is minimal. Many theorists and diversity trainers imply that self-examination or awareness of personal prejudices and biases is an important step in the cognitive process of developing cultural competence (Andrews & Boyle, 2005; Campinha-Bacote, 2006; Giger & Davidhizar, 2008). However, discussions of emotional feelings elicited by this cognitive awareness are somewhat limited, given the potential impact of emotions and conscious feelings on behavioral outcomes.

> In your opinion, why is there conflict about working with culturally diverse clients? What attitudes are necessary to deliver quality care to clients whose culture is different from yours?

Self-awareness in cultural competence is a deliberate and conscious cognitive and emotional process of getting to know yourself: your personality, your values, your beliefs, your professional knowledge standards, your ethics, and the impact of these factors on the various roles you play when interacting with individuals different from yourself. The ability to understand oneself sets the stage for integrating new knowledge related to cultural differences into the professional's knowledge base and perceptions of health interventions.

> What have you done in the last 5 to 10 years to increase your self-awareness? Has increasing your self-awareness resulted in an increased appreciation for cultural diversity? How might you increase your knowledge about the diversity in your community? In your school?

Culture and Essential Terminology

CULTURE DEFINED

Anthropologists and sociologists have proposed many definitions of culture. For the purposes of this book, **culture** is defined as the totality of socially transmitted behavioral patterns, arts, beliefs, values, customs, lifeways, and all other products of human work and thought characteristics of a population of people that guide their worldview and decision making. Health and health-care beliefs and values are assumed in this definition. These patterns may be explicit or implicit, are primarily learned and transmitted within the family, are shared by most (but not all) members of the culture, and are emergent phenomena that change in response to global phenomena. Culture, a combined anthropological and social construct, can be seen as having three levels: (1) a tertiary level that is visible to outsiders, such as things that can be seen, worn, or otherwise observed; (2) a secondary level, in which only members know the rules of behavior and can articulate them; and (3) a primary level that represents the deepest level in which rules are known by all, observed by all, implicit, and taken for granted (Koffman, 2006). Culture is largely unconscious and has powerful influences on health and illness. Health-care providers must recognize, respect, and integrate clients' cultural beliefs and practices into health prescriptions.

An important concept to understand is that cultural beliefs, values, and practices are learned from birth: first at home, then in the church and other places where people congregate, and then in educational settings. Therefore, a 3-month-old male child from Korea adopted by an African American family and reared in an African American environment will have an African American worldview. However, that child's "race" would be Asian, and if that child had a tendency toward genetic/hereditary conditions, they would come from his Korean ancestry, not from African American genetics.

> Who in your family had the most influence in teaching you cultural values and practices? Outside the family, where else did you learn about your cultural values and beliefs? What cultural practices did you learn in your family that you no longer practice?

When individuals of dissimilar cultural orientations meet in a work or a therapeutic environment, the likelihood for developing a mutually satisfying relationship is improved if both parties attempt to learn about each other's culture. Moreover, race and culture are not synonymous and should not be confused. For example, most people who self-identify as African American have varying degrees of dark skin, but some may have white skin. However, as a cultural term, *African American* means that the person takes pride in having ancestry from both Africa and the United States; thus, a person with white skin could self-identify as African American.

IMPORTANT TERMS RELATED TO CULTURE

Attitude is a state of mind or feeling about some matter of a culture. Attitudes are learned; for example, some people think that one culture is better than another. One culture is not better than another; the two are just different, although many patterns are shared among cultures. A **belief** is something that is accepted as true, especially as a tenet or a body of tenets accepted by people in an ethnocultural group. A belief among some cultures is that if a pregnant woman craves a particular food substance, strawberries, for example, and does not satisfy the craving, the baby will be born with a birthmark in the shape of the craving. Attitudes and beliefs do not have to be proven; they are unconsciously accepted as truths. **Ideology** consists of the thoughts and beliefs that reflect the social needs and aspirations of an individual or an ethnocultural group. For example, some people believe that health care is a right of all people, whereas others see health care as a privilege.

The literature reports many definitions for the terms cultural awareness, cultural sensitivity, and cultural competence. Sometimes, these definitions are used interchangeably. However, **cultural awareness** has more to do with an appreciation of the external signs of diversity, such as arts, music, dress, and physical characteristics. **Cultural sensitivity** has more to do with personal attitudes and not saying things that might be offensive to someone from a cultural or ethnic background different from the health-care provider's. **Cultural competence** in health care is having the knowledge, abilities, and skills to deliver care congruent with the client's cultural beliefs and practices. Increasing one's consciousness of cultural diversity improves the possibilities for health-care practitioners to provide culturally competent care.

> What activity have you done to increase your cultural awareness and competence? How do you demonstrate that you are culturally sensitive?

One progresses from unconscious incompetence (not being aware that one is lacking knowledge about another culture), to conscious incompetence (being aware that one is lacking knowledge about another culture), to conscious competence (learning about the client's culture, verifying generalizations about the client's culture, and providing cultural specific interventions), and finally, to unconscious competence (automatically providing culturally congruent care to clients of diverse cultures). Unconscious competence is difficult to accomplish and potentially dangerous because individual differences exist within specific cultural groups. To be even minimally effective, culturally competent care must have the assurance of continuation after the original impetus is withdrawn; it must be integrated into, and valued by, the culture that is to benefit from the interventions.

Developing mutually satisfying relationships with diverse cultural groups involves good interpersonal skills and the application of knowledge and techniques learned from the physical, biological, and social sciences as well as the humanities. An understanding of one's own culture and personal values and the ability to detach oneself from "excess baggage" associated with personal views are essential to cultural competence. Even then, traces of ethnocentrism may unconsciously pervade one's attitudes and behavior. **Ethnocentrism**, the universal tendency of human beings to think that their ways of thinking, acting, and believing are the only right, proper, and natural ways, can be a major barrier to providing culturally competent care. Ethnocentrism, a concept that most people practice to some degree, perpetuates an attitude in which beliefs that differ greatly from one's own are strange, bizarre, or unenlightened and, therefore, wrong. **Values** are principles and standards that are important and have meaning and worth to an individual, family, group, or community. For example, the dominant U.S. culture places high value on youth, technology, and money. The extent to which one's cultural values are internalized influences the tendency toward ethnocentrism. The more one's values are internalized, the more difficult it is to avoid the tendency toward ethnocentrism.

> Given that everyone is ethnocentric to some degree, what do you do to become less ethnocentric? If you were to rate yourself on a scale of 1 to 10, with 1 being less ethnocentric and 10 being very ethnocentric, what score would you give yourself? What score would your friends give you? What score would you give your closest friends?

The Human Genome Project provides evidence that all human beings share a genetic code that is over 99 percent identical. However, the controversial term race must still be addressed when learning about culture. **Race** is genetic in origin and includes physical characteristics that are similar among members of the group, such as skin color, blood type, and hair and eye color. Although there is less than a 1 percent difference, this difference is significant when conducting physical assessments and prescribing medication, as outlined in culturally specific chapters that follow. People from a given racial group may, but do not necessarily, share a common culture. Race as a social concept is just as important, and sometimes more important, than race as a biological concept. Race has social meaning, assigns status, limits or increases opportunities, and influences interactions between patients and clinicians. Racism has been described as prejudice combined with power (Abrums, 2004). The International Convention on the Elimination of All Forms of Racial Discrimination defines racism (1965) as "Any distinction, exclusion, restriction, or preference based on race, colour, descent, or national or ethnic origin which has the purpose or effect of nullifying or impairing the recognition, enjoyment, or exercise, on equal footing, of human rights and fundamental freedoms in the political, economic, social, cultural, or any other field of public life." Racism may be overt or covert. Recent antidiscrimination laws make racism illegal, but the laws do not eliminate racist attitudes; thus, people are just less likely to express racist attitudes openly. Moreover, one must remember that even though one might have a racist attitude, it is not always recognized because it is ingrained during socialization and leads to ethnocentrism.

> How do you define race? What other terms do you use besides race to describe people? In what category did you classify yourself on the last census? What categories would you add to the current census classifications?

Worldview is the way individuals or groups of people look at the universe to form basic assumptions and values about their lives and the world around them. Worldview includes cosmology, relationships with nature, moral and ethical reasoning, social relationships, magicoreligious beliefs, and aesthetics.

Any **generalization**—reducing numerous characteristics of an individual or group of people to a general form that renders them indistinguishable—made about the behaviors of any individual or large group of people is almost certain to be an oversimplification. When a generalization relates less to the actual observed behavior than to the motives thought to underlie the behavior (i.e., the why of the behavior), it is likely to be oversimplified. Thus, generalizations can lead to **stereotyping**, an oversimplified conception, opinion, or belief about some aspect of an individual or group. Generalization and stereotyping are similar, but functionally, they are very different. Stereotyping is an endpoint; generalization is a starting point. For example, knowing whether the person comes from an individualistic versus a collectivistic culture is important. Remember, individualism and collectivism exist to some degree in all cultures, but one pattern tends to dominate. People identifying with a collectivist culture, such as most Asians, are more likely to place a higher value on the family than on the individual, harmony, and solidarity. However, people who identify with an individualistic culture, such as the dominant American and Scandinavian cultures, are more likely to place a higher value on the individual, independence, autonomy, and achievement. The health-care provider must specifically ask questions to determine these values and avoid stereotypical views of clients.

> Everyone engages in stereotypical behavior to some degree. We could not function otherwise. If someone asked you to think of a nurse, what image do you have? Is the nurse male or female? How old is the nurse? How is the nurse dressed? Is the nurse wearing a hat? How do you distinguish a stereotype from a generalization?

Even in relatively homogeneous cultures, subcultures and ethnic groups exist that may not hold all the values of their dominant culture. **Subcultures**, ethnic groups, or ethnocultural populations are groups of people who have experiences different from those of the dominant culture. Some of these differences may include socioeconomic status, ethnic background, residence, religion, education, or other factors that functionally unify the group and act collectively on each member with a conscious awareness of these differences. Subcultures differ from the dominant ethnic group and share beliefs according to the primary and secondary characteristics of culture.

Primary and Secondary Characteristics of Culture

Great diversity exists within a cultural group. Major influences that shape peoples' worldview and the degree to which they identify with their cultural group of origin are called the primary and secondary characteristics of culture. The **primary characteristics** are things that a person cannot easily change, but if they do, a stigma may occur for themselves, their families, or the society in which they live. The primary characteristics of culture include nationality, race, color, gender, age, and religious affiliation. For example, consider two people with these primary characteristics: one is a 75-year-old devout Islamic female from Saudi Arabia; the other is a 19-year-old African American fundamentalist Baptist male from Louisiana. Obviously, the two do not look alike, and they probably have very different worldviews and beliefs, many of which come from their religious tenets and country of origin.

> What are your primary characteristics of culture? How has each one influenced you and your worldview? How has your worldview changed as your primary characteristics have changed? How is each of these a subculture?

The **secondary characteristics** include educational status, socioeconomic status, occupation, military experience, political beliefs, urban versus rural residence, enclave identity, marital status, parental status, physical characteristics, sexual orientation, gender issues, reason for migration (sojourner, immigrant, or undocumented status), and length of time away from the country of origin. For example, the secondary cultural characteristics of being a single transsexual urban business executive will most likely evolve into a different worldview from that of a married heterosexual rural secretary who has two teenagers. In another case, a migrant farm worker from the highlands of Guatemala, who has an undocumented status, has a different perspective than an immigrant from Mexico who has lived in New York City for 10 years. People who live in ethnic enclaves and get their work, shopping, and business needs met without learning the language and customs of their host country may be more traditional than people in their home country. Such was the case for a Japanese man who lived in a Japanese ethnic enclave in San Francisco. When he returned to Japan after 20 years to visit relatives, he was criticized for being too traditional. Japanese society had changed, while he had not.

What are your secondary characteristics of culture? How has each one influenced you and your worldview? How has your worldview changed as your secondary characteristics have changed? How is each of these a subculture?

Immigration status influences a person's worldview. For example, people who voluntarily migrate generally **acculturate** more willingly; that is, they have given up most traits from the culture of origin as a result of contact with another culture. A number of acculturation scales exist; some are generic for any population, whereas others are specific to a particular culture such as Chinese, Korean, or Filipino. Yet, others are specific to an age group such as teenagers and older people. More traditional people adhere, and sometimes tenaciously, to most of the traits of their culture of origin. Similarly, **assimilation** is gradually adopting and incorporating the majority of the characteristics of the prevailing culture. Many people who migrate become bicultural; they are able to function equally well in their dominant and their host cultures. Marginalized people seem to have few traits from their dominant or host culture. People who voluntarily immigrate assimilate and acculturate more easily than people who immigrate unwillingly or as sojourners. Sojourners, who immigrate with the intention of remaining in their new homeland only a short time, or refugees, who think they may return to their home country, may not identify a need to acculturate or assimilate. In addition, undocumented individuals (illegal aliens) may have a different worldview from those who have arrived legally with work visas or as "legal immigrants."

The debate regarding the precise definition and differences among the terms *transcultural, cross-cultural,* and *intercultural* continues. Many authors and texts define the terms differently. This book uses the terms interchangeably to mean "crossing," "spanning," or "interacting" with a culture other than one's own. When people interact with individuals whose cultures are different from their own, they are engaged in cultural diversity. Awareness of the differences and similarities among ethnocultural groups results in a broadened multicultural worldview.

Ethics Across Cultures

As globalization grows and population diversity with nations increases, health-care providers are increasingly confronted with ethical issues related to cultural diversity. At the extremes stand those who favor multiculturalism and postmodernism versus those who favor humanism. Internationally, **multiculturalism** asserts that no common moral principles are shared by all cultures; **postmodernism** asserts a similar claim against all universal standards, both moral and nonmoral. Postmodernism holds the stance that everything is social construction, which leads to the contention that context is all-important (Baker, 1998). The concern is that universal standards provide a disguise whereas dominant cultures destroy or eradicate traditional cultures.

Humanism asserts that all human beings are equal in worth, that they have common resources and problems, and that they are alike in fundamental ways (Macklin, 1999). Humanism does not put aside the many circumstances that make individuals' lives different around the world. Many similarities exist as to what people need to live well. Humanism says that there are human rights that should not be violated. Macklin (1998) asserts that universal applicability of moral principles is required, not universal acceptability. Beaucamp (1998) concurs that fundamental principles of morality and human rights allow for cross-cultural judgments of immoral conduct. Of course, there is a middle ground.

Throughout the world, practices are claimed to be cultural, traditional, and beneficial, even when they are exploitive and harmful. For example, the practice of female circumcision, a traditional cultural practice, is seen by some as exploiting women. In many cases, the practice is harmful and can even lead to death. Whereas empirical anthropological research has shown that different cultures and historical eras contain different moral beliefs and practices, it is far from certain that what is right or wrong can be determined only by the beliefs and practices within a particular culture or subculture. Slavery and apartheid are examples of civil rights violations.

Accordingly, codes of ethics are open to interpretation and are not value-free. Furthermore, ethics belong to the society, not to professional groups. Ethics and ethical decision making are culturally bound. The Western ethical principles of patient autonomy, self-determination, justice, do no harm, truth telling, and promise keeping are not interpreted or shared by some non-Western societies. In the dominant American culture, truth telling, promise keeping, and not cheating on examinations are highly valued. However, not all cultures place such high regard on these values. For example, in Russia, the truth is optional, people are expected to break their promise, and most students cheat on examinations. Cheating on a business deal is not necessarily dishonorable (Birch, 2006).

In health organizations in the United States, advance directives give patients the opportunity to decide about their care, and staff members are required to ask patients about this upon admission to a health-care facility. Western ethics, with its stress on individualism, asks this question directly of the patient. However, in collectivist societies, such as among ethnic Chinese and Japanese, the preferred person to ask may be a family member. In most collectivist societies, a person does not stand alone, but rather is defined in relation to another unit, such as the family or work group. In addition, translating these forms into another language can be troublesome because a direct translation can be confusing. For example, "informed consent" may be translated to mean that the person relinquishes his or her right to decision making.

How do you perceive truth telling? Do you always tell the truth? Do you always tell the whole truth? If a female colleague asks you how you like her new hairstyle, are you completely truthful or are you likely to be a little less than completely truthful and tell her what you think she wants to hear? If a patient asks you how he is doing and if he is going to get better, do you tell him that everything is okay, even if you know he is not?

What practices have you seen that might be considered a cultural imposition?
What practices have you seen that might be considered cultural imperialism?
What practices have you seen that might be considered cultural relativism?
What have you done to address them when you have seen them occurring?

Some cultural situations occur that raise legal issues. For instance, in Western societies, a competent person (or an alternative such as the spouse, if the person is married) is supposed to sign her or his own consent for medical procedures. However, in some cultures, the eldest son is expected to sign consent forms, not the spouse. In this case, both the organization and the family can be satisfied if both the spouse and the son sign the informed consent.

Instead of Western ethics prevailing, some authorities advocate for universal ethics. Each culture has its own definition of what is right or wrong and what is good or bad. Accordingly, some health-care providers encourage international codes of ethics, such as those developed by the International Council of Nurses. These codes are intended to reflect the patient's culture and whether the value is placed on individualism or collectivism. Most Western codes of ethics have interpretative statements based on the Western value of individualism. International codes of ethics do not contain interpretative statements, but rather let each society interpret them according to its culture. As our multicultural society increases its diversity, health-care providers need to rely upon ethics committees that include members from the cultures they serve.

As the globalization of health-care services increases, providers must also address very crucial issues such as cultural imperialism, cultural relativism, and cultural imposition. **Cultural imperialism** is the practice of extending the policies and practices of one group (usually the dominant one) to disenfranchised and minority groups. An example is the U.S. government's forced migration of Native American tribes to reservations with individual allotments of lands instead of group ownership as well as forced attendance of their children at white people's boarding schools. Proponents of cultural imperialism appeal to universal human rights values and standards.

Cultural relativism is the belief that the behaviors and practices of people should be judged only from the context of their cultural system. Proponents of cultural relativism argue that issues such as abortion, euthanasia, female circumcision, and physical punishment in child rearing should be accepted as cultural values without judgment from the outside world. Opponents argue that cultural relativism may undermine condemnation of human rights violations, and family violence cannot be justified or excused on a cultural basis.

Cultural imposition is the intrusive application of the majority group's cultural view upon individuals and families (Universal Declaration of Human Rights, 2001). Prescription of special diets without regard to clients' cultures and limiting visitors to immediate family, a practice of many acute-care facilities, border on cultural imposition.

Health-care professionals must be cautious about forcefully imposing their values regarding genetic testing and counseling. No group is spared from genetic disease. Ashkenazi Jews have been tested for Tay-Sachs disease for many years. Advances in technology and genetics have found that many diseases such as Huntington's chorea have a genetic basis. Some forms of breast and colon cancers, adult-onset diabetes, Alzheimer's disease, and hypertension are some of the newest additions. Currently, only the well-to-do can afford broad testing. Advances in technology will provide the means for access to screening that will challenge genetic testing and counseling. The relationship of genetics to disability, disabled individuals, and the potentially disabled will create moral dilemmas of new complexity and magnitude.

Many questions surround genetic testing. Should health-care providers encourage genetic testing? What is, or should be, done with the results? How do we approach testing for genes that lead to disease or disability? How do we maximize health and well-being without creating a eugenic devaluation of those who are disabled? Should employers and third-party payers be allowed to discriminate based on genetic potential for illness? What is the purpose of prenatal screening and genetic testing? What are the assumptions for state-mandated testing programs? Should parents and individuals be allowed to "opt out" of testing? What if the individual does not want to know the results? What if the results could have a deleterious outcome to the infant or the mother? What if the results got into the hands of insurance companies that then denied payment or refused to provide coverage? Should public policy support genetic testing, which may improve health and health care for the masses of society? Should multiple births from fertility drugs be restricted because of the burden of cost, education, and health of the family? Should public policy encourage limiting family size in the contexts of the mother's health, religious and personal preferences, and the availability of sufficient natural resources (such as water and food) for future survival? What effect do these issues have on a nation with an aging population, a decrease in family size, and decreases in the numbers and percentages of younger people? What effect will these issues have on the ability of countries to provide health care for their citizens? Health-care providers must understand these three concepts and the ethical issues involved because they will increasingly encounter situations in which they must balance the client's cultural practices and behaviors with health promotion and wellness as well as illness, disease, and injury prevention activities for the good of the client, the family, and society. Other international issues that may be less controversial include sustainable environments, pacification, and poverty (Purnell, 2001).

Individual Cultural Competence

Much has been debated, especially since the early 1990s, about objectively measuring individual competence. Most tools for measuring cultural competence are self-reported and subjective in nature. A number of tools have been developed to assess individual and organizational cultural competence. Some have been validated and are specific to a discipline or area of practice, whereas others are more general in nature. To select one that more specifically meets your needs, go to the Internet search engine www.scholar.google.com and type "cultural competence measurement" or "cultural competence assessment tools" in the search field. The Office of Minority Health also has a document on Cultural Competence Standards (www.omhrc.gov). In general, cultural competence is a journey involving the willingness and ability of an individual to deliver culturally congruent and acceptable health and nursing care to the clients to whom one provides care. To these authors, individual cultural competence can be arbitrarily divided among cultural general approaches, the clinical encounter, and language.

> Whose values and beliefs should come first—yours, the organization's, or the client's?

CULTURAL GENERAL APPROACHES

1. Developing an awareness of one's own existence, sensations, thoughts, and environment without letting it have an undue influence on those from other backgrounds.
2. Continuing to learn cultures of clients to whom one provides care.
3. Demonstrating knowledge and understanding of the client's culture, health-related needs, and meanings of health and illness.
4. Accepting and respecting cultural differences in a manner that facilitates the client's and the family's ability to make decisions to meet their needs and beliefs.
5. Recognizing that the health-care provider's beliefs and values may not be the same as the client's.
6. Resisting judgmental attitudes such as "different is not as good."
7. Being open to new cultural encounters.
8. Recognizing that the primary and secondary characteristics of culture determine the degree to which clients adhere to the beliefs, values, and practices of their dominant culture.
9. Having contact and experience with the communities from which clients come.
10. Being willing to work with clients of diverse cultures and subcultures.

11. Accepting responsibility for one's own education in cultural competence by attending conferences, reading literature, and observing cultural practices.
12. Promoting respect for individuals by discouraging racial and ethnic slurs among coworkers.
13. Intervening with staff behavior that is insensitive, lacks cultural understanding, or reflects prejudice.
14. Having a cultural general framework for assessment as well as having cultural specific knowledge about the clients to whom care is provided.

THE CLINICAL ENCOUNTER

1. Adapting care to be congruent with the client's culture.
2. Responding respectively to all clients and their families (includes addressing clients and family members as they prefer, formally or informally).
3. Collecting cultural data on assessments.
4. Forming generalizations as a method for formulating questions rather than stereotyping.
5. Recognizing culturally based health-care beliefs and practices.
6. Knowing the most common diseases and illnesses affecting the unique population to whom care is provided.
7. Individualizing care plans to be consistent with the client's cultural beliefs.
8. Having knowledge of the communication styles of clients to whom you provide care.
9. Accepting varied gender roles and childrearing practices from clients to whom you provide care.
10. Having a working knowledge of the religious and spirituality practices of clients to whom you provide care.
11. Having an understanding of the family dynamics of clients to whom you provide care.
12. Using faces and language pain scales in the ethnicity and preferred languages of the clients.
13. Recognizing and accepting traditional, complementary, and alternative practices of clients to whom you provide care.
14. Incorporating client's cultural food choices and dietary practices into care plans.
15. Incorporating client's health literacy into care plans and health education initiatives.

LANGUAGE

1. Developing skills and using interpreters (includes sign language) with clients and families who have limited English proficiency.
2. Providing clients with educational documents that are translated into their preferred language.

3. Providing discharge instructions at a level the client and the family understand and in the language the client and the family prefer.

4. Providing medication and treatment instruction in the language the client prefers.

5. Using pain scales in the preferred language of the client.

> Look at the list of activities that promote individual cultural competence. Which of these activities have you used to increase your cultural competence? Which ones can you easily add to increase your cultural competence? Which ones are the most difficult for you to incorporate?

Organizational Cultural Competence

Individual cultural competence is not sufficient for culturally competent care. The organization in which the care is delivered must also demonstrate a commitment to cultural competence. Several things must be in place if an organization is to demonstrate cultural competence. A list of attributes of culturally competent organizations, organized arbitrarily by governance and administration, education and orientation, and language follows:

GOVERNANCE AND ADMINISTRATION

1. The organization must have a mission statement and policies that address diversity.

2. The Board of Governance must include members of the ethnicity of the community it serves.

3. A committee for cultural competence exists and includes staff, managers, administrators, chaplains, and members representative of the community.

4. The organization engages in community diversity fairs.

5. The organization seeks resources from federal, state, and private agencies to continually upgrade and integrate cultural competence into care.

6. The organization partners with diverse community agencies.

7. The organization networks with diverse community leaders.

8. Administrators, managers, and staff are encouraged to be active in public policy for the client base to whom they deliver care.

9. Policy statements include efforts to eliminate the bias and prejudice of clients and staff.

10. Programs reflect the needs of the diversity of the community.

11. The organization's programs are advertised in community newspapers and on the radio and television in the languages of the community.

12. The organization is willing to support a mentoring program to entice recruitment into the health professions.

13. Data collected include race, ethnicity, culture, and language preferences of the staff and client base.

14. Patient rights documents are in the major languages served by the community.

15. Cultural and Linguistic Appropriate Services (CLAS) Standards are adhered to.

16. Fiscal resources are available for interpretation.

17. The strategic plan reflects the needs of the community.

18. Input on research priorities is sought from consumers.

19. Researchers are reflective of the staff, clients, and community.

20. Human Resources recruitment and hiring activities reflect the diversity of the community.

21. The job analysis procedure includes scoring for ethnocultural and language ability.

22. Position descriptions and evaluation practices reflect cultural competence.

23. Conflict and grievance procedures reflect the language of the staff.

24. The organization demonstrates active recruitment of bilingual staff.

25. The staff is compensated for bilingual ability and certification.

26. The ethics committee has members reflective of the staff and clients.

27. Hours of operation of clinics are adjusted to meet the needs of the community.

28. Pictures and posters are reflective of the client base.

29. Food choices are reflective of the client and staff.

30. The holiday calendar represents the client population base.

31. Intake forms reflect cultural assessment.

32. Pain scales are in diverse languages of the population served.

33. Culturally appropriate toys are available (Hispanic Santa, black dolls).

34. If staff is used or interpretation is available, a plan is in effect to address their job duties while interpreting for patients and staff (also a Joint Commission on Accreditation of Healthcare Organizations [JCAHO] requirement).

EDUCATION AND ORIENTATION

1. Diversity must be addressed as part of new employees' orientation, in-service, and continuing-education programs.

2. Nursing care delivery systems, the U.S. system of insurance reimbursement, and issues related to culture and autonomy are discussed.

3. Mentoring programs exist for diverse student and staff populations.

4. Diversity of the health professions is included in orientation.

5. All employees must be offered cultural general topics and cultural specific needs of populations for whom they provide care.

6. Cultural celebrations are reflective of the staff and clients.

7. Resources are available to staff on the unit and in the library.

8. The staff is trained in language interpretation.

9. Health classes are offered to clients the community serves.

10. Certification in culture for staff is offered at various levels.

11. Pharmacists, nurses, and physicians are educated in ethnopharmacology.

12. A lunch and learn series that supports the ongoing development of cultural competence can be started.

LANGUAGE

1. Mechanisms must be in place for translation of written materials in the preferred language of the client.

2. Policies must address interpretation services.

3. Resources are available for translation of educational materials and discharge instructions in the languages of the client population.

4. The organization engages in activities that address health literacy of the population it serves.

5. Written documents undergo a cultural sensitivity review.

6. Consent and procedure forms are translated into the languages of the population served.

7. English-as-a-second language classes exist for staff.

8. Language classes are offered to clients and family (English and language of the population served).

9. Waiting areas have literature in the language of the population served.

10. Directions to referral facilities are in the languages of the client base.

11. Videos are in the language of the client and have pictures of the client base.

12. Diverse language includes sign language.

13. Need for interpreters is determined ahead of time.

14. Telephone system is in the languages of the community.

15. Television programs are in the languages of the community.

16. Satisfaction surveys are in the languages of the community.

17. Staff surveys are in the languages of the employees.

18. Audiovisual materials for staff and clients are in their preferred languages.

19. Wellness and health promotion classes are offered in the languages of the client base.

> Look at the list of activities that promote organizational cultural competence. Which of these activities have you used to increase the organization's cultural competence? Which ones can you easily add to increase the organization's cultural competence? Which ones are the most difficult to accomplish?

Evidence-Based Practice: Developing Individual and Organizational Culture

Section written by Susan Salmond

The mandate for evidence-based practice (EBP) to reduce the "know-do" gap (Antes, Sauerland, & Seiter, 2006) between known science and implementation in practice is being driven by the demand for improved safety and quality outcomes for clients. Although a laudable goal, it will require a culture shift. The prevailing culture in health care is an "opinion-based culture" grounded in intuition, clinical experience/expertise, and pathophysiological rationale (DiCenso, Guyatt, & Ciliska, 2005). A culture of EBP calls for the conscientious, explicit, and judicious use of current best evidence in making decisions about the care of individuals or groups of patients. However, evidence alone does not constitute EBP but requires the integration of this evidence with clinical expertise, patient values and preferences, and the clinical context of care (Sackett, Rosenberg, Gray, Haynes, & Richardson, 1996). The achievement of best patient outcomes is not assumed but is continuously evaluated though measurement of outcomes and patient safety (Coopey, Nix, & Clancy, 2006). This evidence is fed back into the system for consideration, and improvement changes at the individual, group, and system levels. Figure 1–1 portrays the components of EBP process, and Table 1–1 examines the components of EBP and the change/resources needed to facilitate its implementation.

BEST EVIDENCE

The best evidence is usually found in clinically relevant research that has been conducted using sound methodology (Sackett, 2000). With more than 1500 new articles per day and 55 new clinical trials per day, individual clinicians cannot hope to locate and read even a small portion of the relevant research published each year to assure best practices (Cilaska, Pinelli, DiCenso, & Cullum, 2001). The

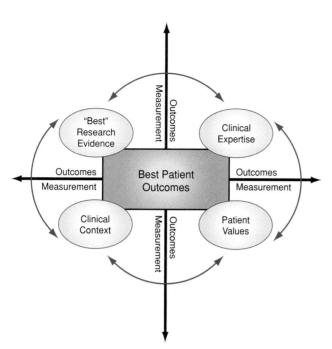

FIGURE 1–1   Components of evidence-based practice.

EBP process presents a more focused way of searching for information. Rather than routinely reviewing the contents of journals for interesting articles, the EBP process targets issues related to specific patient problems and provides clinicians with a set of skills for developing clinical questions related to these problems, searching current databases to keep current with the literature, and appraising the validity of the research on the topic of interest. In this process, the abstract exercise of reading and critically appraising the literature is converted into a pragmatic process of using the literature to benefit individual patients while simultaneously expanding the clinician's knowledge base (Bordley, 1997).

Within EBP, not all evidence is the same. The EBP clinician must know the nature and strength of the evidence found and, therefore, the accompanying degree of certainty/uncertainty with which to make decisions about whether the evidence should be applied to practice (Bhandari, 2003). Because much of research has been focused on the evaluation of "intervention effectiveness," in the evidence pyramid, the gold standard has been the randomized controlled trial followed by cohort studies, case-controlled studies, case series, and qualitative studies (Fig. 1–2). Yet, much of nursing practice and the majority

TABLE 1.1   *The Evidence-Based Practice Process*

	Components	Resources/Change Needed
Identify best evidence	*Clinical inquiry:* What knowledge is needed? *Informed skepticism:* Why are we doing it this way? Is there a better way to do it? What is the evidence for what we do? Would doing this be as effective as doing that? (Salmond, 2007)	• Shift from "know how" and doing to "know why" • Reflect on what information is needed to provide "best" care • Generate questions about practice and care • Role model clinical inquiry at report, rounds, conferences • Use interdisciplinary case reviews to evaluate actual care • Include clinical librarians as members of teams participating in clinical rounds and conferences
	Convert information needs from practice into focused, searchable questions (patient-intervention-comparison-outcome [PICO] framework).	• Differentiate between background and foreground questions • Consider recurring clinical issues, need for information, negative incidents/events as sources for questions or information needs • Identify clinical issues sensitive to nursing interventions • Narrow broad clinical issues/questions into searchable, focused questions • Use the mnemonic PICO to frame questions
	Search databases for highest level of evidence in a timely manner	• Use evidence-searching skills to target relevant focused evidence • Access evidence databases ideally at the point of care. • Understand evidence pyramids • Databases available include pre-appraised literature sources for point-of-care answers regarding intervention • Search strategies: key terms, multiple databases, point-of-care data • Use assistance of clinical librarian

(Continued on following page)

TABLE 1.1   *The Evidence-Based Practice Process (Continued)*

Components		Resources/Change Needed
	Use critical appraisal process to determine strength and validity of evidence and relevance to one's practice	• Clinical Practice Guidelines available at www.clearinghouse.gov • Preappraised sources such as Critically Appraised Topics (CATs) • Demonstrate knowledge of research design • Demonstrate knowledge of statistics • Use critical appraisal tools to guide process of research critique • Utilize journal clubs • Summarize findings from evaluation, resolving conflicting evidence
Clinical experience and expertise	Use clinical expertise to determine how to use evidence in care of patient and how to manage patient in absence of evidence or presence of conflicting evidence	• Consider evidence in relation to own patient population • Consider cost-benefit ratio • Consider multidimensionality of patient and clinical situation in relation to evidence that is often reductionistic
Patient values and preferences	Demonstrate ability to perform a culture assessment and identify client preferences and values that inform the clinical decision.	• Understand culture-general and culture-specific knowledge to guide interactions with client • Use interview skills to avoid culture imposition and seek client's true preferences • Communicate evidence and treatment options considering patient values and preferences • Involve client and family in both information giving and decision making
Translation evidence from total process into clinical decisions and strategies for best patient outcomes	Use all four components in clinical decision-making process and implementation of clinical decision	• Provide plan of care based on evidence, clinical judgment, patient preferences, and organizational context
Monitor patient outcomes	Use outcome tools to track client outcomes	• Develop audit systems to track client outcomes • Make clinical outcomes accessible electronically for analysis • Analyze outcomes and effectiveness of "evidence-based" clinical intervention

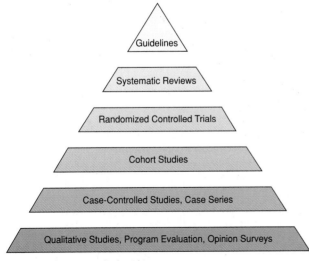

FIGURE 1–2   Pyramid of evidence.

of transcultural nursing knowledge are informed by research approaches that describe and explain an experience or phenomenon. Consequently, the hierarchy of evidence focusing on description of experience is quite different. Here, the lowest tier includes quantitative studies, and the highest tier includes qualitative studies and metasyntheses of qualitative work (Fig. 1–3). Whether working from a quantitative or qualitative perspective, searching should begin from the top of the pyramid, where evidence is presented as systematic reviews or evidence-based guidelines. Systematic reviews are a rigorous research methodology that summarizes the research on a prescribed clinical question. This level of evidence is generally most relevant to the clinical setting but may not be available. If evidence is not found at this level, one should continue searching at each subsequent level, being aware that there may be no good evidence to support clinical judgment (Rychetnik, Frommer, Hawe, & Shiell, 2002).

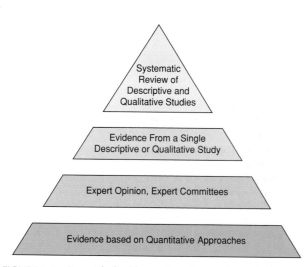

FIGURE 1–3   Pyramid of evidence: Description of experience.

Through consideration of this evidence or lack of evidence, clinicians and their affiliated health-care organizations have increased their awareness of evidence gaps and provided insight into the need for more research into unanswered questions. Ongoing nursing-driven and nursing-conducted research must become part of the evidence-based environment and not an occasional educational program or "window dressing" for the organization (Pravikoff, 2006).

CLINICAL EXPERTISE AND JUDGMENT

The value of expert clinical judgment can never be minimized in the clinical setting. Although drawing from best evidence is the goal, often there is insufficient evidence for the findings to be put into practice. Clinicians use their expertise to thoroughly assess the patient and differentiate nuances that influence treatment perspectives. With this expertise, the usefulness of the evidence in helping to care for a particular patient or patient population must be considered, and decisions about how to use that treatment must be made.

PATIENT VALUES

Combining the evidence with clinical expertise is necessary but not sufficient for driving quality care (Ivers, 2004; Rychetnik et al., 2002; Swales, 1998). Between the science (best evidence) and the final clinical decision, a judgment has to be made based on the values of the patient or group who will be exposed to the intervention (Swales, 1998). Cross-cultural comparisons provide abundant evidence for relativism of value systems. How the individual defines health and perceives the importance of health states such as mobility, freedom from pain, prolonged life expectancy, and preservation of faculties may all be valued differently, and these values influence both clinician recommendations and patient decisions (Swales, 1998). Failure to consider these patient preferences and values leads to "unintentional biasing" toward a professionals' view of the world (Kitson, 2002). If EBP is to be value-added, it is critical to assure that the users of the

knowledge, the clients, become "active shapers" of knowledge and action (Clough, 2005). Clinicians must be prepared to make "real-time" adjustments to their approach to care based on client feedback.

To date, much of the focus on EBP has been on scientism and determination of best evidence. Unfortunately, little science examines intervention efficacy or desirability by cultural group. The study of culture and the individual nature of values is by its very nature holistic and adverse to a reductionistic approach that can be expressed as a population average. Clinicians armed with culture-general knowledge are more open to multiple ways of being. Understanding of culture-specific knowledge can guide clinicians in their assessment approach, leading to a patient-focused discussion of preferred approaches to treatment and care. This critical component of EBP needs to be more fully developed. How is it operationalized in practice? What are the best strategies for integrating patient values? Is there a preferred intervention by cultural group? This information is needed to facilitate best patient outcomes. The goal is not to achieve a single prescriptive system of care but to respect the individual nonuniform values that determine specific patient needs (Swales, 1998).

CLINICAL CONTEXT

The clinical context encompasses the setting in which practice takes place or the environment in which the proposed change is to be implemented (McCormack, Kitson, Harvey, Rycroft-Malone, Titchen, & Seers, 2002). Drennan (1992) argues that culture, or "the way things are done around here" at the individual, team, and organizational levels, creates the context for practice and change. Organizational culture is a paradigm—a way of thinking about the organization, comprising a linkage of basic assumptions, values, and artifacts (Schein, 1992).

Implementation of EBP is not so much about getting trained in the right protocol, although that will be necessary, as it is about changing the culture of the organization or practice to one that is measurement- and outcomes-orientated across all disciplines, not in isolated silos (Morrison, 2004). Implementation of evidence (translation of evidence into practice) is explained as a dynamic, simultaneous relationship between *evidence* (best research evidence, clinical experience, and patient preferences) and *context* (organizational capacity, infrastructure, and culture).

The abundance of new evidence that has *not* been successfully translated into practice is a critical reminder of the importance of context and the strength of the existing culture. Descriptive and qualitative data must be gathered to make an assessment of the likelihood of transferability; organization-specific strategies need to be used to facilitate this process. Best evidence specific to knowledge transfer and practice change needs to be incorporated in the change plan. Measuring clinician, unit, or organizational outcomes and benchmarking these outcomes provide the feedback necessary to effect change. Difficult questions will need to be grappled with. What should be done with clinicians who cannot or will not adapt to EBP? How will lack of interdisciplinary collaboration be approached? How will it be handled if long-standing treatment approaches show no evidence of fostering improvement? What is the individual's responsibility, as compared with the organization's responsibility, in assuring readiness for EBP? How the organization handles these critical questions influences the outcomes of the change process.

FACILITATING THE SHIFT TOWARD EVIDENCE-BASED PRACTICE

Achieving this culture shift requires a commitment and a long-term investment in providing the leadership support, skill development, and infrastructure necessary to advance and sustain this shift.

Leadership Commitment

The transition must begin with a commitment from upper administration at both the nursing and the hospital administration levels to assure that all clinicians develop information literacy or the "ability to recognize that information is needed, find it, evaluate it, and use it in practice" (American Library Association, 2006). This commitment must include an investment of resources as well as a commitment to build EBP into organizational processes, to consistently communicate a vision for EBP, and to role-model and demonstrate ongoing commitment to EBP. A particularly difficult leadership challenge will be to move away from hierarchical, paternalistic processes and facilitate interdisciplinary involvement and commitment in EBP and to deal with the critical questions that emerge when EBP goals are not being met (Cilaska et al., 2001; Stetler, 2003). Clinical management structures must be developed to support effective interdisciplinary clinical decision-making activities (Mallach & Porter-O'Grady, 2006). Mink, Esterhuysen, Mink, and Owen's model (1993) of transformational change is an appropriate implementation model for leaders to remove barriers to EBP and begin the journey to developing an interdisciplinary culture of EBP. The model calls for formation of interdisciplinary teams consisting of a central, transformational team that performs an environmental assessment, sets goals, and guides the practice change as well as unit-based interdisciplinary action teams who develop clinical practice protocols and practices and implement the change at the point of care. Resources include dedicated time for the teams to work and educational support so that the teams can serve as support systems within the organization for implementation of EBP and clinical research.

Developing the Needed Skill Set

Developing the needed skill set begins with a commitment on the part of every individual practitioner to making EBP the framework for clinical decision-making (Mallach & Porter-O'Grady, 2006). In addition to individual responsibilities for developing needed knowledge and skills, an EBP organization has ongoing, leveled, onsite educational programs about information literacy, the EBP process, and research. Initial programs should attempt to

create a sense of urgency by helping clinicians see how science has changed practice, recognize the lag in transferring this knowledge, and understand how outcomes vary based on the differential use of new science. Clinicians need to be helped with the new vocabulary of EBP. This should be done in a format that can be quickly retrieved and understood. Educational content must target information literacy skills—how to access, interpret, synthesize, and apply most current evidence at the point of care. Table 1–1 summarizes educational targets that must be reached. Multiple approaches to learning, such as face-to-face programs, on-line references and modules, and small group learning, should all be used to reach the multiple audiences and multiple levels of learning.

Systematic reviews of traditional forms of continuing education, such as browsing journals, attending conferences, and listening to didactic lectures, have little impact on changing practice (Thomson O'Brien, Freemantle, & Oxman, 2001). Active learning strategies are needed to develop the capacity to engage in EBP. Journal clubs, poster presentations, EBP internships, clinical coaching/mentoring by expert clinical leaders or clinical nurse specialists, evidence-based scholar groups, and evidence-based rounds are all examples of active learning approaches that facilitate development of a culture of inquiry or inquisitiveness, openness, and encouragement of learning new skills (Pravikoff, 2006; Turkel, Reidinger, Ferket, & Reno, 2005).

The expectation for EBP should be articulated at orientation as a universal expectation with differing skill sets evident at differing rungs of the clinical ladder. At the lowest rung, everyone should manifest clinical inquiry or informed skepticism and the ability to ask questions about care and know when information is needed. Incorporating more advanced skills can be integrated into the differing levels of a clinical ladder. These advanced skills include translating clinical questions into patient-intervention-comparison-outcome (PICO) format, searching presynthesized literature, critiquing research for reliability and validity, comparing research findings with actual clinical populations and settings, planning for evidence translation, implementing new EBP interventions, measuring the results of evidence implementation, and planning primary research studies needed to fill in evidence gaps. Integrating EBP into career ladder expectations, different levels of clinicians can be advancing the EBP process for the organization.

Access to Information

In order for nurses to be able to use evidence in their busy clinical routines, there must be a systematic organizational infrastructure to support EBP as a way of delivering care (Mallach & Porter-O'Grady, 2006). This includes access to a digital information framework that provides ready access to real-time information at the point of care delivery that is neither time nor place dependent. The technological/informational infrastructure needed to support EBP includes user-friendly, credible summaries of up-to-date evidence; the informatics structure to integrate EBP data (internal and external) into quality processes (electronic medical records and other clinical databases); access to clinical librarians or others who are expert in information literacy and who can coach staff; electronic library sources to guide the EBP process; and computer experts and technological support (Antes et al., 2006; Mallach & Porter-O'Grady, 2006). This technology must be at the point of care—either on a unit/service area or via hand-held technology to facilitate EBP as a clinical decision process.

The interface among the information infrastructure, performance measurement, and quality patient care outcomes is critical. This requires integration between clinical practice and data management and is ideally tracked through clinical information management systems and/or clinical audits. This component of EBP, in which best practices are implemented and outcomes are tracked, completes the feedback loop needed to modify and adapt evidence in the practice setting. The internal findings can be used for ongoing competency development and performance approval as well as integrated with external evidence and analyzed for needed best practice changes.

SUMMARY

The move to a culture of EBP requires a shift from a culture of doing to a culture of clinical reflection, in which care is evaluated based on the need for evidence and patient preferences. This culture change process must be actively managed so that all members of the health-care team are aware of the expectations regarding EBP, receive appropriate educational and mentor support for information literacy, and are held accountable through audit and performance appraisal for using EBP as a clinical decision model.

REFERENCES

Abrums, M. (2004). Faith and feminism: How African American women from a forefront church resist oppression in health care. *Advances in Nursing Science, 27*, 187–201.

Agency for Healthcare Research and Quality (AHRQ). (2005). Third National Healthcare Disparities Report. U.S. Department of Health and Human Services. AHRQ Publication No. 06-0017.

American Library Association. Presidential Committee on Information Literacy. (2006). Final report. (Vol. 2006). American Library Association, 1989. Retrieved March 14, 2007, from http://www.ala.org/ala/acrl/acrlpubs/whitepapers/presidential.htm

Andrews, M., & Boyle, J. (2005). *Transcultural concepts in nursing.* (4th ed.). Philadelphia: Lippincott.

Antes, G., Sauerland, S., & Seiler, C. M. (2006). Evidence-based medicine—From best research evidence to a better surgical practice and health care. *Archives of Surgery, 391*, 61–67.

Baker, R. (1998). A theory of international bioethics: Multiculturism, post-modernism, and the bankruptcy of fundamentalism. *Kennedy Institute Ethics Journal, 8*(3), 201–231.

Beaucamp, T. (1998). The mettle of moral fundamentalism: A reply to Robert Baker. *Kennedy Institute of Ethics Journal, 8*(4), 389–401.

Bhandari, M. (2003). Evidence-based orthopaedics: A paradigm shift. *Clinical Orthopaedics and Related Research, 413*, 9–10.

Birch, D. (2006, October 27). In Russia, the truth is optional. *Baltimore Sun,* pp. 2F, 6F.

Bordley, D. R. (1997). Evidence-based medicine: A powerful educational tool for clerkship education. *American Journal of Medicine, 102*(5), 427–432.

Campinha-Bacote, J. (2006). *The process of cultural competence in the delivery of health services: A culturally competent approach* (4th ed.). Cincinnati, OH: Transcultural C.A.R.E. Associates.

CIA World Factbook: World. (2007). Retrieved March 28, 2007, from https://www.cia.gov/cia/publications/factbook/geos/xx.html

Cilaska, D. K., Pinelli, J., DiCenso, A., & Cullum, N. (2001). Resources to enhance evidence-based nursing practice. *AACN Clinical Issues, 12*(4), 520–528.

Clough, E. (2005). Foreword. In J. Burr and P. Nicholson (Eds.). *Researching health care consumers, critical approaches* (pp. ix–xi). Basingstoke, UK: Palgrave (MacMillan).

Coopey, M., Nix, M. P., & Clancy, C. M. (2006). Translating research into evidence-based nursing practice and evaluating effectiveness. *Journal of Nursing Care Quality, 21*(3), 195–202.

DiCenso, A., Guyatt, G., & Ciliska, D. (2005). *Evidence-based nursing: A guide to clinical practice.* Philadelphia: Elsevier, Mosby.

Drennan, D. (1992). *Transforming company culture.* London: McGraw-Hill.

Giger, J., & Davidhizar, R. (2008). *Transcultural nursing: Assessment and intervention* (4th ed.). St. Louis: Mosby.

Health Inequities: A Challenge for Europe. (2005, October). Retrieved August 19, 2006, from www.ec.europa.eu/health/ph_determinants/

Healthy People 2010. (2005). Retrieved August 20, 2006, from http://www.healthypeople.gov

Healthy People 2010 Companion Document for Lesbian, Gay, Bisexual, and Transgender Health. (2001). Retrieved September 14, 2006, from http://www.lgbthealth.net

Home Office Study. (2002). Retrieved August 19, 2006, from http://news.google.com/news?q=Home+Office+Study++United+Kingdom&hl=en&lr=&sa=X&oi=news&ct=title.

International Convention on the Elimination of All Forms of Racial Discrimination (1965). Retrieved August 20, 2006, from http://www.unhchr.ch/html/menu3/b/d_icerd.htm

Ivers, R. G. (2004). An evidence-based approach to planning tobacco interventions for Aboriginal people. *Drug and Alcohol Review, 23*, 5–9.

Kitson, A. (2002). Recognizing relationships: Reflections on evidence-based practice. *Nursing Inquiry, 9*(3), 179–186.

Koffman, J. (2006). Transcultural and ethical issues at the end of life. In J. Cooper (Ed.). *Stepping into palliative care* 1 (chap. 15, pp. 171–186). Abington, UK: Radcliffe Publishing Ltd.

Macklin, R. (1998). A defense of fundamental principles and human rights: A reply to Robert Baker. *Kennedy Institute of Ethics Journal, 8*(4), 389–401.

Macklin, R. (1999). *Against relativism: Cultural diversity and the search for ethical universals in medicine.* New York: Oxford University Press.

Mallach, K., & Porter-O'Grady, T. (2006). *Evidence-based practice in nursing and healthcare.* Boston: Jones & Bartlett.

McCormack, B., Kitson, A., Harvey, G., Rycroft-Malone, J., Titchen, A., & Seers, K. (2002). Getting evidence into practice: The meaning of "context." *Journal of Advanced Nursing, 38*(1), 94–104.

Mink, O. G., Esterhuysen, P. W., Mink, B. P., & Owen, K. Q. (1993). *Change at work.* San Francisco: Jossey Bass.

Morrison, D. (2004). Real-world use of evidence-based treatments in community behavioral health care. *Psychiatric Services,* http://ps.psychiatryonline.org, *55*(5), 485–487.

National Healthcare Quality Report. (2006). Retrieved August 24, 2007, from http://www.ahr.gov/qua1/nhqr06/nhqr/06.htm

National Research Council. (1998). Retrieved August 18, 2006, from www.nationalacademies.org/news.nsf/isbn/0309063566?OpenDocument

Perspectives on Disease Prevention and Health Promotion. (1985). Retrieved September 23, 2006, from www.cdc.gov/mmwr/preview/mmwrthml/00000688.htm

Police Unit Reaches Out to Gay Community, Inspires Others. (2006, September 16). *Baltimore Sun,* p. 5A.

Pravikoff, D. S. (2006). Mission critical: A culture of evidence-based practice and information literacy. *Nursing Outlook, 54*(4), 254–255.

Purnell, L. (2001). Cultural competence in a changing health-care environment. In N. L. Chaska (Ed.), *The nursing profession: Tomorrow and beyond* (pp. 451–461). Thousand Oaks, CA: Sage Publications.

Purnell, L. (2003, March–August). Cultural diversity for older Americans. Cultural competence for the physical therapist working with clients with alternative lifestyles. A monograph. American Physical Therapy Association: Author.

Rychetnik, L., Frommer, M., Hawe, P., & Shiell, A. (2002). Criteria for evaluating evidence on public health interventions. *Journal of Epidemiology in Community Health, 56*, 119–127.

Sackett, D. (2000). *Evidence-based medicine: How to practice and teach EB.* (2nd ed.). Amsterdam, The Netherlands: Churchill Livingtone.

Sackett, D. L., Rosenberg, W. M. C., Gray, J. A. M., Haynes, R. B., & Richardson, W. S. (1996). Evidence based medicine: What it is and what it is not. *British Medical Journal, 312*, 71–72.

Schein, E. H. (1992). *Organizational Culture and Leadership.* (2nd ed). San Francisco, CA: Jossey-Bass.

Stetler, C. B. (2003). Role of the organization in translating research into evidence-based practice. *Outcomes Management, 7*(3):97–103.

Swales, J. (1998). Culture and medicine. *Journal of the Royal Society of Medicine, 91,* 118–126.

Thomson O'Brien, M. A., Feemantle, N., & Oxman, A. D. (2001). Continuing education meetings and workshops: Effects on professional practice and health care outcomes. *Cochrane Database Systematic Reviews,* (1), CD003030.

Turkel, M. C., Reidinger, G., Ferket, K., & Reno, K. (2005). An essential component of the magnet journey: Fostering an environment for evi-dence-based practice and nursing research. *Nursing Administration Quarterly, 29*(3), 254–262.

Universal Declaration of Human Rights. (2001). Retrieved March 28, 2007, from www.amnesty.org.

U.S. Bureau of the Census: Demographic Profiles. (2006). Retrieved August 25, 2006, from http://www.census.gov/main/www/cen2000.html

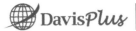

DavisPlus | For case studies, review questions, and additional information, go to http://davisplus.fadavis.com.

Chapter *2*

The Purnell Model for Cultural Competence

LARRY D. PURNELL

This chapter presents the Purnell Model for Cultural Competence, its organizing framework, and the assumptions upon which the model is based. In addition, American cultural values, practices, and beliefs are presented to assist non–native American health-care providers to understand American ways. The American references are meant to describe, not prescribe or predict, behaviors and practices. Although the authors recognize that Canada and Mexico are part of North America, *American,* as used in this chapter, refers to the dominant middle-class values of citizens of the mainland United States. Owing to space limitations, this chapter deals not with the objective culture—arts, literature, humanities, and so on—but rather with the subjective culture. Many Americans are not aware of the subjective culture because they identify differences as individual personality traits and disregard political and social origins of culture. Many view culture as something that belongs only to foreigners or disadvantaged groups. However, when Americans travel abroad, their host country inhabitants many times stereotypically identify them as Americans because of their values, beliefs, attitudes, behaviors, speech patterns, and mannerisms. Some feel that Americans are "fun lovers" and that, for some Americans, violence is a way of life. However, "the right to bear arms" is guaranteed by the Constitution. Most likely, the United States is not any more violent than, or even as violent as, many other societies, but American media coverage may be better than other countries, thereby giving the impression that the United States is more violent than it actually is. Accordingly, these stereotypes are not always accurate or desirable.

Western academic and health-care organizations stress structure, systematization, and formalization when studying complex phenomena such as culture and ethnicity. Given the complexity of individuals, the Purnell Model for Cultural Competence provides a comprehensive, systematic, and concise framework for learning and understanding culture. The empirical framework of the model can assist health-care providers, managers, and administrators in all health disciplines to provide holistic, culturally competent therapeutic interventions; health promotion and wellness; illness, disease, and injury prevention; health maintenance and restoration; and health teaching across educational and practice settings.

The purposes of this model are to

1. Provide a framework for all health-care providers to learn concepts and characteristics of culture.
2. Define circumstances that affect a person's cultural worldview in the context of historical perspectives.
3. Provide a model that links the most central relationships of culture.
4. Interrelate characteristics of culture to promote congruence and to facilitate the delivery of consciously sensitive and competent health care.
5. Provide a framework that reflects human characteristics such as motivation, intentionality, and meaning.
6. Provide a structure for analyzing cultural data.
7. View the individual, family, or group within their unique ethnocultural environment.

Assumptions Upon Which the Model Is Based

The major explicit assumptions upon which the model is based are

1. All health-care professions need similar information about cultural diversity.

2. All health-care professions share the metaparadigm concepts of global society, family, person, and health.

3. One culture is not better than another culture; they are just different.

4. Core similarities are shared by all cultures.

5. Differences exist within, between, and among cultures.

6. Cultures change slowly over time.

7. The primary and secondary characteristics of culture (see Chapter 1) determine the degree to which one varies from the dominant culture.

8. If clients are coparticipants in their care and have a choice in health-related goals, plans, and interventions, their compliance and health outcomes will be improved.

9. Culture has a powerful influence on one's interpretation of and responses to health care.

10. Individuals and families belong to several subcultures.

11. Each individual has the right to be respected for his or her uniqueness and cultural heritage.

12. Caregivers need both culture-general and culture-specific information in order to provide culturally sensitive and culturally competent care.

13. Caregivers who can assess, plan, intervene, and evaluate in a culturally competent manner will improve the care of clients for whom they care.

14. Learning culture is an ongoing process that develops in a variety of ways, but primarily through cultural encounters (Campinha-Bacote, 2006).

15. Prejudices and biases can be minimized with cultural understanding.

16. To be effective, health care must reflect the unique understanding of the values, beliefs, attitudes, lifeways, and worldview of diverse populations and individual acculturation patterns.

17. Differences in race and culture often require adaptations to standard interventions.

18. Cultural awareness improves the caregiver's self-awareness.

19. Professions, organizations, and associations have their own culture, which can be analyzed using a grand theory of culture.

20. Every client encounter is a cultural encounter.

Overview of the Theory, the Model, and Organizing Framework

The Purnell model has been classified as holographic and complexity theory because it includes a model and organizing framework that can be used by all health-care providers in various disciplines and settings. The model is a circle, with an outlying rim representing global society, a second rim representing community, a third rim representing family, and an inner rim representing the person (Fig. 2–1). The interior of the circle is divided into 12 pie-shaped wedges depicting cultural domains and their concepts. The dark center of the circle represents unknown phenomena. Along the bottom of the model, a jagged line represents the nonlinear concept of cultural consciousness. The 12 cultural domains (constructs) provide the organizing framework of the model. A box following the discussion of each domain provides statements that can be adapted as a guide for assessing patients and clients in various settings. Accordingly, health-care providers can use these same questions to better understand their own cultural beliefs, attitudes, values, practices, and behaviors.

MACRO ASPECTS OF THE MODEL

The macro aspects of this interactional model include the metaparadigm concepts of a global society, community, family, person, and conscious competence. The theory and model are conceptualized from biology, anthropology, sociology, economics, geography, history, ecology, physiology, psychology, political science, pharmacology, and nutrition as well as theories from communication, family development, and social support. The model can be used in clinical practice, education, research, and the administration and management of health-care services or to analyze organizational culture.

Phenomena related to a **global society** include world communication and politics; conflicts and warfare; natural disasters and famines; international exchanges in education, business, commerce, and information technology; advances in health science; space exploration; and the expanded opportunities for people to travel around the world and interact with diverse societies. Global events that are widely disseminated by television, radio, satellite transmission, newsprint, and information technology affect all societies, either directly or indirectly. Such events create chaos while consciously and unconsciously forcing people to alter their lifeways and worldviews.

Think of a recent event that has affected global society, such as conflict or war, health advances in technology, or recent travel and possible environmental exposure to health problems. How did you become aware of this event? How has this event altered your views and other people's views of worldwide cultures?

The Purnell Model for Cultural Competence

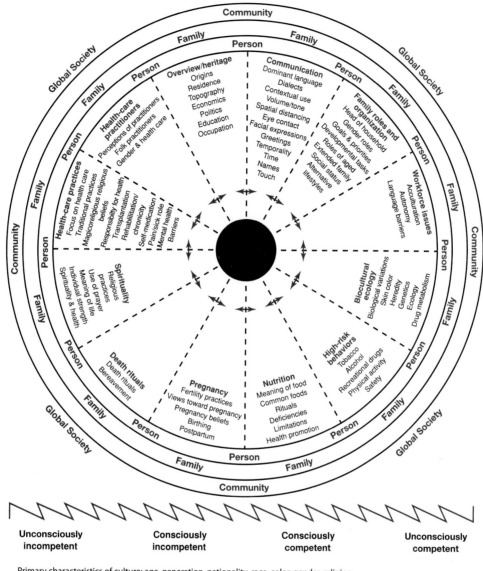

FIGURE 2–1 Purnell's Model for Cultural Competence. (Adapted with permission from Larry Purnell, Newark, DE.)

In the broadest definition, **community** is a group of people having a common interest or identity and goes beyond the physical environment. Community includes the physical, social, and symbolic characteristics that cause people to connect. Bodies of water, mountains, rural versus urban living, and even railroad tracks help people define their physical concept of community.

Today, however, technology and the Internet allow people to expand their community beyond physical boundaries. Economics, religion, politics, age, generation, and marital status delineate the social concepts of community. Symbolic characteristics of a community include sharing a specific language or dialect, lifestyle, history, dress, art, or musical interest. People actively and passively interact with the community, necessitating adaptation and assimilation for equilibrium and homeostasis in their worldview. Individuals may willingly change their physical, social, and symbolic community when it no longer meets their needs.

How do you define your community in terms of objective and subjective cultural characteristics? How has your community changed over the last 5 to 10 years? The last 15 years? The last 20 years? If you have changed communities, think of the community in which you were raised.

A **family** is two or more people who are emotionally connected. They may, but do not necessarily, live in close proximity to each other. Family may include physically and emotionally close and distant consanguineous relatives as well as physically and emotionally connected and distant non–blood-related significant others. Family structure and roles change according to age, generation, marital status, relocation or immigration, and socioeconomic status, requiring each person to rethink individual beliefs and lifeways.

Whom do you consider family? How have they influenced your culture and worldview? Who else has helped instill your cultural values?

A **person** is a biopsychosociocultural being who is constantly adapting to her or his community. Human beings adapt biologically and physiologically with the aging process; psychologically in the context of social relationships, stress, and relaxation; socially as they interact with the changing community; and ethnoculturally within the broader global society. In Western cultures, a person is a separate physical and unique psychological being and a singular member of society. The self is separate from others. However, in Asian and some other cultures, the individual is defined in relation to the family or other group rather than a basic unit of nature.

In what ways have you adapted (1) biologically and physiologically to the aging process, (2) psychologically in the context of social relationships, (3) socially in your community, and (4) ethnoculturally within the broader society?

Health, as used in this book, is a state of wellness as defined by the individual within his or her ethnocultural group. Health generally includes physical, mental, and spiritual states because group members interact with the family, community, and global society. The concept of health, which permeates all metaparadigm concepts of culture, is defined globally, nationally, regionally, locally, and individually. Thus, people can speak about their personal health status or the health status of the nation or community. Health can also be subjective or objective in nature.

How do you define health? Is health the absence of illness, disease, injury, and/or disability? How does your profession define health? How does your nation or community define health? How do these definitions compare with your original ethnic background?

MICRO ASPECTS OF THE MODEL

On a micro level, the model's organizing framework comprises 12 domains and their concepts, which are common to all cultures. These 12 domains are interconnected and have implications for health. The utility of this organizing framework comes from its concise structure, which can be used in any setting and applied to a broad range of empirical experiences and can foster inductive and deductive reasoning in the assessment of cultural domains. Once cultural data are analyzed, the practitioner can fully adopt, modify, or reject health-care interventions and treatment regimens in a manner that respects the client's cultural differences. Such adaptations improve the quality of the client's health-care experiences and personal existence.

The Twelve Domains of Culture

The 12 domains essential for assessing the ethnocultural attributes of an individual, family, or group are

1. Overview, inhabited localities, and topography.
2. Communication.
3. Family roles and organization.
4. Workforce issues.
5. Biocultural ecology.
6. High-risk behaviors.
7. Nutrition.
8. Pregnancy and childbearing practices.
9. Death rituals.
10. Spirituality.
11. Health-care practices.
12. Health-care practitioners.

OVERVIEW, INHABITED LOCALITIES, AND TOPOGRAPHY

This domain, *overview, inhabited localities, and topography,* includes concepts related to the country of origin, the current residence, the effects of the topography of the country of origin and current residence on health, economics, politics, reasons for migration, educational status, and occupations. These concepts are interrelated. For example, economic and political conditions may affect one's reason for migration, and educational attainment is usually interrelated with employment choices and opportunities. Sociopolitical and socioeconomic conditions influence individual behavioral responses to health and illness.

Learning about a culture includes becoming familiar with the heritage of its people and understanding how discrimination, prejudice, and oppression influence value systems and beliefs used in everyday life. Given the primary and secondary characteristics of diversity (see Chapter 1), cultural specific generalizations may not be part of a particular individual's beliefs or value system.

For most Americans, dominant cultural values and beliefs include individualism, free speech, rights of choice, independence and self-reliance, confidence, "doing" rather than "being," egalitarian relationships, nonhierarchal status of individuals, achievement status over ascribed status, "volunteerism," friendliness, openness, futuristic temporality, ability to control the environment, and an emphasis on material things and physical comfort. These concepts are more fully described in other sections of this chapter.

Given the size, population density, and diversity of the United States, one cannot generalize too much about American culture. Every generalization in this chapter is subject to exceptions, although most people will agree with the descriptions to some degree and on some level. Moreover, we believe the descriptions about the dominant American culture are true for white middle-class European Americans (and many other groups as well) who hold the majority of prestigious positions in the United States. The degree to which people conform to this dominant culture depends on the primary and secondary characteristics of culture discussed in Chapter 1 as well as individual personality differences. We recognize that some Americans do not think there is an American culture and resent any attempt at generalizations. Many foreigners believe that all Americans are rich, everyone lives in fancy apartments or houses, crime is everywhere, everyone drives an expensive gasoline-inefficient car, and there is little or no poverty. For the most part, these misconceptions come from the media and Americans who travel overseas.

Heritage and Residence

The United States comprises 3.5 million square miles and a population of nearly 300 million people, making it the world's third most populous country (CIA Factbook, 2006). The United States is mostly temperate but tropical in Hawaii and Florida, arctic in Alaska, semiarid in the great plains west of the Mississippi River, and arid in the Great Basin of the southwest. Low winter temperatures in the northwest are ameliorated in January and February by warm Chinook winds from the eastern slopes of the Rocky Mounatins. There is a vast central plain; mountains in the west; hills and low mountains in the east; rugged mountains and broad river valleys in Alaska; and rugged, volcanic topography in Hawaii.

When Europeans began settling the United States in the 16th century, approximately 2 million American Indians, who mostly lived in geographically isolated tribes, populated the land. The first permanent European settlement in the United States was St. Augustine, Florida, which was settled by the Spanish in 1565. The first English settlement was Jamestown, Virginia, in 1607. By 1610, the nonnative population in the United States was only 350 people. By 1700, the population increased to 250,900; by 1800, to 5.3 million; and by 1900, to 75.9 million (Time Almanac, 2001). From 1607 until 1890, most immigrants to the United States came from Europe and essentially shared a common European culture. The plantation economy of the South paid for the forced relocation of natives from (primarily Western) Africa beginning in 1619 and ending with the American Civil War (1861–1865). This group did not share the common culture, and their acculturation was strongly influenced by their status as slaves.

In the 1830s, a war with Mexico resulted in the annexation of greater Texas. From 1860 until 1865, the North and South fought over the issue of slavery, which resulted not only in the elimination of slavery but also in the industrialization of the North and the establishment of the United States as a major military power. The Spanish-American War (1898) resulted in the United States becoming a colonial power, with the annexation of Spain's last colony in the Western Hemisphere, Cuba, and also its colony in the Philippines. World War I (1914–1918) established the United States as one of the world's superpowers, and World War II (1939–1945) significantly extended U.S. military power. In the postwar period, the ideological differences between the United States and the USSR resulted in the Cold War, which lasted until 1989. Today, U.S. military, cultural, and economic power affect almost every other country on the planet.

The American colonies broke with the parent country, Britain, on July 4, 1776, and were recognized as the new nation of The United States of America with the original 13 colonies following the Treaty of Paris in 1783. During the 19th and 20th centuries, 37 new states were added to the original 13 as the nation expanded across the North American continent and acquired a number of overseas possessions.

The Constitution of the Untied States was ratified in 1789 and included seven articles, which laid the foundation for an independent nation. The Bill of Rights, the first 10 amendments to the Constitution, guarantees freedom of religion, speech, and the press; the right to petition, bear arms; and the right to a speedy trial. Only 17 additional amendments have been made to the Constitution. The 13th Amendment in 1865 prohibited slavery; the 14th Amendment in 1868 defined citizenship and privileges of citizens; the 15th Amendment in 1870 gave suffrage rights regardless of race or color; and the 19th Amendment in 1920 gave women the right to vote.

The United States is the world's oldest constitutional democracy with three branches of government: (1) the executive branch, which includes the Office of the President and the administrative departments; (2) the legislative branch, Congress, which includes both the Senate and the House of Representatives; and (3) the judicial branch, which includes the Supreme Court and the lesser federal courts. The Supreme Court has nine members appointed by the President and approved by Congress. The Justices serve a life term if they so choose. The

President serves a 4-year term and can be reelected only one time. The President is the Commander-in-Chief of the Armed Forces and oversees the executive departments. The members of the House of Representatives are divided among the states based on the population of each state. Members of the House of Representatives serve 2-year terms. Each state has two senators, regardless of the population of the state. Senators serve 6-year terms. Each of the 50 states has its own constitution establishing, for the most part, a parallel structure to the federal government, with the executive branch headed by a governor, a state congress with representatives and senators, and a state court system.

No limitations were placed on immigrants from Europe until the late 1800s. From 1892 to 1952, most European immigrants to America came through Ellis Island, New York, where they had to prove to officials that they were financially independent. More severe restrictions were placed on other immigrant groups, particularly those from Asia. In the 1960s, immigration policy changed to allow immigrants from all parts of the world without favoritism to or restrictions on ethnicity. Today, the United States includes immigrants or descendents from immigrants from almost every nation and culture of the world and is the world's premier international nation. The United States admitted 52,868 refugees during fiscal year 2003–2004, including 13,331 from Somalia, 6000 from Laos, 3482 from Ukraine, 2959 from Cuba, and 1787 from Iran. As of June 2005, 32,229 refugees had been admitted (CIA Factbook, 2006).

The United States has the largest and most technologically powerful economy in the world, with a per capita gross domestic product (GDP) of $42,000. In this market-oriented economy, private individuals and business firms make most of the decisions, and the federal and state governments buy needed goods and services predominantly in the private marketplace. U.S. business firms enjoy greater flexibility than their counterparts in Western Europe and Japan in decisions to expand capital plant, to lay off surplus workers, and to develop new products. At the same time, they face higher barriers to enter their rivals' home markets than foreign firms face entering U.S. markets. U.S. firms are at or near the forefront in technological advances, especially in computers and in medical, aerospace, and military equipment; their advantage has narrowed since the end of World War II.

The on-rush of technology largely explains the gradual development of a "two-tier labor market," in which those at the bottom lack the education and the professional/technical skills of those at the top and, more and more, fail to get comparable pay raises, health insurance coverage, and other benefits. Since 1975, practically all the gains in household income have gone to the top 20 percent of households.

The response to the terrorist attacks of September 11, 2001, showed the remarkable resilience of the economy. The war in March–April 2003 between a U.S.-led coalition and Iraq, and the subsequent occupation of Iraq, required major shifts in national resources to the military. The rise in GDP in 2004 and 2005 was supported by substantial gains in labor productivity. Hurricane Katrina caused extensive damage in the Gulf Coast region in August 2005 but had a small impact on overall GDP growth for the year. Soaring oil prices in 2005 and 2006 threatened inflation and unemployment, yet the economy continued to grow through mid 2006. Imported oil accounts for about two-thirds of U.S. consumption. Long-term problems include inadequate investment in economic infrastructure, rapidly rising medical and pension costs of an aging population, sizable trade and budget deficits, and stagnation of family income in the lower economic groups (CIA Factbook, 2006).

People have been attracted to immigrate to the United States because of its vast resources and economic and personal freedoms, particularly the dogma that "all men are created equal." Immigrants and their descendants achieved enormous material success, which further encouraged immigration.

Reasons for Migration and Associated Economic Factors

The United States has a very large middle-class population and a small, but growing, wealthy population. Approximately 12.7 percent of the population lives in poverty, with higher rates among children (17.8 percent), older persons (20.5 percent), blacks (24.7 percent), and nonwhite Hispanics (21.9 percent) (U.S. Bureau of the Census: Poverty Rates, 2006c). The social, economic, religious, and political forces of the country of origin play an important role in the development of the ideologies and the worldview of individuals, families, and groups and are often a major motivating force for emigration.

The earlier settlers in the United States came for better economic opportunities, because of religious and political oppression and environmental disasters such as earthquakes and hurricanes in their home countries, and by forced relocation such as slaves and indentured servants. Others have immigrated for educational opportunities and personal ideologies or a combination of factors. Most people immigrate in the hope of a better life; however, the individual or group personally defines this ideology.

A common practice for many immigrants is to relocate to an area that has an established population with similar ideologies that can provide initial support, serve as cultural brokers, and orient them to their new culture and health-care system. For example, most people of Cuban heritage live in New York and Florida; French Canadians are concentrated in the Northeast; and the Amish are concentrated in Pennsylvania, Indiana, and Ohio. When immigrants settle and work exclusively in predominantly ethnic communities, primary social support is enhanced, but acculturation and assimilation into the wider society may be hindered. Groups without ethnic enclaves in the United States to assist them with acculturation may need extra help in adjusting to their new homeland's language, access to health-care services, living accommodations, and employment opportunities. People who move voluntarily are likely to experience less difficulty with acculturation than people who are forced to emigrate. Some individuals immigrate with the intention of remaining in this country only a short time, making money, and returning home, whereas others immigrate with the intention of relocating permanently.

> **What is your cultural heritage? How might you find out more about it? Does your cultural heritage influence your current beliefs and values about health and wellness? What brought you/your ancestors to your current country of residence? Why did you/your ancestors emigrate?**

Educational Status and Occupations

The value placed on formal education differs among cultural and ethnic groups and is often related to their socioeconomic status in their homeland and their abilities and reasons for emigrating. The United States places a high value on education, which has recently become a major issue in federal and state elections. Some groups, however, do not stress formal education because it is not needed for employment in their homeland. Consequently, they may become engulfed in poverty, isolation, and enclave identity, which may further limit their potential for formal educational opportunities and planning for the future.

In the United States, preparation in elementary and secondary education varies widely. There is no national curriculum that each school is expected to follow, although there is standardized testing at a national level, which is used in the selection process for admission to institutions of higher education. Most states require children to attend school until the age of 16, although the child can drop out of school at a younger age with parents' signed permission. Overall, the United States has the goal of producing a well-rounded individual with a variety of courses and 100 percent literacy. Theoretically, people have the freedom to choose a profession, regardless of gender and background. Educational attainment in the United States varies by race, gender, and region of the country. Eighty-seven percent of all adults age 25 years and older have completed high school, and 27 percent have completed a bachelor's degree or higher. Of Asians, 87.6 percent have completed high school and 49.8 percent have a bachelor's degree or higher. Of blacks, only 80 percent have completed high school and 17.3 percent have a bachelor's degree or higher. Of Hispanics, only 57 percent have completed high school and only 1.4 percent have a bachelor's degree or higher (U.S. Bureau of the Census, 2006b). In regard to learning styles, the Western system places a high value on the student's ability to categorize information using linear, sequential thought processes. However, not everyone adheres to this pattern of thinking. For example, many Native Americans, Asians, and others have spiral and circular thought patterns that move from concept to concept without being linear or sequential; therefore, they may have difficulty placing information in a stepwise methodology. When someone is unaware of the value given to such behaviors, she or he may see such individuals as disorganized, scattered, and faulty in their cognitive patterns, resulting in increased difficulty with written and verbal communications.

The American educational system stresses application of content over theory. Most European educational programs emphasize theory over practical application, and Arab education emphasizes theory with little attention given to practical application. As a result, Arab students are more proficient at tests requiring rote learning than at those requiring conceptualization and analysis. Being familiar with the individual's personal educational values and learning modes allows health-care providers, educators, and employers to adjust teaching strategies for clients, students, and employees. Educational materials and explanations must be presented at a level consistent with clients' educational capabilities and within their cultural framework and beliefs.

> **How strongly do you believe in the value of education? Who in your life is responsible for instilling this value? Do you consider yourself to be a more linear/sequential learner or a random-patterned learner?**

Immigrants bring job skills from their native homelands and traditionally seek employment in the same or similar trades. Sometimes, these job skills are inadequate for the available jobs in the new society; thus, immigrants are forced to take low-paying jobs and join the ranks of the working poor and economically disadvantaged. Immigrants to America are employed in a broad variety of occupations and professions; however, limited experiential, educational, and language abilities of more recent immigrants often restrict employment possibilities. More importantly, experiential backgrounds sometimes encourage employment choices that are identified as high risk for chronic diseases, such as exposure to pesticides and chemicals. Others may work in factories that manufacture hepatotoxic chemicals, in industries with pollutants that increase the risk for pulmonary diseases, and in crowded conditions with poor ventilation that increase the risk for tuberculosis or other respiratory diseases.

Understanding clients' current and previous work background is essential for health screening. For example, newer immigrants who worked in malaria-infested areas in their native country, such as Egypt, Italy, Turkey, and Vietnam to name a few, may need health screening for malaria. Those who worked in mining, such as in Ireland and Poland, may need screening for respiratory diseases. Those who lived in overcrowded and unsanitary conditions, such as refugees and migrant workers, may need to be screened for infectious diseases such as tuberculosis, parasitosis, and respiratory diseases.

Box 2–1 identifies guidelines for assessing the cultural domain *overview, inhabited localities, and topography.*

COMMUNICATION

Perhaps no other domain has the complexities of communication. Communication is interrelated with all other domains and depends on verbal language skills that include the dominant language, dialects, and the contextual use of the language as well as paralanguage variations, such as voice volume, tone, intonations, reflections, and willingness to share thoughts and feelings. Other important communication characteristics include nonverbal communications such as eye contact, facial

BOX 2.1

Overview, Inhabited Localities, and Topography

Overview, Inhabited Localities, and Topography

1. Identify the part of the world from which this cultural or ethnic group originates and describe the climate and topography of the country.

Heritage and Residence

2. Identify where this group predominantly resides and include approximate numbers.

Reasons for Migration and Associated Economic Factors

3. Identify major factors that motivated this group to emigrate.
4. Explore economic or political factors that have influenced this group's acculturation and professional development in America.

Educational Status and Occupations

5. Assess the educational attainment and value placed on education by this ethnic group.
6. Identify occupations that individuals in this group predominantly seek on immigration.

some other countries; for example, the English spoken in Glasgow, Scotland, is utterly unlike the English spoken in Central London. The Spanish spoken in Spain differs from the versions spoken in Puerto Rico, Panama, or Mexico, which has as many as 50 different dialects within its borders. In such cases, dialects that vary widely may pose substantial problems for health-care providers and interpreters in performing health assessments and in obtaining accurate health data, in turn increasing the difficulty of making accurate diagnoses.

Of the nearly 300 million people in the United States, almost 250 million were born in the United States. When language ability is looked at, 217 million speak only English, 23 million speak English less than very well, and 52 million speak a language other than English (CIA Factbook, 2006).

> What is your dominant language? Do you have difficulty understanding other dialects of your dominant language? Have you traveled abroad where you had difficulty understanding the dialect or accent? What other languages beside your dominant language do you speak?

When speaking in a nonnative language, health-care providers must select words that have relatively pure meanings, be certain of the voice intonation, and avoid the use of regional slang and jargon to avoid being misunderstood. Minor variations in pronunciation may change the entire meaning of a word or a phrase and result in inappropriate interventions.

Given the difficulty of obtaining the precise meaning of words in a language, it is best for health-care providers to obtain someone who can interpret the meaning and message, not just translate the individual words. Remember, *translation* refers to the written word and *interpretation* refers to the spoken word. Children should never be used as interpreters for their family members. Not only does it have a negative bearing on family dynamics, but sensitive information may not be transmitted. California's law Government Code 7290 et seq. prohibits using children as interpreters. Here are some guidelines for communicating with non–English-speaking clients:

expressions, use of touch, body language, spatial distancing practices, and acceptable greetings; temporality in terms of past, present, or future orientation of worldview; clock versus social time; and the degree of formality in the use of names. Communication styles may vary between insiders (family and close friends) and outsiders (strangers and unknown health-care providers). Hierarchical relationships, gender, and some religious beliefs affect communication.

Dominant Language and Dialects

The health-care provider must be aware of the dominant language and the difficulties that dialects may cause when communicating in the client's native language. American English is a monochromic, low-contextual language in which most of the message is in the verbal mode, and verbal communication is frequently seen as being more important than nonverbal communication. Thus, Americans are more likely to miss the more subtle nuances of communication. Accordingly, if a misunderstanding occurs, both the sender and the receiver of the message take responsibility for the miscommunication.

Americans speak *American English*, which differs somewhat in its pronunciation, spelling, and choice of words from English spoken in Great Britain, Australia, and other English-speaking countries. Within the United States, several dialects exist, but generally the differences do not cause a major concern with communications. Aside from people with foreign accents, in certain areas of the United States people speak with a dialect; these include the South and Northeast, in addition to local dialects such as "Elizabethan English" and "western drawl." For the most part, these dialects and accents are not as different as in

1. Use interpreters who can decode the words and provide the meaning behind the message.
2. Use dialect-specific interpreters whenever possible.
3. Use interpreters trained in the health-care field.
4. Give the interpreter time alone with the client.
5. Provide time for translation and interpretation.
6. Use same-gender interpreters whenever possible.
7. Maintain eye contact with both the client and the interpreter to elicit feedback: read nonverbal cues.
8. Speak slowly without exaggerated mouthing, allow time for translation, use the active rather than the passive tense, wait for feedback, and

restate the message. Do not rush; do not speak loudly.

9. Use as many words as possible in the client's language and nonverbal communication when unable to understand the language.

10. Use phrase charts and picture cards if available.

11. During the assessment, direct your questions to the patient, not to the interpreter.

12. Ask one question at a time and allow interpretation and a response before asking another question.

13. Be aware that interpreters may affect the reporting of symptoms, insert their own ideas, or omit information.

14. Remember that clients can usually understand more than they can express; thus, they need time to think in their own language. They are alert to the health-care provider's body language, and they may forget some or all of their English in times of stress.

15. Avoid the use of relatives, who may distort information or not be objective.

16. Avoid using children as interpreters, especially with sensitive topics.

17. Avoid idiomatic expressions and medical jargon.

18. If a certified interpreter is unavailable, the use of a translator may be acceptable. The difficulty with translation is omission of parts of the message, distortion of the message, including transmission of information not given by the speaker and messages not being fully understood.

19. If available, use an interpreter who is older than the patient.

20. Review responses with the patient and interpreter at the end of a session.

21. Be aware that social class differences between the interpreter and the client may result in the interpreter's not reporting information that he or she perceives as superstitious or unimportant.

Those with limited English ability may have inadequate vocabulary skills to communicate in situations in which strong or abstract levels of verbal skills are required, such as in the psychiatric setting. Helpful communication techniques with diverse clients include tact, consideration, and respect; gaining trust by listening attentively; addressing the client by preferred name; and showing genuine warmth and openness to facilitate full information sharing. When giving directions, be explicit. Give directions in sequential procedural steps (e.g., first, second, third). Do not use complex sentences with conjunctions or contractions.

> **Give some examples of problems communicating with patients who did not speak or understand English. What did you do to promote effective communication?**

Before trying to engage in more sensitive areas of the health interview, the health-care practitioner may need to start with social exchanges to establish trust, use an open-ended format rather than yes or no closed-response questions, elicit opinions and beliefs about health and symptom management, and focus on facts rather than feelings. An awareness of nonverbal behaviors is essential to establishing a mutually satisfying relationship.

The context within which a language is spoken is an important aspect of communication. The German, English, and French languages are low in context, and most of the message is explicit, requiring many words to express a thought. Chinese and Native American languages are highly contextual, with most of the information either in the physical context or internalized, resulting in the use of fewer words with more emphasis on unspoken understandings.

Voice volume and tone are important paralanguage aspects of communication. Americans and people of African heritage may be perceived as being loud and boisterous because their volume carries to those nearby. Compared with Chinese and Hindus, Americans and African Americans generally talk loudly. Their loud voice volume may be interpreted by Chinese or Hindus as reflecting anger, when in fact a loud voice is merely being used to express their thoughts in a dynamic manner. In contrast, Westerners witnessing impassioned communication among Arabs may interpret the excited speech pattern and shouting as anger, but emotional communication is part of the Arab culture and is usually unrelated to anger. Thus, health-care providers must be cautious about voice tones when interacting with diverse cultural groups so their intentions are not misunderstood. In addition, the speed at which people speak varies by region; for example, in parts of Appalachia and the South, people speak more slowly than do people in the northeastern part of the United States.

> **On a scale of 1 to 10, with 1 low and 10 high, where do you place yourself in the scale of high-contextual versus low-contextual communication? Do you tend to use a lot of words to express a thought? Do you know family members/friends/acquaintances who are your opposite in terms of low-contextual versus high-contextual communication? Does this sometimes cause concerns in communication? Do you think biomedical language is high or low context?**

Cultural Communication Patterns

Communication includes the willingness of individuals to share their thoughts and feelings. Many Americans are willing to disclose very personal information about themselves, including information about sex, drugs, and family problems. In fact, personal sharing is encouraged in a wide variety of topics, but not religion as in Central America, politics as in Spain, or philosophical things as discussed in most of Europe. In the United States, having well-developed verbal skills is seen as important, whereas in Japan, the person who has very highly developed verbal skills is seen as having suspicious intentions. Similarly, among many Appalachians, the person who has well-developed verbal skills may be seen as a "smooth talker"; and therefore, her or his actions may be suspect. In some cultural groups, such as many Asian cultures, individuals are expected to be shy, withdrawn, and diffident—at least in public—whereas in other cultures, such as Jewish and Italian, individuals are expected to be more flamboyant and expressive. Most Appalachians and Mexicans willingly share their thoughts and feelings among family members and close friends, but they may not easily share thoughts, feelings, and health information with "outside" health-care providers until they get to know them. By engaging in small talk and inquiring about family members before addressing the client's health concerns, health-care providers can help establish trust and, in turn, encourage more open communication and sharing of important health information.

> **How willing are you to share personal information about yourself? How does it differ with family, friends, or strangers? Do you tend to speak faster, slower, or about the same rate as the people around you? What happens when you meet someone who speaks much more rapidly or much more slowly than you do? Do you normally speak in a loud or low voice volume? How do you respond when someone speaks louder or softer than you do?**

Touch, a method of nonverbal communication, has substantial variations in meaning among cultures. For the most part, America is a low-touch society, which has recently been reinforced by sexual harassment guidelines and policies. For many, even casual touching may be seen as a sexual overture and should be avoided whenever possible. People of the same sex (especially men) or opposite sex do not generally touch each other unless they are close friends. However, among most Asian cultures, two people of the same gender can touch each other without it having a sexual connotation. Among Egyptian Americans, touch between opposite sexes is accepted in private and only between husband and wife, parents and children, and adult brothers and sisters; it is less readily accepted from strangers. Mexican Americans, even though they frequently touch family members and friends, tend to be modest during health-care examinations by the opposite gender. Always explain the necessity and ask permission before touching a client for a health examination. Being aware of individual practices regarding touch is essential for effective health assessments.

Personal space needs to be respected when working with multicultural clients and staff. American, Canadian, and British conversants tend to place at least 18 inches of space between themselves and the person with whom they are talking. Arabs require less personal space when talking with each other (Hall, 1990). They are quite com-

fortable standing closer to each other than Americans; in fact, they interpret physical proximity as a valued sign of emotional closeness. Middle Eastern clients, who stand very close and stare during a conversation, may offend health-care practitioners. These clients may interpret American health-care providers as being cold because they stand so far away. An understanding of personal space and distancing characteristics can enhance the quality of communication among individuals.

> **How comfortable are you being touched on the arm or shoulder by friends? By people who know you well? Do you consider yourself to be a "person who touches frequently" or do you rarely touch friends? Can you think of groups in the clinical setting for whom therapeutic touch is not appropriate?**

Regardless of class or social standing of the conversants, Americans are expected to maintain direct eye contact without staring. A person who does not maintain eye contact may be perceived as not listening, not being trustworthy, not caring, or being less than truthful. Among traditional Mexicans, Cubans, Puerto Ricans, Iranians, Egyptians, Italians, and Greeks, sustained eye contact between a child and an older adult may bring on the "evil eye" or "bad eye." In many Asian cultures, a person of lower social class or status should avoid eye contact with superiors or those with a higher educational status. Thus, eye contact must be interpreted within its cultural context to optimize relationships and health assessments.

The use of gestures and facial expressions varies among cultures. Most Americans gesture moderately when conversing and smile easily as a sign of pleasantness or happiness, although one can smile as a sign of sarcasm. A lack of gesturing can mean that the person is too stiff, too formal, or too polite. However, when gesturing to make, emphasize, or clarify a point, one should not raise one's elbows above the head unless saying hello or good-bye. Americans, unlike the Japanese and Chinese, do not normally smile as a form of embarrassment, confusion, or not understanding. For the Japanese and Chinese, happiness hides behind a straight face; if you are truly happy, you do not need to smile.

> **What are your spatial distancing practices? How close do you stand to family? Friends? Strangers? Does this distancing remain the same with the opposite gender? Do you maintain eye contact when speaking with people? Is it intense? Does it vary with the age or gender of the person with whom you are conversing? What does it mean when someone does not maintain eye contact with you? How do you feel in this situation?**

Preferred greetings and acceptable body language also vary among cultural groups. An expected practice for

American men and women in business is to extend the right hand when greeting someone for the first time. In northern European countries, it is considered rude and impolite to converse with one's hands in the pockets. In the United States, confidence and competence are associated with a relaxed posture; however, in Korea and Japan, confidence and competence are more closely associated with slightly tense postures (Krebs & Kunimoto, 1994). More elaborate greeting rituals occur in Asian, Arab, and Latin American countries and are covered in individual chapters.

Although many people consider it impolite or offensive to point with one's finger, many Americans do so, and do not see it as impolite. In Iran, beckoning is done by waving the fingers with the palm down, whereas extending the thumb, like thumbs-up, is considered a vulgar sign. Among the Vietnamese, signaling for someone to come by using an upturned finger is a provocation, usually done to a dog. Among the Navajo, it is considered rude to point; rather, the Navajo shift their lips toward the desired direction.

> Do you tend to use your hands a lot when speaking? Can people tell your emotional state by your facial expressions?

Temporal Relationships

Temporal relationships, people's worldview in terms of past, present, and future orientation, vary among individuals and among cultural groups. The American culture is future-oriented, and people are encouraged to sacrifice for today and work to save and invest in the future. The future is important in that people can influence it. Americans generally see fatalism, the belief that powers greater than humans are in control, as negative; but to many others, it is seen as a fact of life not to be judged. For example, the German culture is regarded as a past-oriented society, in which laying a proper foundation by providing historical background information can enhance communication. Most people of Central American heritage are more present oriented, placing great importance on the here and now, not something that may occur in the future or has occurred in the past. However, for people in many societies, temporality is balanced among past, present, and future in the sense of respecting the past, valuing and enjoying the present, and saving for the future.

Differences in temporal orientation can cause concern or misunderstanding among health-care providers. For example, in a future-oriented culture, a person is expected to delay purchase of nonessential items to afford prescription medications. However, in less future-oriented cultures, the person buys the nonessential item because it is readily available and defers purchasing the prescription medication. The attitude is, why not purchase it now— the prescription medication can be purchased *mañana* (tomorrow or later).

Americans see time as a highly valued resource and do not like to be delayed because it "wastes time." When visiting friends or meeting for strictly social engagements, punctuality is less important, but one is still expected to appear within a "reasonable" time frame. In the health-care setting if an appointment is made for 9 a.m., the person is expected to be there at 8:45 a.m. so she or he is ready for the appointment and does not delay the health-care provider. Some organizations refuse to see the patient if they are more than 15 to 30 minutes late for an appointment; a few charge a fee, even though the patient was not seen, giving the impression that money is more important than the person. In other cultures, patients are seen whenever they arrive.

For immigrants from rural settings, time may be even less important. These individuals may not even own a timepiece or be able to tell time. Expectations for punctuality can cause conflicts between health-care providers and clients, even if one is cognizant of these differences. These details must be carefully explained to individuals when such situations occur. Being late for appointments should not be misconstrued as a sign of irresponsibility or not valuing one's health.

> How timely are you with professional appointments? With social engagements? What does it mean to you when people are chronically late? Can you give examples indicating that you are past oriented? Present oriented? Future oriented? Do you consider yourself more one than the other?

Format for Names

Names are important to individuals, and their format differs among cultures. The American name "David Thomas Jones" denotes a man whose first name is "David," middle name is "Thomas," and family surname is "Jones." Friends would call him by his first name, "David." In the formal setting, he would be called "Mr. Jones." In addition, he could also have a "nickname" that would be used by family and close friends, for example, "Davy" from his first name or "Tom" or "Tommy" from his middle name. Hispanics may have a more complex system for denoting their full name. For example, a married woman may take her husband's surname while maintaining both of her parents' last names, resulting in an extended name such as "La Senora Roberta Rodriguez de Malena y Perez." In this example, Mrs. Rodriguez has the first name of "Roberta," her husband's surname "Rodriguez," her mother's maiden name "Malena," and her father's surname "Perez." Friends would address her as "Roberta," whereas in the formal setting, she would be called "Mrs. Rodriguez." This extended name format may become even more confusing because one's last name can be, for example, "de la Caza." Therefore, a single woman's name might be "Angelica [first name] Elena [middle name] de la Caza [family name] y de la Cruz [mother's maiden name]." She may choose any name she wants for legal purposes. When in doubt, the health-care provider needs to ask which name is used for legal purposes. Such extensive naming formats can create a challenge for health-care workers keeping a medical record when they are unaware of differences in ethnic recording of names.

> How do you prefer to be addressed or greeted? Does this change with the situation? How do you normally address and greet people? Do your responses change with the situation?

Box 2–2 identifies guidelines for assessing the cultural domain *communication*.

BOX 2.2

Communications

Dominant Language and Dialects

1. Identify the dominant and other languages spoken by this group.
2. Identify dialects that may interfere with communication.
3. Explore contextual speech patterns of this group. What is the usual volume and tone of speech?

Cultural Communication Patterns

4. Explore the willingness of individuals to share thoughts, feelings, and ideas.
5. Explore the practice and meaning of touch in their society: within the family, between friends, with strangers, with members of the same sex, with members of the opposite sex, and with health-care providers.
6. Identify personal spatial and distancing characteristics when communicating on a one-to-one basis. Explore how distancing changes with friends versus strangers.
7. Explore the use of eye contact within this group. Does avoidance of eye contact have special meanings? How does eye contact vary among family, friends, and strangers? Does eye contact change among socioeconomic groups?
8. Explore the meaning of various facial expressions. Do specific facial expressions have special meanings? How are emotions displayed or not displayed in facial expressions?
9. Are there acceptable ways of standing and greeting outsiders?

Temporal Relationships

10. Explore temporal relationships in this group. Are individuals primarily past, present, or future oriented? How do individuals see the context of past, present, and future?
11. Identify how differences in the interpretation of social time versus clock time are perceived.
12. Explore how time factors are interpreted by this group. Are individuals expected to be punctual in terms of jobs, appointments, and social engagements?

Format for Names

13. Explore the format for a person's names.
14. How does one expect to be greeted by strangers and health-care practitioners?

FAMILY ROLES AND ORGANIZATION

The cultural domain of *family roles and organization* affects all other domains and defines relationships among insiders and outsiders. This domain includes concepts related to the head of the household, gender roles, family goals and priorities, developmental tasks of children and adolescents, roles of the aged and extended family members, individual and family social status in the community, and acceptance of alternative lifestyles such as single parenting, nontraditional sexual orientations, childless marriages, and divorce. Family structure in the context of the larger society determines acceptable roles, priorities, and the behavioral norms for its members.

Head of Household and Gender Roles

An awareness of family decision-making patterns (i.e., patriarchal, matriarchal, or egalitarian) is important for determining with whom to speak when health-care decisions have to be made. Among Americans, it is acceptable for women to have a career and for men to assist with child care, household domestic chores, and cooking responsibilities. Both parents work in many families, necessitating placing children in child-care facilities.

In some families, fathers are responsible for deciding when to seek health care for family members, but mothers may have significant influence on final decisions. Among many Hispanics, the decisions may be egalitarian, but the male's role in the family is to be the spokesperson for the family. The health-care provider, when speaking with parents, should maintain eye contact and direct questions about a child's illness to both parents.

> How would you classify the decision making in your family—patriarchal, matriarchal, or egalitarian? Does it vary by what decision has to be made? Are gender roles prescribed in your family? Who makes the decisions about health and health care?

Prescriptive, Restrictive, and Taboo Behaviors for Children and Adolescents

Every society has prescriptive, restrictive, and taboo practices for children and adolescents. Prescriptive beliefs are things that children or teenagers *should do* to have harmony with the family and a good outcome in society. Restrictive practices are things that children and teenagers *should not do* to have a positive outcome. Taboo practices are those things that, if done, are likely to cause significant concern or negative outcomes for the child, teenager, family, or community at large.

For most Americans, a child's individual achievement is valued over the family's financial status. This is different from non-Western cultures in which attachment to family may be more important and the need for children to excel individually is not as important. In most middle- and upper-class American families, children have their own room, television, and telephone, and in many homes, their own computer. At younger ages, rather than having group toys each child has his or her own toys and is taught to share them with others. Americans encourage autonomy in children, and after completing homework assignments (with which parents are expected to help), children are expected to contribute to the family by doing chores such as taking out the garbage, washing dishes, cleaning their own room, feeding and caring for pets, and helping with cooking. They are not expected to help with heavy labor at home except in rural farm communities.

Children are allowed and encouraged to make their own choices, including managing their own money allowance and deciding who their friends might be, although parents may gently suggest one friend might be a better choice than another. American children and teenagers are permitted and encouraged to have friends of the same and opposite gender. They are expected to be well behaved, especially in public. They are taught to stand in line—first come, first served—and to wait their turn. As they reach the teenage years, they are expected to refrain from premarital sex, smoking, using recreational drugs, and drinking alcohol until they leave the home. However, this does not always occur and teenage pregnancy and use of recreational alcohol and drugs remains high. When children become teenagers, most are expected to get a job, such as baby sitting, delivering newspapers, or doing yard work to make their own spending money, which they manage as a way of learning independence. The teenage years are also seen as a time of natural rebellion.

In American society, when young adults become 18 or complete their education, they usually move out of their parents' home (unless they are in college) and live independently or share living arrangements with nonfamily members. More single males (59 percent) than single females (48 percent) over the age of 18 years elect to live with their parents (U.S. Bureau of the Census, 2006a). If the young adult chooses to remain in the parents' home, then she or he might be expected to pay room and board. However, young adults are generally allowed to return home when they are needed or for financial or other purposes. Individuals over the age of 18 are expected to be self-reliant and independent, which are virtues in the American culture. This differs from other cultures, such as the Japanese and some Hispanic cultures, in which children are expected to live at home with their parents until they marry, because dependence, not independence, is the virtue.

Adolescents have their own subculture, with its own values, beliefs, and practices that may not be in harmony with those of their major ethnic group. Being in harmony with peers and conforming to the prevalent choice of music, clothing, hairstyles, and adornment may be especially important to adolescents. Thus, role conflicts can become considerable sources of family strain in many more-traditional families who may not agree with the American values of individuality, independence, self-assertion, and egalitarian relationships. Many teens may experience a cultural dilemma with exposure outside the home and family.

As outsiders, health-care practitioners in school health can have a significant role in providing factual informa-tion regarding issues related to sexuality. Expressing an openness to discuss these sensitive issues in a group or one-on-one format within their cultural context may assist teenagers to learn more about sexuality and primary prevention. Health-care providers can assist adolescents and family members to work through these cultural differences by helping them resolve personal conflicts in ways that convey respect for the family's culture. However, in some religions, parental permission may be needed to discuss sexual issues with their children. Discussing personal parenting practices and providing information about disease, illness, and treatment in culturally congruent ways encourage individuals to explore alternative beliefs while continuing to value their own culture.

> **Were you taught to be independent and autonomous or dependent in your family? Was there more emphasis on the individual or on the group?**

Family Goals and Priorities

American family goals and priorities are centered on raising and educating children. During this stage in the American culture, young adults make a personal commitment to a spouse or significant other and seek satisfaction through productivity in career, family, and civic interests. In most societies, young adulthood is the time when individuals work on Erikson's developmental tasks of *intimacy versus isolation* and *generativity versus stagnation*.

The median age at first marriage and unwed pregnancy in the United States has changed significantly over the last century and varies by the part of the country. In the 1890s, the median age at first marriage for men was 21.6 years, and for women, 22.0 years. By the 1920s, the median age at first marriage for men increased to 22.8 years, while it remained relatively stable for women at 20.3 years. By 2004, the age at first marriage for men increased to 26.7 years, and to 25.1 years for women (U.S. Bureau of the Census, 2006a). Southern states and the District of Columbia also tend to have a higher percentage of unwed mothers with infants compared with the national average. These include the District of Columbia, 53.4 percent; Mississippi, 45.7 percent; and Louisiana, 40.2 percent of all mothers. The states with the lowest percentages of unwed mothers with infants were Utah, 14.7 percent; Minnesota, 20.6 percent; and Idaho, 21.6 percent (U.S. Bureau of the Census, 2006a).

The American culture places a high value on children, and many laws have been enacted to protect children who are seen as the "future of the society." In most Asian cultures, children are desirable and highly valued as a source of family strength, and family members are expected to care for each other more so than in the American culture.

The United States has seen an explosion in its older population during the 20th century, up from 3.1 million in 1900 to over 47 million in 2006 being over the age of 65 years. This population is expected to increase by

74 percent by 2030 (U.S. Bureau of the Census, 2006a). The American culture, which emphasizes youth, beauty, thinness, independence, and productivity, contributes to some societal views of the aged as less important members and tends to minimize the problems of older people. A contrasting view among some Americans emphasizes the importance of older people in society.

Chinese and Appalachian cultures have great reverence for the wisdom of older people, and families eagerly make space for them to live with extended families. Children are expected to care for elders when the elders are unable to care for themselves. A great embarrassment may occur to family members when they cannot take care of their older family members. Helping the ethnic family to network and find social support, resources, or acceptable long-term-care facilities within the community is a useful strategy for the health-care provider.

The concept of extended family membership varies among societies. The extended family is extremely important in the Hispanic/Latino/Spanish cultures, and health-care decisions are often postponed until the entire family is consulted. The extended family may include biological relatives and nonbiological members who may be considered brother, sister, aunt, or uncle. In some Asian cultures, the influence of grandparents in decision making is considered more important than that of the parents. An accepted practice among Filipinos is for the grandparents to raise the grandchildren so that the parents can work. Grandparents, aunts, and cousins often assume the parental role in African American families, and fellow church members are frequently considered important members of the extended family. A common practice in such cultures is for several generations of a family to live in the same household, providing an ideal situation for health teaching. The health-care provider can have a significant impact on the health status of the extended family in primary care, home health, acute care, or long-term care.

Americans also place a high value on egalitarianism, nonhierarchical relationships, and equal treatment regardless of their race, color, religion, ethnicity, educational or economic status, sexual orientation, or country of origin. However, these beliefs are theoretical and not always seen in practice. For example, women still have a lower status than men, especially when it comes to prestigious positions and salaries. Most top-level politicians and corporate executive officers are white men. Subtle classism does exist, as evidenced by comments referring to "working-class men and women." Despite the current inequities, Americans value equal opportunities for all and significant progress has been made since about 1980.

Americans are known worldwide for their informality and for treating everyone the same. They call people by their first names very soon after meeting them, whether in the workplace, in social situations, in classrooms, in restaurants, or in places of business. Americans readily talk with waitstaff and store clerks and call them by their first names. Most Americans consider this respectful behavior. Formality can be communicated by using the person's last (family) name and title such as Mr., Mrs., Miss, Ms., or Dr. To this end,

achieved status is more important than ascribed status. What one has accumulated in material possessions, where one went to school, and one's job position and title are more important than one's family background and lineage. However, in some families in the South and the Northeast, one's ascribed status has equal importance to achieved status. The United States does not have a caste or class system, and theoretically, one can move readily from one socioeconomic position to another. To many Americans, if formality is maintained, it may be seen as pompous or arrogant, and some even deride the person who is very formal. However, formality is a sign of respect in many other cultures and is also valued by older Americans.

> What were prescriptive behaviors for you as a child? As a teenager? As a young adult? What were restrictive behaviors for you as a child? As a teenager? As a young adult? What were taboo behaviors for you as a child? As a teenager? As a young adult? How are elders regarded in your culture? In your family?

Alternative Lifestyles

The traditional American family is nuclear, with a married man and woman living together with one or more unmarried children. The American family is becoming a more varied community, including (1) unmarried people, both women and men, living alone; (2) single people of the same or different genders living together with or without children; (3) single parents with children; (4) and blended families consisting of two parents who have remarried, with children from their previous marriages and additional children from their current marriage. However, in some cultures, the traditional family is extended, with parents, unmarried children, married children with their children, and grandparents all sharing the same living space or at least living in very close proximity.

The newest category of family, domestic partnerships, is sanctioned by many cities or counties in the United States and grants some of the rights of traditional married couples to unmarried heterosexual, homosexual, older people, and disabled couples who share the traditional bond of the family. Courts in some states allow gay and lesbian couples to adopt children. Among more rural subcultures, same-sex couples living together may not be as accepted or recognized in the community as they are in larger cities. As gay parents have become more visible, lesbian and gay parenting groups have started in many cities across the United States to offer information, support, and guidance, resulting in more lesbians and gay men considering parenthood through adoption and artificial insemination.

Social attitudes toward homosexual activity vary widely, and homosexual behavior occurs in societies that deny its presence. Homosexual behavior carries a severe stigma in some societies. To discover that one's son or daughter is homosexual is akin to a catastrophic event for Egyptian Americans. In Iran and in some provinces of

China, a lesbian or gay man may be killed. In February 2001, a judge in Somalia sentenced two Somali lesbians to death for "exercising unnatural behavior" (Judge orders Executions, 2001).

> **Do you consider your family nuclear or extended? How close are you to your extended family? How is status measured in your family? By money or by some other attribute? What are your personal views of two people of the same gender living together in a physical relationship? What about heterosexual couples? Does divorce cause a stigma in your culture? In your family?**

When the health-care provider needs to provide assistance and make a referral for a person who is gay, lesbian, bisexual, or transsexual, a number of options are available. Some referral agencies are local, whereas others are national, with local or regional chapters. Many are ethnically or religiously specific. Some national groups that have links to local and regional organizations include the following:

Gay, Lesbian, and Straight Education Network, *http://www.glsen.org*

National Latino(a) Lesbian, Gay, Bisexual, and Trans-gender Organization, *http://www.lego.org*

Parents, Families, and Friends of Lesbians and Gays, *http://www.pflag.org*

National Center for Lesbian Rights, *http://www.info @nclrights.org*

Log Cabin Republicans, *http://www.lcr.org*

National Stonewall Democratic Federation, *http://www.stonewalldemocrats.org*

National Youth Advocacy Coalition, *http://www.nyacyouth.org*

Family Pride Coalition, *http://www.familypride.org*

It's Time, America, *http://www.gender.org*

BINET U.S., *http://www.binetUS.org*

National Black, Lesbian, and Gay Leadership Forum, *http://www.nblglf.org*

Box 2–3 identifies guidelines for assessing the cultural domain *family roles and organization*.

WORKFORCE ISSUES

Culture in the Workplace

A fourth domain of culture is *workforce issues*. Differences and conflicts that exist in a homogeneous culture may be intensified in a multicultural workforce. Factors that affect these issues include language barriers, degree of assimilation and acculturation, and issues related to autonomy. Moreover, concepts such as gender roles, cultural communication styles, health-care practices of the country of origin, and selected concepts from all other domains affect workforce issues in a multicultural work environment.

Americans are expected to be punctual on their job, with formal meetings, and with appointments. If one is

---

BOX 2.3

Family Roles and Organization

Head of Household and Gender Roles

1. Identify which family members make which types of decisions in the household. Is the overall decision-making pattern patriarchal, matriarchal, or egalitarian?
2. Describe gender-related roles of men and women in the family system.

Prescriptive, Restrictive, and Taboo Behaviors

3. Identify prescriptive, restrictive, and taboo behaviors for children.
4. Identify prescriptive, restrictive, and taboo behaviors for adolescents.

Family Roles and Priorities

5. Describe family goals and priorities emphasized by this culture.
6. Explore developmental tasks in this group.
7. Explore the status and role of the aged in the family.
8. Explore the roles and importance of extended family members.
9. Describe how one gains social status in this cultural system. Is there a caste system?

Alternative Lifestyles

10. Describe how alternative lifestyles and nontraditional families, such as single parents, blended families, communal families, same-sex families, are viewed by this society.

---

more than a minute or two late, an apology is expected, and if one is late by more than five or 10 minutes, a more elaborate apology is expected. When people know they are going to be late for a meeting, the expectation is that they call or send a message indicating that they will be late. The convener of the meeting or teacher in a classroom is expected to start and stop on time out of respect for the other people in attendance. This is in contrast to practices in many other cultures, for example, Panama, where a meeting or class starts when the majority of people arrive. However, in social situations in the United States, a person can be 15 or more minutes late, depending on the importance of the gathering. In this instance, an apology is not really necessary or expected; however, most Americans will politely provide a reason for the tardiness.

The American workforce stresses efficiency (time is money), operational procedures on how to get things done, task accomplishment, and proactive problem solving. Intuitive abilities and common sense are not usually valued as much as technical abilities. The scientific method is valued, and everything has to be proven. Americans want to know *why*, not *what*, and will search for a single factor that is the cause of the problem and the reason why something is to be done in a specific way. Many are obsessed with collecting facts and figures before they make decisions. Pragmatism is valued. In the United States, everyone is expected to have a job description, meetings are to have a predetermined agenda (although items can be added at the beginning of the meeting), and the agenda is followed throughout the meeting. Americans prefer to vote on almost every item on an agenda, including approving the agenda itself. Everything is given a time frame, and deadlines are expected to be respected. In these situations, American values expect that the needs of individuals are subservient to the needs of the organization. However, with the postmodernist movement, greater credibility and recognition have been given to approaches other than the scientific method.

> How timely are you in reporting to work? Do you see others in the workforce who do not report to work on time? What problems does it cause if they are not on time? What would you do as a supervisor to encourage people to report to work on time?

Most Americans place a high value on "fairness" and rely heavily on procedures and policies in the decision-making process. However, Americans' value for individualism, in which the individual is seen as the most important element in society, favors a person's decision to further her or his own career over the needs or wants of the employer. Therefore, individuals frequently demonstrate little loyalty to the organization and leave one position to take a position with another company for a better opportunity. In organizations in which people generally conform because of the fear of failure, there is a hierarchical order for decision making, and the person who succeeds is the one with strong verbal skills who conforms to the hierarchy's expectations. This person is well liked and does not stand out too much from the crowd. Frequently, others view as a threat the person with a high level of competence who stands out. Thus, to be successful in the highly technical American workforce, get the facts, control your feelings, have precise and technical communication skills, be informal and direct, and clearly and explicitly state your conclusion.

> How important are technical skills and verbal skills in your work environment? Does your organization encourage more formal or more informal communication? Why? Do you believe that everything needs to be proven scientifically? Do you value a more direct or indirect style of communication?

Clinical professionals trained in their home countries now occupy a significant share of technical and laboratory positions in U.S. health-care facilities. Service employees such as food preparation workers, nurse aides, orderlies, housekeepers, and janitors represent the most culturally diverse component of hospital workforces.

These unskilled and semiskilled positions are among the most attainable for new immigrants.

Minority groups employed as professionals are underrepresented among all health-care professions. According to the American Physical Therapy Association, only 0.5 percent of U.S. physical therapists are American Indian or Alaskan Native, 4.6 percent are African American or black, 1.8 percent are Hispanic/Latino, 3.3 percent are Asian/Pacific Islander, and the remainder (81.8 percent) are white (American Physical Therapy Association, 2006). The American Nurses Association found that only 0.5 percent of U.S. registered nurses are Native American or Alaskan Native, 4.2 percent are black, 1.6 percent are Hispanic/Latino, 3.4 percent are Asian/Pacific Islander, and the remainder (89.7 percent) are white (National Sample Survey of Registered Nurses, 2006). According to the American Medical Association (2006), of physicians in the United States, 0.7 percent are Native American or Alaskan Native, 7.9 percent are black, 6.9 percent are Hispanic, 19.4 percent are Asian/Pacific Islander, and 65 percent are white.

The educational preparation of health-care professionals in some countries is not comparable with that in the United States. The vast array of health-care providers in the United States—radiology technicians, physical therapists, occupational therapists, social service workers, electrocardiogram technicians, respiratory therapists, and so on—may not exist in other countries. In Mexico, some Latin American countries, and some other developing countries, nursing education is offered primarily at the high school level. Concerns surface about the amount of additional training needed for some emigrating foreign graduates before sitting for American licensing examinations.

During nursing workforce shortages, American health-care facilities rely on emigrating nurses from the Philippines, Canada, England, Ireland, and other countries to supplement their numbers. Some foreign nurses, such as British and Australian, culturally assimilate into the workforce more easily than others but still have difficulty with *defensive* charting as is required in the United States. In their socialized health-care system, clients are not likely to initiate litigation (Purnell & Galloway, 1995). Others may have difficulty with the assertiveness expected from American nurses.

Timeliness and punctuality are two culturally based attitudes that can create serious problems in the multicultural workforce. In some situations, conflicts may arise over the issue of reporting to work on time or on an assigned day. The lack of adherence to meeting time demands in other countries is often in direct opposition to the American ethic for punctuality.

> Does your workforce (class) reflect the ethnic and racial diversity of the community? Why? Why not? What might you do to increase this diversity?

Issues Related to Autonomy

Cultural differences related to assertiveness influence how health-care practitioners view each other. Specifically, some Asian nurses may not be as assertive with physicians as American nurses are. The concept of nurses being dependent on physicians and male administrators is inseparable from the Muslim concept of women being subject to the authority of husbands, fathers, and elder brothers. Polish nursing is seen as a vocation; therefore, Polish nurses may be unprepared for the level of sophistication and autonomy of American nursing. Educational training for nurses in Pakistan is culturally different from training in America.

The Commission on Graduates of Foreign Nursing Schools administers a screening examination for temporary work visas to foreign graduate nurses seeking work. This examination assesses the ability to write and comprehend the English language, but it cannot examine the specific nuances of selected language barriers that may cause difficulties in the workplace. One area in which problems typically develop is in taking physicians' prescription instructions over the telephone. The newer immigrant health-care professional may have passed the state's professional licensing examination but still need extra time in translating messages and formulating replies.

When individuals speak in their native language at work, it may become a source of contention for both clients and health-care personnel. For example, most non–English-speaking employees do not want to exclude or offend others, but it is easier to speak in their native language to articulate ideas, feelings, and humor among themselves. Negative interpretations of behaviors can be detrimental to working relationships in the health-care environment. Some foreign graduates, with limited aural language abilities, may need to have care instructions written or procedures demonstrated.

> **Does your profession encourage autonomy in the workforce? Does your current work (class) encourage autonomy and independence? Do you see any cultural or gender differences in autonomy? Do people speak different languages at work? What difficulty does this cause?**

Diversity and Inclusion in the Workforce

Although many organizations focus on race and ethnicity, to these authors, diversity includes religion, gender, sexual orientation, and age. The Human Resource Institute (2005) addresses diversity and inclusion issues globally and reports the following global concerns:

1. In France, women's salaries are 33 percent less than men's salaries given the same employment characteristics.
2. Ethnic minorities in Wales are five times more likely to express workplace bullying resulting in burnout, increased stress, and depression and anxiety.
3. The Roma "gypsies" in Slovakia have an 87 percent unemployment rate.
4. In Canada, nearly 350,000 Aboriginals are slated to enter the workforce in the next few years.

5. Northern Ireland has now banned religious discrimination in employment, something the United States has done for many years. However, this does not mean that religious discrimination on an individual basis can not occur given the setting.
6. The Hispanic workforce in the United States is growing by almost 10 percent a year, while the non-Hispanic workforce is growing at a rate of only 1 percent a year.
7. Whereas 78 percent of people with a disability work at least part-time, 26% of them live in poverty. However, only 22 percent report experiencing discrimination.
8. Religious preferences and sexual orientation continue to cause discrimination, especially from religious groups whose beliefs reject homosexuality.
9. Acknowledging workers' sexual orientation improves productivity because employees feel more comfortable knowing there is no criticism of their lifestyles. However, 22 percent of heterosexual employees admit being uncomfortable working with gay, lesbian, bisexual, or transgender individuals.
10. The European Union's Equal Treatment Framework Directive (2000/78C) prohibits discrimination on the basis of age, religion, belief, disability, or sexual orientation, the latter of which has not yet occurred in the United States.

Generational Differences in the Workforce

Not only is the U.S. workforce becoming more multicultural, but the last decade has seen an increase in the professional literature regarding generational differences in our workforce. Most of the literature on generational differences describes the dominant culture, with little mention as to how these differences might coincide with the multiethnic workforce. These authors believe that these descriptions do not "fit" the generalizations as well as they do for the dominant, nonethnic, nonimmigrant populations. However, these descriptions do have value and are briefly described here.

For the first time in U.S. history, we now have four generations working together, recognizing some general but overlapping differences among the groups. Much can be gained in teamwork when these four generations are working together, especially when it is combined with ethnic and cultural diversity. At the same time, if administration does not effectively manage these diverse groups, interpretations, misunderstandings, and potential uncontrolled conflict can occur in the work environment. These four groups are (1) traditionalists, (2) baby boomers, (3) generation Xers, and (4) millennials. Each group brings a different worldview, different perspectives, and varied strengths to the workforce. A brief description of each group follows.

The traditionalists were born prior to 1945 and are characterized as being loyal, patriotic, and hard working. Many from this group worked under "control and command" styles of management and may perceive changes in the health-care field as being too radical. They are an invaluable resource with the history of the organization and the profession and have a wealth of practical expertise to share. Most have also developed conflict resolution and negotiation skills. Many who retired have now returned to new professions or returned to work part-time (Anthony, 2006; Kupperschmidt, 2006; Sherman, 2006, Weston, 2006).

The baby boomers, born between 1945 and 1965, currently account for almost half the workforce. Most are seen as idealistic, optimistic, competitive, and community focused. They are also considered the "sandwich generation" because they are often caring for their children and their parents. They are also "sandwiched" between the traditionalist with whom they have worked for many years and the generation Xers. This group also has a wealth of practical expertise to share and has developed conflict resolution and negotiation skills (Anthony, 2006; Kupperschmidt, 2006; Sherman, 2006, Weston, 2006).

Generation Xers, born between 1966 and 1980, compose about 30 percent of the workforce. They are characterized as being highly dependent and skeptical and have a "free-agent" mentality and will change jobs easily to meet family and personal needs. Most are looking for experience rather than job security (Anthony, 2006; Kupperschmidt, 2006; Sherman, 2006, Weston, 2006).

Millennials, born between after 1981, compose only about 15 percent of the population. Born of the baby boomers, they like new ideas and change. Technology use is a given, and most are comfortable with diversity. This group has travel and educational experiences that previous generations did not have (Anthony, 2006; Kupperschmidt, 2006; Sherman, 2006, Weston, 2006).

> How many generations are in your work group (class)? Are their beliefs and practices similar to or different from what is reported in the literature? Do the generational differences cause conflict? Which generation takes the lead in resolving conflicts when they arise?

Box 2–4 identifies guidelines for assessing the cultural domain *workforce issues*.

BIOCULTURAL ECOLOGY

The domain *biocultural ecology* identifies specific physical, biological, and physiological variations in ethnic and racial origins. These variations include skin color and physical differences in body habitus; genetic, hereditary, endemic, and topographic diseases; psychological makeup of individuals; and differences in the way drugs are metabolized by the body. No attempt is made here to explain or justify any of the numerous, conflicting, and highly controversial views and research about racial variations in drug metabolism and genetics.

Skin Color and Other Biological Variations

Skin coloration is an important consideration for health-care providers because anemia, jaundice, and rashes

---

BOX 2.4

Workforce Issues

Culture in the Workplace

1. Identify specific workforce issues affected by immigration, for example, education.
2. Describe specific multicultural considerations when working with this culturally diverse individual or group in the workforce.
3. Explore factors influencing patterns of acculturation in this cultural group.
4. Explore native health-care practices and their influence in the workforce.

Issues Related to Autonomy

5. Identify cultural issues related to professional autonomy, superior or subordinate control, religious issues, and gender in the workforce.
6. Identify language barriers with concrete interpretations of the language.

---

require different assessment skills in dark-skinned people than in light-skinned people. To assess for oxygenation and cyanosis in dark-skinned people, the practitioner must examine the sclera, buccal mucosa, tongue, lips, nail beds, palms of the hands, and soles of the feet rather than relying on skin tone alone. Jaundice is more easily determined in Asians by assessing the sclera rather than relying on the overall change in skin color. Health-care providers must establish a baseline skin color (by asking a family member or someone known to the individual), use direct sunlight if possible, observe areas with the least amount of pigmentation, palpate for rashes, and compare skin in corresponding areas. With people who are generally fair-skinned, such as Germans, Polish, Irish, and British, to name a few, prolonged exposure to the sun places them at an increased risk for skin cancer.

> Do you have difficulty assessing rashes, bruises, and sunburn in people with dark skin? Do you have difficulty assessing jaundice and oxygenation in people with dark skin? How does your assessment of skin differ between clients with light versus dark skin? Do you take precautions and protect yourself against the sun? Why? Why not?

Variations in body habitus occur among ethnic and racially diverse individuals. For example, the long bones of many blacks are significantly longer and narrower than those of whites (Giger & Davidhizar, 2004). Asians have narrower shoulders and wider hips than other ethnic/racial groups. Additional racial variations include flat nose bridges among Asians, which may be overlooked by opticians when fitting and dispensing eyeglasses. Many Vietnamese children are small by American standards and do not fall within normal ranges on standardized American growth charts. Mandibular tori occur more frequently among Asians, making fitting dentures more difficult. Bone density is greater in whites than in Chinese, Japanese, and Eskimos, whereas osteoporosis is lowest in black males and highest in white females. Other musculoskeletal variations such as the ulna and radius are equal among most Swedes. Other musculoskeletal variations such as the number of vertebrae, thickness of the frontal bone, and rotation of the humerus exist among ancestry groups and are listed in the Appendix. Such biocultural data provide important information for healthcare practitioners when assessing health problems geared to the unique attributes of people of diverse cultures. Given diverse gene pools, this type of information is often difficult to obtain, and much of the research is inconclusive.

Diseases and Health Conditions

Some diseases are more prevalent and endemic in certain racial or ethnic groups than in others. The incidence varies somewhat among the different ethnic groups. Specific health problems are covered in individual chapters in this book. Cardiovascular disease is the leading killer of both men and women in all racial and ethnic groups in the United States. The causative factors that contribute to the development of cardiovascular disease include obesity, 54.9 percent; lack of physical activity, 27.7 percent; and smoking, 22.9 percent (Centers for Disease Control and Prevention [CDC], 2006a). The leading sites for cancer for white male Americans are lung (74.2 percent), prostate (24.4 percent), colon and rectum (23.4 percent), pancreas (9.8 percent), and blood/leukemia (8.6 percent). The most common sites for white female Americans are lung (32.9 percent), breast (27.7 percent), colon and rectum (15.6 percent), ovary (8.2 percent), and pancreas (7.0 percent). Although these same sites account for most cancers in other ethnic and racial groups, the order of occurrence differs. For example, prostate cancer is the highest reported cancer among American Indians, blacks, Filipinos, Japanese, and non-white Hispanic men. In women, breast cancer incidence rates are higher in all groups except Vietnamese, for whom cervical cancer rates rank highest. Stomach cancer appears in the top cancers for men and women in Asian populations except for Filipinos and Chinese women (National Cancer Institute 2006). A more thorough description of the variations in the sites and incidence of cancer among racial and ethnic groups in the United States can be obtained from the National Cancer Institute (CDC, 2006a) and the CDC.

Almost 16 million Americans have been diagnosed with diabetes mellitus (DM), and the disease is undiagnosed in an additional 5.4 million people. More women than men suffer from DM. In addition, the prevalence of DM varies by race and ethnicity. The prevalence of DM among whites is 7.8 percent. However, blacks are 1.7 times as likely to have diabetes as whites; Mexican Americans, 1.9 times as likely; and American Indians and Alaskan Natives, 2.8 times as likely. Prevalence rates for Asian and Pacific Islanders in the United States are limited, but DM among Native Hawaiians is twice that of white Americans in Hawaii (CDC, 2006b).

HIV continues as a pandemic trend. An estimated 36 million people are living with HIV/AIDS; 16.4 million are women and 1.4 million are children under the age of 15 years. Worldwide, HIV is increasingly affecting women. The overwhelming majority of people with HIV (95 percent) are from developing countries. Latin America accounts for 1.4 million people with HIV. Brazil has the highest rate in South America, and Honduras has the highest rate in Central America. Nearly 1 million people in the United States have HIV, with the highest concentration in large urban areas. The Caribbean has approximately 390,000 people with HIV; the most affected country is Haiti (CDC, 2006b). International health agencies, such as the World Health Organization (WHO), Pan American Health Organization (PAHO), CDC, and Joint United Nations Programme on HIV/AIDS (UNAIDS), have joined together in partnership for global HIV prevention efforts, with specific programs for selected countries, populations, and cultural groups. A number of world religions, among them Roman Catholicism and Islam, do not believe in the use of condoms because they are contraceptives and because they may encourage promiscuity and sex outside marriage. To them, abstinence is the only option for the control of HIV and AIDS. For more information on AIDS prevention, contact CDC National AIDS Hotline at 1-800-342-AIDS; Spanish 1-800-344-SIDA; Deaf, 1-800-243-7889. The CDC National Prevention Information Network can be contacted at 1-800-458-5231.

In the United States, more than 65 million people are currently living with an incurable sexually transmitted infection (STI). Although extremely common, STIs are difficult to track, and many people are not aware they have these infections, resulting in hidden epidemics. Although syphilis is at an all-time low in the United States, other STIs such as gonorrhea, chlamydia, genital herpes, trichomoniasis, human papillomavirus, hepatitis B, and bacterial vaginosis continue to surge through the population. Women bear the greatest burden of STIs, suffering more frequent and more serious complications than men. Roughly one-fourth of these diseases occur in teenagers, with chlamydia and gonorrhea the most prevalent STIs among teenagers and young adults under the age of 25. STIs affect all racial, ethnic, and cultural groups. Each population needs culturally specific, relevant, and congruent education to decrease the incidence of these diseases. The middle socioeconomic white groups in the United States have responded favorably to educational programs geared to age-specific groups through media and school campaigns. Likewise, other communities have been successful with educational programs geared to the unique needs of the population. Some comparisons of each STI with ethnospecific populations, age groups, and gender can be obtained from the CDC (2006a) or the Institute of Medicine (2006).

Illnesses and diseases with an increased incidence in white ethnic groups in the United States include appendicitis, diverticular disease, cancer of the colon, hemorrhoids, varicose veins, cystic fibrosis, rosacea, osteoporosis and osteoarthritis, and phenylketonuria. Many immigrant groups have higher rates of some infectious diseases and illnesses that are not common in the United States. Accordingly, health-care providers should assess newer immigrants for diseases that are common in their homelands. An awareness of populations at risk for specific endemic diseases allows the health professional to provide culturally appropriate screening and education for disease prevention and health promotion. See Appendix for illnesses and diseases and their causes for specific ethnic and cultural groups common in the United States.

The topography of a given country or region may provide the health-care practitioner with essential clues to symptoms requiring investigation. People who have been working in coal mines are at inceased risk for pulmonary illnesses, even though they have been retired for many years. Thus, previous occupations should be included as part of the health assessment, not just indicating that they are retired.

People who emigrate from mosquito-infested tropical areas such as Brazil, Mexico, Central America, Turkey, and Vietnam may present with chills, fever, lassitude, and splenic enlargement, which are consistent with malaria. Air pollution, which increases the risk for respiratory diseases, may be a significant risk factor for any group who emigrates from or lives in a large city. Knowledge of specific risk factors related to the topography of the client's country of origin and current residence enhances the diagnostic process and ensures accurate assessments.

> **What are the most common illnesses and diseases in your family? In your community? What might you do to decrease the incidence of illness and diseases in your family? In your community?**

Since the late 1990s, every continent has had outbreaks of new or re-emerging diseases. North America has had outbreaks of bubonic plague, campylobacteria, cyclospora, salmonella, e coli in spinach, and Legionnaire's disease. Central and South America have been particularly affected by cholera, yellow fever, malaria, dengue fever, and rabies. Europe has had outbreaks of shigella in Paris, *Escherichia coli* and mad cow disease in Great Britain, and leptospirosis in the Ukraine. Asia has had an increase in dengue fever; anthrax has been seen in Russia and the United States; and avian flu has occurred in Hong Kong and other places. Africa has had meningitis in Chad, endemic rates of ebola in Zaire and Sudan, and bubonic plague in Malawi and Mozambique. To this end, educators in colleges and health-care organizations need to educate students, staff, and the community about new and re-emerging illnesses as a public health concern.

> **Are you aware of any outbreaks of new illnesses or diseases in your community? In other parts of the world? How might these outbreaks have been prevented?**

Variations in Drug Metabolism

Information regarding drug metabolism among racial and ethnic groups has important implications for health-care practitioners when prescribing medications. Besides the effects of (1) smoking, which accelerates drug metabolism; (2) malnutrition, which affects drug response; (3) a high-fat diet, which increases absorption of antifungal medication, whereas a low-fat diet renders the drug less effective; (4) cultural attitudes and beliefs about taking medication; and (5) stress, which affects catecholamine and cortisol levels on drug metabolism, studies have identified some specific alterations in drug metabolism among diverse racial and ethnic groups. For instance, the Chinese are more sensitive to the cardiovascular effects of propranolol and have an increased absorption of antipsychotics, some narcotics, and antihypertensives than their white American counterparts. Eskimos, American Indians, and Hispanics have an increased risk for developing peripheral neuropathy while taking the drug isoniazid, compared with white Americans, who inactivate the drug more rapidly. African Americans respond better to diuretic therapy than do white ethnic groups (Aschenbrenner, 2005; GenSpec, 2006; Kudzma, 1999; Lavizzo-Mourey & Mackenzie, 2006; Levy, 1993; Munoz & Hilgenberg, 2005; Prows & Prows, 2004; U.S. Food and Drug Administration, 2006). The difference in the way physicians prescribe medications in various countries is an additional cultural consideration. For example, in most Asian countries and Great Britain, the preferred practice is to start out with low dosages of medicines and adjust upward until side effects or therapeutic responses are reached. In the United States, most clinicians start with the maximum dosage and adjust downward as side effects occur (Levy, 1993). Health-care providers need to investigate the literature for ethnic-specific studies regarding variations in drug metabolism, communicate these findings to other colleagues, and educate their clients regarding these side effects. Medication administration is one area in which health-care providers see the importance of culture, ethnicity, and race.

> **Why is it important for health-care providers to be aware of variations in drug metabolism in the body? What conditions besides genetics have an influence on drug metabolism?**

Box 2–5 identifies guidelines for assessing and the cultural domain *biocultural ecology*.

HIGH-RISK BEHAVIORS

High-risk behaviors include use of tobacco, alcohol, or recreational drugs; lack of physical activity; increased calorie consumption; unsafe driving practices; failure to use seat belts and helmets; failure to take precautions against HIV and STIs; and high-risk recreational activities. Johnson's research (2000) found that barriers to exercise among South Asians included unsafe neighborhoods and lack of gender-specific facilities. High-risk behaviors occur in all ethnocultural groups; the degree and types of high-risk behaviors vary.

The steady decline in smoking prevalence has been observed nationally, but in some segments of the

Biocultural Ecology

Skin Color and Biological Variations

1. Identify the skin color and physical variations for this group.
2. Explore any special problems or concerns skin color may pose for health-care practitioners.
3. Identify biological variations in body habitus or structure.

Diseases and Health Conditions

4. Identify specific risk factors for individuals related to the topography or climate.
5. Identify hereditary or genetic diseases or conditions that are common within this group.
6. Identify endemic diseases specific to this cultural or ethnic group.
7. Identify any diseases or health conditions for which this group has increased susceptibility.

Variations in Drug Metabolism

8. Identify specific variations in drug metabolism, drug interactions, dosages, and related side effects.

population, smoking prevalence remains high, highlighting the need for expanded interventions that can better reach persons of low socioeconomic status and populations living in poverty. In 2004, 44.5 million adults in the United States were current smokers—23.4 percent of men and 18.5 percent of women. Among racial and ethnic groups, smoking prevalence was highest among American Indians/Alaska Natives (33.4 percent) and lowest among Hispanics (15 percent) and Asians (11.3 percent). Among income groups, smoking prevalence was higher among adults living below the poverty level (29.1 percent) than among those at or above the poverty level (20.6 percent). Smoking prevalence was highest among those aged 18 to 24 years (23.6 percent) and 25 to 44 years (23.8 percent) and lowest among those aged 65 years and older (8.8 percent). Whereas from 1993 to 2004 the proportion of heavy smokers and the overall number of cigarettes smoked among daily smokers declined, the percentage of daily smokers who smoked 1 to 4 cigarettes and 5 to 14 cigarettes per day increased. Middle school and high school student smoking rates have remained steady at 15 and 21 percent (CDC, 2005).

Alcohol consumption crosses all cultural and socioeconomic groups. Enormous differences exist among ethnic and cultural groups around use of and response to alcohol. Even in cultures in which alcohol consumption is taboo, it is not ignored. However, alcohol problems are not simply a result of how much people drink. When drinking is culturally approved, it is typically done more by men than women and is more often a social, rather than a solitary, act. The group in which drinking is most frequently practiced is usually composed of same-age social peers (Peele & Brodsky, 2001). Studies on increasing controls on the availability of alcohol to decreasing alcohol consumption, with the premise that alcohol-related

problems occur in proportion to per capita consumption, has not been supported. Furthermore, countries with temperance movements have greater alcohol-related behavior problems than do countries without temperance movements (Purnell & Foster, 2003a, 2003b).

Countries in which drinking alcoholic beverages is integrated into rites and social customs, and in which one is expected to have self-control and sociability have lower rates of alcohol-related problems than those of countries and cultures in which ambivalent attitudes toward drinking prevail (Purnell & Foster, 2003a; 2003b). In addition, Hilton's (1987) study demonstrated a clear and distinct difference in alcohol abuse rate by socioeconomic status. Higher–socioeconomic status Americans were more likely to drink but also more likely to drink without problems. The conclusion of many studies suggests that alcohol-related violence is a learned behavior, not an inevitable result of alcohol consumption (Purnell & Foster, 2003a; 2003b). Other studies have correlated per capita alcohol consumption rates with the number of Alcoholics Anonymous (AA) groups per million population. Countries with the lowest per capita consumption rate of alcohol had higher numbers of AA groups. Countries with the highest per capita consumption rate of alcohol had lower numbers of AA groups; for example, Iceland, with a low per capita alcohol consumption rate of 3.9 L, had 784 AA groups, whereas France, with a per capital alcohol consumption rate of 13.2 L, had 7 AA groups (Table 2–1).

TABLE 2.1 *Alcohol Consumption by Country*

Country	Alcohol Consumption (L/capita)	Number of Alcoholics Anonymous Groups (per million population)
Iceland	3.9	784
Norway	4.0	28
Sweden	5.5	33
Canada	7.1	177
Ireland	7.2	210
United States	7.2	164
United Kingdom	7.6	51
Finland	7.8	110
New Zealand	7.8	102
Australia	8.3	56
Netherlands	8.4	12
Italy	8.6	6
Denmark	9.8	22
Belgium	9.9	53
Portugal	9.9	1
Spain	10.4	8
Switzerland	10.8	22
Austria	11.5	92
Germany	12.6	26
France	13.2	7
Luxembourg	13.6	0

Source: The Stanton Peale Addiction Center. Http://www.stantonpeele.net

No information was found about the number of people in each group.

Of world drinking patterns, Luxembourg has the highest yearly consumption of alcohol per individual at 11.9 L, followed by Hungary at 11.1 L, and the Czech Republic and Ireland at 10.8 L each. The United States did not rank in the top 20 (Pocket World in Figures, p. 98).

When assessing clients' alcohol and recreational drug use, the health-care provider must place these high-risk behaviors within the context of their cultural group. Health-care providers can have a significant impact on behavior-related health problems of alcohol by encouraging moderate drinking, providing educational and counseling materials in their preferred language, working with the regulators of alcohol manufacturing as well as the beverage industry, and working with elementary and secondary school teachers to promote responsible drinking.

Health-Care Practices

In 2003 to 2004, 17.1 percent of children and adolescents 2 to 19 years of age were overweight, and 32.2% of adults were obese. Significant differences in obesity among racial and ethnic groups remain. The prevalence of overweight in Mexican American and non-Hispanic black girls was higher than among non-Hispanic white girls. Among boys, the prevalence of overweight was significantly higher among Mexican Americans than among either non-Hispanic black or white boys. Among adults, similar differences existed. Approximately 30 percent of non-Hispanic white adults were obese, and 45 percent of non-Hispanic black adults and 36.8 percent of Mexican American adults were obese (National Center for Health Statistics, 2004).

Significant differences existed by age. Adolescents were more likely to be overweight than younger children, and older adults were more likely to be obese than younger adults. The only exception was among adults 80 years and over who were no different than adults 20 to 39 years of age. Between 1999 and 2004, there was a significant increase in the prevalence of overweight among girls—3.8 percent in 1999 to 16.0 percent in 2004. Similarly, among boys, the prevalence increased significantly from 14.0 percent in 1999 to 18.2 percent in 2004. The prevalence of obesity among men also increased significantly from 27.5 percent to 31.1 percent. There was no change in obesity among women—33.4 percent in 1999 to 33.2 percent in 2004 (National Center for Health Statistics, 2004).

Obesity and overweight are a result of an imbalance between food consumed and physical activity. National data have shown an increase in the calorie consumption of adults and no change in physical activity patterns. But obesity is a complex issue related to lifestyle, environment, and genes. Many underlying factors have been linked to the increase in obesity, such as increased portion sizes; eating out more often; increased consumption of sugar-sweetened drinks; increased television, computer, electronic gaming time; changing labor markets; and fear of crime, which prevents outdoor exercise. Obese adults are at increased risk of type 2 diabetes, hypertension, stroke, certain cancers, and other conditions. Overweight

adolescents often become obese adults. Although the United States has the highest prevalence of obesity among the more developed nations, it is not alone in terms of trends. Increases in the prevalence of overweight and obesity among children and adults have been observed throughout the world (National Center for Health Statistics, 2004).

Health-care providers can assist overweight clients in reducing calorie consumption by identifying healthy choices among culturally preferred foods, altering preparation practices, and reducing portion size.

The ethnocultural practice of self-care using folk and magicoreligious practices before seeking professional care may also have a negative impact on the health status of some individuals. Overreliance on these practices may mean that the health problem is in a more advanced stage when a consultation is sought. Such delays make treatment more difficult and prolonged. Selected complementary and alternative health-care practices are addressed in this chapter under the domain *healthcare practices* and in each culture-specific chapter.

The cultural domain of *high-risk behaviors* is one area in which health-care providers can make a significant impact on clients' health status. High-risk health behaviors can be controlled through ethnic-specific interventions aimed at health promotion and health-risk prevention through educational programs in schools, business organizations, churches, and recreational and community centers, as well as through one-on-one and family counseling techniques. Taking advantage of public communication technology can enhance participation in these programs if they are geared to the unique needs of the individual, family, or community.

> In which high-risk health behaviors do you engage? What do you do to control or reduce your risk? Which high-risk health behaviors do you see most frequently in your family? In your community? What might you do to help decrease these high-risk behaviors?

Box 2–6 identifies guidelines for assessing the cultural domain *high-risk behaviors*.

NUTRITION

The cultural domain of *nutrition* includes more than having adequate food for satisfying hunger. This domain also comprises the meaning of food to the culture; common foods and rituals; nutritional deficiencies and food limitations; and the use of food for health promotion and wellness, illness and disease prevention, and health maintenance and restoration. Understanding a client's food patterns is essential for providing culturally competent dietary counseling. Health-care practitioners may be considered professionally negligent when prescribing, for example, an American diet to a Hispanic or an Asian client whose food choices and mealtimes may be different from American food patterns.

High-Risk Behaviors

High-Risk Behaviors

1. Identify specific high-risk behaviors common among this group.
2. Explore behaviors related to the use of alcohol, tobacco, and recreational drugs and other substances among this group.
3. Explore beliefs and practices related to safe sex.

Health-Care Practices

4. Identify the typical health-seeking behaviors of this group.
5. Assess the level of physical activity in their lifestyle.
6. Assess the use of safety measures such as seat belts and helmets.

Meaning of Food

Food and the absence of food—hunger—have diverse meanings among cultures and individuals. Cultural beliefs, values, and types of foods available influence what people eat, avoid, or alter to make food congruent with cultural lifeways; and food offers cultural security and acceptance. Food plays a significant role in socialization; has symbolic meaning for peaceful coexistence; denotes caring or lack of caring, closeness, kinship, and solidarity; and may be used as an expression of love or anger (Leininger, 1988). When Americans invite a guest to dinner for the first time, the guest frequently brings a gift, although this is not required, and one of the choices is often food. There are no specific rules as to what type of food to bring, but wine, cheese baskets, and candy are usually appropriate. Bread (unless it is a very special bread) and soft drinks are not usually appropriate unless specifically requested.

What are your personal beliefs about weight and health? Do you agree with the dominant American belief that thinness correlates with desirability and beauty? What does food mean in your culture besides satisfying hunger?

Common Foods and Food Rituals

American food and preparation practices reflect traditional food habits of early settlers who brought their unique cuisines with them. Accordingly, the "typical American diet" has been brought from elsewhere. Americans vary their mealtimes and food choices according to the region of the country, urban versus rural residence, and weekdays versus weekends. In addition, food choices vary by marital status, economic status, climate changes, religion, ancestry, availability, and personal preferences.

Overall, the typical American diet is high in fats and cholesterol and low in fiber, according to the U.S.

Department of Agriculture (USDA). The USDA recommends the Food Pyramid for Americans, originally adapted in 1950, and revised in 1992, and again in 2005. This food pyramid is commonly taught in elementary and secondary education and is used as a guide for teaching healthy eating to the public. Daily recommendations include 6 to 11 servings of bread, cereal, rice, or pasta; 3 to 5 servings of vegetables; 2 to 4 servings of fruit, 2 to 3 servings of milk, yogurt, or cheese; 2 to 3 servings of meat, poultry, fish, dry beans, eggs, and nuts; and limited use of fats, oils, and sweets. However, it has been recognized that specific foods in this pyramid must be adapted for non-American food preferences. Specific food pyramids have been developed by several organizations and are available for Vietnamese, African American, Chinese, Puerto Rican, Navajo, Jewish, and Asian Indians. They are included in culture-specific chapters and can also be found on the Web by going to a search engine and typing in "multicultural food pyramid."

Many older people and people living alone do not eat balanced meals, stating they do not take the time to prepare a meal, even though most American homes have labor-saving devices such as stoves, microwave ovens, refrigerators, and dishwashers. For those who are unable to prepare their own meals because of disability or illness, most communities have a Meals on Wheels program through which community and church organizations deliver, usually once a day, a hot meal along with a cold meal for later and food for the following morning's breakfast. Other community and church agencies prepare meals for the homeless or collect food, which is delivered to those who have none. When people are ill, they generally prefer toast, tea, juice, and other easily digested foods.

Socioeconomic status may dictate food selections: for example, hamburger instead of steak, canned or frozen vegetables and fruit rather than fresh, and fish instead of shrimp or lobster. Given the size of the United States and its varied terrain, food choices differ by region: beef in the Midwest, fish in coastal areas, poultry in the South and along the Eastern seaboard. Vegetables vary by season, climate, and altitude, although larger grocery stores have a wide variety of all types of American and international meats, fruits, and vegetables. Many television stations and major newspapers have large sections devoted to foods and preparation practices, a testament to the value that Americans place on food and diversity in food preparation.

Special occasions and holidays are frequently associated with ethnic-specific foods. For example, in the United States, hot dogs are consumed at sports events, and turkey is served at Thanksgiving. Many religious groups are required to fast during specific holiday seasons, such as Ramadan for Muslims and Lent for Catholics. However, health-care providers may need to remind clients that fasting is not required during times of illness or pregnancy.

Given the intraethnic variations of diet, it is important for health professionals to inquire about the specific diets of their clients. Expecting the client to eat according to an American mealtime schedule and to select American foods from an exchange list may be unrealistic for clients of different cultural backgrounds. Counseling about food-group requirements, intake restrictions, and exercise must respect cultural behaviors and individual lifeways. Culturally congruent dietary counseling, such as changing amounts and preparation practices while including preferred ethnic food choices, can reduce the risk for obesity, cardiovascular disease, and cancer. Whenever possible, determining a client's dietary practices should be started during the intake interview.

> In what food rituals does your family engage? Do you have specific foods and rituals for holidays? What would happen if you changed these rituals? Do food patterns change for you by the season? During the week versus the weekend?

Dietary Practices for Health Promotion

The nutritional balance of a diet is recognized by most cultures throughout the world. Most cultures have their own distinct theories of nutritional practices for health promotion and wellness, illness and disease prevention, and health maintenance and restoration. Common folk practices and selected diets are recommended during periods of illness and for prevention of illness or disease. For example, many societies such as Iranian, Mexican, Puerto Rican, Chinese, and Vietnamese subscribe to the hot-and-cold theory of food selection to prevent illness and maintain health. Although each of these ethnic groups has its own specific name for the hot-and-cold theory of foods, the overall belief is that the body needs a balance of opposing foods. These practices are covered in culture-specific chapters.

A thorough history and assessment of dietary practices can be an important diagnostic tool to guide health promotion. Although school lunch programs, Meals on Wheels, and church meal plans, to name a few, are programs through which the health-care provider can encourage and support families in attaining better nutrition, these may not provide optimal nutritional selections.

> What do you eat to maintain your health? What does a healthy diet mean to you? Do you agree with the U.S. Department of Agriculture Food Pyramid? Why? Why not? What do you eat when you are ill?

Nutritional Deficiencies and Food Limitations

Because of limited socioeconomic resources or limited availability of their native foods, immigrants may eat foods that were not available in their home country. These dietary changes may result in health problems when they arrive in a new environment. This is more likely to occur when individuals immigrate to a country where they do not have native foods readily available and do not know which new foods contain the necessary and comparable nutritional ingredients. Consequently, they do not know which foods to select for balancing their diet. Widespread nutritional deficiencies of many types have occurred with recent immigrants from Southeast Asia, in part because of the time spent in refugee camps, but also because of changes in food habits when immigrating to America. Among the Hindu, the consumption of a single grain such as rice may result in a poor intake of lysine and other essential amino acids.

Enzyme deficiencies exist among some ethnic and racial groups. For example, many Vietnamese Americans are lactose-intolerant and are unable to drink milk or eat dairy products to maintain their calcium needs. By consuming soups and stews made with pureed bones and cooked to an edible consistency, this deficiency can be overcome. In general, the wide availability of foods in this country reduces the risks of these disorders as long as people have the means to obtain culturally nutritious foods. Recent emphasis on cultural foods has resulted in larger grocery stores having sections designated for ethnic goods and in small businesses selling ethnic foods and spices to the general public. The health-care provider's task is to determine how to assist the client and identify alternative foods to supplement the diet when these stores are not financially or geographically accessible.

> What enzyme deficiencies run in your family? Do you have any difficulty getting your preferred foods? What other food limitations do you have?

Box 2–7 identifies guidelines for assessing the cultural domain *nutrition*.

BOX 2.7

Nutrition

Meaning of Food

1. Explore the meaning of food to this group.

Common Foods and Food Rituals

2. Identify foods, preparation practices, and major ingredients commonly used by this group.
3. Identify specific food rituals.

Dietary Practices for Health Promotion

4. Identify dietary practices used to promote health or to treat illness in this cultural group.

Nutritional Deficiencies and Food Limitations

5. Identify enzyme deficiencies or food intolerances commonly experienced by this group.
6. Identify large-scale or significant nutritional deficiencies experienced by this group.
7. Identify native food limitations in their new country that may cause special health difficulties.

PREGNANCY AND CHILDBEARING PRACTICES

The cultural domain *pregnancy and childbearing practices* includes culturally sanctioned and unsanctioned fertility practices; views toward pregnancy; and prescriptive, restrictive, and taboo practices related to pregnancy, birthing, and the postpartum period.

Many traditional, folk, and magicoreligious beliefs surround fertility control, pregnancy, childbearing, and postpartum practices. The reason may be the mystique that surrounds the processes of conception, pregnancy, and birthing. Ideas about conception, pregnancy, and childbearing practices are handed down from generation to generation and are accepted without validation or being completely understood. For some, the success of modern technology in inducing pregnancy in postmenopausal women and others who desire children through in vitro fertilization and the ability to select a child's gender raises serious ethical questions about parenting.

Fertility Practices and Views Toward Pregnancy

Commonly used methods of fertility control in the United States include natural ovulation methods, birth control pills, foams, Norplant, the morning-after pill, intrauterine devices, sterilization, vasectomy, prophylactics, and abortion. Although not all of these methods are acceptable to all people, many women use a combination of fertility control methods. The most extreme examples of fertility control are sterilization and abortion. Sterilization in the United States is now strictly voluntary; however, some countries still perform involuntary sterilization to control birth rates and to control conception in people with mental retardation or deformities. Abortion remains a controversial issue in the United States and in other countries. For example, in some countries, women are encouraged to have as many children as possible, and abortion is illegal. However, in China, abortion is commonly used as a means of limiting family size because of China's one-couple, one-child law. Many women in China have 5 or 6 abortions in their lifetime because they lack other birth control methods (personal communications with Chinese women in Beijing and Xian, China, 1998). The "morning-after pill" also continues to be controversial to some. Anyone, male or female, over the age of 18 years can purchase the drug without a prescription. Those under the age of 18, whether male or female, must have a prescription.

A current literature search did not reveal any recent and dependable data on fertility control used by select cultural or ethnic groups. One notable study by Herold, Westhoff, Warren, and Seltzer (1989) studied the use of fertility control methods among Catholic Puerto Rican women and found that the incidence of pregnancy is higher for Catholic Puerto Ricans than for non-Catholic Puerto Ricans. However, contraceptive use is widespread among the Puerto Rican population regardless of social contexts such as socioeconomic levels, rural versus urban residence, and educational level. Other studies report fertility control from decades past and are deemed too dated to be accurate. Although some men have vasectomies, the literature is also scarce on the number of families who use vasectomy as a method of birth control.

Fertility practices and sexual activity, sensitive topics for many, is one area in which "outside" health-care practitioners may be more effective than health-care providers known to the client because of the concern about providing intimate information to someone they know. Some of the ways health-care providers can promote a better understanding of practices related to family planning include using videos in the native language and videos and pictures of native ethnic people, using material written at the individual's level of education, and providing written instructions in both English and the native language. Health-care providers should avoid family planning discussions on the first encounter; such information may be better received on subsequent visits when some trust has developed. Approaching the subject of family planning obliquely may make it possible to discuss these topics more successfully.

> Does pregnancy have a special meaning in your culture? Is fertility control acceptable in your culture? Do most people adhere to fertility control practices in your culture? What types of fertility control are acceptable? Unacceptable?

Prescriptive, Restrictive, and Taboo Practices in the Childbearing Family

Most societies have prescriptive, restrictive, and taboo beliefs for maternal behaviors and the delivery of a healthy baby. Such beliefs affect sexual and lifestyle behaviors during pregnancy, birthing, and the immediate postpartum period. Prescriptive practices are things that the mother should do to have a good outcome (healthy baby and pregnancy). Restrictive belief practices are those things that the mother should not do to have a positive outcome (healthy baby and delivery). Taboo practices are those things that, if done, are likely to harm the baby or mother.

A prescriptive belief among Americans is that women are expected to seek preventive care, eat a well-balanced diet, and get adequate rest to have a healthy pregnancy and baby. The American health-care system encourages women to breastfeed, and many places of employment have made arrangements for women to breastfeed while working. A restrictive belief among Americans is that pregnant women should refrain from being around loud noises for prolonged periods of time. Taboo behaviors during pregnancy among Americans are smoking, drinking alcohol, drinking large amounts of caffeine, and taking recreational drugs—practices that are sure to cause harm to the mother or baby.

A taboo belief common among many cultures is that a pregnant woman should not reach over her head because the baby may be born with the umbilical cord around its neck. A restrictive belief among Indians in Belize and Panama is that permitting the father to be present in the delivery room and seeing the mother or baby before they have been cleaned can cause harm to the baby or mother. Because the father is absent from the delivery room or does not want to see the mother or baby immediately after birth does not mean that he does not care about them. However, in the American culture, in which the father is often encouraged to take prenatal classes with the expectant mother and provide a supportive role in the delivery process, fathers with opposing beliefs may feel guilty if they do not comply. The woman's female relatives provide assistance to the new mother until she is able to care for herself and baby. Additional cultural beliefs carried over from cultural migration and American diversity include

> If you wear an opal ring during pregnancy, it will harm the baby.
>
> Birth marks are caused by eating strawberries or seeing a snake and being frightened.
>
> Congenital anomalies can occur if the mother sees or experiences a tragedy during her pregnancy.
>
> Nursing mothers should eat a bland diet to avoid upsetting the baby.
>
> The infant should wear a band around the abdomen to prevent the umbilicus from protruding and becoming herniated.
>
> A coin, key, or other metal object should be put on the umbilicus to flatten it.
>
> Cutting a baby's hair before baptism can cause blindness.
>
> Raising your hands over your head while pregnant may cause the cord to wrap around the baby's neck.
>
> Moving heavy items can cause your "insides" to fall out.
>
> If the baby is physically or mentally abnormal, God is punishing the parents.

In some other cultures, the postpartum woman is prescribed a prolonged period of recuperation in the hospital or at home, something that may not be feasible in the United States because of the shortened length of confinement in the hospital after delivery. Among the Vietnamese, the head is considered sacred, and it is taboo to touch the head of the mother or the infant. Even removal of vernix from the infant's head can cause distress.

The health-care provider must respect cultural beliefs associated with pregnancy and the birthing process when making decisions related to the health care of pregnant women, especially those practices that do not cause harm to the mother or baby. Most cultural practices can be integrated into preventive teaching in a manner that promotes compliance.

What are some prescriptive practices for pregnant women in your culture? What are some restrictive practices for pregnant women in your culture? What are some taboo practices for pregnant women in your culture? What special foods should a woman eat to have a healthy baby in your culture? What foods should be avoided? What foods should a nursing mother eat postpartum? What foods should she avoid?

Box 2–8 identifies guidelines for assessing the cultural domain *pregnancy and childbearing practices*.

BOX 2.8

Pregnancy and Childbearing Practices

Fertility Practices and Views Toward Pregnancy

1. Explore cultural views and practices related to fertility control.
2. Identify cultural practices and views toward pregnancy.

Prescriptive, Restrictive, and Taboo Practices in the Childbearing Family

3. Identify prescriptive, restrictive, and taboo practices related to pregnancy, such as foods, exercise, intercourse, and avoidance of weather-related conditions.
4. Identify prescriptive, restrictive, and taboo practices related to the birthing process, such as reactions during labor, presence of men, position for delivery, preferred types of health practitioners, or place of delivery.
5. Identify prescriptive, restrictive, and taboo practices related to the postpartum period, such as bathing, cord care, exercise, foods, and roles of men.

DEATH RITUALS

The cultural domain *death rituals* includes how the individual and the society view death and euthanasia, rituals to prepare for death, burial practices, and bereavement. Death rituals of ethnic and cultural groups are the least likely to change over time and may cause concerns among health-care personnel. Some staff may not understand the value of customs with which they are not familiar, such as the ritual washing of the body. Death practices, beliefs, and rituals vary significantly among cultural and religious groups. To avoid cultural taboos, health-care professionals must become knowledgeable about unique practices related to death, dying, and bereavement.

Death Rituals and Expectations

For many American health-care providers educated in a culture of mastery over the environment, death is seen as one more disease to conquer, and when this does not happen, death becomes a personal failure. Thus, for many, death does not take a natural course because it is "managed" or "prolonged," making it difficult for some to die with dignity. Moreover, death and responses to death are not easy topics for many Americans to verbalize. Instead, many euphemisms are used rather than verbalizing that the person died: for example, "He passed on or passed away," "She is no longer with us," and "He went to visit the Grim Reaper." The American cultural belief in self-determination and autonomy extends to people making their own decisions about end-of-life care. Mentally competent adults have the right to refuse or decide what medical treatment and interventions they wish to extend life, such as artificial life support and artificial feeding and hydration.

What terms do you use when referring to death? Why do you use these terms? What specific burial practices do you have in your family/culture?

Among most Americans, the belief is that a dying person should not be left alone, and accommodations are usually made for a family member to be with the dying person at all times. Health-care personnel are expected to care for the family as much as for the patient during this time. Most people are buried or cremated within 3 days of the death, but extenuating circumstances may lengthen this period to accommodate family and friends who must travel a long distance to attend a funeral or memorial service. The family can decide whether the deceased will have an open casket, for viewing the deceased by family or friends, or whether the casket will remain closed. Significant variations in burial practices occur with other ethnocultural groups in the United States.

The tradition among Orthodox Jews is to bury their deceased before sundown the next day and have post-death rituals that last for several days. Other groups have elaborate ceremonies in commemoration of the dead, such as a *velorio* among Mexican Americans, which may last for days. To some people, these rituals look like a celebration; in reality, it is a celebration of the person's life. In Greek Orthodox culture, successive stages of mourning include memorial services 40 days after burial and then at 3 months and 6 months, with yearly rituals thereafter. When Muslims approach death, they may wish to face Mecca and recite passages from the Qur'an; the health-care provider needs to determine the direction of Mecca and position the bed accordingly. Whether in the hospital, in an extended-care facility, or at home in the community, the furniture may need to be rearranged to accomplish this important ritual.

Responses to Death and Grief

American society has been launching major initiatives to help patients die as comfortably as possible without pain. As a result, more people are choosing to remain at home or to enter a hospice for end-of-life care where their comfort needs are better met. One of the requirements for entering a hospice in the United States is that the patient must sign documents indicating that he or she does not want extensive life-saving measures performed. When death does occur, most Americans conservatively control their grief, although women are usually more expressive than men. For many, especially men, they are expected to be stoic in their reactions to death, at least in public. Generally, tears are shed, but loud wailing and uncontrollable sobbing rarely occur. The belief is that the person has progressed to a better existence and does not have to undergo the pressures of life on Earth.

Bereavement time for Chinese people may be a week or longer, depending on the relationship of the family member to the deceased and the degree of acculturation. The family of a deceased Chinese American may need extra leave time to fulfill their cultural obligations. These variations in the grieving process may cause confusion for health-care providers, who may perceive some clients as overreacting and others as not caring. The behaviors associated with the grieving process must be placed in the context of the specific ethnocultural belief system in order to provide culturally competent care. Caregivers should accept and encourage ethnically specific bereavement practices when providing support to family and friends. Bereavement support strategies include being physically present, encouraging a reality orientation, openly acknowledging the family's right to grieve, accepting varied behavioral responses to grief, acknowledging the patient's pain, assisting them to express their feelings, encouraging interpersonal relationships, promoting interest in a new life, and making referrals to other resources such as a priest, minister, rabbi, or pastoral care.

> How do men grieve in your culture? How do women grieve in your culture? Do you have a living will or advance directive? Why? Why not? Are you an organ donor? Why? Why not? Is there a specific time frame for bereavement?

Box 2–9 identifies guidelines for assessing the cultural domain *death rituals*.

SPIRITUALITY

The domain *spirituality* involves more than formal religious beliefs related to faith and affiliation and the use of prayer. For some people, religion has a strong influence over and shapes nutrition practices, health-care practices, and other cultural domains. Spirituality includes all behaviors that give meaning to life and provide strength to the individual. Furthermore, it is difficult to distinguish religious beliefs from cultural beliefs because for some, especially the very devout, religion guides the dominant beliefs, values, and practices even more than their culture.

Spirituality, a component of health related to the essence of life, is a vital human experience that is shared by all humans. Spirituality helps provide balance among the mind, body, and spirit. Trained and traditional religious leaders provide comfort to both the patient and the family. Spirituality does not have to be scientifically proven and is patterned unconsciously from a person's worldview. Accordingly, people may deviate somewhat from the majority view or position of their formally recognized religion.

Dominant Religion and Use of Prayer

Of the major religions in the world, 33 percent of people are Christians; 21 percent are Islamic; 16 percent are atheist,

---

BOX 2.9

Death Rituals

Death Rituals and Expectations

1. Identify culturally specific death rituals and expectations.
2. Explain death rituals and mourning practices.
3. What are specific burial practices, such as cremation?

Responses to Death and Grief

4. Identify cultural responses to death and grief.
5. Explore the meaning of death, dying, and the afterlife.

agnostic, or nonreligious; and 14 percent are Hindu (Major Religions, 2006). In the United States, the three major religious groups are Christians, 76.5 percent; nonreligious/secular, 13.2 percent; Judaism, 2.3 percent. Hindu, Islam, Agnostic, and Buddhist are each 0.5 percent and are increasing more rapidly than other groups (Top Twenty Religions, 2001). Obviously, the United States does not mirror the world in terms of religious affiliation. Immigration to the United States is increasing the nation's religious diversity.

Many groups settled in America for religious freedom. Furthermore, specific religious groups are concentrated regionally in the United States, with Baptists in the South, Lutherans in the North and Midwest, and Catholics in the Northeast, East, and Southwest. Within this context, there is a separation of church and state, and the U.S. government cannot support any particular religion or prevent people from practicing their chosen religion. However, this does not include cults or extremist groups, which usually devote themselves to esoteric ideals and fads. Even though there is a separation of church and state in the United States, many public events and ceremonies open with a prayer, and phrases such as "one nation under God" are often heard. American money still has the phrase "in God we trust." Most people see these religious symbols as harmless rituals. Instead of speaking to "religious values," politicians speak to "family values" as a way of getting around religious principles. However, these issues are subject to debate from time to time. Unlike in many countries that support a specific church or religion and in which people discuss their religion frequently and openly, religion is not an everyday topic of conversation for most Americans.

The health-care practitioner who is aware of the client's religious practices and spiritual needs is in a better position to promote culturally competent health care. The practitioner must demonstrate an appreciation of and respect for the dignity and spiritual beliefs of clients by avoiding negative comments about religious beliefs and practices. Clients may find considerable comfort in speaking with religious leaders in times of crisis and serious illness.

Prayer takes different forms and different meanings. Some people pray daily and may have altars in their homes. Others may consider themselves devoutly religious and say prayers only on special occasions or in times of crisis or illness. Among the Amish, faith-related behavior includes corporate (group) worship, prayer, and singing, which help build conformity and maintain harmony within the group. Prayer is a significant source of strength for many including devout Muslims, who pray five times a day. Health-care providers may need to make special arrangements for individuals to say prayers in accordance with their belief systems.

> With what religion do you identify? Do you consider yourself devout? Do you need anything special to pray? When do you pray? Do you pray for good health? How do religiosity and spirituality differ for you? What gives meaning to your life? How are spirituality, religiosity, and health connected for you?

Meaning of Life and Individual Sources of Strength

What gives meaning to life varies among and within cultural groups. To some people, their formal religion may be the most important facet of fulfilling their spirituality needs, whereas for others, religion may be replaced as a driving force by other life forces and worldviews. Among other people, family is the most important social entity and is extremely important in helping meet their spiritual needs. For others, what gives meaning to life is good health and well-being. For a few, spirituality may include work or money.

A person's inner strength comes from different sources. Among the Navajo, the inner self is dependent on being in harmony with one's surroundings. For Christians, a belief in God may give personal strength. For most people, spirituality includes a combination of these factors. Knowing these beliefs allows health-care providers to assist individuals and families in their quest for strength and self-fulfillment.

Spiritual Beliefs and Health-Care Practices

Spiritual wellness brings fulfillment from a lifestyle of purposeful and pleasurable living that embraces free choices, meaning in life, satisfaction in life, and self-esteem. For example, when Navajo Indians are not in harmony with their surroundings and experience insomnia from anxieties, the Blessing Way Ceremony, ritual dancing, and herbal treatments, combined with prayers and songs, are performed for total body healing and the return of spirits to the body. Practices that interfere with a person's spiritual life can hinder physical recovery and promote physical illness.

Health-care providers should inquire whether the person wants to see a member of the clergy even if she or he has not been active in church. Religious emblems should not be removed as they provide solace to the person and removing them may increase or cause anxiety. A thorough assessment of spiritual life is essential for the identification of solutions and resources that can support other treatments.

Box 2–10 identifies guidelines for assessing the cultural domain *spirituality*.

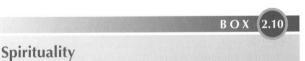

Spirituality

Religious Practices and Use of Prayer

1. Identify the influence of the dominant religion of this group on health-care practices.
2. Explore the use of prayer, meditation, and other activities or symbols that help individuals reach fulfillment.

Meaning of Life and Individual Sources of Strength

3. Explore what gives meaning to life for individuals.
4. Identify the people's sources of strength.

Spiritual Beliefs and Health-Care Practices

5. Explore the relationship between spiritual beliefs and health practices.

HEALTH-CARE PRACTICES

Another domain of culture is *health-care practices*. The focus of health care includes traditional, magicoreligious, and biomedical beliefs; individual responsibility for health; self-medicating practices; and views toward mental illness, chronicity, rehabilitation, and organ donation and transplantation. In addition, responses to pain and the sick role are shaped by specific ethnocultural beliefs. Significant barriers to health care may be shared among cultural and ethnic groups.

Health-Seeking Beliefs and Behaviors

For centuries, people's health has been maintained by a wide variety of healing and medical practices. Currently, the United States is undergoing a paradigm shift: from one that places high value on curative and restorative medical practices with sophisticated technological care to one of health promotion and wellness; illness, disease, and injury prevention; health maintenance and restoration; and increased personal responsibility. Most believe that the individual, the family, and the community have the ability to influence their health. However, among other populations, good health may be seen as a divine gift from God, with individuals having little control over health and illness.

The primacy of patient autonomy is generally accepted as an enlightened perspective in American society. To this end, advance directives such as "durable power of attorney" or a "living will" are an important part of medical care. Accordingly, patients can specify their wishes concerning life and death decisions before entering an inpatient facility. The durable power of attorney for health care allows the patient to name a family member or significant other to speak for the patient and make decisions when or if the patient is unable to do so. The patient can also have a living will that outlines the person's wishes in terms of life-sustaining procedures in the event of a terminal illness. Each inpatient facility has these forms available and will ask the patient what his or her wishes are. Patients may sign these forms at the hospital or elect to bring their own forms, many of which are on the Internet.

The acceptance of advanced directives and living wills is not uniform across ethnocultural groups. A study in New Jersey found that non-Hispanic whites were more than six times more likely to have advance directives than either Hispanics or Asians, and nearly three times more likely than African Americans (Advance Care Planning, 2004). People born in the United States were more than three times more likely than people who wore not born in the United States to have advanced directives. People who speak English at home were 10 times more likely to have advanced directives than people who do not speak English at home (Advance Care Planning, 2004). What is not known is what influence religion has on advance directives.

Most countries and cultural groups engage in preventive immunization for children. Guidelines for immunizations were developed largely as a result of the influence of WHO. Specific immunization schedules and the ages at which they are prescribed vary widely among countries and can be obtained from the Web site of WHO (http://www.who.int.gov). Campaigns since the early 1970s in the United States have resulted in an increase in immunization rates for children. In 1999, 78 percent of children age 19 to 35 months had completed the combined series of vaccinations for diphtheria-pertussis-tetanus (DPT), polio, measles, and *Haemophilus* influenza type b (Hib), up from 69 percent in 1994. Some still consider this unsatisfactory because other countries have higher immunization rates (Federal Interagency Forum, 2006). However, some religious groups, such as Christian Scientists, do not believe in immunizations. Beliefs like this, which restrict optimal child health, have resulted in court battles with various outcomes.

Some societies do not have the sophisticated technology and resources needed to facilitate health promotion. For example, Pap smears are relatively new in Egypt, and mammograms are either not offered or unavailabe. Thus, the health-care provider's first step may be to assess a person's previous knowledge and experience related to preventive and acute-care practices.

Responsibility for Health Care

The United States is moving to a paradigm in which people take increased responsibility for their health. In a society in which individualism is valued, people are expected to be self-reliant. In fact, people are expected to exercise some control over disease, including controlling the amount of stress in their lives. If someone does not maintain a healthy lifestyle and then gets sick, some believe it is the person's own fault. Unless someone is very ill, she or he should not neglect social and work obligations.

The health-care delivery system of the country of origin may shape the client's and employee's beliefs regarding personal responsibility for health care. In the United States, everyone, regardless of socioeconomic or immigration status, can receive acute-care services. However, they will be charged a fee for the service, and they may not be able to get nonacute follow-up care unless they can prove they are able to pay for the service. Even if they are covered by health insurance, an insurance company representative may need to approve the visit and then have a list of procedures, medicines, and treatments for which it will pay. Individuals who did not need health insurance in their native country may not realize the importance of having health insurance in the United States.

A large number of the working poor cannot afford to purchase basic economic essentials for the family and, thus, cannot even consider the purchase of health insurance. As of 2004, 46 million people living in the United States were not covered by health insurance and were unevenly distributed. Almost 30 percent of Hispanics and Native Americans/Alaskan Natives and 20 percent of African Americans are not covered by health insurance, compared with 11 percent of whites (U.S. Bureau of the Census, 2004). Considering that a family insurance plan averaged $10,800 a year in 2006, which is higher than the salary of a person making minimum wage, it is understandable why so many are uninsured. In most countries in the more developed world as well as in the less developed world, citizens have free access to care at the point of entry. Of the more developed nations, only the United States and South Africa do not have free access to care at the point of entry (Dagmara & Hopkins, 2003). Health-care providers should not assume that clients who do not have health insurance or practice health prevention do not care about their health. The health-care provider must assess clients individually and provide culturally congruent education regarding health promotion and wellness and illness, disease, and injury prevention activities.

What do you do to take responsibility for your health? Do you take vaccines yearly to prevent the flu or other illnesses? Do you have adequate health insurance? Do you have regular checkups with your health-care practitioner?

A potential high-risk behavior in the self-care context includes self-medicating practices. Self-medicating behavior in itself may not be harmful, but when combined with or used to the exclusion of prescription medications, it may be detrimental to the person's health. A common practice with prescription medications is for people to take medicine until the symptoms disappear and then discontinue the medicine prematurely. This practice commonly occurs with antihypertensive medications and antibiotics. No culture is immune to self-medicating practices; almost everyone engages in it to some extent.

Each country has some type of control over the purchase and use of medications. The United States is more restrictive than many countries and provides warning labels and directions for the use of over-the-counter medications. In many countries, pharmacists may be consulted before physicians for fever-reducing and pain-reducing medicines. In parts of Central America, a person can purchase antibiotics, intravenous fluids, and a variety of medications over the counter; most stores sell medications, and vendors sell drugs in street corner shops and on public transportation systems. People who are accustomed to purchasing medications over the counter in their native country frequently see no problem in sharing their medications with family and friends. To help prevent contradictory or exacerbated effects of prescription medication and treatment regimens, health-care providers should ask about clients' self-medicating practices. One cannot ignore the ample supply of over-the-counter medications in American pharmacies, the numerous television advertisements for self-medication, and media campaigns for new medications, encouraging viewers to ask their doctor or health-care provider about a particular medication such as the "purple pill."

In what self-medicating practices do you engage? What makes you decide when to see your health-care practitioner when you have an illness?

Folk and Traditional Practices

Some societies favor traditional, folk, or magicoreligious health-care practices over biomedical practices, and use some or all of them simultaneously. For many, what are considered alternative or complementary health-care practices in one country may be mainstream medicine in another society or culture. In the United States, interest has increased in alternative and complementary health practices. The U.S. government has an Office of Alternative Medicine at the National Institutes of Health that has awarded millions of dollars in grants to bridge the gap between traditional and nontraditional therapies.

In the context of Western medicine, in what complementary and alternative practice have you practiced? For what conditions have you used them? Were they helpful? How willingly do you accept other people's traditional practices?

As an adjunct to biomedical treatments, many people use acupuncture, acupressure, acumassage, herbal therapies, and other traditional treatments. Some cultural groups, for example, Hispanics, commonly visit traditional healers because modern medicine is viewed as inadequate. Examples of folk medicines include covering a boil with axle grease, wearing copper bracelets for arthritis pain, mixing wild turnip root and honey for sore throat, and drinking herbal teas. Native American traditions include ceremonial dances and songs. The Chinese subscribe to the yin-and-yang theory of treating illnesses, and Hispanic groups believe in the hot-and-cold theory of foods for treating illnesses and disease. Traditional schools of pharmacy in Brazil grow, sell, and teach courses on folk remedies. Most Americans practice folk medicine in some form; they may use family remedies passed down from previous generations.

An awareness of combined practices when treating or providing health education to individuals and families helps ensure that therapies do not contradict each other, intensify the treatment regimen, or cause an overdose. At other times, they may be harmful, conflict with, or potentiate the effects of prescription medications. Many times, these traditional, folk, and magicoreligious practices are and should be incorporated into the plans of care for clients. Inquiring about the full range of therapies being used, such as food items, teas, herbal remedies, nonfood substances, over-the-counter medications, and medications prescribed or loaned by others, is essential so that conflicting treatment modalities are not used. If clients perceive that the health-care provider does not accept their beliefs, they may be less compliant with prescriptive treatment and less likely to reveal their use of these practices.

Barriers to Health Care

In order for people to receive adequate health care, a number of considerations need to be addressed. Several studies have identified that a lack of fluency in language is the primary barrier to receiving adequate health care in the United States (U.S. Department of Health and Human Services, 2004). One can only deduce that this is true for other countries as well.

Availability: Is the service available and at a time when needed? For example, no services exist after 6 p.m. for someone who needs suturing of a minor laceration. Clinic hours coincide with clients' work hours, making it difficult to schedule appointments for fear of work reprisals.

Accessibility: Transportation services may not be available, or rivers and mountains may make it difficult for people to obtain needed health-care services when no health-care provider is available in their immediate region. It can be difficult for a single parent with four children to make three bus transfers to get one child immunized.

Affordability: The service is available, but the client does not have financial resources.

Appropriateness: Maternal and child services are available, but what might be needed are geriatric and psychiatric services.

Accountability: Are health-care providers accountable for their own education and do they learn about the cultures of the people they serve? Are they culturally aware, sensitive, and competent?

Adaptability: A mother brings her child to the clinic for an immunization. Can she get a mammogram at the same time or must she make another appointment?

Acceptability: Are services and client education offered in a language preferred by the client?

Awareness: Is the client aware that needed services exist in the community? The service may be available, but if clients are not aware of it, the service will not be used.

Attitudes: Adverse subjective beliefs and attitudes from caregivers means that the client will not return for needed services until the condition is more compromised. Do health-care providers have negative attitudes about patients' home-based traditional practices?

Approachability: Do clients feel welcomed? Do health-care providers and receptionists greet patients in the manner in which they prefer? This includes greeting patients with their preferred names.

Alternative practices and practitioners: Do biomedical providers incorporate clients' alternative or complementary practices into treatment plans?

Additional services: Are child- and adult-care services available if a parent must bring children or an aging parent to the appointment with them?

Health-care providers can help reduce some of these barriers by calling an area ethnic agency or church for assistance, establishing an advocacy role, involving professionals and laypeople from the same ethnic group as the client, using cultural brokers, and organizationally providing culturally congruent and linguistically appropriate services. If all of these elements are in place and used appropriately, they have the potential of generating culturally responsive care.

> **Looking at the list of barriers to health care, which apply to you? How can you decrease these barriers? What are the barriers to health care in your community?**

Cultural Responses to Health and Illness

Significant research has been conducted on patients' responses to pain, which has been called the "fifth vital sign." Most Americans believe that patients should be made comfortable and not have to tolerate high levels of pain. Accrediting bodies, such as the Joint Commission for Accreditation of Healthcare Organizations (JCAHO), survey organizations to assure that patients' pain levels are assessed and that appropriate interventions are instituted.

Beliefs regarding pain are one of the oldest culturally related research areas in health care. A 1969 study revealed that Irish Americans are stoic in their responses to pain, whereas Jewish Americans and Italian Americans are more vocal (Zborowski, 1969). A number of studies related to pain and the ethnicity/culture of the patient have been completed. Most of the studies have come from end-of-life care. Some of the salient research findings follow:

- Sixty-five percent of "minority" patients have inadequate pain control versus 30 percent of "nonminority" patients (Anderson, Richman, Hurley, et al., 2000; Cleeland et al., 1994; Cleeland, Gonin, Baez, Loeher, & Pandya, 1997; Foley, 2000).

- A patient's ethnicity has a greater influence on the amount of opioid prescribed by the clinician than on the amount of opioid self-administered by the patient (Ng, Dimsdale, Rollnik, & Shapiro, 1996).

- Communication between patient and health-care provider influences pain diagnosis and treatment (American Academy of Pain Medicine, 2004; Purnell & Paulanka, 2005).

- The brain's pain-processing and pain-killing systems vary by race and ethnicity (American Academy of Pain Medicne, 2004).

- Few minority patients are told in advance about possible side effects of pain medicine and how to manage them (Anderson et al., 2002).

- African American and Hispanic patients with severe pain are less likely than white patients to be able to obtain needed pain medicine because pharmacies do not carry the medicines (Morrison, Wallenstein, Natale, Senzel, & Huang, 2001).

- African Americans are less likely to have their pain recorded (Bernabei et al., 1998).

- Inadequate education of pain and analgesia expectations may contribute to poor pain relief in the Asian populations (Kuhn, Cooke, Collins, Jones, & Mucklow, 1990).

- Disparities in pain management and quality care at end of life exist among African American women in general and specifically with breast cancer (Payne, Medina, & Hampton, 2003).

- Hispanic patients are more likely to describe pain as "suffering," the emotional component. African Americans are more likely to describe pain as "hurts," the sensory component (Anderson et al., 2002).
- Socioeconomic factors negatively influence prescribing pain medicine.
- Pain does not have the same debilitating effect for patients from Eastern cultures as it does for patients from Western cultures (Kodiath & Kodiath, 1992).
- Stoicism, fatalism, family, and spirituality have a positive impact on Hispanics and pain control (Duggleby, 2003; Purnell & Paulanka, 2005; Zoucha & Purnell, 2003).
- Chinese, Korean, and Vietnamese patients do not favor taking pain medicine over a long period of time.
- Vietnamese Canadians prefer herbal therapies over prescription pain medicine (Voyer, Rail, Laberge, & Purnell, 2005).
- Haitians, Haitian Americans, and Haitian Canadians combine herbal therapies with prescription medicine without telling the health-care provider (Voyer et al., 2005).
- Black, Hispanic, and Asian women receive less epidural analgesia than do white women (Rust et al., 2004).
- Cultural background, worldview, and primary and secondary characteristics of culture profoundly influence the pain experience.
- The greater the language differences, the poorer the pain control.
- For Asians, tolerating pain may be a way of atoning for past sins.

Astute observations and careful assessments must be completed to determine the level of pain a person can and is willing to tolerate. Some recommendations: (1) **Always** ask about preferred treatment and **integrate** complementary alternative medicine (CAM) into pain/symptom control and management; (2) review the literature of the ethnicity of the patients for whom you provide care; (3) discover your own ethnocentrism and stereotyping of various ethnocultural groups (Mann, 2006); (4) observe for verbal and nonverbal responses to pain; and (5) have pain scales in different languages and with ethnic faces appropriate to the language and ethnicity of the patient (Pain Source Book, 2005). Additional resources for pain are the American Pain Foundation, The American Pain Society, the Boston Cancer Pain Education Center (in 11 languages), and the OUCHER Pain scale for children, all of which are available on the Internet. Health-care practitioners must investigate the meaning of pain to each person within a cultural explanatory framework to interpret diverse behavioral responses and provide culturally competent care. The health-care provider may need to offer and encourage pain medication and explain that it will help the healing progress. Research needs to be conducted in the areas of ethnic pain experiences and management of pain.

> **What is your first line of intervention when you are having pain? When do you decide to see a health-care practitioner when you are in pain? What differences do you see between yourself and others when they are in pain? Where did you learn your response to pain? Do you see any difference in the clinical setting in response to pain among ethnic and cultural groups? Between men and women?**

The manner in which mental illness is perceived and expressed by a cultural group has a direct effect on how individuals present themselves and, consequently, on how health-care providers interact with them. In some societies, such as American and Asian, mental illness may be seen by many as not being as important as physical illness. Mental illness is culture-bound; what may be perceived as a mental illness in one society may not be considered a mental illness in another. For some, mental illness and severe physical handicaps are considered a disgrace and taboo. As a result, the family is likely to keep the mentally ill or handicapped person at home as long as they can. This practice may be reinforced by the belief that all individuals are expected to contribute to the household for the common good of the family, and when a person is unable to contribute, further disgrace occurs. In Korea, mentally disturbed children are stigmatized, and the lack of supportive services may cause families to abandon their loved ones because of the cost of long-term care and the family's desire and desperate need for support. Such children are kept from the public eye in hope of saving the family from stigmatization. Koreans in the United States may hold these same values.

> **What are your perceptions about mental illness? Does mental illness have the same value as physical illness and disease? When you are having emotional difficulties, what is your first line of defense? Have you observed different attitudes/responses from providers regarding physical and mental illnesses?**

The physically and mentally handicapped may be treated differently in diverse cultures. In previous decades, physically handicapped individuals in the United States were seen as less desirable than those who did not have a handicap. If the handicap was severe, the person was sometimes hidden from the public's view. In 1992, the Americans with Disabilities Act went into effect, protecting handicapped individuals from discrimination.

In the United States, rehabilitation and occupational health services focus on returning individuals with handicaps to productive lifestyles in society as soon as possible.

The goal of the American health-care system is to rehabilitate everyone: convicted criminals, people with alcohol and drug problems, as well as those with physical conditions. Rehabilitation seems to now be well established in the United States. To establish rapport, health-care practitioners working with clients suffering from chronic disease must avoid assumptions regarding health beliefs and provide rehabilitative health interventions within the scope of cultural customs and beliefs. Failure to respect and accept clients' values and beliefs can lead to misdiagnosis, lack of cooperation, and alienation of clients from the health-care system.

Do you see physically challenged individuals as important as nonphysically challenged individuals in terms of their worth to society? What are your beliefs about rehabilitation? Should everyone have the opportunity for rehabilitation?

Sick role behaviors are culturally prescribed and vary among ethnic societies. Traditional American practice calls for fully disclosing the health condition to the client. However, traditional Filipino families prefer to be informed of the bad news first, and then slowly break the news to the sick family member. The sick role may not be readily accepted by Italian Americans and Polish Americans; some individuals may keep an illness hidden from the family until it reaches a more advanced stage. Given the ethnocultural acceptance of the sick role, health-care providers must assess each client and family individually and incorporate culturally congruent therapeutic interventions to return the client to an optimal level of functioning.

What do you normally do when you have a minor illness? Do you go to work (class) anyway? What would make you decide to not go to work or class? Does the sick role have a specific meaning in your culture?

Blood Transfusions and Organ Donation

Most Americans and most, but not all, religions favor organ donation and transplantation and transfusion of blood or blood products. Jehovah's Witnesses do not believe in blood transfusions. Christian Scientists, Orthodox Jews, Greeks, and some Spanish-speaking societies choose not to participate in organ donation or autopsy because of their belief that they will suffer in the afterlife or that the body will not be whole on resurrection. Because organ and tissue donation rates are lower among African Americans and Hispanics, some donor organizations have started to target specific campaigns to these communities. Information about kidney transplants and ethnicity can be found at the National Kidney Foundation's Website, http://www.kidney.org, and in indiviual chapters in this book. Health-care providers may need to assist clients in obtaining a religious leader to support them in making decisions regarding organ donation or transplantation.

Some people will not sign donor cards because the concept of organ donation and transplantation is not customary in their homelands. Health-care professionals should provide information regarding organ donation on an individual basis, be sensitive to individual and family concerns, explain procedures involved with organ donation and procurement, answer questions factually, and explain involved risks. A key to successful marketing approaches for organ donation is cultural awareness.

Are you averse to receiving blood or blood products? Why? Why not? Are you an organ donor? Why? Why not?

Box 2–11 identifies guidelines for assessing the cultural domain *health-care practices*.

BOX 2.11

Health-Care Practices

Health-Seeking Beliefs and Behaviors

1. Identify predominant beliefs that influence health-care practices.
2. Describe health promotion and prevention practices.

Responsibility for Health Care

3. Describe the focus of acute-care practice (curative or fatalistic).
4. Explore who assumes responsibility for health care in this culture.
5. Describe the role of health insurance in this culture.
6. Explore practices associated with the use of over-the-counter medications.

Folklore Practices

7. Explore combinations of magicoreligious, folk, and traditional beliefs that influence health-care behaviors.

Barriers to Health Care

8. Identify barriers to health care such as language, economics, accessibility and geography for this group.

Cultural Responses to Health and Illness

9. Explore cultural beliefs and responses to pain that influence interventions. Does pain have a special meaning?
10. Describe beliefs and views about mental illness in this culture.
11. Differentiate between the perceptions of mentally and physically handicapped in this culture.
12. Describe cultural beliefs and practices related to chronicity and rehabilitation.
13. Identify cultural perceptions of the sick role in this group.

Blood Transfusion and Organ Donation

14. Describe the acceptance of blood and blood products, organ donation, and organ transplantation among this group.

HEALTH-CARE PRACTITIONERS

The domain *health-care practitioners* includes the status, use, and perceptions of traditional, magicoreligious, and biomedical health-care providers. It is interconnected with communications, family roles and organization, and spirituality. In addition, the gender of the health-care provider may be significant for some people.

Traditional Versus Biomedical Practitioners

Most people combine the use of biomedical health-care practitioners with traditional practices, folk healers, and magicoreligious healers. The health-care system abounds with individual and family folk practices for curing or treating specific illnesses. A significant percentage of all care is delivered outside the perimeter of the formal health-care arena. Many times herbalist-prescribed therapies are handed down from family members and may have their roots in religious beliefs. Traditional and folk practices often contain elements of historically rooted beliefs.

What alternative practitioners do you see for your health-care needs besides traditional allopathic-care practitioners? For what conditions do you use nonallopathic practitioners? Do you think traditional practitioners are as valuable as allopathic practitioners?

The American practice is to assign staff to patients regardless of gender differences, although often an attempt is made to provide a same-gender health-care provider when intimate care is involved, especially when the patient and caregiver are of the same age. However, health-care providers should recognize and respect differences in gender relationships when providing culturally competent care, because not all ethnocultural groups accept care from someone of the opposite gender. For example, many Hispanics are traditionally quite modest, even with health-care providers and, as a result, may feel uncomfortable and refuse care provided by someone of the opposite gender unless it is an emergency. Health-care providers need to respect clients' modesty by providing adequate privacy and assigning a same-gender caregiver whenever possible. In providing care to a Hasidic male client, a female caregiver should touch him only when providing care, and then preferably with gloves. Therapeutic touch is inappropriate with these clients.

Do you prefer a same-gender practitioner for your general health care? Do you mind having an opposite gender practitioner for intimate care? Why? Why not? Do you prefer Western-trained health-care providers or does it not make any difference?

Status of Health-Care Providers

Health-care practitioners are perceived differently among ethnocultural groups. Individual perceptions of selected practitioners may be closely associated with previous contact and experiences with health-care providers. In many Western societies, health-care providers, especially physicians, are viewed with great respect, although recent studies show that this is declining among some groups. Although many nurses in the United States do not believe they have respect, public opinion polls usually place clients' respect of nurses higher than that of physicians. The advanced practice role of registered nurses is gaining respect as more of them have successful careers and the public sees them as equal or preferable to physicians and physician assistants in many cases.

Does one type of health-care practitioner have increased status over another type? Should all health-care practitioners receive equal respect, regardless of educational requirements? Does the ethnicity or race of a provider make any difference to you? Why? Why not?

Within Arab cultures, the physician may rely more on physiological cues than technology for a diagnosis. When physicians order many tests or ask clients what they think the problem is, the client may view them as incompetent (Lipson & Meleis, 1985). Immigrant physicians from Iran may misunderstand the assertive behavior of American nurses, and immigrant Iranian nurses may be considered not as assertive as they should be in the American culture. Many people from the Middle East perceive older male physicians as being of higher rank and more trustworthy than younger health professionals. Chinese Americans, as well as many other people from collectivest societies especially, are taught from a very early age to respect elders and to show deference to nurses and physicians, regardless of gender or age.

Evidence suggests that respect for professionals is correlated with their educational level. In Australia, rather than equal respect, paramedics and police officers are often held in higher regard than nurses. In most cultures, the nurse is expected to defer to physicians. In many countries, the nurse is viewed more as a domestic than as a professional person, and only the physician commands respect.

Nurses in the United States, however, are held in high regard. This may be related to factors such as the completion of high school or an equivalency examination before entering a nursing program; the rigorous licensing examination required before practicing the profession; baccalaureate-, master's-, and doctoral-level programs of study; and the impact of nursing interventions on health-care outcomes. Some countries do not have programs leading to a master's or doctorate in nursing but they are in the initial stages of starting them.

In some cultures, folk and magicoreligious health-care providers may be deemed superior to biomedically educated

Health-Care Practitioners

Traditional Versus Biomedical Care

1. Explore the roles of traditional, folk/traditional, and magicoreligious practitioners and their influence on health practitioners.
2. Describe the acceptance of health-care practitioners in providing care to each gender. Does the age of the practitioner make a difference?

Status of Health-Care Providers

3. Explore perceptions of health-care practitioners with this group.
4. Identify the status of health-care providers in this society.
5. Describe how different health-care practitioners view each other.

physicians and nurses. It may be that folk, traditional, and magicoreligious health-care providers are well known to the family and provide more individualized care. In such cultures, practitioners take time to get to know clients as individuals and engage in small talk totally unrelated to the health-care problem to accomplish their objectives. Establishing satisfactory interpersonal relationships is essential for improving health care and education in these ethnic groups.

Throughout the world, except for Francophone Africa where the number of men and women in nursing are equal, a gender disparity exists between men and women in nursing. In Spain and Portugal, 20 to 23 percent of nurses are men because during communist times, if a man agreed to go to nursing school, he did not have to serve in the military. Twenty percent of nurses in Italy are men, 16.5 percent of nurses in Israel are men, and 10 percent of nurses in the Scandanavian countries and Great Britain are men. In the United States approximately 10 percent of nurses are men, with very active campaigns in some areas of the country to recruit men and other underrepresented groups into nursing (Purnell, 2007). Iceland did an effective major recruitment effort to enroll men. In 1999, 30 percent of the student nurses were men. However, because they lacked a program to support men who faced bias and stigma from faculty and other students, only one man completed the program 3 years later. Currently, less than 1 percent of nurses in Iceland are men (Kristinsson, 2001).

Box 2–12 identifies the guidelines for assessing the cultural domain *health-care practitioners*.

REFERENCES

Advance Care Planning in New Jersey. (2004). Retrieved September 5, 2006, from www.cshp.rutgers.edu/downloads/3450.pdf
American Academy of Pain Medicine. (2004). Retrieved September 9, 2006, from www.painmed.org
American Medical Association. (2006). http://www.ama-assn.org.
American Physical Therapy Association. (2006). *Demographics.* Retrieved August 30, 2006, from http://www.apta.org.
Anderson, K., Richman, S., Hurley, J., Palos, G., Valero, V., Mendoza, T., et al. (2002). Cancer pain management among underserved minority outpatients: Perceived needs and barriers to optimal control. *Cancer, 94*(8), 2295–2304.
Anthony, M. K. (2006). Overview and summary: The multigenerational workforce: boomers and Xers and nets, oh my. [Electronic Version]. *Online Journal of Issues in Nursing,* (11), 2.
Aschenbrenner, D. S. (2005). First drug targeted for use in an ethnic group. *American Journal of Nursing,* (105), 10, 58.
Bates, M., & Rankin-Hill, L. (1994). Culture, control and chronic pain. *Social Science Medicine, 39*(5), 629–645.
Bernabei, R., Gambassi, G., Lapane, K., Landi, F., Gasonis, C., Dunlop, R., et al. (1998). Management of pain in elderly patients with cancer. *Journal of the American Medical Association, 279*(23), 1877–1882.
Campinha-Bacote, J. (2006). *The process of cultural competence in the delivery of health-care services: A culturally competent model of care* (3rd ed.). Cincinnati, OH: Transcultural C.A.R.E. Associates. Retrieved September 9, 2006, from www.transculturalcare.net
Centers for Disease Control and Prevention. (2001). *Sexually transmitted disease surveillance.* Retrieved August 7, 2001, from http://www.cdc.gov.
Centers for Disease Control and Prevention (CDC). (2005, November 11). Cigarette smoking among adults: United States. *MMWR. Morbidity and Mortality Weekly Report.*
Centers for Disease Control and Prevention (CDC). (2006a). *Cardiovascular disease.* Retrieved September 9, 2006, from http://www.cdc.gov.
Centers for Disease Control and Prevention (CDC). (2006b). *National diabetes fact sheet.* Retrieved September 9, 2006, from http://www.cdc.gov.
Chung, D. (1992). Asian cultural communications: A comparison with mainstream American culture. In D. K. Chung, et al. (Eds.). *Social work practice with Asian Americans* (pp. 27–44). Newbury Park, CA: Sage.
CIA Factbook: United States. (2006). Retrieved September 9, 2006, from https://www.cia.gov/cia/publications/factbook/index.html
Cleeland, C., Gonin, R., Baez, L., Loehrer, P., & Pandya, K. (1997). Pain and treatment of pain in minority patients with cancer: The Eastern Cooperative Oncology Group Minority Outpatient Pain Study. *Annals of Internal Medicine, 127*(9), 813–816.
Cleeland, C., Gonin, R., Hatfield, A., Edmonson, J., Blum, R., Steward, J., et al. (1994). Pain and its treatment in outpatients with metastatic cancer. *New England Journal of Medicine, 330,* 592–596.
Corneilson, A. (2001). Cultural barriers to compassionate care—Patients' and health professionals' perspectives. *Bioethics Forum, 17*(1), 7–17.
Crawley, L., Marshall, P., & Koening, B. (2002). Strategies for culturally effective end-of-life-care. *Annals of Internal Medicine, 136*(9), 673–679.
Dagmara, S., & Hopkins, K. (2003, July). Global health report. *Hospitals and Health Networks,* 52–65.
Duggleby, E. (2003). Helping Hispanic/Latino home health patients manage their pain. *Home Healthcare Nurse, 21*(3), 174–179.
Federal Interagency Forum on Child and Family Statistics. (2006). *America's children: Key national Indicators of well-being.* Retrieved September 9, 2006, from http://www.childstats.gov/americaschildren
Foley, K. (2000). Controlling cancer pain. *Hospital Practice, 35*(4), 111–112.
Freeman, H., & Payne, R. (2000). Racial injustice in health care. *New England Journal of Medicine, 342*(14), 1045–1047.
Fujii, J., Fukushima, S., & Yamamoto, J. (1993). Psychiatric care of Japanese Americans. In A. Gaw (Ed.). *Culture, ethnicity, and mental illness* (pp. 305–345). Washington, DC: American Psychiatric Press.
Fulton, J., Rakowski, W., & Jones, A. (1995). *Public Health Reports, 110,* 476–482.
Gaw, C. (1993). Psychiatric care of Chinese Americans. In A. Gaw (Ed.). *Culture, ethnicity, and mental illness* (pp. 245–280). Washington, DC: American Psychiatric Press.
GenSpec. (2006). Retrieved August 31, 2006, from www.4genspec.com.
Giger, J. N., & Davidhizar, R. E. (2004). *Transcultural nursing: Assessment and intervention* (3rd ed.). St. Louis, MO: Mosby.
Hall, E. (1990). *The silent language.* New York: Anchor Books.
Hanson, L., & Rogdman, E. (1996). The use of living wills at the end of life: A national study. *Archives of Internal Medicine, 156,* 1018–1022.
Herold, J. M., Westhoff, C. F., Warren, D. W., & Seltzer, J. (1989). Catholicism and fertility in Puerto Rico. *American Journal of Public Health, 79*(9), 1258–1262.
Hill, R. (1995). *We Europeans.* Brussels, Belgium: Europublications.
Hilton, M. (1987). Demographic characteristics and the frequency of heavy drinking as predictors of drinking problems. *British Journal of Addiction, 82,* 913–925.
Ho, M. (1992). *Minority children and adolescents in therapy.* Newbury Park, CA: Sage.

Hughes, C. (1993). Culture in clinical psychiatry. In A. Gaw (Ed.). *Culture, ethnicity, and mental illness* (pp. 347–357). Washington, DC: American Psychiatric Press.

Human Resource Institute. (2005). *Diversity and inclusion.* Tampa, FL: University of Tampa.

Institute of Medicine. (2006). Retrieved September 9, 2006, from http://www.iom.org.

Johnson, M. R. D. (2000). Perceptions of barriers to health physical activity among Asian communities. *Sport, Education, and Society, 1*(5), 51–70.

Juarez, G., Ferrell, B., & Bourneman, T. (1998). Influence of culture on cancer pain management in Hispanic patients. *Cancer Practitioner, 6*(5), 262–269.

Judge orders executions for lesbian duo. (2001, February 23). *Washington Blade.*

Kim, L. (1993). Psychiatric care of Korean Americans. In A. Gaw (Ed.). *Culture, ethnicity, and mental illness* (pp. 347–357). Washington, DC: American Psychiatric Press.

Kodiath, M., & Kodiath, A. (1992). A comparative study of patients with chronic pain in India and the United States. *Clinical Nursing Research, 3,* 278–291.

Krebs, G., & Kunimoto, Y. (1994). *Effective communication in multicultural health-care settings.* Thousand Oaks, CA: Intercultural Press.

Kristinsson, P. (2001). *Fields of masculinity; Icelandic men in nursing.* Retrieved August 24, 2007, from http://ankavefir.hjvkrus.is/veistv/

Kudzma, E. E. (1999). Culturally competent drug administration. *American Journal of Nursing, 99*(8), 46–51.

Kuhn, S., Cooke, K., Collins, M., Jones, J., & Mucklow, J. (1990). Perceptions of pain relief after surgery. *British Medical Journal, 300,* 1687–1690.

Kupperschmidt, B. R. (2006). Addressing multigenerational conflict: Mutual respect and care fronting as strategy. [Electronic Version]. *Online Journal of Issues in Nursing,* (11), 2.

Lasch, K. (2000). Culture, pain, and culturally sensitive pain care. *Pain Management Nursing, 3*(Suppl. 1), 16–22.

Lashe, K., Wilkes, G., Montuori, L., Chew, P., Leonard, C., & Hilton, S. (2000). Using focus group methods to develop multicultural cancer pain education materials. *Pain Management Nursing, 1*(4), 129–138.

Lavizzo-Mourey, R., & Mackenzie, E. R. (1996). Cultural competence: Essential measurements of quality for managed care organizations. *Annals of Internal Medicine, 10*(124), 919–921.

Leininger, M. E. (1988). Transcultural eating patterns and nutrition: Transcultural nursing and anthropological perspectives. *Holistic Nursing Practice, 3*(1), 16–25.

Levy, R. (1993). Ethnic and racial differences in response to medications: Preserving individualized therapy in managed pharmaceutical programmes. *Pharmaceutical Medicine, 7,* 139–165.

Lipson, J. G., & Meleis, A. I. (1985). Culturally appropriate care: The case of immigrants. *Topics in Clinical Nursing, 7*(3), 48–56.

Major religions of the world. (2006). Retrieved September 4, 2006, from http://www.adherents.com/Religions_By_Adherents.html

Mann, A. (2006). Manage the power of pain. *Men in Nursing, 1*(4), 20–30.

Mattson, S., & Lew, L. (1991). Culturally sensitive prenatal care for Southeast Asians. *Journal of Obstetric, Gynecological, and Neonatal Nursing, 12*(1), 48–54.

McKinley, E., Garrett, J., Evans, A., & Danis, M. (1996). Differences in end-of-life decision-making among black and white ambulatory cancer patients. *Journal of General Internal Medicine, 11,* 651–656.

Miller, W. S., & Supersad, J. W. (1991). East Hindu Americans. In J. N. Giger & R. E. Davidhizar (Eds.). *Transcultural nursing: Assessment and intervention* (pp. 437–464). St. Louis, MO: Mosby.

Morgan, C., Park, E., & Cortes, D. (1995). Beliefs, knowledge, and behavior about cancer among urban Hispanics. *Journal of the National Cancer Institute, 18,* 57–63.

Mosher, W. D., & Goldscheider, C. (1984). *Studies in Family Planning, 15*(3), 101–111.

Morrison, R. S., Wallenstein, S., Natale, D. K., Senzel, R. S., & Huang, L. L. (2001). "We don't carry that"—Failure of pharmacies in predominantly nonwhite neighborhoods to stock opioid analgesics. *New England Journal of Medicine, 342*(14), 1023–1026.

Munoz, C., & Hilgenberg, C. (2005). Ethnopharmacology. *American Journal of Nursing, 105*(8), 40–49.

National Cancer Institute. (2006). Current and accurate cancer information. Retrieved September 9, 2006, from http://www.cancernet.nci.nih.gov.

National Center for Health Statistics (2004). Retrieved September 1, 2006, from http://www.cdc.gov/nchs/pressroom/06facts/obesity03_04.htm

National Center for HIV, STD, and TB Prevention. (2006). Centers for Disease Control and Prevention. http://www.cdc.gov.

National Sample Survey of Nurses. (2006). Retrieved September 9, 2006, from http://bhpr.hrsa.gov/nursing/

Newbauer, B., & Hamilton, C. (1990). Racial differences in attitudes toward hospice care. *Hospice Journal, 16,* 37–48.

Ng, B., Dimsdale, J., Rollnik, J., & Shapiro, H. (1996). The effect of ethnicity on prescriptions for patient-controlled analgesia for post-operative pain. *Pain, 66*(1), 9–12.

Ngo-Metzger, Q., Massagli, M., Clarridge, B., Manocchia, M., Davis, R., Lezzoni, L., & Phillips, R. (2003). Linguistic and cultural barriers to care. *General Internal Medicine, 18*(1), 44–52.

O'Brien, L., Siegert, E., & Grisso, J. (1997). Tube feeding among nursing home residents. *Journal of General Internal Medicine, 12,* 354–371.

Pain Source Book. (2005). Retrieved September 9, 2006, from www.painsourcebook.ca

Payne, R., Medina, E., & Hampton, J. (2003). Quality of life concerns in patients with breast cancer: Evidence for disparity of outcomes and experiences in pain management and palliative care among African-American Women. *Cancer, 97*(1 Suppl), 311–317.

Peele, S., & Brodsky, A. (2001). *Alcohol and society.* Retrieved September 9, 2006, from http://www.peele.net.

Perez-Stable, E., Herrera, B., Jacob, P., & Benowitz, M. (1998). Nicotine metabolism and intake in Black and White smokers. *Journal of the American Medical Association, 280*(2), 152–156.

Pocket world in figures: Alcohol consumption. (2005). *The economist.* London, Profile Books Ltd.

Prows, C. A., & Prows, D. R. (2004). Tailoring drug therapy with pharmacogenetics. *American Journal of Nursing, 104*(5), 60–71.

Purnell, L. (2007). Men in nursing: An international perspective. In C. O'Lynn & R. Tranbarger (Eds), *Men in nursing,* pp, 219–235. New York: Springer Publishing.

Purnell, L., & Galloway, W. (1995). What to do if called upon to testify. *Accident and Emergency Nursing, 17*(4), 246–249.

Purnell, L., & Foster, J. (2003a). Cultural aspects of alcohol use: Part I. *The Drug and Alcohol Professional, 3*(3), 17–23.

Purnell, L., & Foster, J. (2003b). Cultural aspects of alcohol use: Part II. *The Drug and Alcohol Professional, 2*(3), 3–8.

Purnell, L. & Paulanka, B. (2005). *Guide to culturally competent health care.* Philadelphia: F. A. Davis Company.

Rust, G., Nembhard, W., Nichols, M., Omole, R., Minor, P., et al. (2004). Racial and ethnic disparities in the provision of epidural analgesia to Georgia Medicaid beneficiaries during labor and delivery. *American Journal of Obstetrics and Gynecology, 191,* 456–462.

Sherman, R. O. (2006). Leading multigenertaional nursing workforce: Issues, challenges, and strategies. [Electronic Version] *Online Journal of Issues in Nursing,* (11),2.

Sue, D. W., & Sue, D. (1990). *Counseling the culturally different: Theory and practice* (2nd ed.). New York: John Wiley.

Top twenty religions in the United States. (2001). Retrieved September 4, 2006, from http://www.adherents.com/rel_USA.html#religions

U.S. Bureau of the Census. (2001). *Median age at first marriage.* Retrieved September 9, 2006 from http://www.census.gov.

U.S. Bureau of the Census. (2004). *Income, poverty, and health insurance coverage in the United States.* Retrieved September 9, 2006, from www.census.gov/prod/2004pubs/

U.S. Bureau of the Census. (2006a). *American factfinder: Social.* Retrieved September from http://www.census.gov/

U.S. Bureau of the Census. (2006b). *Educational attainment.* Retrieved September from http://www.census.gov/

U.S. Bureau of the Census. (2006c). *Poverty rates.* Retrieved September from http://www.census.gov/

U.S. Department of Agriculture (USDA). (2006). *My food pyramid.* Retrieved September 9, 2006, from http://www.nal.usda.gov

U.S. Food and Drug Administration. (2006). *Drugs.* Retrieved September 9, 2006, from http://www.fda.gov/cder/

U.S. Department of Health and Human Services Office of Minority Health. (2004). *Physician toolkit and curriculum.* Retrieved September 5, 2006, from http://www.onhrc.gov/assets/pdf/checked/toolkit.pdf

Voyer, P., Rail, G., Laberge, S., & Purnell, L. (2005). Cultural minority older women's attitudes toward medication and implications for adherence to a drug regimen. *Journal of Diversity in Health and Social Care, 2*(1), 47–61.

Warren, J., et al. (1995). Organ-limited autopsies: Obtaining permission for postmortem examination of the urinary tract, *Archives of Pathology Laboratory Medicine, 119,* 440–443.

Wenger, A. F. Z. (1991). The culture care theory and the Old Order Amish. In M. M. Leininger (Ed.). *Culture care diversity and universality: A theory of nursing* (pp. 147–178). New York: National League for Nursing.

Weston, M. J. (2006). Integrating generational perspectives in nursing. [Electronic Version]. *Online Journal of Issues in Nursing,* (11), 2.

Yamamoto, J. (1986). Therapy for Asian Americans and Pacific Islanders. In C. Wilkinson (Ed.). *Ethnic psychiatry* (pp. 89–141). New York: Plenum.

Yamamoto. J., et al. (1993). Cross-cultural psychotherapy. In A. Gaw (Ed.). *Culture, ethnicity, and mental illness* (pp. 101–124). Washington, DC: American Psychiatric Press.

Zborowski, M. (1969). *People in pain.* San Francisco: Jossey-Bass.

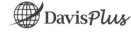

For case studies, review questions and additional information, go to
http://davisplus.fadavis.com.

Chapter 3

People of African American Heritage

JOSEPHA CAMPINHA-BACOTE

Overview, Inhabited Localities, and Topography

OVERVIEW

African Americans are one of the largest ethnic groups in the United States. Statistics from the U.S. Census Bureau reveal that there are more than 37 million African Americans in the United States, which represents 12.1 percent of the total population (U.S. Department of Commerce, Bureau of the Census, 2006). The African American population is expected to increase to 40.2 million by 2010 (American Demographics, 1991). African Americans are mainly of African ancestry; however, many have non-African ancestors as well. In fact, African Americans encompass a gene pool of over 100 racial strains. Because there is much diversity among African Americans, health-care providers must be aware of the intracultural variations that exist within this ethnic group.

African Americans have been identified as "Negro," "colored," "black," "black American," "Afro-American," and "people of color." Depending on their cohort group, some African Americans may prefer to identify themselves differently. For example, younger blacks may prefer the term *African American*, whereas elderly African Americans may use the terms *Negro* and *colored*. In contrast, middle-aged African Americans refer to themselves as *black* or *black American*. These different descriptors can cause confusion for those who are attempting to use the politically correct term for this ethnic group. In addition, we still see such organizational titles as the National Black Nurses Association, National Center for the Advancement of Blacks in the Health Professions, and the National Association for the Advancement of Colored People, which clearly depict the differences in how African Americans prefer to be identified. Therefore, it is culturally sensitive to ask African Americans what they prefer to be called.

HERITAGE AND RESIDENCE

African Americans are largely the descendants of Africans who were brought forcibly to this country as slaves between 1619 and 1860. The literature contains many conflicting reports of the exact number of slaves that arrived in this country. Varying estimates reveal that from 3.5 to 24 million slaves landed in the Americas during the slave trade era. Many slaves who were brought to the American colonies and early United States came from the west coast of Africa, from the Kwa- and Bantu-speaking people. The legacy of African American heritage and history of slavery is often passed on from generation to generation through African American folk tales and lived experiences (Taulbert, 1969).

African American slaves were settled mostly in Southern states, and currently, over 50 percent of African Americans still live in the South; 19 percent live in the North and Northeast, 9 percent in the West, and 19 percent in the Midwest. The highest concentration of African Americans can be found in metropolitan areas, with over 2 million in New York City and over 1 million in Chicago (U.S. Department of Commerce, Bureau of the Census, 2006). Major African-American communities are also found in 11 other cities: Atlanta, Georgia; Washington, D.C.; Baltimore, Maryland; Jackson, Mississippi; Gary, Indiana; Newark, New Jersey; Detroit, Michigan;

Memphis, Tennessee; Birmingham, Alabama; Richmond, Virginia; and New Orleans, Louisiana (Louisiana Department of Health and Hospitals, 2001).

Watts (2003) contended that race is an issue for African Americans, and "the black experience" in America is markedly different from that of other immigrants, specifically in terms of the extended period of the institution of slavery and the issue of skin color as a means for dehumanization of black persons. Watts concluded that matters of race, racism, and racial discrimination persist throughout contemporary American life.

REASONS FOR MIGRATION AND ASSOCIATED ECONOMIC FACTORS

The Civil War ended slavery in 1865, and particularly in the state of South Carolina, the Reconstruction Act allowed blacks the right to vote and participate in state government. However, most African Americans in the South were denied their civil rights and were segregated. Thus, African Americans lived in poverty and encountered many hardships. After the Civil War, more African Americans migrated from southern rural areas to northern urban areas. Blacks migrated because of a lack of security for life and property. They were unable to get out of debt and support their families in spite of having good crops. Also, World War II was a major catalyst in fostering migration to urban and northern areas, which provided greater economic opportunities and brought African Americans and European Americans into close contact for the first time. Jaynes and Williams (1989) reported that during the 1940s, a net outmigration from the South totaled approximately 1.5 million African Americans (15 percent of the South's black population). Although the migration was viewed as a positive move, many African Americans encountered all the problems of fragmented urban life, racism, poverty, and covert segregation.

EDUCATIONAL STATUS AND OCCUPATIONS

Before 1954, educational opportunities for African Americans were compromised. School systems were segregated, and blacks were victims of inferior facilities. In fact, in 1910, almost one-third of all blacks were illiterate (Blum, Morgan, Rose, Schleisinger, Stampp, & Woodward, 1981). However, in 1954, the Supreme Court decision in *Brown v. Board of Education of Topeka* ruled against the segregation of blacks and whites in the public school systems. Conant (1961) described the plight of African Americans in segregated schools and, to some extent, predicted the long-term social consequences of such a system. His predictions have been borne out as inadequate job opportunities and poor wages, resulting in poverty. Poverty has had a ripple effect on African American communities, often leading to poorly educated individuals, high dropout rates from school, and drug and alcohol misuse (Ladner & Gourdine, 1992). In many African American communities, this oppressive environment contributes to the existing alcohol and drug problems and the high dropout rate among African Americans,

which has been reported as high as 61 percent (Braithwaite, Taylor, & Austin, 2000).

Despite these devastating occurrences, most African American families place a high value on education. The African American family views education as the process most likely to ensure work security and social mobility. Families often make great sacrifices so at least one child can go to college. In African American families, it is not uncommon to see cooperative efforts among siblings to assist each other financially to obtain a college education. For example, as the older child graduates and becomes employed, that child then assists the next sibling who, in turn, assists the next one. This continues until all of the children who attend college have graduated. Before the civil rights movement, a major emphasis for African Americans in higher education was vocational. The thinking was that if African Americans could learn a trade or vocation, they could become self-sufficient and improve their economic well-being. Preparation for vocational careers is evidenced in the name, mission, and goals of two of the renowned, historically black institutions, Hampton University and Tuskegee University, formerly known as Hampton Institute and Tuskegee Normal and Industrial Institute.

Although African Americans have successfully completed a variety of majors in universities, significant differences exist in the ethnic, racial, and gender makeup of those obtaining higher degrees. For example, between 1977 and 1993, 55 percent of African Americans awarded doctorates were women. In 1995, there were a disproportionately higher number of African American women than African American men in the labor force (Albers, 1999). Today, African Americans continue to be underrepresented in managerial and professional positions. In addition, the representation of many African Americans and other ethnic groups within the health professions is far below their representation in the general population (Sullivan, 2004). Increasing racial and ethnic diversity among health professionals is critical because evidence indicates that diversity is associated with improved access to care for racial and ethnic minority patients, greater patient choice and satisfaction, and better educational experiences for all students (Institute of Medicine [IOM], 2004).

African Americans represent a large segment of blue-collar workers employed in service occupations (Low-wage labor market, 2006). One reason for this disproportionate representation in professional and managerial positions is believed to be discrimination in employment and job advancement. In 1961, President Kennedy established the Committee on Equal Employment Opportunity to protect minorities from discrimination in employment. However, most African Americans still believe that job discrimination is a major variable contributing to problems they encounter in obtaining better jobs or successful career mobility. With the dismantling of affirmative-action programs, based on misinterpretation of their purpose, this view will, perhaps, continue to gain support.

Most working-class African Americans do not typically advance to the higher socioeconomic levels. Because they are overrepresented in the working class, they are more likely to be employed in hazardous occupations, resulting in occupation-related diseases and illness. For example, Michaels (1993) reported that African American males are at a higher risk for developing cancer, which is related to their high representation in the steel and tire industries. According to Clark (1999), genetic factors of greatest importance in the work environment are probably race and gender. Implications are that health-care providers must not only assess African American clients for occupation-related diseases such as cancer and stress-related diseases such as hypertension but must also be familiar with the government's *Healthy People 2010* goals for the health and safety of individuals in the work environment (U.S. Department of Health and Human Services, 1997).

⊙— VIGNETTE 3.1

Miss Keesiah Young, a 19-year-old African American, presents to the emergency room (ER) with her 3-year-old son who is experiencing an exacerbation of his asthma. In reviewing her son's records, you find that Miss Young is unemployed and lives with her son and grandmother in a substandard housing project. The medical records reveal that she doubts the usefulness of medication for the treatment of her son's asthma, is concerned about possible side effects of prescribed medications, has failed to keep many of her scheduled outpatient clinic visits, and has a high frequency of ER visits related to his asthma.

1. What are some of the environmental factors that may have an impact on her son's asthma?
2. What are the cultural factors you must consider in providing culturally relevant care to Miss Young and her son?
3. What are some of the challenges you might encounter in providing care?

Communication

DOMINANT LANGUAGE AND DIALECTS

The dominant language spoken among African Americans is English. In addition, there is a way of speaking among some African Americans that sociolinguists refer to as *African American English (AAE)*. The two main hypotheses about the origin of AAE are the dialect hypothesis and the Creole hypothesis. The dialect hypothesis supports the position that African slaves, upon arriving in the United States, picked up English very slowly and learned it incorrectly. In turn, these inaccuracies have been passed down through generations. The Creole hypothesis maintains that AAE is the result of a Creole derived from English and various West African Languages.

The major problem that AAE speakers face is prejudice. Most people believe that AAE is inferior to Standard American English (SAE). At times, African Americans who use AAE are misinterpreted as being uneducated. However, it is common for educated African Americans who are extremely articulate in SAE to use AAE when conversing with each other. Thompson, Craig, and Washington (2004) referred to this ability as *dialect-shifting*. The literature suggests that AAE provides African Americans with a framework for communicating unique cultural ideas as well as serves as a way to symbolize racial pride and identity (Allender & Spradley, 2001; Murray & Zentner, 2001).

Over the years, a number of names have been used to describe the different varieties or dialects of AAE. Some of the more common terms are *Black English, Ebonics, Black Vernacular English (BEV),* and *African American Vernacular English (AAVE)* (Bland-Stewart, 2005). Much controversy exists regarding the use of these labels. In December 1996, the Oakland School Board in Oakland, California, passed a resolution to recognize Ebonics as the primary language of African American children and take it into account in their Language Arts lessons and classrooms (Rickford, 1999). This resolution sparked national debate and in April 1997, Oakland School Board dropped the word "Ebonics" from their implementation proposals. Obvious problems occur with defining a language racially because not all African Americans speak these varieties and some non–African Americans speak them as well.

CULTURAL COMMUNICATION PATTERNS

African American communication has been described as high-context (Cokley, Cooke, & Nobles, 2005). These people tend to rely on fewer words and use more nonverbal messages than what is actually spoken. The volume of African Americans' voices is often louder than those in some other cultures; therefore, health-care practitioners must not misunderstand this attribute and automatically assume this increase in tone is reflecting anger. African American speech is dynamic and expressive. Body movements are involved when communicating with others. Facial expressions can be very demonstrative. African Americans are reported to be comfortable with a closer personal space than other ethnic groups. Touch is another form of nonverbal communication seen when African Americans are interacting with relatives and extended family members. When interacting with African Americans, the power of touching should not be underestimated for its healing powers (Cokley et al., 2005).

Many African Americans mistrust health-care practitioners and express their feelings only to trusted friends or family. What transpires within the family is viewed as private and not appropriate for discussion with strangers. A common phrase that reflects this perspective is, "Don't air your dirty laundry in public." Health-care practitioners must be sensitive to this form of communication in that older and more traditional African Americans may not embrace "talk therapy."

Humor is a form of communication that can serve as a tool to release angry feelings and to reduce stress and ease racial tension. The *dozens*, a social game in which African Americans use humor, is a joking relationship between two African Americans in which each in turn is, by custom, permitted to tease or make fun of the other (Campinha-Bacote, 1993). Frequently, humor is used among the African American population as a preventive mechanism to ward off an anticipated attack. Often, the joking is loud and can be mistaken for aggressive communication if not understood within the context of the African American culture. Knowledge and understanding the function that humor serves within the African American culture can assist health-care practitioners to formulate culturally responsive health-care interventions. For example, Campinha-Bacote (1993, 1997) documented the effective use of culturally specific humor groups with African American patients with psychiatric disorders.

TEMPORAL RELATIONSHIP

In general, African Americans are more present- than past- or future-oriented. However, the past or future may be valued in specific subgroups of African Americans, such as the elderly, who place greater emphasis on the past than on the present. In contrast, younger and middle-aged African Americans are more present-oriented, with evidence of becoming more future-oriented, as indicated by the value placed on education.

Some African Americans are more relaxed about time and may not be prompt for their appointment. Within this context, it is more important for them to show up at an appointment than to be on time for the appointment. What they see as important is the fact that they are there, even though they may arrive 1 to 2 hours late. Therefore, flexibility in timing appointments may be necessary for African Americans, who have a circular sense of time rather than the dominant culture's categorically imperative linear sense of time (Murray & Zentner, 2001).

FORMAT FOR NAMES

Most African Americans prefer to be greeted formally as Dr., Rev., Pastor, Mr., Mrs., Ms., or Miss. They prefer their surname because the "family name" is highly respected and connotes pride in their family heritage. However, African Americans do not use such formal names when they interact among themselves. An African American youth commonly addresses an unrelated African American who lives in the community as Uncle, Aunt, or cousin. Adult African Americans may also be called names different from their legal name. Until invited to do otherwise, greet African American patients by using their last name and appropriate title.

Family Roles and Organization

HEAD OF HOUSEHOLD AND GENDER ROLES

Although today it is common to find a patriarchal system in African American families, a high percentage of families still have a matriarchal system. The head of the household can be a single mother, grandmother, or aunt. A single head of household is accepted without associated stigma in African American families. When women are unable to provide emotional and physical support for their children, grandmothers, aunts, the church, and extended or augmented families readily provide assistance or take responsibility for the children. One impor-

tant trend noted today is that a growing number of African American grandparents are functioning in primary parental roles. For example, 44 percent of all children living with grandparents today are African American. Approximately 66 percent of these children have grandparents as the primary caregivers.

Ladner and Gourdine (1992) contended, "single parenting and poverty are viewed as the causal factor in destabilizing the African-American family" (p. 208). Other contributing factors are the absence (Heady, 1996) and plight of black males, who have high unemployment rates and low life expectancy. Poverty and incarceration are three times higher among black males than among their white counterparts. Furthermore, a number of incarcerated black males have left children behind, thus increasing the number of black children who lack male role models and must be cared for by the mother.

Gender roles and child-rearing practices in the African American family vary widely depending on ethnicity, socioeconomic class, rural versus urban location, and educational achievement. The diverse family structure extends the care of family members beyond the nuclear family to include relatives and nonrelatives. Similar to the pattern in the general society, dual employment of many middle-class African American families requires cooperative teamwork. Many family tasks such as cooking, cleaning, childcare, and shopping are shared, requiring flexibility and adaptability of roles.

Because many African American families, especially those with a single head of household, are matrifocal in nature, the health-care practitioner must recognize women's importance in decision making and disseminating health information. Also, the health-care practitioner must focus on, and work with, the strengths of African American families, especially single-parent families. Hill (1997) stated that, although many African American families headed by single women are economically disadvantaged, they should not be compared or equated with broken or intact families.

PRESCRIPTIVE, RESTRICTIVE, AND TABOO ROLES FOR CHILDREN AND ADOLESCENTS

Given African Americans' strong work and achievement orientation, they value self-reliance and education for their children. A dichotomy might exist here, because many parents do not expect to get full benefit from their efforts because of discrimination. Thus, families tend to be more protective of their children and act as a buffer between their children and the outside world.

Respectfulness, obedience, conformity to parent-defined rules, and good behavior are stressed for children. The belief is that a firm parenting style, structure, and discipline is necessary to protect the child from danger outside of the home. In violence-ridden communities, mothers try to keep young children off the streets and encourage them to engage in productive activities. Adolescents are assigned household chores as part of their family responsibility or seek employment for pay when they are old enough, thus learning "survival skills."

By 1999, the rate of teen pregnancy dropped from 15 percent in 1981 to approximately 12.5 percent (National

Center for Health Statistics [NCHS], 1999). Although there has been a decline in the incidence of teen pregnancy, it continues to be a problem in the African American community because of poor pregnancy outcomes such as premature and low-birth-weight infants and obstetric complications. Furthermore, the teenage mother is expected to assume primary responsibility for her child, whereas the extended family becomes a strong support system. Premarital teenage pregnancy is not condoned in African American families; rather, it is accepted after the fact. In other instances, the infant may be informally adopted, and someone other than the mother may become the primary caregiver.

FAMILY ROLES AND PRIORITIES

African American families share a wide range of characteristics, family values, goals, and priorities. An example of a strong family value is the level of respect bestowed upon the elders within the African American community. Within this community, the elders, especially grandmothers, are respected for their insight and wisdom. The role of the grandmother is one of the most central roles in the African American family. Grandmothers are frequently the economic support of African American families, and they often play a critical role in childcare. It is common to see African American children raised by grandparents; this has contributed to an increase in the number of skipped-generational families seen in the African American community.

Understanding the role of the extended family in the lives of African Americans is essential. Several African American extended-family models exist. Billingsley (1968) divided them into four major types: subfamilies, families with secondary members, augmented families, and nonblood relatives. Subfamily members include nieces, nephews, cousins, aunts, and uncles. Secondary members consist of peers of the primary parents, older relatives of the primary parents, and parents of the primary parents. In an augmented family, the head of household raises children who are not his or her own relatives. Nonblood relatives are individuals who are unrelated by blood ties but who are closely involved with the family functioning.

Social status is important within the African American community. Certain occupations receive higher esteem than others. For example, African American physicians and dentists tend to have privileged positions. Ministers and clergy also receive respect within the African American community. They have historically held a high status in African American communities and are critical "First Responders" for the African American community (Cokley et al., 2005).

African Americans who move up the socioeconomic ladder often find themselves caught between two worlds. They have their roots in the African American community, but at times, they find themselves interacting more within the European American community. Other African Americans refer to these individuals as *"oreos"*—a derogatory term that means "black on the outside, but white on the inside." In Frazier's (1957) seminal and controversial publication, *Black Bourgeoisie,* he highly criticized the middle-class blacks. He argued that African American families who achieve upper-middle-class and middle-class status—the so-called black bourgeoisie—perpetuate a myth of "Negro society." According to Frazier, this term describes behavior, attitudes, and values of a make-believe world created by middle- and upper-class African Americans in order to escape feelings of inferiority in American society.

ALTERNATIVE LIFESTYLES

Lesbian and gay relationships undoubtedly occur as frequently among African Americans as in other ethnic groups. Acceptance of same-sex relationships varies between and among families. Personal disclosure to friends and family may jeopardize relationships, thereby forcing some to remain closeted. Debate is ongoing about the pros and cons of legitimizing lesbian and gay families, especially when children are involved. Opponents of this family form believe that parental behavior has a profound effect on children's gender identities and establishing family values (Bender, 1998). Single parenting and other alternative lifestyles are discussed in other sections in this chapter.

VIGNETTE 3.2

John Franks, a 66-year-old African American, has been admitted to the hospital to rule out a myocardial infarction. He is a minister in his church. When you conduct an initial assessment, he is very reluctant to share any personal information about himself or his family. He speaks in a loud manner and moves in close to your personal space as he answers your questions in short, abrupt responses. Although he speaks English, you are having some difficulty understanding his dialect.

1. What may be some possible reasons for his reluctance to share personal information?
2. What is the culturally appropriate way to greet this patient?
3. How do you interpret his loud speech and dialect?

Workforce Issues

CULTURE IN THE WORKPLACE

Although the African American value system reflects a strong emphasis on spirituality, there is also an economic-driven emphasis on materialism. African Americans feel a need to acculturate into mainstream society in order to successfully survive in the workforce. However, this survival is often met with ethnic or racial tension. *Ethnic* or *racial tension* can be defined as a negative workplace atmosphere motivated by prejudicial attitudes about cultural background and/or skin color.

Research reveals that African Americans have a long history of workforce disadvantage. They are underrepresented in highly skilled and managerial positions and overrepresented in low-status positions. Middle-class African Americans who hold higher paying jobs often experience the "glass ceiling" effect, in which access to higher positions is blocked (Bigler & Averhart, 2003). Health-care practitioners must increase their sensitivity and awareness of cultural nuances and issues that create ethnic or racial tension in the workplace environment, for these factors can have an impact on such stress-related conditions as mental health disorders and hypertension.

ISSUES RELATED TO AUTONOMY

Some African American men may experience a difficult time in taking direction from European American supervisors or bosses. This difficulty stems from the era of slavery when African Americans were considered the property of their master. Many African Americans continue to be frustrated at their lower-level positions and the absence of African American leadership in many workplaces. Lowenstein and Glanville (1995) found that along with historical circumstances, culture and politics affect the employment of African Americans in the health-care industry, often relegating African Americans to non-skilled roles. Today, a large number of African Americans continue to work as nursing assistants, licensed practical nurses (LPNs), or technicians. Thus, if the professional nurse who directs and supervises nonprofessional workers lacks cultural sensitivity toward other ethnic groups, the stage is set for cultural conflict.

Because the dominant language of African Americans is English, they usually have no difficulty communicating verbally with others in the workforce. However, some people may inaccurately view African Americans who exclusively speak AAE as poorly educated or unintelligent. This misinterpretation may affect employment and job promotion where verbal skills are more valued. In addition, the nonverbal communication style (e.g., strong intonation and animated body movements) of some African Americans is often misunderstood and labeled as more aggressive than assertive in comparison with that of other cultural groups.

Biocultural Ecology

VIGNETTE 3.3

Cory Moore, a 15-year-old African American adolescent, has been recently diagnosed with schizophrenia. Health-care practitioners are in the process of deciding what antipsychotic drug will be used to effectively treat Cory.

1. What knowledge about neuroleptic and antipsychotic drugs do you need to know in order to effectively treat Cory's psychiatric disorder?
2. What are some of the cultural beliefs of health-care practitioners that may influence the quality of psychiatric care given to this patient?

SKIN COLOR AND OTHER BIOLOGICAL VARIATIONS

African Americans encompass a gene pool of over 100 racial strains. Therefore, skin color among African Americans can vary from light to very dark. As health-care practitioners, we are trained in the art of using alterations in skin color and deviations from an individual's normal skin tone to aid in our diagnoses. For example, jaundice is a sign of a liver disorder; pink and blue skin changes are associated with pulmonary disease; ashen or gray color signals possible cardiac disease; copper skin tone indicates Addison's disease; and a nonblanchable erythema response signifies the presence of a stage I pressure ulcer (Salcido, 2002). We commonly use these alterations in skin color as potential signals of pathology because we can visualize changes such as the increased blood flow (erythema) that signals such problems as inflammation. However, these acquired assessment skills are based on a Eurocentric rather than a melanocentric approach to skin assessment.

Assessing the skin of most African American clients requires clinical skills different from those for assessing people with white skin. For example, pallor in dark-skinned African Americans can be observed by the absence of the underlying red tones that give the brown and black skin its "glow" or "living color." Lighter-skinned African Americans appear more yellowish-brown, whereas darker-skinned African Americans appear ashen. To assess such conditions as inflammation, cyanosis, jaundice, and petechiae in African Americans may require natural light and the use of different assessment skills. African Americans exhibiting inflammation or petechiae must be assessed by palpation of the skin for warmth, edema, tightness, or induration. To assess for cyanosis in dark-skinned African Americans, the health-care practitioner needs to observe the oral mucosa or conjunctiva. Jaundice is assessed more accurately in dark-skinned persons by observing the sclera of the eyes, the palms of the hands, and the soles of the feet, which may have a yellow discoloration.

The literature confirms that health-care practitioners are not doing an adequate job of detecting and reducing pressure ulcer risk in African Americans. According to recent studies, African Americans are at higher risk for developing more severe pressure ulcers and associated mortality and morbidly (Salcido, 2002). The *National Healthcare Disparities Report* (Agency for Healthcare Research and Quality [AQHR], 2005) revealed that in both 2002 and 2003, the proportion of high-risk, long-stay and short-stay residents who had pressure sores was higher among African Americans and Hispanics when compared with non-Hispanic whites. Salcido (2002) asserted that it may be due to our lack of ability to make an early diagnosis of skin in jeopardy of breaking down. Currently, researchers are testing a variety of devices that could be used to detect and diagnose alterations in blood flow, regardless of the color of the patient's skin. These devices include visible and near-infrared spectroscopy, pulse oximetry, laser Doppler, and ultrasound (Matas, Sowa, Taylor, Taylor, Schattka, & Mantsch, 2001; Salcido, 2002; Sowa, Matas, Schattka, & Mantsch, 2002).

Several skin disorders are found among the African American population. The major skin disorder is post-inflammatory hyperpigmentation, which is the darkening of the skin after resolution of skin trauma, lesions of a dermatosis, or as a result of treatments administered for skin disorders. Hypopigmentary changes have also been noted in these instances. African Americans also have a tendency toward the overgrowth of connective tissue associated with the protection against infection and repair after injury. Keloid formation is one example of this tendency. Diseases such as lymphoma and systemic lupus erythematosus occur in African Americans secondary to this overgrowth of connective tissue.

Certain skin conditions are gender-specific among some African Americans. Pseudofolliculitis barbae ("razor bumps") is more common among African American males. This skin condition results from curved hairs growing back into the skin, causing itchy and painful bumps. African American males should be counseled regarding the best shaving method to keep this disorder to a minimum. Suggestions include the use of electric clippers, a triple-bladed razor, a depilatory, or laser therapy. Melasma ("the mask of pregnancy") is more common among darker-skinned African American females during pregnancy. This condition is characterized by brown spots or patches on the face. Also noted among African American women is alopecia (hair loss) related to the use of chemicals to straighten/relax the hair or braiding.

African Americans, in general, also experience a disproportionate amount of pigment discoloration, with vertiligo (white patches) being the most common. This autoimmune disease manifests as white patches on the skin and causes skin discoloration and is also associated with diabetes and thyroid disorders. Birthmarks are more prevalent in African Americans. Birthmarks occur in 20 percent of the African American population compared with 1 to 3 percent in other ethnic groups. One example is mongolian spots, which are found more often in African American newborns but disappear over time.

African Americans must also be screened for skin cancer. Whereas squamous cell carcinoma is the second most common type of skin cancer in white patients, it is the most common type in patients of African and Asian Indian descent. Basal cell cancer is the second most common skin cancer of African Americans and is associated with chronic sun exposure. This type of skin cancer is more aggressive in African Americans than in whites. Many African Americans believe that they are not at risk for skin cancer because of their higher concentration of melanin; however, health-care practitioners must help to dispel this myth and educate African Americans regarding skin cancer protection.

DISEASES AND HEALTH CONDITIONS

Underwood et al. (2005) asserted that African Americans experience an "excessive burden of disease." When examining the relationship of social characteristics such as education, income, and occupation to health indicators, African Americans have worse indicators when compared with those of whites (Navarro, 1997). African Americans are at greater risk for many diseases, especially those associated with low income, stressful life conditions, lack of access to primary health care, and negating health behaviors. Examples of such behaviors are violence, poor dietary habits, lack of exercise, and lack of importance placed on seeking primary health care early. In terms of primary health care, the delays in seeking early treatment

may be associated with perceived health status or perceived risk of acquiring a particular disease (Edleman & Mandle, 1998).

The recent IOM report provides health-care practitioners with overwhelming evidence documenting the severity of health disparities found among African Americans (Smedley, Stith, & Nelson, 2002). Whereas previous research attributed the problem of health disparities among African Americans and other minority groups to access-related factors, income, age, comorbid conditions, insurance coverage, socioeconomic status, and expressions of symptoms; the IOM's report cites racial prejudice and differences in the quality of health as possible reasons for increased disparities (Burroughs, Mackey, & Levy, 2002). Health disparities among the African American population include decreased life expectancy and increased heart disease, hypertension, infant mortality and morbidity rates, cancer, HIV/AIDS, violence, type 2 diabetes, and asthma.

Although progress had been noted regarding an increase in the life expectancy among African Americans, they continue to fall behind statistics of whites. African American men's life expectancy is 68.2 years compared with 74.8 years for white men (American Public Health Association, 2004). African American women's life expectancy is 74.9 years compared with 80 years for white women. In 2000, approximately 8 percent of whites were considered to be in fair or poor health compared with nearly 14 percent of African Americans (NCHS, 2003).

Heart disease is more prevalent among African Americans. In 1999, African American death rates for heart disease were 29 percent higher than those of whites, and African American men were twice as likely as Hispanic men to die of heart disease (American Public Health Association, 2004). The literature cites unequal care, diet, income, education, and risk factors such as hypertension and obesity as potential reasons for the disparity in heart disease.

Hypertension is the single largest risk factor for cardiovascular disease and heart attack among African Americans. Compared with hypertension in other ethnic groups, hypertension among African Americans is more severe, is more resistant to treatment, and begins at a younger age, and the consequence is significantly worst target organ damage (Brewster, van Montfrans, & Kleijinen, 2005; Moore, 2005). The literature suggests that the pathophysiology of hypertension in African Americans is related to volume expansion, decreased renin, and increased intracellular concentration of sodium and calcium. Genetic cardiovascular researchers have hypothesized that there might be a "hypertensive-heart failure genotype" (Moore, 2005). However, it is more likely that the etiology of hypertension among African Americans is multifaceted, including genetics, diet, lifestyle, environment, and socioeconomic status (Moore, 2005; Saunders, 1997).

Although death rates from cardiovascular disease have decreased in the general population since the early 1980s, they have remained somewhat unchanged among African American women (National Women's Health Report, 2005). Of the 34 million African Americans living in the United States, 55 percent are women. Thirty percent of this female population lives in poverty and has limited access to health care because of a lack of health insurance. Poor nutrition, smoking, and alcohol and drug misuse occur more commonly among African American women (Drayton-Brooks & White, 2004). The leading causes of death among African American women are cancer, stroke, chronic obstructive pulmonary disease, pneumonia, unintentional injuries, diabetes, suicide, and HIV/AIDS. African American women also face greater disparities in incidence of infant mortality and morbidity. They have higher rates of delivering premature/low-birth-weight infants, and the rate of death due to prematurity/low birth weight for black infants is almost four times that for whites (March of Dimes, 2003).

African Americans also experience higher rates of diabetes. The incidence of type 2 diabetes in African Americans is among the highest in the world (Sowers, Ferdinand, Bakris, & Douglas, 2002). African Americans experience double the prevalence of complications related to their diabetes. These complications include higher occurrence of lower-limb amputations, end-stage renal disease, and eye disease and higher rates of hospitalization for diabetes when compared with whites. African Americans also have a higher rate of obesity, which puts them at risk for diabetes. African Americans tend to carry upper-body obesity, an additional risk factor for diabetes (Base-Smith, Grootegooed, & Campinha-Bacote, 2003).

African Americans experience higher overall cancer incidence and mortality rates and lower 5-year survival rates compared with non-Hispanic white, Native American, Hispanic, Alaskan Native, Asian American, and Pacific Islander population groups (Underwood & Powell, 2006). Specifically, African Americans' cancer death rate is approximately 35 percent higher than that of whites (American Public Health Association, 2004). African American males have a cancer death rate 50 percent higher than that of European American men, with a higher incidence of lung, prostate, colon, and rectal cancers. Although African American women have a slightly lower incidence of breast cancer than that of white women, their mortality rate is 32 percent higher (Morgan et al., 2006). African American women are less likely to participate in regular breast cancer screening, which is a major factor for this disparity (Spurlock & Cullins, 2006). Unfortunately, this results in breast cancer being discovered in the later stages when it is less responsive to treatment. Once African American women are diagnosed with breast cancer, Morgan et al. (2006) reported that they cope with the diagnosis by relying on God and seeking help from informal supportive networks such as family members and friends. Health-care practitioners must recognize the role of spirituality and informal support systems when developing intervention strategies to have an impact on breast cancer treatment among African American women.

Because African Americans are concentrated in large inner cities, they are at risk for being victims of violence. Violence is the sixth leading cause of death among African Americans (NCHS, 2003). Homicide is the leading cause of death among young African American males between the ages of 15 and 34. Brownstein (1995)

indicated that young black men are murdered by other black men at 10 times the rate of white men between the ages of 20 and 29. This violence has been referred to as "black-on-black" violence. Gangs may be more prevalent in larger cities, which only increases the likelihood of the occurrence of violence in African American communities.

Living in urban industrial or substandard housing also exposes African Americans at risk for developing diseases associated with environmental hazards. For example, the risk of asthma and allergies is increased by such environmental factors as exposure to house dust mite allergen and cockroach allergen. These allergens and respiratory tract irritants are commonly found in substandard housing, which has been related to the development of asthma in children (Asthma and Allergy Foundation, 2006). African Americans have a disproportionately higher rate of poor asthma outcomes, including hospitalizations and deaths. Deaths due to asthma are three times more common among African Americans than among whites (Asthma and Allergy Foundation, 2006).

Lead exposure is another environmental threat for poorer African American communities. African American and urban children are the most exposed to this environmental hazard. Specifically, African American and low-income children suffer lead poisoning at highly disproportionate rates and are at higher risk of exposure to unsafe levels of lead in the home environment. The American Academy of Pediatrics (1998) reported that the prevalence of elevated blood lead levels for African American children ages 1 to 5 years is approximately five times higher than the prevalence among white children. During the 1990s, high lead blood levels were found in 4.4 percent of all U.S. children; however, these blood levels were found in 22 percent of African American children (American Public Health Association, 2004).

Seemingly, minorities suffer the most from environmental pollution and benefit the least from environmental cleanup programs. In 1993, the federal Environmental Protection Agency found evidence that racial and ethnic minorities were disproportionately located near superfund sites, areas where hazardous waste and chemicals deleteriously affect people's health and the local ecosystem. Currently, efforts are directed toward environmental justice in order to ensure that no particular part of the population is burdened by negative effects of pollution (American Public Health Association, 1999).

In addition to the exposure to harmful environmental conditions, African Americans suffer from certain genetic conditions. Sickle cell disease is the most common genetic disorder among the African American population, affecting 1 in every 500 African Americans, and represents several hemoglobinopathies including sickle cell anemia, sickle cell hemoglobin C disease, and sickle cell thalassemia. Sickle cell disease is also found among people from geographic areas in which malaria is endemic, such as the Caribbean, the Middle East, the Mediterranean region, and Asia. In addition to sickle cell disease, glucose-6-phosphate dehydrogenase deficiency, which interferes with glucose metabolism, is another genetic disease found among African Americans.

Finally, in addition to environmental hazards and genetic conditions, AIDS contributes to the lower life expectancy of African Americans compared with that of European Americans. In 2003, African Americans, who make up approximately 12 percent of the U.S. population, accounted for half of the HIV/AIDS cases diagnosed. Although only 16 percent of children in the United States are African American, 62 percent of children reported with AIDS in 2003 are African American. In a national study concerning African Americans' views of the HIV/AIDS epidemic, African Americans were asked why they were not tested for this disease. Fifty-four percent responded that they felt they were not at risk for HIV/AIDS, and 11 percent stated that they did not know where to go to get tested (Kaiser Family Foundation, 2001). A knowledge deficit of HIV/AIDS was also revealed in this report. African Americans shared that such activities as kissing, sharing a drinking glass, and touching a toilet seat posed a risk of infection.

In summary, health conditions and health status for most African Americans are well below average. Health-care practitioners must provide culturally relevant health education, prevention practices, and screening aimed at improving the disparities in their health status and reducing their risks.

VARIATIONS IN DRUG METABOLISM

Research conducted at the University of Maryland revealed that African Americans and other minorities do not always respond to drugs in the same manner as European Americans (Saunders, 1997). Examples of drugs that African Americans respond to or metabolize differently are psychotropic drugs, immunosuppressants, antihypertensives, cardiovascular drugs, and antiretroviral medications.

Glazer, Morganstern, & Douchette (1993) reported from their research that African Americans are twice as likely to develop tardive dyskinesia than their white counterparts when placed on specific neuroleptics. For example, Campinha-Bacote (1991) reported that African American psychiatric clients experience a higher incidence of extrapyramidal effects with haloperidol decanoate than that found in European Americans. African Americans are also more susceptible to tricyclic antidepressant (TCA) delirium than are European Americans. Strickland, Lin, Fu, Anderson, and Zheng (1991) reported that for a given dose of a TCA, African Americans show higher blood levels and a faster therapeutic response. As a result, African Americans experience more toxic side effects from a TCA than do European Americans. In addition, African Americans have a higher risk of lithium toxicity and side effects related to less efficient cell membrane lithium-sodium transport and increased lithium red blood cell to plasma ratio (Herrera, Lawson, & Sramek, 1999). Some African Americans have a lower baseline leukocyte count (benign leukopenia), which puts them at risk for side effects of specific antipsychotic drugs, such as clozapine, which can cause agranulocytosis. Health-care practitioners must make extended efforts to observe African American clients for side effects related to TCAs and other psychotropic medications.

Dirks, Huth, Yates, and Melbohm (2004) reported ethnic differences in the pharmacokinetics of immunosuppressants among African Americans and European Americans. They found that the oral bioavailability of these drugs in African Americans was 20 and 50 percent lower than in non-African Americans. This finding suggests that there is a need for higher dose requirements in African Americans to maintain average concentrations of specific immunosuppressants. Dirk et al. (2004) maintained that recognition of these findings has the potential to improve post-transplant immunosuppressant therapy among African Americans.

African Americans may differ in their response to beta-blockers, angiotensin-converting enzyme (ACE) inhibitors, angiotensin receptor blocking agents, and diuretics used either alone or in combination for the treatment of hypertension (Burroughs, Maxey, & Levy, 2002). Studies report that African Americans do not respond as readily to the beta-blocker propanolol as European Americans do. However, their response to the diuretic hydrochlorothiazide is greater when taken alone or with a calcium channel blocker. Diuretics, alone or in combination with another antihypertensive agent, are reported to counteract increases in salt retention noted among African Americans. Although there has been much discussion about the best type of antihypertensive drug to administer in African Americans, health-care practitioners must remember, "there is no specific class of antihypertensive drugs that categorically should not be used based on race" (Burroughs, Maxey, & Levy, 2002, p. 18).

In 2005, the Food and Drug Administration (FDA) approved the drug BiDil (NitroMed) as adjunct standard therapy in self-identified black patients for heart failure (Ferdinand, 2006). This drug is based on the chemical nitric oxide, found naturally in the body, which dilates the blood vessels allowing blood to flow more easily, easing the burden on the heart. Although this drug was initially considered a drug failure in 2003, when the results were re-examined by race, it was found that a significant percentage of the 400 black patients in the trial seemed to respond. It was postulated that heart failure in African Americans is somehow associated with how they produce and metabolize nitric oxide. Specifically, African Americans may produce less nitric oxide and destroy it too quickly (National Women's Health Report, 2005). The approval of BiDil for "blacks only" is a highly controversial subject. Schwartz (2001) argued that labeling a drug based on race is "racial profiling" and is of no proven value in treating an individual patient. However, Ferdinand (2006) contended, ". . . while controversial, the FDA approval of BiDil does offer evidence that this therapy may be useful in the black population" (p. 157). An obvious question is, In a world of mixed heritages, how do health-care practitioners determine a person's race? Many contend that racial categories are more a societal construct than a scientific one. Health-care practitioners must be cautious in promoting drugs for specific ethnic groups, for it could easily lead to stereotyping and discrimination. Whereas race and ethnicity are important for public health issues, they are not true biological or genetic categories (Ferdinand, 2006). One solution is the designing of drugs that target specific genes, eliminating the need to rely on race.

Research has identified the possibility that a genetic mutation may make antiretroviral treatment less effective in Africans and African Americans (Schaeffeler et al., 2001). The P-glycoprotein (PGP) membrane protein appears to transport antiretroviral drugs out of cells, thus making the drugs less effective. A double mutation of the gene that encodes this protein (C/C genotype) leads to an increased amount of the PGP protein. Schaeffeler et al. (2001) examined the frequency of the C/C genotype in 537 Caucasians, 142 Ghanians (from West Africa), 50 Japanese, and 41 African Americans. The C/C genotype was found in 83 percent of the Ghanians and 61 percent of the African Americans, and only 34 percent of the Japanese and 26 percent of the Caucasians. It was hypothesized that certain antiretroviral drugs may not be as effective in people with the C/C genotype. Considering African Americans account for half of the diagnosed HIV/AIDS cases, this finding has serious implications in efforts to treat the AIDS epidemic among the African American population.

Cultural factors, such as a health-care practitioner's personal beliefs and biases about a specific ethnic group, may lead to unequal treatment, misdiagnosis and overmedication (Levy, 1993; Smedley et al., 2002). For example, African Americans are at a higher risk of misdiagnosis for psychiatric disorders and, therefore, may be treated inappropriately with drugs. Studies have found that African Americans are more likely to be overdiagnosed with having a psychotic disorder and more liable to be treated with antipsychotic drugs, regardless of diagnosis. DelBello et al. (1999) found that in a study with adolescents, although there were no differences in psychotic symptoms (14 percent of the African Americans and 18 percent of the whites were diagnosed as having psychotic symptoms), those who were African American, despite not being more psychotic, received more antipsychotic medications. Specifically, among white patients, 43 percent received antipsychotic medications. Among nonwhite patients, 68 percent received antipsychotic medications. There are several possible explanations. DelBello et al. (1999) contended that one plausible explanation is that clinicians perceived African Americans to be more aggressive and, thus, as more psychotic, and prescribed the antipsychotics.

Studies by Lawson (1999), Strakowski, McElroy, Keck, and West, (1996), and Strickland, Lin, Fu, Anderson, and Zheng (1995) also found that African Americans were more likely to be diagnosed with schizophrenia and more likely to be prescribed antipsychotics.

Access to pain medication is an issue for African Americans and other minority groups. African Americans with severe pain are less likely than whites to be able to obtain commonly prescribed pain medication because pharmacies in predominantly nonwhite communities do not sufficiently stock opiates (Burroughs et al., 2002). Morrison, Wallenstein, Natale, Senzel, and Huang (2000) examined the percentage of pharmacies in New York City stocked with adequate opioid medications and found that pharmacies in predominantly minority neighborhoods were much less likely to stock opioid medications. Only 25 percent of the pharmacies in minority neighborhoods had an ample supply of opioid medications to treat severe pain, compared with 72 percent of pharmacies in predominantly white neighborhoods.

Eye color is another genetic variation related to difference in response to a specific drug. For example, light eyes dilate wider in response to mydriatic drugs than do dark eyes. This difference in response to a mydriatic drug must be taken into consideration when treating African Americans.

High-Risk Behaviors

High-risk health behaviors among African Americans can be inferred from the high incidences of HIV/AIDS and other sexually transmitted diseases, teenage pregnancy, violence, unintentional injuries, smoking, alcoholism, drug abuse, sedentary lifestyle, and delayed seeking of health care. Community health workers can have a significant impact on these detrimental practices by providing health education at community affairs located in African American communities. The goals of health education are to change high-risk health behaviors and improve decision making (Edleman & Mandel, 1998). Examples of effective methods for changing behaviors are mutual goal setting and behavior contracts. Another strategy for changing high-risk behaviors is a teaching module using a culturally appropriate Afrocentric approach to early screening for breast and cervical cancer (Baldwin, 1996).

Efforts to change high-risk behaviors are not always successful. According to Edleman and Mandel (1998), health-care professionals must understand influential factors affecting decision-making regarding health behaviors. These factors include values, attitudes, beliefs, religion, previous experiences with the health-care system, and life goals.

HEALTH-CARE PRACTICES

Because a significant proportion of African Americans are poor and live in inner cities, they tend to concentrate on day-to-day survival. Health care often takes second place to basic needs of the family, such as food and shelter. In addition, the role of the family has an impact on the health-seeking behaviors of African Americans. African Americans have strong family ties; when an individual becomes ill, that individual is frequently taught to seek health care from the family rather than from health-care professionals. This cultural practice may contribute to the failure of African Americans to seek treatment at an early stage. Screening programs may best be initiated in community and church activities in which the entire family is present.

Nutrition

VIGNETTE 3.4

Mrs. Woods, a 28-year-old African American, is 28 weeks' pregnant. She is a master's prepared social worker and works as a case manager at a large medical center. She is married to a family physician resident, and this is their first child. She presents to the outpatient obstetric unit for her regularly scheduled clinic appointment. In reviewing her laboratory work, the complete blood count (CBC) reveals a significantly low hemoglobin and hematocrit, suggesting anemia. In your interview with Mrs. Woods, she states that she is taking her iron pills as prescribed. She is complaining of being fatigued, some infrequent headaches, and loss of appetite, which is consistent with being anemic. She also tells you that she is very anxious about having a baby and seeks a lot of advice from her mother, who resides in rural South Carolina.

1. What are some of the differential diagnoses for her anemia?
2. What cultural factors, related to her dietary habits, may account for Mrs. Woods' anemia?
3. What other cultural factors may be important for you to know when caring for Mrs. Woods.

MEANING OF FOOD

Historically, African American rites revolved around food. Eating foods identified with slavery has provided many African Americans with a sense of their identity and tradition. Special meaning is attached to the soul food diet, a Southern tradition handed down from generation to generation. The term *soul food* comes from the need for African Americans to express the group feeling of soul, and as a result, soul foods are seen to nourish not only the body but also the spirit. Although African Americans have incorporated soul foods into their diets, these foods are more commonly consumed for occasions such as special events, holidays, and birthdays. Therefore, the everyday diet of African Americans may more closely resemble the "American" diet, based on convenience and cost.

COMMON FOODS AND FOOD RITUALS

Chitterlings (pig intestines often either fried or boiled with hot peppers, onions, and spices), okra, ham hocks, corn, pork fat, and sweet potato pie are foods uniquely identified as Southern African American foods. Common ways for African Americans to prepare food include frying, barbecuing, and using gravy and sauces. African American diets are typically high in fat, cholesterol, and sodium. African Americans eat more animal fat, less fiber, and fewer fruits and vegetables than the rest of American society. Traditional breads of Southern African Americans are cornbread and biscuits, and the most popular vegetables are greens such as mustard, collard, or kale. Vegetables are preferred cooked, rather than raw, with some type of fat, such as salt pork, fatback, and bacon or fat meat. Salt pork is a key ingredient in the diet of many African Americans. Salt pork is inexpensive and, therefore, more frequently purchased.

Infant feeding methods may vary among African Americans. African American parents may be encouraged by their elders to begin feeding solid foods, such as cereal, at an early age (usually before 2 months). The cereal is mixed with the formula and given to the infant in a bottle. African Americans believe that giving only formula is starving the baby and that the infant needs "real food" to sleep through the night. Health-care practitioners working with family planning and child-care clinics can pro-

vide knowledge regarding the potential harmful effects of giving infants solid foods at an early age.

DIETARY PRACTICES FOR HEALTH PROMOTION

Some African Americans believe that a healthy person is one who has a good appetite. Foods such as milk, vegetables, and meat are referred to as *strength foods*. In the African American community, individuals who are at an ideal body weight are commonly viewed as "not having enough meat on their bones" and, therefore, unhealthy. African Americans believe that it is important to carry additional weight in order to be able to afford to lose weight during times of sickness. Therefore, being slightly overweight is seen as a sign of good health.

One common belief among Southern African Americans is the concept of "high blood" and "low blood." The healthy state is when the blood is in balance; not too high nor too low. High blood is viewed as more serious than low blood. High blood is often interchanged with high blood pressure. High blood is believed to be a condition in which the blood expands in volume or moves higher in the body, usually to the head. Some African Americans believe that rich foods or foods red in color, especially red meat, are considered the primary cause of high blood. Some African Americans believe that the treatment of high blood is to drink vinegar or eat pickles to "thin" the blood. Garlic is also seen as a health food. Garlic water is consumed to treat hypertension as well as hyperlipidemia in the African American population. In contrast, low blood is believed to be caused by eating too many acidic foods. Low blood is believed to be the cause of anemia. Treatment is aimed at trying to thicken the blood by eating rich foods and red meats. Another treatment for anemia, as well as for malnutrition, is to drink "pot liquor," the liquid that remains after a pot of greens has been cooked.

NUTRITIONAL DEFICIENCIES AND FOOD LIMITATIONS

The calcium consumption in African American women is particularly low. Williams (2005) cites that older African Americans' diets are also extremely low in calcium. The National Health and Nutrition Examination Surveys (NHANES II) reported that the intake levels for African American women 55 to 74 years of age were 460/mg, the lowest among all age and ethnic groups (Williams, 2005, p. 89). One factor that may explain the low calcium intake among African Americans is the lack of awareness of the health risks associated with this deficiency. Another factor is the high level of lactose intolerance in this population. Lactose intolerance occurs in 75 percent of the African American population. Low levels of thiamine, riboflavin, vitamins A and C, and iron are noted among African Americans and are mostly associated with a poor diet secondary to a low socioeconomic status.

Many African Americans are Protestant and have no specific food restrictions. However, a significant number of African Americans are members of religious groups who have dietary restrictions. These may include Seventh-Day Adventists, Muslims, and Jehovah's Witnesses. For example, a Muslim *halal* diet forbids pork or pork products. Muslims also refuse pork-based insulin. They consider these products to be filthy. In addition, some African Americans, especially those from Jamaica and other parts of the Caribbean, may be Rastafarians. Their religious beliefs mandate that they follow a clear dietary restriction, which includes eating fresh foods of vegetable origin and avoiding meat, salt, and alcohol. The health-care provider must always ask about any religious or cultural prohibitions on types of food consumed.

Pregnancy and Childbearing Practices

FERTILITY PRACTICES AND VIEWS TOWARD PREGNANCY

Historically, African American families have been large, especially in rural areas. A large family was viewed as an economic necessity, and African American parents depended on their children to support them when they could no longer work. However, as families moved to cities, they soon found that large families could become an economic burden. To some extent, this shifted attention to family planning.

Although oral contraceptives may be the most popular choice of birth control among African Americans who use birth control, religious beliefs also play a role in choices made. For example, African American Catholics may choose the rhythm method over other forms of birth control. African American communities also hold many views on the issue of pregnancy versus abortion. Many African Americans who oppose abortion do so because of religious or moral beliefs. Others oppose abortion because of moral, cultural, or Afrocentric beliefs. Such beliefs may cause a delay in making a decision so that having an abortion is no longer safe.

PRESCRIPTIVE, RESTRICTIVE, AND TABOO PRACTICES IN THE CHILDBEARING FAMILY

African American women usually respond to pregnancy in the same manner as women in other ethnic groups, based on their satisfaction with self, economic status, and career goals. The elders in the family provide advice and counseling about what should and should not be done during pregnancy. The African American family network guides many of the practices and beliefs of the pregnant woman, including *pica*.

Pica is the eating of nonnutritive substances such as clay, dirt (*geophagia*), sand, laundry starch, burnt matches, plastic, paint chips and plaster, light bulbs, needles, coffee grounds, and string. Women have reported that these items reduce nausea and cause an easy birth. One theory of geophagia is that this natural craving alleviates several mineral deficiencies and that the unborn child "needs" this supplement. However, geophagia can lead to a potassium deficiency, constipation, and anemia. Although it is a common practice among many African Americans, independent of socioeconomic or educational level, some are unaware that the practice exists.

Certain practices are believed to be taboo during pregnancy. For example, some African Americans believe that pregnant women should not take pictures because it may cause a stillbirth; nor should they have their picture taken because it captures their soul. Some also believe that it is not wise to reach over their heads if they are pregnant because the umbilical cord will wrap around the baby's neck. Another taboo concerns the purchase of clothing for the infant. It is thought to be bad luck to purchase clothes for the unborn baby.

Many African American women expect to experience cravings during pregnancy. Several beliefs related to the failure to satisfy this food craving exist. Some African Americans claim that if the mother does not consume the specific food craving, the child can be birth-marked, or more seriously, it can result in a stillbirth. Caribbean food beliefs during pregnancy focus on pregnancy outcomes and eating specific food groups. For example, consuming milk, eggs, tomatoes, and green vegetables is believed to result in a large baby; whereas drinking too many liquids will drown the baby.

Snow (1993) reported several home practices related to initiating labor in pregnant African American women. Taking a ride over a bumpy road, ingesting castor oil, eating a heavy meal, or sniffing pepper are all thought to induce labor. If a baby is born with the amniotic sac (referred to as a "veil") over its head or face, the neonate is thought to have special powers. In addition, certain children are thought to have received special powers from God: those born after a set of twins, those born with a physical problem or disability, or a child who is the seventh son in a family.

The postpartum period for the African American woman can be greatly extended. Some believe that during the postpartum period, the mother is at greater risk than the baby. She is cautioned to avoid cold air and is encouraged to get adequate rest to restore the body to normal. Postpartum practices for child care can involve the use of a bellyband or a coin. These objects, when placed on top of the infant's umbilical area, are believed to prevent the umbilical area from protruding outward.

Death Rituals

VIGNETTE 3.5

Mr. Grant, an 84-year-old African American, has been diagnosed with end-stage renal failure. His health has drastically failed during the past 3 days, and all clinical parameters confirm that death is imminent. Mr. Grant is not conscious, and the family is making the decisions for his end-of-life care. Mr. Grant's daughter, Grace, has medical power of attorney. Despite Mr. Grant's acute clinical condition, family members insist that "everything" must be done to keep him alive. Grace refuses to give permission for a "do not resuscitate" (DNR) order and is offended that doctors and staff would even discuss such a topic. Family members continue to be at his bedside praying and tell you "God answers prayers and will heal him."

1. What are some of the important cultural factors that must be considered in caring for Mr. Grant?
2. How would you incorporate culturally relevant interventions in responding to the family's needs to keep Mr. Grant alive at any cost?

DEATH RITUALS AND EXPECTATIONS

Death rituals for African Americans may vary owing to the diversity in their religious affiliations, geographic location, educational level, and socioeconomic background. African Americans are very family-oriented, and it is important that family members and extended family stay at the bedside of the dying patient in the hospital. They desire to hold on to their loved ones for as long as possible, and as a result may avoid signing Do Not Resuscitate (DNR) orders or making preparations for death (Lobar, Youngblut, & Brooten, 2006, p. 47). Lobar et al. (2006) conducted a qualitative study regarding cross-cultural beliefs, ceremonies, and rituals surrounding death of a loved one and found that African American participants described the importance of giving their loved one a "big send off." This practice involved elaborate financial decisions concerning the type of coffin to buy and the vehicle for carrying the coffin.

Johnson, Elbert-Avila, and Tulsky (2005, p. 711) maintained that spirituality is an important part of African American culture and is often the rationale for more aggressive treatment preferences of some African Americans at the end of life. Specifically, Americans are more likely to prefer life-sustaining treatments than do other ethnic groups (Fairrow, McCallum, & Messinger-Rapport, 2004; Welch, Teno, & Mor, 2005). African Americans do not believe in rushing to bury the deceased. Therefore, it is common to see the burial service held 5 to 7 days after death. Allowing time for relatives who live far away to attend the funeral services is important. Visual display of the body is also important. Southern and rural blacks observe the custom of having the corpse remain at the house the evening before the funeral (Lobar et al., 2006). This practice allows the extended family time to "pay respect" to their deceased loved one.

African Americans believe that the body must be kept intact after death. For example, it is common to hear an African American say, "I came into this world with all my body parts, and I'll leave this world with all my body parts!" Based on this belief, African Americans are less likely to donate organs or consent to an autopsy. Health-care practitioners must be aware that talking about organ donation may be considered an insult to the family.

For most African Americans, death does not end the connection among people, especially family. They believe the deceased is in God's hand and they will be reunited in heaven after death. Relatives communicating with the deceased's spirit is one example of this endless connection. Snow (1993) studied African American families in the southern United States and noted interesting rituals regarding spirits of the deceased. For example, if one passes an infant over the casket of the deceased who has died a sudden or violent death, this protects the infant from the deceased's "haunting spirits."

RESPONSES TO DEATH AND GRIEF

Grieving and death rituals of African Americans are often influenced by religion. Descendants from the Caribbean may practice a blend of Catholicism and African religion

known as *Voudoun,* and spelled alternately as *Voodoo, Vodoun,* and *Vodun.* The name has its roots in an ancient African Yoruban word for "spirit." Some African Americans believe in "voodoo death," which is a belief that illness or death may come to an individual via a supernatural force (Campinha-Bacote, 1992). Voodoo is more commonly known as "root work," "hex," "fix," "conjuring," "tricking," "mojo," "witchcraft," "spell," "black magic," or "hoodoo."

One response to hearing about a death of a family member or close member in the African American culture is "falling out," which is manifested by sudden collapse, paralysis, and the inability to see or speak. However, the individual's hearing and understanding remain intact. Health-care practitioners must understand the African American culture to recognize this condition as a cultural response to the death of a family member or other severe emotional shock and not as a medical condition requiring emergency intervention. Some African Americans are less likely to express grief openly and publicly. However, they do express their feelings openly during the funeral. Funeral services encourage emotional expression, such as crying, screaming, and wailing.

Waters (2000) conducted a research study examining end-of-life directives among African Americans. Findings suggest that African Americans are less likely to know about or complete advance directives. This is attributed, in part, to the fact that end-of-life decisions are usually made by the family. African Americans may also hold mistrust of health-care systems regarding advanced directives and end-of-life care as a family and, therefore, may be less likely to complete advanced directives. Implications of these findings suggest a need for culturally relevant discussion and education in the African American community regarding advance directives.

Spirituality

VIGNETTE 3.6

Dr. Patricia Waits, a 54-year-old African American, presents for a routine physical examination. During the breast examination, the health-care practitioner palpates a suspicious lump in Dr. Waits' right breast. When questioned, she shares with the health-care practitioner that she does not do regular *breast* self-examinations and has had one mammogram, about 4 years ago, which was "fine." She is reluctant to get the suggested mammogram and tells the health-care-practitioner that she needs to pray for healing before she even thinks about further testing.

1. What role does spirituality play in caring for Dr. Waits?
2. How do you provide patient education about the incidence of breast cancer among African Americans in a culturally sensitive manner?

DOMINANT RELIGION AND USE OF PRAYER

Religion and religious behavior is an integral part of the African American community (Fig. 3–1). African American

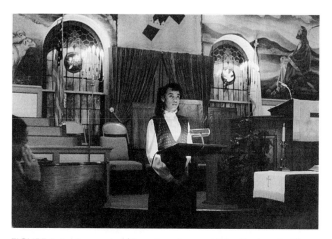

FIGURE 3–1   For many African Americans, spirituality is a significant force for promoting well-being.

churches have played a major role in the development and survival of African Americans. As eloquently stated by Lincoln (1974, pp. 115–116):

> To understand the power of the black Church, it must first be understood that there is no disjunction between the black Church and the black community . . . whether one is a church member or not is beside the point in any assessment of the importance and meaning of the black Church.

African Americans take their religion seriously, and they expect to receive a message in preaching that helps them in their daily lives. Brown and Gary (1994) found that religious involvement is associated with positive mental health. Furthermore, most African Americans expect to take an active part in religious activities. In reviewing the literature, Johnson et al. (2005, p. 712) found that African Americans "participate more often in organizational (attendance at religious services) and nonorganizational (prayer or religious study) religious activities and endure higher levels of intrinsic religiosity (personal religious commitment) than do Caucasians."

Most African American Christians are affiliated with the Baptist and Methodist denominations. However, many other denominations and distinct religious groups are represented in African American communities within the United States. These include African Methodist, Episcopalian, Jehovah's Witnesses, Church of God in Christ, Seventh-Day Adventists, Pentecostal, Apostolic, Presbyterian, Lutheran, Roman Catholic, Nation of Islam, and other Islamic sects (Boyd-Franklin, 1989).

African Americans strongly believe in the use of prayer for all situations they may encounter. They also pray for the sake of others who are experiencing problems. "Prayers reflect the trust and faith one has in God" (Roberson, 1985, p. 106). African Americans also believe in the laying on of hands while praying. The belief is that certain individuals have the power to heal the sick by placing hands on them. African Americans may pray in a language that is not understood by anyone but the person reciting the prayer. This expression of prayer is referred to as *speaking in tongues*.

MEANING OF LIFE AND INDIVIDUAL SOURCES OF STRENGTH

Most African Americans' inner strength comes from trusting in God and maintaining a biblical worldview of health and illness. Some African Americans believe that whatever happens is "God's will." Because of this belief, African Americans may be perceived to have a fatalistic view of life. For example, Snow (1993) reported that African Americans trust in "Doctor Jesus," and some believe that sickness and pain are forms of weakness that come directly from Satan. Therefore, for African Americans, having faith in God is a major source of inner strength. Frameworks such as Campinha-Bacote's (2005) Biblically Based Model of Cultural Competence in the Delivery of Healthcare Services can provide health-care practitioners with strategies for implementing culturally specific interventions for African Americans who share a biblical worldview of health and illness.

SPIRITUAL BELIEFS AND HEALTH-CARE PRACTICES

Spiritual beliefs strongly direct many African Americans as they cope with illness and the end of life. In a review of the literature on spiritual beliefs and practices of African Americans, Johnson et al. (2005, p. 711) noted the following recurrent themes; "spiritual beliefs and practices are a source of comfort, coping, and support and are the most effective way to influence healing; God is responsible for physical and spiritual health; and the doctor is God's instrument." African Americans consider themselves spiritual beings, and God is thought to be the supreme healer. Health-care practices center on religious and spiritual activities such as going to church, praying daily, laying on of hands, and speaking in tongues. Drayton-Brooks and White (2004) conducted a qualitative study to explore health-promoting behaviors among African American women with faith-based support. They concluded that "health beliefs, attitudes, and behaviors are not developed outside of social systems; therefore, the facilitation of healthy lifestyle behaviors may be best addressed and influenced within a context of reciprocal social interaction such as a church" (p. 84).

As health-care practitioners develop culturally specific interventions for African Americans, it is important to understand that the church community can serve as a viable support system in developing health-promoting behaviors. Underwood and Powell (2006) further added that considerable improvements can occur in the health status of African Americans if health education and outreach efforts are presented and promoted through religious, spiritual and faith-based efforts (p. 20). Musgrave, Allen, and Allen (2002) cautioned public health not to "use" faith communities or the spirituality of individuals to its own end. Instead, there must be a partnership between public health and faith communities in which the central undertaking of faith is respected.

Health-Care Practices

VIGNETTE 3.7

Ms. Barrett, a 72-year-old female of Haitian descent, lives alone in the inner city of New York. She works as a housekeeper and receives minimum wages. She has difficulty making most of her clinic appointments and has missed the past two scheduled appointments. She has a history of hypertension, which has not been successfully controlled during the past year. She has been given several types of educational resources for managing her hypertension, including brochures, books, and Internet resources. When you speak with Ms. Barrett, she appears to be very angry as well as very defensive in responding to questions regarding the management of her hypertension. She makes such remarks as, "You people really don't care about me!" and "None of these medications even work!"

1. What are some of the cultural responses to health and illness of Ms. Barrett that may have an impact on uncontrolled hypertension?
2. What are some of the barriers that Ms. Barrett may experience in receiving adequate health-care services to address her hypertension?

HEALTH-SEEKING BELIEFS AND BEHAVIORS

According to Snow (1974), many African Americans are pessimistic about human relationships and believe that it is more natural to do evil than to do good. Snow concluded that some African Americans' belief systems emphasize three major themes:

1. The world is a very hostile and dangerous place to live.
2. The individual is open to attack from external forces.
3. The individual is considered to be a helpless person who has no internal resources to combat such an attack and, therefore, needs outside assistance.

Because most African Americans tend to be suspicious of health-care professionals, they may see a physician or nurse only when absolutely necessary. Some older African Americans continue to use the *Farmers' Almanac* to choose what are thought to be good times for medical and dental procedures.

Some African Americans, particularly those of Haitian background, may believe in sympathetic magic. *Sympathetic magic* assumes everything is interconnected and includes the practice of imitative and contagious magic. *Contagious magic* is the belief that once an entity is physically connected to another, it can never be separated; what one does to a specific part, they also do to the whole. This type of belief is seen in the practice of voodoo. An individual will take a piece of the victim's hair or fingernail and place a hex, which they believe will cause the person to become ill (voodoo illness). *Imitative magic* is the belief that "like follows like" (Campinha-Bacote, 1992). For example, a pregnant woman may sleep with a knife under her pillow to "cut" the pains of labor. Another example is the use of a doll or a picture of an individual to inflict harm on that person. Whatever harm is done to the picture is also simultaneously done to the person.

RESPONSIBILITY FOR HEALTH CARE

The African American population believes in natural and unnatural illnesses. *Natural illness* occurs in response to normal forces from which individuals have not protected themselves. *Unnatural illness* is the belief that harm or sickness can come to you via a person or spirit. In treating an unnatural illness, African Americans seek clergy or a folk healer or pray directly to God. In general, health is viewed as harmony with nature, whereas illness is seen as a disruption in this harmonic state owing to demons, "bad spirits," or both.

African Americans may use home remedies to maintain their health and treat specific health conditions as well as seek health care from Western health-care practitioners. When taking prescribed medications, African Americans commonly take the medications differently from the way prescribed. For example, in treating hypertension, African Americans may take their antihypertensive medication on an "as-needed" basis. To provide services that are effective and culturally acceptable to African Americans, health-care practitioners must conduct thorough cultural assessments and become partners with the African American community. Strategies such as focus groups can provide health-care practitioners with insight into health-care practices acceptable to African Americans.

FOLK AND TRADITIONAL PRACTICES

African Americans, like most ethnic groups, engage in folk medicine. The history of African American folk medicine has its origin in slavery. Slaves had a limited range of choices in obtaining health care. Although they were expected to inform their masters immediately when they were ill, slaves were reluctant to submit themselves to the harsh prescriptions and treatments of 18th- and 19th-century European American physicians (Savitt, 1978). They preferred self-treatment or treatment by friends, older relatives, or "folk doctors." This led to a dual system: "white medicine" and "black medicine" (Savitt, 1978). Snow (1993) studied hundreds of folk practices used by African Americans. One example is the belief that drinking a glass half-filled with an alcoholic beverage and half-filled with fish blood can cure alcoholism. This is believed to give an undesirable taste and cause nausea and vomiting when subsequent alcoholic drinks are taken.

BARRIERS TO HEALTH CARE

Healthy People 2010 defined health literacy as "the degree to which individuals have the capacity to obtain, process, and understand basic health information and services needed to make appropriate health decisions" (U.S. Department of Health and Human Services, 2002). Research shows that health literacy is the single best predictor of health status. Low health literacy affects older people, immigrants, the impoverished, and minorities.

Low health literacy affects 40 percent of African Americans and is considered a barrier to receiving optimal health care. Low health literacy is also driven by poor patient-provider communication. Health-care practitioners can reduce low health literacy by limiting the amount of information provided at each visit, avoiding medical jargon, using pictures or models to explain important health concepts, assuring understanding with the "show-me" technique, and encouraging patients to ask questions.

Negative attitudes from health-care professionals can greatly affect African Americans decision to seek medical attention (McNeil, Campinha-Bacote, Tapscott, & Vample, 2002). McNeil et al. (2002) maintained that the attitude of the health-care practitioner is one of the most significant barriers to the care of African Americans (p. 132). One study reported that 12 percent of African Americans, compared with 1 percent of whites, felt that health-care practitioners treated them unfairly or disrespectfully because of their race (Kaiser Family Foundation, 2001).

Some African Americans may experience economic and geographic barriers to health-care services. Needed health-care services may not be accessible or affordable for African Americans in lower socioeconomic groups. Although some services may be available, accessible, and affordable for other African Americans, they may not be culturally relevant. For example, a health-care practitioner may prescribe a strict American Diabetic Association diet to a newly diagnosed diabetic African American client without taking into consideration this person's dietary habits. Therefore, therapeutic interventions developed by health-care practitioners may be underused or ignored.

Underrepresentation of ethnic minority health-care practitioners is an additional barrier to health care for many minorities. In the absence of adequate representation, minority populations are less likely to access and use health-care services. Research investigated doctor-patient race concordance and its impact in predicting greater health-care utilization and satisfaction among minorities (LaVeist & Carroll, 2002; LaVeist & Nuru-Jeter, 2002). LaVeist and Nuru-Jeter (2002) found that patients who were race concordant with their physician reported greater satisfaction with their physician compared with respondents who were not race concordant. These authors concluded that there must be continuing efforts to increase the number of minority physicians, as well as improving the ability of physicians to interact with patients who are not of their own race. These findings are relevant for all health-care practitioners.

CULTURAL RESPONSES TO HEALTH AND ILLNESS

African Americans often perceive pain as a sign of illness or disease. Therefore, it is possible that if they are not experiencing severe and/or immediate pain, a regimen of regularly prescribed medicine may not be followed. For example, African Americans may take their antihypertensive drugs or diuretics only when they experience head or neck pain. This cultural practice interferes with successful and effective treatment of hypertension. In other cases, some African Americans believe, as part of their spiritual and religious foundation, that suffering and pain are inevitable and must be endured, thus contributing to their high tolerance levels for pain. Prayers and the laying on of hands are thought to free the person from all suffering and pain, and people who still experience pain are considered to have little faith.

In addition to religious beliefs, low educational levels among African Americans may limit their access to information about the etiology and treatment of mental illness. Some African Americans hold a stigma against mental illness. The high frequency of misdiagnosis among African Americans contributes to their reluctance to trust mental health professionals. For example, Adebimpe (1981) reported that over the years, a major diagnostic issue has been the high frequency of the diagnosis of schizophrenia among African American clients. Specifically, African Americans are more likely to report hallucinations when suffering from an affective disorder, which may lead to the misdiagnosis of schizophrenia.

Close family and spiritual ties within the African American family allow one to enter the sick role with ease. Extended and nuclear family members willingly care for sick individuals and assume their role responsibilities without hesitation. Sickness and tragedy bring African American families together, even in the presence of family conflict.

BLOOD TRANSFUSIONS AND ORGAN DONATION

Blood transfusions are generally accepted in the African American patient. However, some religious groups, such as Jehovah's Witnesses, do not permit this practice. In addition, Jehovah's Witnesses believe that any blood that leaves the body must be destroyed and, therefore, do not approve of an individual storing her or his own blood for a later autologous transfusion.

A low level of organ donation among African Americans has been cited (Plawecki & Plawecki, 1992). This reluctance is associated with a lack of information about organ donation, religious fears and beliefs, distrust of health-care practitioners, fear that organs will be taken before the patient is dead, and concern that proper medical attention will not be given to patients if they are organ donors. However, in regard to kidney donations, it must be noted that African Americans donate in proportion to their share of the population. African Americans, for example, represent about 13 percent of the population and account for 12 percent of kidney donors. It may appear that there is a low level of kidney donation among the African American community for they are disproportionately represented (35 percent) on the kidney waiting list. Their rate of organ donation does not keep pace with the number of those needing transplants. This increased need for organ donors led the Congress of National Black Churches to make organ and tissue donation a top-priority health issue.

Health-Care Practitioners

TRADITIONAL VERSUS BIOMEDICAL PRACTITIONERS

Physicians are recognized as heads of the health-care team, with nurses having lesser importance. However, as nurses are becoming more educated, African Americans are holding them in higher regard. Whereas some African Americans may prefer a health-care practitioner of the same gender for urological and gynecological conditions, generally gender is not a major concern in the selection of health-care practitioners. Men and women can provide personal care to the opposite sex. On occasion, young men may prefer that another man or an older women give personal care. With the current emphasis on women's health and the responses of women to illness and treatment regimens, some African American women prefer female primary-care practitioners. Health-care practitioners should respect these wishes when possible.

Among the African American community, traditional/folk practitioners can be spiritual leaders, grandparents, elders of the community, voodoo doctors, or priests. For example, the pastor in the African American church is noted to be "a healer of the sick" (Drayton-Brooks & White, 2004, p. 86).

STATUS OF HEALTH-CARE PROVIDERS

Western health-care providers do not generally regard folk practitioners with high esteem. However, as homeopathic and alternative medicine increases in importance in preventive health, these practitioners are gaining more recognition, respect, and utilization. Folk practitioners are respected and valued in the African American community and frequently used by African Americans of all socioeconomic levels. Many African Americans perceive health-care practitioners as outsiders, and they resent them for telling them what their problems are or telling them how to solve them (Underwood, 1994). Generally, most African Americans are suspicious and cautious of health-care practitioners they have not heard of or do not know. Because interpersonal relationships are highly valued in this group, it is important to initially focus on developing a sound, trusting relationship.

REFERENCES

Adebimpe, V. (1981). Overview: White norms in psychiatric diagnosis of black American patients. *American Journal of Psychiatry, 138*(3), 279–285.

Agency for Healthcare Research and Quality (AHRQ). (2005, December). *National Healthcare Disparities Report.* AHRQ Publication No. 06-0017. Retrieved September 25, 2006, from http://www.ahrq.gov/qual/nhdr05/nhdr05.pdf

Albers, C. (1999). *Sociology of families.* Thousand Oaks, CA: Pine Forge Press.

Allender, J., & Spradley, B. (2001). *Community health nursing: Concepts and practice.* Philadelphia: Lippincott.

America, Demographics, Inc. (1991). American diversity. What the 1990 Census reveals about population growth of blacks, Hispanics, Asians, ethnic diversity, and children—and what it means to you. *American Demographics Desk Reference Series, No.1.*

American Academy of Pediatrics. (1998). Screening for elevated blood levels. *Pediatrics, 101*(6), 1072–1078.

American Public Health Association. (1999). More research needed to guide policy on environmental justice. *Nation's Health, 29*(3), 4.

American Public Health Association. (2004). *Disparities: Communities moving from statistics to solutions—Toolkit.* National Public Health Week, April 5–11, 2004. Washington, DC: Author. Retrieved September 20, 2006, from http://www.apha.org/legislative/legislative/disparities.htm#factsheets_disparities

The Asthma and Allergy Foundation of America and the National Pharmaceutical Council. (2006). *Ethnic disparities in the burden and treatment of asthma.* Washington, DC: Author. Retrieved September 25, 2006, from http://www.npcnow.org/resources/PDFs/AsthmaEthnicDis05.pdf

Baldwin, D. (1996). Model for describing low-income African-American women's participation in breast and cervical cancer early detection and screening. *Advances in Nursing Science 19*(2), 21–42.

Base-Smith, V., & Campinha-Bacote, J. (2003). The culture of obesity. *Journal of the National Black Nurses Association, 14*(1), 52–56.

Bender, D. (1998). *The family: Opposing viewpoints.* San Diego, CA: Greenhaven Press.

Bigler, R., & Averhart, C. (2003). Race and the workforce: Occupational status, aspirations, and stereotyping among African American children. *Developmental Psychology, 39*(3), 572–580.

Billingsley, A. (1968). *Black families in White America.* Upper Saddle River, NJ: Prentice Hall.

Bland-Stewart, L. (2005). Difference or deficit in speakers of African American English. What every clinician should know. *ASHA Leader, 10*(6), 6–7, 30–31.

Blum, J., Morgan, E., Rose, W., Schlesinger, A., Stampp, K., & Woodward, C. (1981). *The national experience.* New York: Harcourt Brace Jovanovich.

Boyd-Franklin, N. (1989). *Black families in therapy.* New York: Guilford Press.

Braithwaite, R., Taylor, S., & Austin, J. (2000). *Building health coalitions in the black community.* Thousand Oaks, CA: Sage Publications.

Brewster, L., van Montfrans, G., & Kleijnen, J. (2005). Systematic review: Antihypertensive drug therapy in Black patients. *Annals of Internal Medicine, 14*(18), 614–627.

Brown, D., & Gary, L. (1994). Religious involvement and health status among African-American males. *Journal of the National Medical Association, 86*(11), 825–831.

Brownstein, R. (1995, November 6). Why are so many black men in jail? Numbers in debate equal a paradox. *Los Angeles Times,* p. A5.

Burroughs, V., Mackey, M., & Levy, R. (2002). Racial and ethnic differences in response to medicines: Towards individualized pharmaceutical treatment. *Journal of the National Medical Association, 94*(10), 1–20.

Campinha-Bacote, J. (1991). Community mental health services for the underserved: A culturally specific model. *Archives of Psychiatric Nursing, 5*(4), 29–35.

Campinha-Bacote, J. (1992). Voodoo illness. *Perspectives in Psychiatric Nursing, 28*(1), 11–19.

Campinha-Bacote, J. (1993). Soul therapy: Humor and music with African American clients. *Journal of Christian Nursing, 10*(2), 23–26.

Campinha-Bacote, J. (1997). Humor therapy for culturally diverse psychiatric patients. *Journal of Nursing Jocularity, 7*(1), 38–40.

Campinha-Bacote, J. (2005). *A biblically based model of cultural competence in the delivery of healthcare services.* Cincinnati, OH: Transcultural C.A.R.E. Associates.

Clark, M. J. (1999). *Nursing in the community: Dimensions of community health nursing.* Stamford, CT: Appleton & Lange.

Cokley, K., Cooke, B., & Nobles, W. (2005, September 29). *Guidelines for providing culturally appropriate services for people of African ancestry exposed to the trauma of Hurricane Katrina.* Washington, DC: The Association of Black Psychologists. Retrieved September 23, 2006, from http://www.abpsi.org/special/hurricane-info1.htm

Conant, J. (1961). *Slums and suburbs.* New York, NY: New American Library Publishers.

DelBello, M., Soutullo, C., Ochsner, J., McElroy, J., Keck, P., Strakowski, S., et al. (1999, May 18). Racial differences in the treatment of adolescents with bipolar disorder, *New Research 379.* Presented at the 152nd annual meeting of the American Psychiatric Association. Washington, DC.

Dirks, N., Huth, B., Yates C., & Melbohm, B. (2004). Pharmacokinetics of immunosuppressants: A perspective on ethnic difference. *International Journal of Clinical Pharmacology and Therapeutics, 42*(12), 719–723.

Drayton-Brooks, S., & White, N. (2004). Health promoting behaviors among African American women with faith-based support. *The ABNF Journal, 15*(5), 84–90.

Edleman, C., & Mandel, C. (1998). *Health promotion throughout the lifespan* (3rd ed.). St. Louis, MO: C. V. Mosby.

Fairrow, A., McCallum, T., & Messinger-Rapport, B. (2004). Preferences of older African-Americans for long-term tube feeding at end of life. *Aging & Mental Health, 8*(6), 530–534.

Ferdinand, K. (2006). The isosorbide-hydralazine story: Is there a case for race-based cardiovascular medicine? *The Journal of Clinical Hypertension, 8*(3), 156–158.

Frazier, E. (1957). *Black bourgeoisie.* New York: Collier Books.

Glazer, W. M., Morganstern, H., & Doucette, J. T. (1993). Predicting the long-term risk of tardive dyskinesia in outpatients maintained on neuroleptic medications. *Journal of Clinical Psychiatry, 54*(4), 133–139.

Heady, M. (1996, May 15). Holistic plan urged to aid black males. *Los Angeles Times*, p. A12.

Herrera, J., Lawson, W., & Sramek, J. (1999). *Cross-cultural psychiatry*. New York: John Wiley & Sons.

Hill, R. (1997, July 7). Sociologist taught strength of black family. *Baltimore Sun Times*, p. 2B.

Institute of Medicine (IOM). (2004). *In the nation's compelling interest: Ensuring diversity in the health care workforce*. Washington, DC: Author.

Jaynes, D., & Williams, R. (1989). *A common destiny: Blacks and American society*. Washington, DC: National Academy Press.

Johnson, K., Elbert-Avila, K., & Tulsky, J. (2005). The influence of spiritual beliefs and practices on the treatment preferences of African Americans: A review of the literature. *Journal of the American Geriatrics Society, 53*(4), 711–719.

Kaiser Family Foundation. (2001). *African Americans view of the HIV/AIDS epidemic at 20 years*. Menlo Park, CA: Author.

Ladner, J., & Gourdine, R. (1992). Adolescent pregnancy in the African-American community. In R. Braithwaite & S. Taylor (Eds.), *Health issues in the black community* (pp. 206–221). San Francisco, CA: Josey-Bass.

LaVeist, T., & Carroll, T. (2002). Race of physician and satisfaction with care among African American patients. *The Journal of the National Medical Association, 94*(11), 937–943.

LaVeist, T., & Nuru-Jeter, A. (2002). Is doctor-patient concordance associated with greater satisfaction with care? *Journal of Health and Social Behavior, 43*(3), 296–306.

Lawson, W. (1999, May 19). *Ethnicity and treatment of bipolar disorder*. Presented at the 152nd annual meeting of the American Psychiatric Association. Washington, DC.

Levy, R. (1993). Ethnic and racial differences in response to medicines: Preserving individualized therapy in managed pharmaceutical programmes. *Pharmaceutical Medicine, 7*, 139–165.

Lincoln, C. (1974). *The black church since Frazier*. New York: Schocken Books.

Lobar, S., Youngblut, J., & Brooten, D. (2006). Cross-cultural beliefs, ceremonies, and rituals surrounding death of a loved one. *Pediatric Nursing, 32*(1), 44–55.

Louisiana Department of Health and Hospitals. (2001). *Louisiana Health Report Card*. New Orleans, LA: Louisiana Auxiliary Enterprises.

Low-wage labor market. (2006). Retrieved September 28, 2006, from http://aspe.hhs.gov/hsp/lwlm99/henly.htm

Lowenstein, A., & Glanville, C. L. (1995). Cultural diversity and conflict in the health care workplace. *Nursing Economics, 13*(4) 203–209.

March of Dimes. (2003). *March of Dimes data book for policy maker: Material, infant, and child health in the United States, 2003*. White Plains, NY: Author.

Matas, A., Sowa, M., Taylor, V., Taylor, G., Schattka, B., & Mantsch, H. (2001). Eliminating the issue of skin color in assessment of the blanch response. *Advances in Skin Wound Care,14*, 180–8.

McNeil, J., Campinha-Bacote, J., Tapscott, E., & Vample, G. (2002). *BESAFE: National minority AIDS education and training center cultural competency model*. Washington, DC: Howard University Medical School.

Michaels, D. (1993). Occupational cancer in the black population: The health effects of job discrimination. *Journal of the National Black Medical Association, 75*, 1014–1018.

Minorities get inferior care, even if insured. (2002, March 21). *New York Times*. Retrieved March 21, 2001, from http://www.nytimes.com

Moore, J. (2005). Hypertension: Catching the silent killer. *Nurse Practitioner, 30*(10), 16–18, 23–24, 26–27.

Morgan, P., Barnett, K., Perdue, B., Fogel, J., Underwood, S., Gaskins, M., & Brown-Davis, C. (2006). African American women with breast cancer and their spouses' perception of care received from physicians. *The ABNF Journal, 17*(1), 32–37.

Morrison, R., Wallenstein, S., Natale, D., Senzel, R., & Huang L. (2000). "We don't carry that"—failure of pharmacies in predominantly nonwhite neighborhoods to stock opioid analgesics. *New England Journal of Medicine, 342*:1023-1026

Murray, R., & Zentner, J. (2001). *Health promotion strategies through the lifespan*. Upper Saddle River, NJ: Prentice Hall.

Musgrave, C., Allen, C., & Allen, G. (2002). Rural health and women of color: Spirituality and health for women of color. *American Journal of Public Health, 92*(4), 557–560.

National Center for Health Statistics (NCHS). (1999). *Health US 1999, with socioeconomic status and health chartbook*. Hyattsville, MD: Author.

National Center for Health Statistics (NCHS). (2002). *Socioeconomic status and health chartbook*. Hyattsville, MD: U.S. Department of Human Services, Centers for Disease Control and Prevention, National Center for Health Statistics.

National Center for Health Statistics (NCHS). (2003). *Socioeconomic status and health chartbook*. Hyattsville, MD: U.S. Department of Human Services, Centers for Disease Control and Prevention, National Center for Health Statistics.

National Women's Health Report. (2005). African-American women & heart health. *National Women's Health Report, 27*(10), 6.

Navarro, V. (1997). Race or class versus race and class: Mortality differentials in the US. In P. R. Lee & C. L. Estes (Eds.), *The nation's health* (pp. 32–36). Sudbury, MA: Jones & Barlett.

Plawecki, H., & Plawecki, J. (1992). Improving organ donation rates in the black community. *Journal of Holistic Nursing, 10*(1), 34–46.

Rickford, J. (1999). The Ebonics controversy in my backyard: A sociologist's experiences and reflections. *Journal of Sociolinguistics, 3*(2), 267.

Roberson, M. (1985). The influence of religious beliefs on health choices of Afro-Americans. *Topics in Clinical Nursing, 7*(3), 57–63.

Salcido, S. (2002). Finding a window into the skin. *Advances in Skin and Wound Care, 15*(3), 100.

Saunders, E. (1997). High blood pressure: A call to action for African-Americans. *Baltimore Sun*, p. A3.

Savitt, T. (1978). *Medicine and slavery*. Chicago: University of Illinois Press.

Schaeffeler, E., Eichelbaum, M., Brinkmann, U., Penger, A., Asante-Poku, S., Zanger, U., & Schwab, M. (2001, August 4). Frequency of C3435T polymorphism of gene in African people. *The Lancet, 358*(9279), 383–384.

Schwartz, R. (2001). Racial profiling in medical research. *New England Journal of Medicine, 344*, 1392–1393.

Smedley, B., Stith, A., & Nelson, A. (2002). Unequal treatment: Confronting racial and ethnic disparities in healthcare. Washington, DC: National Academy Press.

Snow, L. (1974). Folk medical beliefs and their implications for care of patients. *Annals of Internal Medicine, 81*, 82–96.

Snow, L. (1993). *Walkin' over medicine*. Boulder, CO: Westview Press.

Sowa, M., Matas, A., Schattka, B., & Mantsch, H. (2002). Spectroscopic assessment of cutaneous hemodynamics in the presence of high epidermal melanin concentration. *Clinica Chimica Acta, 317*, 203–212.

Sowers, J., Ferdinand, K., Bakris, G., & Douglas, J. (2002). Hypertension-related disease in African Americans. *Postgraduate Medicine, 112*(4). Retrieved September 21, 2006, from http://www.postgradmed.com/issues/2002/10_02/sowers1.hn

Spurlock, W., & Cullins, L. (2006). Cancer fatalism and breast cancer screening in African American women. *The ABNF Journal, 17*(10), 38–43.

Strakowski, S., McElroy, S., Keck P., & West, S. (1996). Racial influence on diagnosis in psychotic mania. *Journal of Affect Disorders, 39*(2), 157–162.

Strickland, T. I., Lin, K. M., Fu, P., Anderson, D., & Zheng, Y. (1995). Comparison of lithium ratio between African-American and Caucasian bipolar patients. *Biological Psychiatry, 37*(5), 325–330.

Strickland, T. L., Ranganath, V., Lin, K. M., Poland, R. E., Mendoza, R., & Smith, M. W. (1991). Psychopharmacologic considerations in the treatment of black American populations. *Psychopharmacology Bulletin, 27*(4), 441–448.

Sullivan, L. (2004). *Missing persons: Minorities in the health professions: A report of the Sullivan Commission on diversity in the healthcare workforce*. Battle Creek, MI: W. K. Kellogg Foundation.

Taulbert, C. (1969). *Once upon a time when we were colored*. Tulsa, OK: Counsel Oak Books.

Thompson, C., Craig, H., & Washington, J. (2004). Variable production of African American English across oral and literary contexts. *Language, Speech, and Hearing in Schools, 35*(3), 269–282.

Underwood, S. (1994). Increasing the participation of minorities and other at-risk groups in clinical trials. *Innovations in Oncology Nursing, 10*(4), 106.

Underwood, S., Buseh, A., Canales, M., Powe, B., Dockery, B, Kather, T., & Kent, N. (2005). Nursing contributions to the elimination of health disparities among African Americans: Review and critique of a decade of research (part II). *Journal of National Black Nurses Association, 16*(10), 31–47.

Underwood, S., & Powell, R. (2006). Religion and spirituality: Influence on health/risk behavior and cancer screening behavior of African Americans. *The ABNF Journal, 17*(10), 20–31.

U.S. Department of Commerce, Bureau of the Census. (1993). *We the American blacks*. Washington, DC: U.S. Government Printing Office.

U.S. Department of Commerce, Bureau of the Census. (2006). www.census.gov.

U.S. Department of Health and Human Services. (1997). *Healthy people 2010: National health promotion and disease prevention objectives.* Washington, DC: Author.

U.S. Department of Health and Human Services. (2002). *Healthy people 2010: Understanding and improving health* (2nd ed.). Washington, DC: Author.

Waters, C. (2000). End-of-life directives among African Americans: A need for community-centered discussion and education. *Journal of Community Health Nursing, 17*(1), 25–37.

Watts, R. (2003, January). Race consciousness and the health of African Americans. *Online Journal of Nursing, 8*(1), Manuscript 3. Retrieved September 22, 2006, from http://nursingworld.org/ojin/topic20_3.htm.

Welch, L., Teno, J., & Mor, V. (2005). End-of-life care in black and white: Race matters for medical care of dying patients and their families. *Journal of the American Geriatrics Society, 53*(7), 11154–11161.

Williams, B. (2005). Older African Americans and calcium-deficient diets: What rehabilitation specialists need to know. *Topic in Geriatric Rehabilitation, 21*(1), 88–92.

Davis*Plus*

For case studies, review questions, and additional information, go to http://davisplus.fadavis.com.

Chapter *4*

The Amish

ANNA FRANCES Z. WENGER and MARION R. WENGER

Overview, Inhabited Localities, and Topography

OVERVIEW

As dusk gathers on the hospital parking lot, a man first ties his horse to the hitching rack and then helps a matronly figure wrapped in a shawl as dark as his own greatcoat down from the carriage. On their mother's heels, a flurry of children dressed like undersized replicas of their parents turn their wide eyes toward the fluorescent-lit glass façade of the reception area, a glimmering beacon from the world of high-technology health care. Their excitement is muted by their father's soft-spoken rebuke in a language more akin to German than English, and in a hush, the Amish family crosses a cultural threshold—into the workaday world of health-care professionals.

This Amish family appears to come from another time and place. Those familiar with the health-care needs of the Amish know the profound cultural distance they have bridged in seeking professional help. Others, only marginally acquainted with Amish ways, may ask why this group dresses, acts, and talks like visitors to the North American cultural landscape of the 21st century. Amish are "different" by intention and by conviction. That is to say, for most of the ways in which they depart from the norm for contemporary American culture, they cite a reason related to their understanding of the biblical mandate to live a life separated from a world they see as unregenerate or sinful.

As noted in the primary and secondary characteristics of culture in the introduction to cultural diversity in Chapter 1, dissimilar appearance, behavior, or both may signal deeper underlying differences in the Amish culture.

Noting these differences does not, of necessity, lead to better acceptance or deeper understanding of attitudes and behaviors. Appearances can be misleading. For example, the Amish family's arrival at the hospital by horse and carriage might suggest a general taboo against modern technological conveniences. In fact, most Amish homes are not furnished with electric and electronic labor-saving devices and appliances. But that does not preclude the Amish's openness to using state-of-the-art medical technology if it is perceived as necessary to promoting their health.

This minority group's exotic features of dress and language may disguise true motivations regarding health-seeking behaviors, which they share in common with the larger, or majority, culture. To enable such clients to attain their own standard of health and well-being, health-care professionals need to look beyond the superficial appearance and to listen more carefully to the cues they provide.

HERITAGE AND RESIDENCE

It is as important to locate the Amish topographically according to cultural and religious coordinates as well as to the geographical areas they inhabit. The hospital visit scene just portrayed could have taken place in any one of a number of towns spanning the American Midwest from the eastern seaboard, but the basic circumstances surrounding the interaction with professional caregivers and the cultural assumptions underlying it are basically similar. For the Amish, seeking help from health-care professionals requires them to go outside their own people and, in so doing, to cross over a significant "permeable boundary" that delimits their community in cultural-geographic terms.

Today's Amish live in rural areas in a band of over 20 states stretching westward from Pennsylvania, Ohio, and Indiana as far as Montana, with some scattered **settlements** as far south as Florida and as far north as the province of Ontario, Canada (Huntington, 2001). About 75 percent of their estimated total population of over 175,000 is concentrated in Pennsylvania, Ohio, and Indiana (Kraybill & Hostetter, 2001; C.N. Hostetter, personal communication, January 5, 2007). The **Old Order Amish**, so-called for their strict observance of traditional ways that distinguishes them from other, more progressive "plain folk," are the largest and most notable group among the Amish. As such, they constitute an ethnoreligious cultural group in modern America with roots in Reformation-era Europe.

REASONS FOR MIGRATION AND ASSOCIATED ECONOMIC FACTORS

The Amish emerged after 1693 as a variant of one stream of the **Anabaptist** movement that originated in Switzerland in 1525 and spread to neighboring German-speaking lands. The Amish embraced, among other essential Anabaptist tenets of faith, the baptism of adult believers as an outward sign of membership in a voluntary community with an inner commitment to live peaceably with all. The Amish parted ways with the larger Anabaptist group, now known as *Mennonites*, over the Amish propensity to strictly avoid community members whom they excluded from fellowship in their church (Hostetler, 1993). The *Amish* name is derived from the surname of Jacob Ammann, a 17th-century Anabaptist who led the Amish division from the Anabaptists in 1693 (Hüppi, 2000). Similarly, the name *Mennonite* is derived from the given name of Menno Simons, a former Catholic priest, who was a key leader of the Anabaptist movement in Europe.

Anabaptists were disenfranchised and deported, and their goods expropriated for their refusal to bear arms as a civic service and to accept the authority of the state church in matters of faith and practice. Their attempts at radical discipleship in a "free church," following the guidelines of the early church as set forth in the New Testament, resulted in conflict with Catholic and Protestant leaders. After experiencing severe persecution and martyrdom in Europe, the Amish and related groups emigrated to America in the 17th and 18th centuries. No Amish live in Europe today, the last survivors having been assimilated into other religious groups (Hostetler, 1993). As a result, the Amish, unlike many other ethnic groups in the United States, have no larger reference group in their former homeland to which their customs, language, and lifeways can be compared.

Denied the right to hold property in their homelands, the Amish sought not only religious freedom but also the opportunity to buy farmland where they could live out their beliefs in peace. In their communities, the Amish have transplanted and preserved a way of life that bears the outward dress of preindustrial European peasantry. In modern industrial America, they have persisted in social isolation based on religious principles, a paradoxically separated life of Christian altruism. Living for others entails a caring concern for members of their in-group, a community of mutuality, but it also calls them to reach out to others in need outside their immediate Amish household of faith (Hostetler, 1993).

Although the Amish value inner harmony, mutual caring, and a peaceable life in the country, it would be a mistake to see Amish society as an idyllic, pastoral folk culture, frozen in time and serenely detached from the dynamic developments all around them. Since the mid-19th century, Amish communities have experienced inner conflicts and dissension as well as outside pressures to conform and modernize. Over time, the Amish have continued to adapt and change, but at their own pace, accepting innovations selectively.

One cost of controlled, deliberate change has been the loss of some members through factional divisions over "progressive" motivations, both religious and material. The influence of revivalism led to religious reform variants, which introduced Sunday schools, missions, and worship in meetinghouses instead of homes. Others who were impatient to use modern technology such as gasoline-powered farm machinery, telephones, electricity, electronic devices, and automobiles also split off from the main body of the most conservative traditionalists, now called the *Old Order Amish*. Some variant groups were named after their factional leaders (e.g., Egli and Beachy Amish); some were called *Conservative Amish Mennonites*; and others, *The New Order Amish*. Today, these progressives stand somewhere between the parent body, the Mennonites, and the Old Order Amish (technically Old Order Amish Mennonites), hereafter simply referred to as the Amish (Hostetler, 1993). This latter group, the (Old Order) Amish, which has been widely researched and reported on, provides the observational basis for this present culture study.

EDUCATIONAL STATUS AND OCCUPATIONS

The controversy over schooling of Amish children is a good example of a policy issue that attracts public attention. Amish parents assume primary responsibility for child rearing, with the constant support of the extended family and the church community to reinforce their teaching. On the family farm, parents and older siblings model work roles for younger siblings. Corporate worship and community religious practices nurture and shape their faith. Learning how to live and to prepare for death is more important in the Amish tradition than acquiring special skills or knowledge through formal education or training (Hostetler & Huntington, 1992).

The mixed-grade, one-room schoolhouses (Fig. 4–1), typical of rural America before 1945, were acceptable to the Amish because the schools were more amenable to local control. With the introduction of consolidated high schools, however, the Amish resisted secondary education, particularly compulsory schooling mandated by state and federal agencies, and raised objections both on principle and on scale. To illustrate the latter, the amount of time required by secondary education and the distances required to bus students out of their home communities were cited as problems. But probably more crucial was the understanding that the high school promised

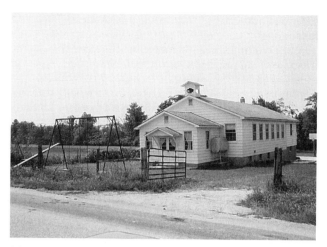

FIGURE 4–1 A one-room Amish schoolhouse in Indiana. (Photograph by Joel Wenger.)

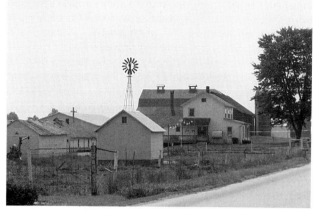

FIGURE 4–2 An Amish farm. The windmill in the background is usually used to pump water. (Photograph by Joel Wenger.)

to socialize and instruct the young in a value system that was antithetical to the Amish way of life. For example, in the high school, individual achievement and competition were promoted, rather than mutuality and caring for others in a communal spirit. On pragmatic grounds, Amish parents objected to "unnecessary" courses in science, advanced math, and computer technology, which seemed to have no place and little relevance in their tradition (Meyers, 1993).

The Amish response to this perceived threat to their culture was to build and operate their own private elementary schools. Their right to do so was litigated but finally upheld in the U.S. Supreme Court in the 1972 *Wisconsin v. Yoder* ruling. Today, school-aged children are encouraged to attend only eight grades, but Amish parents actively support local private and public schools.

The Amish rejection of higher learning for their children means that only the rare individual may pursue professional training and still remain Amish. Health-care professionals, by definition, are seen as outsiders who mediate information on health promotion, make diagnoses, and propose therapies across cultural boundaries. To the extent that they do so with sensitivity and respect for Amish cultural ways, they are respected, in turn, and valued as an important resource by the Amish.

As the 20th century drew to a close, important changes were underway among Amish in North America, whose principal and preferred occupations have long been agricultural work and farm-related enterprises (Fig. 4–2). They had typically settled on good farmland from their earliest immigration some 250 years ago. As cultivable land at an affordable price became an increasingly scarce commodity near centers of Amish settlements, the trend toward other work away from home led to a reshaping of the Amish family. Income from goods and services once delivered for internal domestic consumption came increasingly from cottage industry production for the retail market and wage-earning with nearby employers. The alternative, seeking new farmland at a distance, has led to community resettlement as far away from Philadelphia as Montana.

Young women who have learned quantity cookery at the many church and family get-togethers may find jobs in restaurants and catering or skills learned in household chores may be exchanged for wages in child care or housecleaning. Young men who bring skills from the farm may practice carpentry or cabinetmaking in the trades and construction industry. This, in turn, brings a change in family patterns, as "lunchbox daddies" are absent during daylight workday hours and the burden for parenting is borne more by stay-at-home mothers. The bonds of family and church have proved resilient but are clearly experiencing more tension in the current generation.

In summary, jobs away from home, an established majority culture pattern, and increased contacts with non-Amish people test the strength of sociocultural bonds that tie young people to the Amish culture. Given the enticements of the majority culture to change and to acculturate, it is noteworthy that so many young Amish find their way back to full membership in the ethnoreligious culture that nurtured them.

Communication

DOMINANT LANGUAGES AND DIALECTS

Like most people, the Amish vary their language usage depending on the situation and the individuals being addressed. American English is only one of three language varieties in their repertoire. For the Amish, English is the language of school, of written and printed communications, and above all, the language used in contacts with most non-Amish outsiders, especially business contacts. Because English serves a useful function as the contact language with the outside world, Amish schools all use English as the language of instruction, with the strong support of parents, because elementary schooling offers the best opportunity for Amish children to master the language. But within Amish homes and communities, use of English is discouraged in favor of the vernacular **Deitsch**, or Pennsylvania German. Because all Amish except preschool children are literate in their second language, American English, language usage helps to define their cultural space (Hostetler, 1993).

The first language of most Amish is *Deitsch,* an amalgamation of several upland German dialects that emerged from the interaction of immigrants from the Palatinate and Upper Rhine areas of modern France, Germany, and Switzerland. Their regional linguistic differences were resolved in an immigrant language better known in English as "Pennsylvania German." Amish immigrants who later moved more directly from the Swiss Jura and environs to Midwestern states (with minimal mixing in transit with *Deitsch*-speakers) call their home language *Düütsch,* a related variety with marked Upper Alemannic features. Today, *Deitsch* and *Düütsch* both show a strong admixture of vocabulary borrowed from English, whereas the basic structure remains clearly nonstandard German. Both dialects have practically the same functional distribution (Meyers & Nolt, 2005; Wenger, 1970).

Deitsch is spoken in the home and in conversation with fellow Amish and relatives, especially during **visiting**, a popular social activity by which news is disseminated orally. It is important to note that *Deitsch* is primarily a spoken language. Some written material has been printed in Pennsylvania German, but Amish seldom encounter it in this form. Even Amish publications urging the use of *Deitsch* in the family circle are printed in English, by default the print replacement for the vernacular, the spoken language (What is in a language?, 1986).

Health-care providers can expect all their Amish clients of school age and older to be fluently bilingual. They can readily understand spoken and written directions and answer questions presented in English, although their own terms for some symptoms and illnesses may not have exact equivalents in *Deitsch* and English. Amish clients may be more comfortable consulting among themselves in *Deitsch,* but generally, they intend no disrespect for those who do not understand their mother tongue.

Although of limited immediate relevance for health-care considerations, the third language used by the Amish deserves mention in this cultural profile to complete the scope of their linguistic repertoire. Amish proficiency in English varies according to the type and frequency of contact with non-Amish, but it is increasing. The use of Pennsylvania German is in decline outside the Old Order Amish community. Its retention by Amish, despite the inroads of English, has been related to their religious communities' persistent recourse to *Hochdeitsch,* or Amish High German, their so-called third language, as a sacred language (Huffines, 1994).

Amish do not use Standard Modern High German, but an approximation, which gives access to texts printed in an archaic German with some regional variations. Rote memorization and recitation for certain ceremonial and devotional functions, and for selected printed texts from the Bible, from the venerable "Ausbund" hymnbook, and from devotional literature are a part of public and private prayer and worship among the Amish. Such restricted and nonproductive use of a third language hardly justifies the term "trilingual" because it does not encompass a fully developed range of discourse. However, Amish High German does provide a situational-functional complement to their other two languages (Enninger & Wandt, 1982). Its retention is one more symbol of a consciously separated way of life that reaches back to its European heritage.

Within a highly contextual subculture like the Amish, the base of shared information and experience is proportionately larger. As a result, less overt verbal communication is required than in the relatively low-contextual American culture, and more reliance is placed on implicit, often unspoken understandings. Amish children and youth may learn adult roles in their society more through modeling, for example, than through explicit teaching. The many and diverse kinds of multigenerational social activities on the family farm provide the optimal framework for this kind of enculturation. Although this may facilitate the transmission of traditional, or accepted, knowledge and values within a high-context culture, this same information network may also impede new information imparted from the outside, which entails some behavior changes. Wenger (1988, 1991c) suggested that nurses and other health-care providers should consider role modeling as a teaching strategy when working with Amish clients. Later on, a brief example of the promotion of inoculation is presented to illustrate how public-health workers can use culture-appropriate information systems to achieve fuller cooperation among the Amish.

In a final note on language and the flow of verbal information, health-care providers should be aware that much of what passes for "general knowledge" in our information-rich popular culture is screened, or filtered out of, Amish awareness. The Amish have severely restricted their own access to print media, permitting only a few newspapers and periodicals. Most have also rejected the electronic media, beginning with radio and television, but also including entertainment and information applications of film and computers. Conversely, the Amish are openly curious about the world beyond their own cultural horizons, particularly regarding a variety of literature that deals with health and quality-of-life issues. They especially value the oral and written personal testimonial as a mark of the efficacy of a particular treatment or health-enhancing product or process. Wenger (1988, 1994) identified testimonials from Amish friends and relatives as a key source of information in making choices about health-care providers and products.

CULTURAL COMMUNICATION PATTERNS

Fondness and love for family members is held deeply but privately. Some nurses have observed the cool, almost aloof behavior of Amish husbands who accompany their wives to a maternity center, but it would be premature to assume that it reflects a lack of concern. The expression of joy and suffering is not entirely subdued by dour or stoic silence, but Amish are clearly not outwardly demonstrative or exuberant. Amish children, who can be as delightfully animated as any other children at play, are taught to remain quiet throughout a worship service lasting more than 2 hours. They grow up in an atmosphere of restraint and respect for adults and elders. But privately, Amish are not so sober as to lack a sense of humor and appreciation of wit.

Beyond language, much of the nonverbal behavior of Amish is also symbolic. Many of the details of Amish garb and customs were once general characteristics without any particular religious significance in Europe, but in the American setting, they are closely regulated and serve to distinguish the Amish from the dominant culture as a self-consciously separate ethnoreligious group (Kraybill, 2001).

It is precisely in the domain of ideas held to be normative for the religious aspects of Amish life that they find their English vocabulary lacking. The key source texts in *Hochdeitsch* and the oral interpretation of them in *Deitsch* are crucial to an understanding of two German values, which have an important impact on Amish nonverbal behavior. **Demut**, German for *humility*, is a priority value, the effects of which may be seen in details such as the height of the crown of an Amish man's hat as well as in very general features such as the modest and unassuming bearing and demeanor usually shown by Amish people in public. This behavior is reinforced by frequent verbal warnings against its opposite, **Hochmut**, *pride* or *arrogance*, which is to be avoided (Hostetler, 1993).

The second term, **Gelassenheit**, is embodied in behavior more than it is verbalized. *Gelassenheit* is treasured not so much for its contemporary German connotations of passiveness, even of resignation, as for its earlier religious meanings, denoting quiet acceptance and reassurance, encapsulated in the biblical formula "godliness with contentment" (1 Tim. 6:5). The following Amish paradigm for the good life flows from the calm assurance found through inner yielding and foregoing one's ego for the good of others:

1. One's life rests secure in the hands of a higher power.
2. A life so divinely ordained is therefore a good gift.
3. A godly life of obedience and submission will be rewarded in the life hereafter (Kraybill, 2001).

A combination of these inner qualities, an unpretentious, quiet manner, and modest outward dress in plain colors lacking any ornament, jewelry, or cosmetics presents a striking contrast to contemporary fashions, both in clothing styles and in personal self-actualization. Amish public behavior is consequently seen as deliberate, rather than rash, deferring to others instead of being assertive or aggressive, avoiding confrontational speech styles and public displays of emotion in general.

Health-care workers should greet Amish clients with a handshake and a smile. Amish use the same greeting both among themselves and with outsiders, but little touching follows the handshake. Younger children are touched and held with affection, but older adults seldom touch socially in public. Therapeutic touch, conversely, appeals to many Amish and is practiced informally by some individuals who find communal affirmation for their gift of **warm hands**. This concept is discussed further in the section on health-care practices.

In public, the avoidance of eye contact with non-Amish may be seen as an extension, on a smaller scale, of the general reserve and measured larger body movements related to a modest and humble being. But in one-on-one clinical contacts, Amish clients can be expected to express openness and candor with unhesitating eye contact.

Among their own, Amish personal space may be collapsed on occasions of crowding together for group meetings or travel. In fact, Amish are seldom found alone, and a solitary Amish person or family is the exception rather than the rule. But Amish are also pragmatic, and in larger families, physical intimacy cannot be avoided in the home where childbearing and care of the ill and dying are accepted as normal parts of life. Once health-care professionals recognize that Amish prefer to have such caregiving within the home and family circle, professionals will want to protect modest Amish clients who feel exposed in the clinical setting.

TEMPORAL RELATIONSHIPS

So much of current Amish life and practice has a traditional dimension reminiscent of a rural American past that it is tempting to view the Amish culture as "backward-looking." In actuality, Amish self-perception is very much grounded in the present, and historical antecedents or reasons for current consensus have often been lost to common memory. Conversely, the Amish existential expression of Christianity focused on today is clearly seen as a preparation for the afterlife. So one may say that Amish are also future-oriented, at least in a metaphysical sense, although not as it relates to modern, progressive, or futuristic thought.

After generations of rural life guided by the natural rhythms of daylight and seasons, the Amish manage the demands of clock time in the dominant culture. They are generally punctual and conscientious about keeping appointments, although they may seem somewhat inconvenienced by not owning a telephone or car. These communication conveniences, deemed essential by the dominant American culture, are viewed by the most conservative Amish as technological advances that could erode the deeply held value of community, in which face-to-face contacts are easily made. Therefore, telephones and automobiles are generally owned by nearby non-Amish neighbors and used by Amish only when it is deemed essential, such as for reaching health-care facilities.

Because the predominant mode of transportation for the Amish is horse and carriage, travel to a doctor's office, a clinic, or a hospital requires the same adjustment as any other travel outside their rural community to shop, trade, or attend a wedding or funeral. The latter three reasons for travel are important means of reinforcing relationship ties, and on these occasions, the Amish may use hired or public transportation, excluding flying. Taking time out of normal routines for extended trips related to medical treatments is not uncommon, such as a visit to radioactive mines in the Rocky Mountains or to a laetrile clinic in Mexico to cope with cancer (Wenger, 1988).

FORMAT FOR NAMES

Using first names with Amish people is appropriate, particularly because generations of intermarriage have resulted in a large number of Amish who share only a limited number of surnames. So it is preferable to use John or Mary during personal contacts rather than Mr. or Mrs. Miller, for example. In fact, within Amish communities, with so many Millers, Lapps, Yoders, and Zooks, given names like Mary and John are overused to the extent that individuals have to be identified further by nicknames, residence, a spouse's given name, or a patronymic, which may reflect three or more generations of patrilineal descent. For example, a particular John Miller may be known as "Red John," or "Gap John," or "Annie's John," or "Sam's Eli's Roman's John" (Hostetler, 1993).

During an interview with an Amish mother and her 5-year-old son, Wenger (1988) asked the child where he was going that day. The boy replied that he was going to play with Joe Elam John Dave Paul, identifying his age-mate Paul with four preceding generations. This little boy was giving useful everyday information while at the same time, unbeknownst to him, keeping oral history alive. The patronymics also illustrate the cultural value placed on intergenerational relationships and help to create a sense of belonging that embraces several generations and a broad consanguinity. Thus, one can see that medical record keeping can be a challenge when an extensive Amish clientele is served.

Family Roles and Organization

HEAD OF HOUSEHOLD AND GENDER ROLES

From the time of marriage, the young Amish man's role as husband is defined by the religious community he belongs to. Titular patriarchy is derived from the Bible: Man is the head of the woman as Christ is the head of the church (I Cor. 3). This patriarchal role in Amish society is balanced or tempered by realities within the family, in which the wife and mother is accorded high status and respect for her vital contributions to the success of the family. Practically speaking, husband and wife may share equally in decisions regarding the family farming business. In public, the wife may assume a retiring role, deferring to her husband, but in private, they are typically partners. However, it is best to listen to the voices of Amish women themselves as they reflect on their values and roles within Amish family and their shared ethnoreligious cultural community.

Traditionally, the highest priority for the parents is child rearing, an ethnoreligious expectation in the Amish culture. With a completed family averaging seven children, the Amish mother contributes physically and emotionally to the burgeoning growth in Amish population. She also has an important role in providing family food and clothing needs, as well as a major share in child nurturing. Amish society expects the husband and father to contribute guidance, serve as a role model, and discipline the children. This shared task of parenting takes precedence over other needs, including economic or financial success in the family business. On the family farm, all must help as needed, but in general, field and barn work and animal husbandry are primarily the work of men and boys, whereas food production and preservation, clothing production and care, and management of the household are mainly the province of women.

PRESCRIPTIVE, RESTRICTIVE, AND TABOO BEHAVIORS FOR CHILDREN AND ADOLESCENTS

Children and youth represent a key to the vitality of the Amish culture. Babies are welcomed as a gift from God,

and the high birth rate is one factor in their population growth. Another is the surprisingly high retention of youth, an estimated 75 percent or more, who choose as adults to remain in the Amish way. Before and during elementary school years, parents are more directive as they guide and train their children to assume responsible, productive roles in Amish society.

Young people over age 16 may be encouraged to work away from home to gain experience or because of insufficient work at home or on the family farm, but their wages are still usually sent home to the parental household because of the cultural value that the whole family contributes to the welfare of the family. Some experimentation with non-Amish dress and behavior among Amish teenagers is tolerated during this period of relative leniency, but the expectation is that an adult decision to be baptized before marriage will call young people back to the discipline of the church, as they assume adult roles.

In recent years, the media have been fascinated with this period of Amish teenage life as Americans in general have learned more about the Amish as a distinctive culture. Meyers and Nolt (2005) contended that although some Amish teenagers do experiment with behaviors that are incongruent with Amish beliefs and values, they do so in a distinctive Amish way. Amish teenagers are aware of the dominant American culture and when they choose to participate in behaviors, some of which may involve the legal system, they do so in distinctive Amish ways, not in ways more common to American teenagers in general. For example, Amish youth will usually experiment within an Amish context and with other Amish youth, rather than with non-Amish teenagers.

FAMILY GOALS AND PRIORITIES

VIGNETTE 4.1

Elmer and Mary Miller, both 35 years old, live with their five children in the main house on the family farmstead in one of the largest Amish settlements in Indiana. Aaron and Annie Schlabach, aged 68 and 70, live in the attached grandparents' cottage. Mary is the youngest of their eight children, and when she married, she and Elmer moved into the grandparents' cottage with the intention that Elmer would take over the farm when Aaron wanted to retire.

Eight years ago, they traded living space, and now Aaron continues to help with the farm work, despite increasing pain in his hip, which the doctor advises should be replaced. Most of Mary's and Elmer's siblings live in the area, though not in the same church district or settlement. Two of Elmer's brothers and their families recently moved to Tennessee, where farms are less expensive and where they are helping to start a new church district.

1. Develop three open-ended questions or statements you would use in learning from Mary and Elmer what health and caring mean to them and to the Amish culture.
2. How might health-care providers use the Amish values of the three-generational family and their visiting patterns in promoting health in the Amish community?

The Amish family pattern is referred to as the **freind-schaft**, the dialectical term used for the three-generational family structure. This kinship network includes consanguine relatives consisting of the parental unit and the households of married children and their offspring. All members of the family personally know their grandparents, aunts, uncles, and cousins, with many Amish knowing their second and third cousins as well.

Individuals are identified by their family affiliation. Children and young adults may introduce themselves by giving their father's first name or both parents' names so they can be placed geographically and geneologically. Families are the units that make up church districts, and the size of church districts are measured by the number of families rather than by the number of church members. This extended family pattern has many functions. Families visit together frequently, thus learning to anticipate caring needs and preferences. Health-care information often circulates through the family network, even though families may be geographically dispersed. Wenger (1988) found that informants referred to *freindschaft* when discussing the factors influencing the selection of health-care options. "The functions of family care include maintaining *freindschaft* ties, bonding family members together intergenerationally, and living according to God's will by fulfilling the parental mandate to prepare the family for eternal life" (Wenger, 1988, p. 134).

As grandparents turn over the primary responsibility for the family farm to their children, they continue to enjoy respected status as elders, providing valuable advice and sometimes material support and services to the younger generation. Many nuclear families live on a farm with an adjacent grandparent's cottage, which promotes frequent interactions across generations. Grandparents provide child care and help in rearing grandchildren and, in return, enjoy the respect generally paid by the next generations. This emotional and physical proximity to older adults also facilitates elder care within the family setting. In an ethnonursing study on care in an Amish community, Wenger (1988) reported that an informant discussed the reciprocal benefits of having her grandparents living in the attached **daadihaus** and her own parents living in a house across the road. Her 3-year-old daughter could go across the hall to spend time with her great-grandfather, which, the mother reported, was good for him in that he was needed, whereas the small child benefited from learning to know her great-grandfather, and the young mother gained some time to do chores. There is no set retirement age among the Amish, and grandmothers also continue in active roles as advisers and assistants to younger mothers.

Assuming full adult membership and responsibility means the willingness to put group harmony ahead of personal desire. In financial terms, it also means an obligation to help others in the brotherhood who are in need. This mutual aid commitment also provides a safety net, which allows Amish to rely on others for help in emergencies. Consequently, the Amish do not need federal pension or retirement support; they have their own informal "social security" plan. Amish of varying degrees of affluence enjoy approximately the same social status, and extremes of poverty and wealth are uncommon. Property damage or loss and unusual health-care expenses are also covered to a large extent by an informal brotherhood alternative to commercial insurance coverage. The costs of high-technology medical care present a new and severe test of the principle of mutual aid or "helping out," which is almost synonymous with the Amish way of life.

ALTERNATIVE LIFESTYLES

There is little variation from the culturally sanctioned expectations for parents and their unmarried children to live together in the same household while maintaining frequent contact with the extended family. Unmarried children live in the parents' home until marriage, which usually takes place between the ages of 20 and 30. Some young adults may move to a different community to work and live as a boarder with another Amish family. Being single is not stigmatized, although almost all Amish do marry. Single adults are included in the social fabric of the community with the expectation that they will want to be involved in family-oriented social events.

Individuals of the same gender do not live together except in situations in which their work may make it more convenient. For example, two female schoolteachers may live together in an apartment or home close to the Amish school where they teach. There are no available statistics on the incidence of homosexuality in Amish culture. Isolated incidents of homosexual practice may come to the attention of health professionals, but homosexual lifestyles do not fit with the deeply held values of Amish family life and procreation.

Pregnancy before marriage does not usually occur, and it is viewed as a situation to be avoided. When it does occur, in most Amish families, the couple would be encouraged to consider marriage. If they are not yet members of the church, they need to be baptized and to join the church before being married. Although not condoning pregnancy before marriage, the families and the Amish community support the young couple about to have a child. If the couple chooses not to marry, the young girl is encouraged to keep the baby and her family helps raise the child. Abortion is an unacceptable option. Adoption by an Amish family is an acceptable alternative.

Workforce Issues

CULTURE IN THE WORKPLACE

In every generation except the present one, the Amish have worked almost exclusively in agriculture and farm-related tasks. Their large families were ideally suited to labor-intensive work on the family farm. As the number of family farms has been drastically reduced because of competition from agribusinesses that use mechanized and electronically controlled production methods, few options are available for Amish youth.

Traditionally, the Amish have placed a high value on hard work, with little time off for leisure or recreation.

Productive employment for all is the ideal, and the intergenerational family provides work roles appropriate to the age and abilities of each person. But prospects began to narrow with the increased concentration of family farms in densely settled Amish communities as their population increased.

In addition, several cultural factors combine to limit the opportunities for young Amish to adapt to new work patterns. Amish children, who are encouraged to attend school through only eight grades, lack a basis for vocational training in work areas other than agriculture. Amish avoidance of compromising associations with "worldly" organizations, such as labor unions, restricts them to nonunion work, which often pays lower hourly rates. Work off the family farm, at one time a good option for unmarried youth, has become an economic necessity for some parents, although it is considered less acceptable for social reasons. Fathers who "work away," sometimes called "lunchpail daddies," have less contact with children during the workday, which in turn has an impact on the traditional father's modeling role and places more of the responsibility for child rearing on stay-at-home mothers. This shift in traditional parental roles is a source of some concern, although the effects are not yet clear.

ISSUES RELATED TO AUTONOMY

As described previously, external and internal factors have converged in the early 21st century to cause doubt about the continued viability of compact Amish farming communities. Exorbitant land prices triggered group out-migrations and resettlement in states to the west and south. The declining availability of affordable prime arable land in and around the centers of highest Amish population density is due in part to their non-Amish neighbors' land-use practices, especially in areas of suburban sprawl. A powerful internal force is at work as well in the population growth rate among the Amish, now well above the national average. So, contrary to popular notions that such a "backward" subculture is bound to die out, the Amish today are thriving. Population growth continues even without a steady influx of new immigrants from the European homeland or significant numbers of new converts to their religion or way of life (Kraybill, 2001).

The resulting pressures to control the changes in their way of life while maintaining its religious basis, particularly the high value placed on in-group harmony, have challenged the Amish to develop adaptive strategies. One outcome is an increasingly diversified employment base, with a trend toward cottage industries and related retail sales, as well as toward wage labor to generate cash needed for higher taxes and increasing medical costs. Another recent development includes a shift from traditional multigenerational farmsteads, as some retirees and crafts workers employed off the farm have begun to relocate to the edges of country towns. In summary, pressures to secure a livelihood within the Amish tradition have heightened awareness of the tension field within which the Amish coexist with the surrounding majority American culture.

Because English is the language of instruction in schools and is used with business contacts in the outside world, there is generally no language barrier for the Amish in the workplace. English vocabulary that is lacking in their normative ideas for religious aspects of Amish life is rarely a concern in the workplace.

Biocultural Ecology

SKIN COLOR AND OTHER BIOLOGICAL VARIATIONS

Most Amish are descendants of 18th-century Southern German and Swiss immigrants; therefore, their physical characteristics vary, as do those of most Europeans, with skin variations ranging from light to olive tones. Hair and eye colors vary accordingly. No specific health-care precautions are relevant to this group.

DISEASES AND HEALTH CONDITIONS

Since 1962, several hereditary diseases have been identified among the Amish. The major findings of the genetic studies have been published by Dr. Victor McKusick of the Johns Hopkins University (McKusick, 1978). Because Amish tend to live in settlements with relatively little domiciliary mobility, and because they keep extensive genealogical and family records, genetic studies are more easily done than with more mobile cultural groups. Many years of collaboration between the Amish and a few geneticists from the Johns Hopkins Hospital have resulted in mutually beneficial projects (Hostetler, 1993). The Amish received printed community directories, and geneticists compiled computerized genealogies for the study of genetic diseases that continue to benefit society in general.

The Amish are essentially a closed population with exogamy occurring very rarely. However, they are not a singular genetically closed population. The larger and older communities are consanguineous, meaning that within the community the people are related through bloodlines by common ancestors. Several consanguine groups have been identified in which relatively little intermarriage occurs between the groups. "The separateness of these groups is supported by the history of the immigration into each area, by the uniqueness of the family names in each community, by the distribution of blood groups, and by the different hereditary diseases that occur in each of these groups" (Hostetler, 1993, p. 328). These diseases are one of the indicators of distinctiveness among the groups.

Hostetler (1993) cautioned that although inbreeding is more prevalent in Amish communities than in the general population, it does not inevitably result in hereditary defects. Through the centuries in some societies, marriages between first and second cousins were relatively common without major adverse effects. However, in the Amish gene pool are several recessive tendencies that in some cases are limited to specific Amish communities in which the consanguinity coefficient (degree of relatedness) is high for the specific genes. Of at least 12 recessive diseases, 4 should be noted here (Hostetler, 1993; McKusick, 1978; Troyer, 1994).

Dwarfism has long been recognized as obvious in several Amish communities. Ellis–van Creveld syndrome, known in Europe and named for Scottish and Dutch physicians, is especially prevalent among the Lancaster County, Pennsylvania, Amish (McKusick, Egeland, Eldridge, & Krusen, 1964). This syndrome is characterized by short stature and an extra digit on each hand, with some individuals having a congenital heart defect and nervous system involvement resulting in a degree of mental deficiency. The Lancaster County Amish community, the second largest Amish settlement in the United States, is the only one in which Ellis–van Creveld syndrome is found. The lineage of all affected people has been traced to a single ancestor, Samuel King, who immigrated in 1744 (Troyer, 1994).

Cartilage hair hypoplasia, also a dwarfism syndrome, has been found in nearly all Amish communities in the United States and Canada and is not unique to the Amish (McKusick, Eldridge, Hostetler, Ruanquit, & Egeland, 1965). This syndrome is characterized by short stature and fine, silky hair. There is no central nervous system involvement and, therefore, no mental deficiency. However, most affected individuals have deficient cell-mediated immunity, thus increasing their susceptibility to viral infections (Troyer, 1994).

Pyruvate kinase anemia, a rare blood cell disease, was described by Bowman and Procopio in 1963. The lineage of all affected individuals can be traced to Jacob Yoder (known as "Strong Jacob"), who immigrated to Mifflin County, Pennsylvania, in 1792 (Hostetler, 1993; Troyer, 1994). This same genetic disorder was found later in the Geauga County, Ohio, Amish community. Notably, the families of all those who were affected had migrated from Mifflin County, Pennsylvania, and were from the "Strong Jacob" lineage. Symptoms usually appear soon after birth, with the presence of jaundice and anemia. Transfusions during the first few years of life and eventual removal of the spleen can be considered cures.

Hemophilia B, another blood disorder, is disproportionately high among the Amish, especially in Ohio. Ratnoff (1958) reported on an Amish man who was treated for a ruptured spleen. It was discovered that he had grandparents and 10 cousins who were hemophiliacs; 5 of the cousins had died from hemophilia. Research studies on causative mutations indicated a strong probability that a specific mutation may account for much of the mild hemophilia B in the Amish population (Ketterling, Bottema, Koberl, Setsuko, & Sommer., 1991).

Through the vigilant and astute observations of some public-health nurses known to these authors, a major health-care problem was noted in a northern Indiana Amish community. A high prevalence of phenylketonuria (PKU) was found in the Elkhart-Lagrange Amish settlement (Martin, Davis, & Askew, 1965). Those affected are unable to metabolize the amino acid phenylalanine, resulting in high blood levels of the substance and, eventually, severe brain damage if the disorder is untreated. Through epidemiological studies, the health department found that 1 in 62 Amish were affected, whereas the ratio in the general population was 1 in 25,000 at that time.

Through the leadership of these nurses, the county and the state improved case funding for PKU and health-care services for affected families throughout Indiana, which was followed by improved health services in Amish communities in other states as well.

In recent years, a biochemical disorder called *glutaric aciduria* has been studied by Dr. Holmes Morton, a Harvard-educated physician who has chosen to live and work among the Amish in Lancaster County, Pennsylvania. Morton made house calls, conducted research at his own expense because funding was not forthcoming, and established a clinic in the Amish community to screen, diagnose, and educate people to care for individuals afflicted with the disease (Allen, 1989). By observing the natural history of glutaric aciduria type I, the researchers postulated that the onset or progression of neurological disease in Amish clients can be prevented by screening individuals at risk; restricting dietary protein; and thus limiting protein catabolism, dehydration, and acidosis during illness episodes.

Dr. Morton was well received in the Amish community, with many people referring friends and relatives to him. When he noted the rapid onset of the symptoms and the high incidence among the Amish, he did not wait for them to come to his office. He went to their homes and spent evenings and weekends driving from farm to farm, talking with families, running tests, and compiling genealogical information (Wolkomir & Wolkomir, 1991). In 1991, he built a clinic with the help of donations, in part the result of an article in the *Wall Street Journal* about the need for this nonprofit clinic. Hewlett-Packard donated the needed spectrometer that cost $80,000; local companies provided building materials, and an Amish couple donated the building site. Although volunteers helped to build the clinic, a local hospital provided temporary clinic space lease-free because the community recognized the very important contribution Morton was making, not only to the Amish and the advancement of medical science but also to the public health of the community.

A countywide screening program is now in place. Health-care professionals are able to recognize the onset of symptoms. Research continues on this metabolic disorder, its relationship to cerebral palsy in the Amish population, and the biochemical causes and methods of preventing spastic paralysis in the general population. However, education remains a highly significant feature of any community health program. Nurses and physicians need to plan for family and community education about genetic counseling, screening of newborns, recognition of symptoms during aciduric crises in affected children, and treatment protocols. In *The New York Times Magazine* (Belkin, 2005), Dr. Morton was called "a doctor for the future" because he practices what is now referred to as "genetic medicine," which recognizes genetics as part of all medicine. But to the Amish, he is their friend who cares about their children, knows their families by name, and comes to their homes to see how they are able to cope with the manifestations of these genetically informed diseases.

Extensive studies of manic-depressive illnesses have been conducted in the Amish population. At first, there seemed to be evidence of a link between the Harvey-*ras*-1 oncogene and the insulin locus on chromosome 11. Studies on non-Amish families (Foroud, Casteluccio, Kollar, Edenberg, 2000) and more extensive studies on Amish families have revealed new information on the genome, although the locus for the bipolar disorder has not yet been found (Ginns, Egeland, Allen, Pauls, & Falls, 1992; Kelsoe, Ginns, & Egeland, 1989; Kelsoe, Kristobjanarson, Bergesch, Shiling, Hutch, et al., 1993; Law, Richard, Cottingham, Lathrop, Cox, & Meyers, 1992; Myers, 1992; Pauls, Morton, & Egeland, 1992). Attempts have been made to gain knowledge about the affective response the Amish have to their ethnoreligious cultural identity and experience. Reiling (1998) studied the relationship between Amish self-identity and mental health.

The incidence of alcohol and drug abuse, which can complicate psychiatric diagnoses, is much lower among the Amish than in the general North American population, thus contributing to the importance of the Amish sample. Although the incidence of bipolar affective disorder is not found to be higher in the Amish, some large families with several affected members continue to contribute to medical science by being subjects in the genetic studies. Because the Old Order Amish descend from 30 pioneer couples whose descendants have remained genetically isolated in North America, have relatively large kindred groups with multiple living generations, and generally live in close geographic proximity, they are an ideal population for genetic studies (Kelsoe et al., 1989).

VARIATIONS IN DRUG METABOLISM

No drug studies specifically related to the Amish were found in the literature. However, given the genetic disorders common among selected populations of Amish, this is one area in which more research needs to be conducted.

High-Risk Behaviors

Amish are traditionally agrarian and prefer a lifestyle that provides intergenerational and community support systems to promote health and mitigate against the prevalence of high-risk behaviors. Genetic studies using Amish populations are seldom confounded by use of alcohol and other substances. However, health professionals should be alert to potential alcohol and recreational drug use in some Amish communities, especially among young unmarried men. Young adult men straying from the Amish way of life and "sowing their wild oats" before becoming baptized church members and before marriage is tolerated. Although this may be considered a high-risk behavior, it is not prevalent in all communities, nor is it promoted in any. Parents confide in each other and sometimes in trusted outsiders that this errant behavior causes many heartaches, although at the same time, they try to be patient and keep contact with the youth so the latter may choose to espouse the Amish lifeways.

Another lifestyle pattern that poses potential health risks is nutrition. Amish tend to eat high-carbohydrate and high-fat foods with a relatively high intake of refined sugar. Wenger (1994) reported that in an ethnonursing study on health and health-care perceptions, informants talked about their diet being too high in "sweets and starches" and knowing they should eat more vegetables. The prevalence of obesity was found to be greater among Amish women than for women in general in the state of Ohio (Fuchs, Levinson, Stoddard, Mullet, & Jones, 1990). In this major health-risk survey of 400 Amish adults and 773 non-Amish adults in Ohio, the authors found that the pattern of obesity in Amish women begins in the 25-year-old and older cohort, with the concentration occurring between the ages of 45 and 64. An explanation for the propensity for weight gain among the Amish may be related to the central place assigned to the consumption of food in their culture and the higher rates of pregnancy throughout their childbearing years (Wenger, 1994). However, in recent studies related to eating behaviors, obesity, and diabetes, the Old Order Amish cohorts showed some significant differences from other Caucasians in the majority culture. Hsueh et al. (2002) reported in the Third National Health and Nutrition Examination Survey that the Old Order Amish sample evidenced diabetes approximately half as frequently as did other Caucasians in the survey. Another important difference was the level of daily physical activity, which was reported to be higher among both Amish men and women than among other Caucasian cohorts (Bassett, 2004).

HEALTH-CARE PRACTICES

Most Amish are physically active, largely owing to their chosen agrarian lifestyle and farming as a preferred occupation. Physical labor is valued, and men as well as women and children help with farm work. Household chores and gardening, generally considered to be women's work, require physical exertion, particularly because the Amish do not choose to use electrically operated appliances in the home or machinery, such as riding lawn mowers, that conserve human energy. Nevertheless, many women do contend with a tendency to be overweight. In recent years, it is not uncommon to find Amish women seeking help for weight control from Weight Watchers and similar weight control support groups.

Farm and traffic accidents are an increasing health concern in communities with a dense Amish population. In states such as Indiana, with relatively high concentrations of Amish who drive horse-drawn vehicles (Fig. 4–3), blinking red lights and large red triangles are required by law to be attached to their vehicles. Jones (1990) reported on a study of trauma by examining hospital records of Amish clients admitted to one hospital in mideastern Ohio. Transportation-related injuries were the largest group, with many of those involving farm animals. Falls from ladders and down hay holes resulted in orthopedic injuries, but no deaths. Amish families need to be encouraged to monitor their children who operate farm equipment and transportation vehicles and to teach them about safety factors. Concern about accidents is evident in Amish newsletters, many of which have a regular column reporting accidents and asking for prayers or expressing gratitude that the injuries were not more

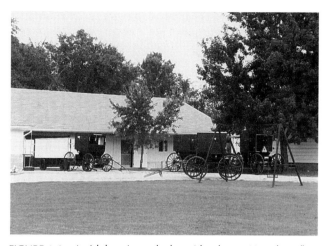

FIGURE 4–3   Amish buggies parked outside a home. Note the reflective safety triangle attached to the back of the rightmost buggy in the picture. These are usually required by law in areas that have large Amish populations. (Photograph by Joel Wenger.)

severe, that God had spared the person, or that the community had responded in caring ways (Wenger, 1988).

Nutrition

MEANING OF FOOD

Among the Amish, food is recognized for its nutritional value. Most Amish prefer to grow their own produce for economic reasons and because for generations they have been aware of their connections with the earth. They believe that God expects people to be the caretakers of the earth and to make it flourish.

The Amish serve food in most social situations because food also has a significant social meaning. Because visiting has a highly valued cultural function, occasions occur during most weeks for Amish to visit family, neighbors, and friends, especially those within their church district. Some of these visits are planned when snacks or meals are shared, sometimes with the guests helping to provide the food. Even if guests come unexpectedly, it is customary in most Amish communities for snacks and drinks to be offered.

COMMON FOODS AND FOOD RITUALS

Typical Amish meals include meat; potatoes, noodles, or both; a cooked vegetable; bread; something pickled (e.g., pickles, red beets); cake or pudding; and coffee. Beef is usually butchered by the family and then kept in the local commercially owned freezer for which they pay a rental storage fee. Some families also preserve beef by canning, and most families have chickens and other fowl, such as ducks or geese, which they raise for eggs and for meat. Amish families still value growing their own foods and usually have large gardens. A generation ago, this was an unquestioned way of life, but an increasing number of families living in small towns and working in factories and construction own insufficient land to plant enough food for the family's consumption.

Snacks and meals in general tend to be high in fat and carbohydrates. A common snack is large, home-baked cookies about 3 inches in diameter. Commercial non-Amish companies have recognized large soft cookies as a marketable commodity and have advertised their commercially made products as "Amish" cookies, even though no Amish are involved in the production. Other common snacks are ice cream (purchased or home-made), pretzels, and popcorn.

When Amish gather for celebrations such as weddings, birthdays, work bees, or quiltings, the tables are usually laden with a large variety of foods. The selection, usually provided by many people, includes several casseroles, noodle dishes, white and sweet potatoes, some cooked vegetables, few salads, pickled dishes, pies, cakes, puddings, and cookies. Hostetler (1993) provided a detailed ethnographic description of the meaning and practices surrounding an Amish wedding, including the food preparation, the wedding dinner and supper, and the roles and functions of various key individuals in this most important rite of passage that includes serving food.

In communities in which tourists flock to learn about the Amish, many entrepreneurs have used the Amish love of wholesome simple foods to market their version of Amish cookbooks, food products, and restaurants that more aptly reflect the Pennsylvania German, commonly referred to as *Pennsylvania Dutch*, influence of communities such as Lancaster County, Pennsylvania. Many of these bear little resemblance to authentic Amish foods, and some even venture to sell "Amish highballs" or "Amish sodas" (Hostetler, 1993). Some Amish families help to satisfy the public interest in their way of life by serving meals in their homes for tourists and local non-Amish. But most Amish view their foods and food preparation as commonplace and functional, not something to be displayed in magazines and newspapers. Because many Amish are wary of outsiders' undue interest, health professionals need to discuss nutrition and food as a part of their lifeways to promote healthy nutritional lifestyles.

In Amish homes, a "place at the table" is symbolic of belonging (Hostetler, 1993). Seating is traditionally arranged with the father at the head and boys seated youngest to oldest to his right. The mother sits to her husband's left with the girls also seated youngest to oldest or placed so that an older child can help a younger one. The table is the place where work, behavior, school, and other family concerns are discussed. During the busy harvesting season, preference is given to the men and boys who eat and return to the fields or barn. At mealtimes, all members of the household are expected to be present unless they are working away from home or visiting at a distance, making it difficult to return home.

Sunday church services, which for the Old Order Amish are held in their homes or barns, are followed by a simple meal for all who attended church (Fig. 4–4). The church benches, which are transported from home to home wherever the church service is to be held, are set up with long tables for serving the food. In many communities, some of the benches are built so they can quickly be converted into tables. Meals become ritualized so the focus is not on what is being served but rather on the opportunity to visit together over a simple meal. In

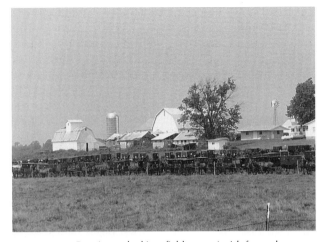

FIGURE 4–4   Buggies parked in a field on an Amish farm where people have gathered for a Sunday church service and noon meal. (Photograph by Joel Wenger.)

one community, an Amish informant who had not attended services because of a complicated pregnancy told the researcher that she missed the meal, which in that community consisted of bread, butter, peanut butter mixed with marshmallow crème and honey, apple butter, pickles, pickled red beets, soft sugar cookies, and coffee (Wenger, 1988).

Pregnancy and Childbearing Practices

FERTILITY PRACTICES AND VIEWS TOWARD PREGNANCY

Children are viewed as a gift from God and are welcomed into Amish families. Estimates place the average number of live births per family at seven (Hostetler & Huntington, 1992). The Amish fertility pattern has remained constant during the past 100 years, while many others have declined. Household size varies from families with no children to couples with 15 or more children (Huntington, 1988, Meyers & Nolt, 2005). Even in large families, the birth of another child brings joy because of the core belief that children are "a heritage from the Lord," and another member of the family and community means another person to help with the chores (Hostetler, 1993).

Having children has a different meaning in Old Order Amish culture than in the dominant American culture. In a study on women's roles and family production, the authors suggested that women in Amish culture enjoy high status despite the apparent patriarchal ideology because of their childbearing role and their role as producers of food (Lipon, 1985). A large number of children benefit small labor-intensive farms and with large families comes an apparent need for large quantities of food. Interpretation of this pragmatic view of fertility should always be moderated with recognition of the moral and ethical core cultural belief that children are a gift from God, given to a family and community to nurture in preparation for eternal life.

Scholars and researchers of long-term acquaintance with Old Order Amish agree that the pervasive Amish perception of birth control is that it interferes with God's will and thus should be avoided (Kraybill, 2001). Nevertheless, fertility control does exist, although the patterns are not well known and very few studies have been reported. Wenger (1980) discussed childbearing with two Amish couples in a group interview, and they conceded that some couples do use the rhythm method. In referring to birth control, one Amish father stated, "It is not discussed here, really. I think Amish just know they shouldn't use the pill" (Wenger, 1980, p. 5). Three physicians and three nurses were interviewed, and they reported that some Amish do ask about birth control methods, especially those with a history of difficult perinatal histories and those with large families. Some Amish women do use intrauterine devices, but this practice is uncommon. Most Amish women are reluctant to ask physicians and nurses and, therefore, should be counseled with utmost care and respect because this is a topic that generally is not discussed, even among themselves. Approaching the subject obliquely may make it possible for the Amish woman or man to sense the health professional's respect for Amish values and thus encourage discussion. "When you want to learn more about birth control, I would be glad to talk to you" is a suggested approach.

PRESCRIPTIVE, RESTRICTIVE, AND TABOO PRACTICES IN THE CHILDBEARING FAMILY

VIGNETTE 4.2

Mary and Elmer's fifth child, Melvin, was born 6 weeks prematurely and is 1 month old. Sarah, age 13, Martin, age 12, and Wayne, age 8, attend the Amish elementary school located 1 mile from their home. Lucille, age 4, is staying with Mary's sister and her family for a week because baby Melvin has been having respiratory problems, and their physician told the family he will need to be hospitalized if he does not get better within 2 days.

1. Choose two or three areas of perinatal care that you would want to discuss with Mary, and then write brief notes about what you know and/or need to learn about Amish values in order to discuss perinatal care in a way that is culturally congruent.
2. Discuss three Amish values, beliefs, or practices to consider when preparing to do prenatal education classes with Amish clients.

Amish tend to have their first child later than do non-Amish. In a retrospective chart review examining pregnancy outcomes of 39 Amish and 145 non-Amish women at a rural hospital in southern New York State, it was found that Amish had their first child an average of 1 year later than non-Amish couples (Lucas, O'Shea, Zielezny, Freudenheim, & Wold, 1991). The Amish had a narrower range of maternal ages and had proportionately fewer teenage pregnancies. All subjects received prenatal care, with the Amish receiving prenatal care from Amish lay midwives during the first trimester.

In some communities, Amish have been reputed to be reluctant to seek prenatal health care. Professionals who gain the trust of the Amish learn that they want the best perinatal care, which fits with their view of children being a blessing (Miller, 1997). However, they may choose to use Amish and non-Amish lay midwives who promote childbearing as a natural part of the life cycle. In a study of childbearing practices as described by Amish women in Michigan, Miller (1997) learned that they prefer home births, they had "limited formal knowledge of the childbirth process" (p. 65), and health-care professionals were usually consulted only when there were perceived complications. Although many may express privately their preference for perinatal care that promotes the use of nurse-midwifery and lay midwifery services, home deliveries, and limited use of high technology, they tend to use the perinatal services available in their community. In ethnographic interviews with informants, Wenger (1988) found that grandmothers and older women reported greater preference for hospital deliveries than did younger women. The younger women tend to have been influenced by the increasing general interest in childbirth as a natural part of the life cycle and the deemphasis on the medicalization of childbirth. Some Amish communities, especially those in Ohio and Pennsylvania, have a long-standing tradition of using both lay midwifery and professional obstetric services, often simultaneously.

In Ohio, the Mt. Eaton Care Center developed as a community effort in response to retirement of an Amish lay midwife known as Bill Barb (identified by her spouse's name, as discussed in the section on communication). She provided perinatal services, including labor and birth, with the collaborative services of a local Mennonite physician who believed in providing culturally congruent and safe health-care services for this Amish population. At one point in Bill Barb Hochstetler's 30-year practice, the physician moved a trailer with a telephone onto Hochstetler's farm so that he could be called in case of an emergency (Huntington, 1993). Other sympathetic physicians also delivered babies at Bill Barb's home. After state investigation, which coincided with her intended retirement, Hochstetler's practice was recognized to be in a legal gray area. The Mt. Eaton Care Center became a reality in 1985 after careful negotiation with the Amish community, Wayne County Board of Health, Ohio Department of Health, and local physicians and nurses. Physicians and professional nurses and nurse-midwives, who are interested in Amish cultural values and health-care preferences, provide low cost, safe, low-technology perinatal care in a homelike atmosphere. In 1997, the New Eden Care Center, modeled after the Mt. Eaton Care Center in Ohio, was built in LaGrange County in northern Indiana and, in recent years, has had more than 400 births per year (Meyers & Nolt, 2005).

Because the Amish want family involvement in perinatal care, outsiders may infer that they are open in their discussion of pregnancy and childbirth. In actuality, most Amish women do not discuss their pregnancies openly and make an effort to keep others from knowing about them until physical changes are obvious. Mothers do not inform their other children of the impending birth of a sibling, preferring for the children to learn of it as "the time comes naturally" (Wenger, 1988). This fits with the Amish cultural pattern of learning through observation that assumes intergenerational involvement in life's major events. Anecdotal accounts exist of children being in the house, though not physically present, during birth. Fathers are expected to be present and involved, although some may opt to do farm chores that cannot be delayed, such as milking cows.

Amish women do participate in prenatal classes, often with their husbands. The women are interested in learning about all aspects of perinatal care but may choose not to participate in sessions when videos are used. Prenatal class instructors should inform them ahead of time when videos or films will be used, so they can decide whether to attend. For some Amish in which the **Ordnung** (the set of unwritten rules prescribed for the church district) is more prescriptive and strict, the individuals may be concerned about being disobedient to the will of the community. Even though the information on the videos may be acceptable, the type of media is considered unacceptable.

Amish have no major taboos or requirements for birthing. Men may be present, and most husbands choose to be involved. However, they are likely not to be demonstrative in showing affection verbally nor physically. This does not mean they do not care; it is culturally inappropriate to show affection openly in public. The laboring woman cooperates quietly, seldom audibly expressing discomfort.

Given the Amish acceptance of a wide spectrum of health-care modalities, the nurse or physician should be aware that the woman in labor might be using herbal remedies to promote labor. Knowledge about and a respect for Amish health-care practices alerts the physician or nurse to a discussion about simultaneous treatments that may be harmful or helpful. It is always better if these discussions can take place in a low-stress setting before labor and birth.

As in other hospitalizations, the family may want to spend the least allowable time in the hospital. This is generally related to the belief that birth is not a medical condition and because most Amish do not carry health insurance. In their three-generational family, and as a result of their cultural expectations for caring to take place in the community, many people are willing and able to assist the new mother during the postpartum period. Visiting families with new babies are expected and generally welcomed. Older siblings are expected to help care for the younger children and to learn how to care for the newborn. The postpartum mother resumes her family role managing, if not doing, all the housework, cooking, and child care within a few days after childbirth. For a primiparous mother, her mother often comes to stay with the new family for several days to help with care of the infant and give support to the new mother.

The day the new baby is first taken to church services is considered special. People who had not visited the baby in the family's home want to see the new member of the community. The baby is often passed among the women to hold as they become acquainted and admire the newcomer.

Death Rituals

DEATH RITUALS AND EXPECTATIONS

Amish customs related to death and dying have dual dimensions. On the one hand, they may be seen as holdovers from an earlier time when, for most Americans, major life events such as birth and death occurred in the home. On the other hand, Amish retention of such largely outdated patterns is due to distinctively Amish understandings of the individual within and as an integral part of the family and community. Today, when 70 percent of elderly Americans die in hospitals and nursing homes, some still reflect nostalgically on death as it should be and as, in fact, it used to be, in the circle of family and friends, a farewell with familiarity and dignity. In Amish society today, in most cases, this is still a reality. As physical strength declines, the expectation is that the family will care for the aging and the ill in the home. Hostetler's brief observation that Amish prefer to die at home (1993) is borne out by research findings. Tripp-Reimer and Schrock (1982) reported from their comparative study of the ethnic aged that 75 percent of the Amish surveyed expressed a preference for living with family, 25 percent preferred living at home with assistance, and none would choose to live in a care facility, even if bedridden.

Clearly, these preferences are motivated by more than a wish to dwell in the past or an unwillingness to change with the times. The obligation to help others, in illness as in health, provides the social network that supports Amish practices in the passage from life to death. In effect, it is a natural extension of caregiving embraced as a social duty with religious motivation. The Amish accept literally the biblical admonition to "bear one another's burdens," and this finds expression in communal support for the individual, whether suffering, dying, or bereaved. Life's most intensely personal and private act becomes transformed into a community event.

Visiting in others' homes is, for the Amish, a normal and frequent reinforcement of the bonds that tie individuals to extended family and community. As a natural extension of this social interaction, visiting the ill takes on an added poignancy, especially during an illness believed to be terminal. Members of the immediate family are offered not only verbal condolences but many supportive acts of kindness as well. Others close to them prepare their food and take over other routine household chores to allow them to focus their attention and energy on the comfort of the ailing family member.

RESPONSES TO DEATH AND GRIEF

Ties across generations, as well as across kinship and geographic lines, are reinforced around death as children witness the passing of a loved one in the intimacy of the home. Death brings many more visitors into the home of the bereaved, and the church community takes care of accommodations for visitors from a distance as well as funeral arrangements. The immediate family is thus relieved of responsibility for decision making, which otherwise may add distraction to grief. In some Amish settlements, a wakelike "sitting up" through the night provides an exception to normal visiting patterns. The verbal communication with the bereaved may be sparse, but the constant presence of supportive others is tangible proof of the Amish commitment to community. The return to normal life is eased through these visits by the resumption of conversations.

Apart from the usual number of visitors who come to pay their respect to the deceased and survivors, the funeral ceremony is as simple and unadorned as the rest of Amish life. A local Amish cabinetmaker frequently builds a plain wooden coffin. In the past, interment was in private plots on Amish farms, contrasting with the general pattern of burial in a cemetery in the churchyard of a rural church. Because Amish worship in their homes and have no church buildings, they also have no adjoining cemeteries. An emerging pattern is burial in a community cemetery, sometimes together with other Mennonites.

Grief and loss are keenly felt, although verbal expression may seem muted, as if to indicate stoic acceptance of suffering. In fact, the meaning of death as a normal transition is embedded in the meaning of life from the Amish perspective. Parents are exhorted to nurture their children's faith because life in this world is seen as a preparation for eternal life.

Spirituality

DOMINANT RELIGION AND USE OF PRAYER

Amish religious and cultural values include honesty; order; personal responsibility; community welfare; obedience to parents, church, and God; nonresistance or nonviolence; humility; and the perception of the human body as a temple of God.

Amish settlements are subdivided into church districts similar to rural parishes with 30 to 50 families in each district. Local leaders are chosen from their own religious community and are generally untrained and unpaid. Authority patterns are congregationalist, with local consensus directed by local leadership, designated as bishops, preachers, and deacons, all of whom are male. No regional or national church hierarchy exists to govern internal church affairs, although a national committee may be convened to address external institutions of government regarding issues affecting the broader Amish population.

In addition to prayer in church services, silent prayer is always observed at the beginning of a meal, and in many families, a prayer also ends the meal. Children are taught to memorize prayers from a German prayer book for beginning and ending meals and for silent prayer. The father may say an audible amen or merely lift his bowed head to signal the time to begin eating.

MEANING OF LIFE AND INDIVIDUAL SOURCES OF STRENGTH

Outsiders, who are aware of the Amish detachment from the trappings of our modern materialistic culture, may be disappointed to discover in their "otherworldliness" something less than a lofty spirituality. Amish share the earthy vitality of many rural peasant cultures and a pragmatism born of immediate life experiences, not distilled from intellectual pursuits such as philosophy or theology. Amish simplicity is intentional, but even in austerity, there is a relish of life's simpler joys rather than a grim asceticism.

If death is a part of life and a portal to a better life, then individuals are well advised to consider how their lives prepare them for life after death. Amish share the general Christian view that salvation is ultimately individual, preconditioned on one's confession of faith, repentance, and baptism. These public acts are undertaken in the Amish context as part of preparing to fully assume one's adult role in a community of faith. In contrast with the ideals of American individualism, however, the Amish surrender much of their individuality as the price of full acceptance as members of a community. In practical, everyday terms, the religiously defined community is inextricably intertwined with a social reality, which gives it its distinctive shape.

For the Amish, the importance of conformity to the will of the group can hardly be exaggerated. To maintain harmony within the group, individuals often forgo their own wishes. In terms of faith-related behavior, outsiders sometimes criticize this "going along with" the local congregational group as an expression of religiosity, rather than spirituality. The frequent practice of corporate worship, including prayer and singing, helps to build this conformity. It is regularly tested in "counsel" sessions in the congregational assembly in which each individual's commitment to the corporate religious contract is reviewed before taking communion (Kraybill, 2001).

Non-Amish occasionally are baffled at reports of the Amish response to grave injury or even loss of life at the hands of others. Owing to deeply held community values, and especially constrained by love for others, Amish often eschew retaliatory or vengeful attitudes and actions when the majority culture might justify such means. Amish are socialized to sustain such injuries, grieve, and move on without fixing blame or seeking redress or punishment for the perpetrator. The felt need to forgive is for the Amish as strong as others perceive a need to bring wrongdoers to justice. The need to forgive is considered to be "second nature" in the Amish community. It does not indicate moral superiority or a heroic strength of forbearance in the face of adversity, but flows consistently from a biblical mandate to express love, even for an apparent adversary, as a practical application of the "The Golden Rule" (Matt. 7:12). A current example, claiming both national and international attention, was the Amish response of forgiveness in the face of the Nickel Mines, Pennsylvania, tragedy when 10 Amish school girls were held hostage and 5 of the girls were shot to death on October 2, 2006 (Complete Coverage of Nickel Mines Tragedy website at http://local.lancasteronline.com/1/91).

SPIRITUAL BELIEFS AND HEALTH-CARE PRACTICES

As seen in earlier sections on communication among Amish and their socioreligious provenance, many symbols of Amish faith point to the separated life, which they live in accordance with God's will. Over time, they have chosen to embody their faith rather than verbalize it. As a result, they seldom proselytize among non-Amish and nurture among themselves a noncreedal, often-primitive form of Christianity that emphasizes "right living." Their untrained religious leaders offer unsophisticated views of what that entails based on their interpretation of the Bible. Most members are content to submit to the congregational consensus on what right living means, with the assumption that it is based on submission to the will of a loving, benevolent God, an aspect of their spirituality that is seldom articulated (Kraybill, 2001).

Although the directives of religious leaders are normative for many types of decisions, this appears not to be the case for health-care choices (Wenger, 1991a). When choosing among health-care options, families usually seek counsel from religious leaders, friends, and extended family, but the final decision resides with the immediate family. Health-care providers need to be aware of the Amish cultural context and may need to adjust the normal routines of diagnosis and therapy to fit Amish clients' socioreligious context.

Health-Care Practices

HEALTH-SEEKING BELIEFS AND BEHAVIORS

Amish believe that the body is the temple of God and that human beings are the stewards of their bodies. This fundamental belief is based on the Genesis account of creation. Medicine and health care should always be used with the understanding that it is God who heals. Nothing in the Amish understanding of the Bible forbids them from using preventive or curative medical services. A prevalent myth among health-care professionals in Amish communities is that Amish are not interested in preventive services. Although it is true that many times the Amish do not use mainstream health services at the onset of recognized symptoms, they are highly involved in the practices of health promotion and illness prevention.

Although the Amish, as a people, have a reputation for honesty and forthrightness, they may withhold important medical information from medical professionals by neglecting to mention folk and alternative care being pursued at the same time. When questioned, some Amish admit to being less than candid about using multiple therapies, including herbal and chiropractic remedies, because they believe that "the doctor wouldn't be interested in them." Making choices among folk, alternative, and professional health-care options does not necessarily indicate a lack of confidence or respect for the latter, but rather reflects the belief that one must be actively involved in seeking the best health care available (Wenger, 1994).

RESPONSIBILITY FOR HEALTH CARE

The Amish believe that it is their responsibility to be personally involved in promoting health. As in most cultures, health-care knowledge is passed from one generation to the next through women. In the Amish culture, men are involved in major health-care decisions and often accompany the family to the chiropractor, physician, or hospital. Grandparents are frequently consulted about treatment options. In one situation, a scheduled consultation for a 4-year-old was postponed until the maternal grandmother was well enough after a cholecystectomy to make the 3-hour automobile trip to the medical center.

A usual concern regarding responsibility for health care is payment for services. Many Amish do not carry any insurance, including health insurance. However, in most communities, there is some form of agreement for sharing losses caused by natural disasters as well as catastrophic illnesses. Some have formalized mutual aid, such as the Amish Aid Society. Wenger (1988) found that her informants were opposed to such formalized agreements and wanted to do all they could to live healthy and safe lives, which they believed would benefit their community in keeping with their Christian calling. Many hospitals have been astounded by the Amish practice of paying their bills despite financial hardship. Because of this generally positive community reputation, hospitals have been willing to set up payment plans for the larger bills.

Active participation was found to be a major theme in Wenger's (1991a, 1994, 1995) studies on cultural context, health, and care. The Amish want to be actively involved in health-care decision making, which is a part of daily living. "To do all one can to help oneself" involves seeking advice from family and friends, using herbs and other home remedies, and then choosing from a broad array of folk, alternative, and professional health-care services. One informant, who visited an Amish healer while considering her physician's recommendation that she have a computerized axial tomography (CAT) scan to provide more data on her continuing vertigo, told the researcher, "I will probably have the CAT scan, but I am not done helping myself and this [meaning the healer's treatment] may help and it won't hurt." In this study, health-care decision making was found to be influenced by three factors: (1) type of health problem, (2) accessibility of health-care services, and (3) perceived cost of the service. When the Amish use professional health-care services, they want to be partners in their health care and want to retain their right to choose from all culturally sanctioned health-care options.

Caring within the Amish culture is synonymous with being Amish. "It's the Amish way" translates into the expectation that members of the culture be aware of the needs of others and thus fulfill the biblical injunction to bear one another's burdens. Caring is a core value related to health and well-being. Care is expressed in culturally encoded expectations that they can best describe in their dialect as **abwaarde**, meaning "to minister to someone by being present and serving when someone is sick in bed." A more frequently used term for helping is **achtgewwe**, which means "to serve by becoming aware of someone's needs and then to act by doing things to help." Helping others is expressed in gender-related and age-related roles, *freindschaft* (the three-generational family), church district, community (including non-Amish), Amish settlements, and worldwide. No outsiders or

health-care providers can be expected to fully understand this complex caring network, but health-care providers can learn about it in the local setting by establishing trust in relationships with their Amish clients.

When catastrophic illness occurs, the Amish community responds by being present, helping with chores, and relieving family members so that they can be with the afflicted person in the acute-care hospital. Some do opt to accept medical advice regarding the need for high-technology treatment, such as transplants or other high-cost interventions. The client's family seeks prayers and advice from the bishop and deacons of their church and their family and friends, but the decision is generally a personal or family one.

Amish engage in self-medication. Although most Amish regularly visit physicians and use prescription drugs, they also use herbs and other nonprescription remedies, often simultaneously. When discussing the meaning of health and illness, Wenger (1988, 1994) found that her Amish informants considered it their responsibility to investigate their treatment options and to stay personally involved in the treatment process rather than to relegate their care to the judgment of the professional physician or nurse. Consequently, they seek testimonials from other family members and friends about what treatments work best. They may also seek care from Amish healers and other alternative-care practitioners, who may suggest nutritional supplements. One informant told how she would take "blue cohosh" pills with her to the hospital when she was in labor because she believed that they would speed up the labor.

Because of the Amish practice of self-medication, it is essential that health-care providers inquire about the full range of remedies being used. For the Amish client to be candid, the provider must develop a context of mutual trust and respect. Within this context, the Amish client can feel assured that the professional wants to consider and negotiate the most advantageous yet culturally congruent care.

FOLK AND TRADITIONAL PRACTICES

VIGNETTE 4.3

At the doctor's office, Mary suggested to one nurse, who often talks with Mary about "Amish ways," that Menno Martin, an Amish man who "gives treatments," may be able to help. He uses "warm hands" to treat people and is especially good with babies because he can feel what is wrong. The nurse noticed that Mary carefully placed the baby on a pillow as she prepared to leave. The nurse also noticed that Mary is quite overweight and remembered that at a previous office visit, Mary had mentioned shyly that she would like to lose some weight.

1. Why did Mary place the baby on a pillow as she was leaving the doctor's office?
2. Develop a nutritional guide for Amish women who are interested in losing weight. Consider Amish values, daily lifestyle, and food production and preparation patterns.

The Amish, like many other cultures, have an elaborate health-care belief system that includes traditional remedies passed from one generation to the next. They also use alternative health care that is shared by other Americans, though often not sanctioned by medical and other health-care professionals. Although the prevalence of specific health-care beliefs and practices, such as use of chiropractic, Western medical and health-care science, reflexology, iridology, osteopathy, homeopathy, and folklore, is influenced mainly by *freindschaft* (Wenger, 1991b), variations depend on geographic region and the conservatism of the Amish community.

Herbal remedies include those handed down by successive generations of mothers and daughters. One elderly grandmother showed the researcher the cupboard where she kept some cloths soaked in a herbal remedy and shared the recipe for it. She stated that the cupboard was where she remembers her grandmother keeping those same remedies when her grandmother lived in the *daadihaus,* the grandparents' cottage attached to the family farmhouse where her daughter and son-in-law live. She also confided that, although she prepared the herb-soaked cloths for her daughters when they married, she thinks they opt for more modern treatments, such as herb pills and prescription drugs. This is a poignant example of the effect of modern health care on a highly contextual culture.

"Of all Amish folk health care, **brauche** has claimed the most interest of outsiders, who are often puzzled by its historical origins and contemporary application" (Wenger, 1991b, p. 87). *Brauche* is a folk-healing art that was practiced in Europe around the time of the Amish immigration to North America and is not unique to the Amish, but is a common healing art used among Pennsylvania Germans. As with some other European practices, the Amish have retained *brauche* in some communities. In other communities, the practice is considered suspect, and it has been the focus of some church divisions.

Brauche is sometimes referred to as sympathy curing or powwowing. It is unrelated to American Indian powwowing, and the use of this English term to refer to the German term *brauche* is unclear. In most literary descriptions of sympathy curing, it refers to the use of words, charms, and physical manipulations for treating some human and animal maladies. In some communities, the Amish refer to *brauche* as "warm hands," the ability to feel when a person has a headache or a baby has colic. Informants describe situations in which some individuals can "take" the stomachache from the baby into their own bodies in what is described by researchers as *transference.* Wenger (1991a, 1994) stated that all informant families volunteered information about *brauche,* using that term or "warm hands" to describe folk healing. One informant asked the author if she could "feel" it, too.

A few folk illnesses have no Western scientific equivalents. The first is **abnemme**, which refers to a condition in which the child fails to thrive and appears puny. Specific treatments given to the child may include incantations. Some of the older people remember these treatments, and some informants remember having been taken to a healer for the ailment. The second is **aagwachse**, or *livergrown,* meaning "hide-bound" or "grown together," once a common ailment among Pennsylvania Germans (Hostetler, 1993). Symptoms include crying and abdominal discomfort that is believed to be caused by jostling in rough buggy rides. Wenger (1988) reported accompanying an informant with her newborn baby to an Amish healer, and the woman carried the baby on a pillow because she believed the baby to be suffering from *aagwachse.* As stated previously, Amish clients are more likely to discuss folk beliefs and practices with professionals if the nurse or physician gives cues that it is acceptable to do so.

BARRIERS TO HEALTH CARE

VIGNETTE 4.4

Elmer and Mary do not carry any health insurance and are concerned about paying the doctor and hospital bills associated with this complicated pregnancy. In addition, they have an appointment for Wayne to be seen at the Children's Hospital, 3 hours away at the University Medical Center in Indianapolis, for a recurring cyst located behind his left ear. Plans are being made for a driver to take Mary, Elmer, Wayne, Aaron, Annie, and two of Mary's sisters to Indianapolis for the appointment. Because it is on the way, they plan to stop near Fort Wayne to see an Amish healer who gives nutritional advice and does "treatments." Aaron, Annie, and Elmer have been there before, and the other women are considering having treatments, too. Many Amish and non-Amish go there and tell others how much better they feel after the treatments.

They know their medical expenses seem minor in comparison to the family who last week lost their barn in a fire and to the young couple whose 10-year-old child had brain surgery after a fall from the hayloft. Elmer gave money to help with the expenses of the child and will go to the barn raising to help rebuild the barn. Mary's sisters will help to cook for the barn raising, but Mary will not help this time because she needs to care for her newborn.

1. If you were the health-care professional to whom Mrs. Miller confided her interest in taking the baby to the folk healer, how would you learn more about their simultaneous use of folk and professional health services?
2. How might you use role play or some other culturally appropriate way to prepare the Millers for their consultation at the Medical Center?
3. If you were preparing the reference for consultation, what would you mention about the Millers that would help to promote culturally congruent care at the Medical Center?

Barriers to health care include delay in seeking professional health care at the onset of symptoms, occasional overuse of home remedies, and a prevailing perception that health-care professionals are not interested in, or may disapprove of, the use of home remedies and other alternative treatment modalities. In addition, some families may live far from professional health-care services, making travel by horse and buggy difficult or inadvisable. Because in some Amish communities, such as the Old Order Amish, telephones are not permitted in the home, there may be delays in communication with Amish clients. Finally, the cost of health care without health insurance can deter early access to professional care, which could result in more complex treatment regimens.

CULTURAL RESPONSES TO HEALTH AND ILLNESS

The Amish are unlikely to display pain and physical discomfort. The health-care provider may need to remind the Amish client that medication is available for pain relief if they choose to accept it.

Community for the Amish means inclusion of people who are chronically ill or "physically or mentally different." Amish culture approaches these differences as a community responsibility. Children with mental or physical differences are sometimes referred to as "hard learners," who are expected to go to school and be incorporated into the classes with assistance from other student "scholars" and parents. A culturally congruent approach is for the family and others to help engage those with differences in work activities, rather than to leave them sitting around and getting more anxious or depressed.

Hostetler (1993) stated that "Amish themselves have developed little explicit therapeutic knowledge to deal with cases of extreme anxiety" (p. 332). They do seek help from trusted physicians, and some are admitted to mental health centers or clinics. However, the mentally ill are generally cared for at home whenever possible. Studies of clinical depression and manic-depressive illness were discussed in the section on Biocultural Ecology.

As previously mentioned, when individuals are sick, other family members take on additional responsibilities. Little ceremony is associated with being sick, and members know that to be healthy means to assume one's role within the family and community. Caring for the sick is highly valued, but at the same time, receiving help is accompanied by feelings of humility. Amish newsletters abound with notices of thanks from individuals who were ill. A common expression is, "I am not worthy of it all." A care set identified in one research study is that "giving care involves privilege and obligation and receiving care involves expectation and humility" (Wenger, 1991a). The sick role is mediated by very strong values related to giving and receiving care.

The Amish culture also sanctions time out for illness when the sick are relieved of their responsibilities by others who minister to their needs. A good analogy to the communal care of the ill is found in the support offered by family and church members at the time of bereavement, as noted in the section on dying. The informal social support network is an important factor in the individual's sense of well-being. An underlying expectation, however, is that healthy individuals will want to resume active work and social roles as soon as their recovery permits. With reasonable adjustments for age and physical ability, it is understood that a healthy person is actively engaged in work, worship, and social life of the family and community (Wenger, 1994). Work and rest are kept in balance, but for the Amish, the accumulation of days or weeks of free time or time off for vacation outside the framework of normal routines and social interactions is a foreign idea.

In a study of Amish women's construction of health narratives, Nelson (1999) found that the "collective descriptions [of] health included a sense of feeling well and the physical ability to complete one's daily work responsibilities" (p. vi). Women's health traditions included the use of herbal and other home remedies and consulting lay practitioners. In general, health values and beliefs are influenced by cultural group membership and personal developmental history.

BLOOD TRANSFUSIONS AND ORGAN DONATION

No cultural or religious rules or taboos prohibit Amish from accepting blood transfusions or organ transplantation and donation. In fact, with the genetic presence of hemophilia, blood transfusion has been a necessity for some families. Anecdotal evidence is available regarding individuals who have received heart and kidney transplants, although no research reports or other written accounts were found. Thus, some Amish may opt for organ transplantation after the family seeks advice from church officials, extended family, and friends, but the patient or immediate family generally makes the final decision.

Health-Care Practitioners

VIGNETTE 4.5

The state health department is concerned about the low immunization rates in the Amish communities. One community health nurse, who works in the area where Elmer and Mary live, has volunteered to talk with Elmer, who is on the Amish school board. The nurse wants to learn how the health department can work more closely with the Amish and also learn more about what the people know about immunizations. The county health commissioner thinks this is a waste of time and that what they need to do is let the Amish know that they are creating a health hazard by neglecting or refusing to have their children immunized. In addition, the county health commissioner is concerned about the incidence of phenylketonuria (PKU) and glutaric aciduria in the Amish communities.

1. Imagine yourself participating in a meeting with state and local health department officials and several local physicians and nurses to develop a plan to increase the immunization rates in the counties with large Amish populations. What would you suggest as ways to accomplish this goal?
2. Name three health problems with genetic links that are prevalent in some Amish communities and then discuss how health-care professionals can influence incidence and surveillance.

TRADITIONAL VERSUS BIOMEDICAL PRACTITIONERS

Amish usually refer to their own healers by name rather than by title, although some say *brauch-doktor* or **braucher**. In some communities, both men and women provide these services. They may even specialize, with some being especially good with bed wetting, nervousness, women's problems, or livergrown. Some set up treatment rooms, and people come early in the morning and wait long hours to be seen. They do not charge fees but do accept donations. A few also treat non-Amish clients. In some communities, Amish folk healers use a combination of treatment modalities, including physical manipulation, massage, *brauche*, herbs and teas, and reflexology. A few have taken short courses in reflexology, iridology, and various types of therapeutic massage. In a few cases, their practice has been reported to the legal authorities by individuals in the medical profession or others who were concerned about the potential for illegal practice of medicine. Huntington (1993) chronicled several cases, including those of Solomon Wickey and Joseph Helmuth, both in Indiana. Both men continue to practice with some carefully designed restrictions.

STATUS OF HEALTH-CARE PROVIDERS

For the Old Order Amish, health-care practitioners are always outsiders because, thus far, this sect has been unwilling to allow their members to attend medical, nursing, or other health-related professional schools or to seek higher education in general. Therefore, the Old Order Amish must learn to trust individuals outside their culture for health care and medically related scientific knowledge. Hostetler (1993) contended that the Amish live in a state of flux when securing health-care services. They rely on their own tradition to diagnose and sometimes treat illnesses, while simultaneously seeking technical and scientific services from health-care professionals.

Most Amish consult within their community to learn about physicians, dentists, and nurses with whom they can develop trusting relationships. For more information on this practice, see the Amish informants' perceptions of caring physicians and nurses in Wenger's (1994, 1995) chapter and article on health and health-care decision making. Amish prefer professionals who discuss their health-care options, giving consideration to cost, need for transportation, family influences, and scientific information. They also like to discuss the efficacy of alternative methods of treatment, including folk care. When asked, many Amish, like others from diverse cultures, claim that professionals do not want to hear about nontraditional health-care modalities that do not reflect dominant American health-care values.

Amish hold all health-care providers in high regard. Health is integral to their religious beliefs, and care is central to their worldview. They tend to place trust in people of authority when they fit their values and beliefs. Because Amish are not sophisticated in their knowledge of physiology and scientific health care, the health-care professional who gains their trust should bear in mind that because the Amish respect authority, they may unquestioningly follow orders. Therefore, health-care providers should make sure that their clients understand instructions. Role modeling and other concrete teaching strategies are recommended to enhance understanding.

REFERENCES

Allen, F. (1989, September 20). Country doctor: How a physician solved the riddle of rare disease in children of Amish. *Wall Street Journal*, pp. 1, A16.

Bassett, D. R. (2004, January). Old-Time fitness in Old-Order Amish: Why are we less fit than our ancestors? Amish offer clues. *Medicine and Science in Sports and Exercise*, (36), 79–85.

Belkin, L. (2005, November 6). A doctor for the future. *Wall Street Journal Magazine*, pp 68–115.

Bowman, H. S., & Procopio, J. (1963). Hereditary non-sperocytic hemolytic anemia of the pyruvate kinase deficient type. *Annals of Internal Medicine, 58*, 561–591.

Enninger, W., & Wandt, K.-H. (1982). Pennsylvania German in the context of an Old Order Amish settlement. *Yearbook of German-American Studies, 17*, 123–143.

Foroud, T., Casteluccio, P., Kollar, D., Edenberg, H., Miller, M., Boman, L. (2000). Suggestive evidence of a locus on chromosome 10p using the NIMH genetics initiative bipolar affective disorder pedigrees. *American Journal of Medical Genetics, 96*(1), 18–23.

Fuchs, J. A., Levinson, R., Stoddard, R., Mullet, M., & Jones, D. (1990). Health risk factors among Amish: Results of a survey. *Health Education Quarterly, 17*(2), 197–211.

Ginns, E. D., Egeland, J., Allen, C., Pauls, D., & Falls, K. (1992). Update on the search for DNA markers linked to manic-depressive illness in the Old Order Amish. *Journal of Psychiatric Research, 26*(4), 305–308.

Hostetler, J. A. (1993). *Amish society* (4th ed.). Baltimore, MD: Johns Hopkins University Press.

Hostetler, J. A., & Huntington, G. E. (1992). *Amish children: Education in the family, school, and community* (2nd ed.). Dallas, TX: Harcourt Brace Jovanovich.

Hsueh W. C., Mitchell B. D., Aburomia R., Pollin T., Sakul, H., Gelder Ehm M., Michelsen B. K., Wagner, M. J., St. Jean, P. L., Knowler, W. C., Burns, D. K., Bell, C. J. & Shuldine A. R. (2002). Diabetes in the Old Order Amish: Characterization and heritability analysis of the Amish Family Diabetes Study. *American Journal of Clinical Nutrition, 75*(6), 1098–1106.

Huffines, M. L. (1994). Amish languages. In J. R. Dow, W. Enninger, & J. Raith (Eds.), *Internal and external perspectives on Amish and Mennonite life. 4: Old and new world Anabaptist studies on the language, culture, society and health of Amish and Mennonites* (pp. 21–32). Essen, Germany: University of Essen.

Huntington, G. E. (1988). The Amish family. In C. Mindel & R. Haberstein (Eds.), *Ethnic families in America* (3rd ed.). (pp. 367–399). New York: Elsevier.

Huntington, G. E. (1993). Health care. In D. B. Kraybill (Ed.), *The Amish and the state*. Baltimore, MD: Johns Hopkins University Press.

Huntington, G. E. (2001). *Amish in Michigan*. East Lansing, MI: Michigan State University Press.

Hüppi, J. (2000). Research note: Identifying Jacob Ammann. *Mennonite Quarterly Review, 74*(10), 329–339.

Jones, M. W. (1990). A study of trauma in an Amish community. *Journal of Trauma, 30*(7), 899–902.

Kelsoe, J. R., Ginns, E. D., & Egeland, J. A. (1989). Re-evaluation of the linkage relationship between chromosome 11p loci and the gene for bipolar affective disorder in the Old Order Amish. *Nature, 342*, 338–342.

Kelsoe, J. R., Kristobjanarson, H., Bergesch, P., Shilling, S., Attirad, S., Mirow, A., Moises, H., Gillin, J., & Egeland, J. (1993). A genetic linkage study of bipolar disorder and 13 markers on chromosome 11 including the D2 dopamine receptor. *Neuropsychopharmocology, 9*(4), 293–307.

Ketterling, R. P., Bottema, C. D., Koberl, D. D., Setsuko. I, & Sommer, S. S. (1991). T^{296}M, a common mutation causing mild hemophilia B in the Amish and others: Founder effect, variability in factor IX activity assays, and rapid carrier detection. *Human Genetics, 87*, 333–337.

Kraybill, D. B. (2001). *The riddle of Amish culture* (rev. ed.). Baltimore, MD: Johns Hopkins University Press.

Kraybill, D. B., & Hostetter, C. N. (2001). *Anabaptist World USA*. Scottdale, PA: Herald Press.

Law, A., Richard, C. W., Cottingham, R. W., Lathrop, M. G., Cox, D. R., & Meyers, R. M. (1992). Genetic linkage analysis of bipolar affective disorder in an Old Order Amish pedigree. *Human Genetics, 88*, 562–568.

Lipon, T. (1985). Husband and wife work roles and the organization and operation of family farms. *Journal of Marriage and the Family, 47*(3), 759–764

Lucas, C. A., O'Shea, R. M., Zielezny, M. A., Freudenheim, J. L., & Wold, J. F. (1991). Rural medicine and the closed society. *New York State Journal of Medicine, 91*(2), 49–52.

Martin, P. H., Davis, L., & Askew, D. (1965). High incidence of phenylketonuria in an isolated Indiana community. *Journal of the Indiana State Medical Association, 56,* 997–999.

McKusick, V. A. (1978). *Medical genetics studies of the Amish: Selected papers assembled with commentary.* Baltimore, MD: Johns Hopkins University Press.

McKusick, V. A., Egeland, J. A., Eldridge, D., & Krusen, E. E. (1964). Dwarfism in the Amish I. The Ellis-van Creveld syndrome. *Bulletin of the Johns Hopkins Hospital, 115,* 306–330.

McKusick, V. A., Eldridge, D., Hostetler, J. A., Ruanquit, U., & Egeland, J. A. (1965). Dwarfism in the Amish II. Cartilage hair hypoplasia. *Bulletin of the Johns Hopkins Hospital, 116,* 285–326.

Meyers, T. J. (1993). Education and schooling. In D. Kraybill (Ed.), *The Amish and the state* (pp. 87–106). Baltimore, MD: Johns Hopkins University Press.

Meyers, T. J., & Nolt, S. M. (2005). *An Amish patchwork: Indiana's Old Orders in a modern world.* Bloomington, IN: QuarryBooks, Indiana University Press.

Miller, N. L. (1997). Childbearing practices as described by Old Order Amish women. Doctoral dissertation, Michigan State University. *Dissertation Abstracts International,* UMI 1388555.

Myers, R. M. (1992). Genetic linkage analysis of bipolar affective disorder in an Old Order Amish pedigree. *Human Genetics, 88,* 562–568.

Nelson, W. A. (1999). *A study of Amish women's construction of health narratives.* Unpublished doctoral dissertation, Kent State University, Kent, Ohio.

Pauls, D. L., Morton, L. A., & Egeland, J. A. (1992). Risks of affective illness among first-degree relatives of bipolar and Old Order Amish probands. *Archives of General Psychiatry, 49,* 703–708.

Ratnoff, O. D. (1958). Hereditary defects in clotting mechanisms. *Advances in Internal Medicine, 9,* 107–179.

Reiling, D. M. (1998). An explanation of the relationship between Amish identity and depression among Old Order Amish. Doctoral dissertation, Michigan State University. *Dissertation Abstracts International,* UMI 9985454.

Tripp-Reimer, T., & Schrock, M. (1982). Residential patterns of ethnic aged: Implications for transcultural nursing. In C. Uhl & J. Uhl (Eds.), *Proceedings of the Seventh Annual Transcultural Nursing Conference* (pp. 144–153). Salt Lake City, UT: University of Utah, Transcultural Nursing Society.

Troyer, H. (1994). Medical considerations of the Amish. In J. R. Dow, W. Enninger, & J. Raith (Eds.), *Internal and external perspectives on Amish and Mennonite life 4: Old and new world Anabaptist studies on the language, culture, society and health of the Amish and Mennonites* (pp. 68–87). Essen, Germany: University of Essen.

Wenger, A. F. (1980, October). *Acceptability of perinatal services among the Amish.* Paper presented at a March of Dimes symposium, Future Directions in Perinatal Care, Baltimore, MD.

Wenger, A. F. Z. (1988). The phenomenon of care in a high-context culture: The Old Order Amish. Doctoral dissertation, Wayne State University. *Dissertation Abstracts International,* 50/02B.

Wenger, A. F. Z. (1991a). The culture care theory and the Old Order Amish. In M. M. Leininger (Ed.), *Cultural care diversity and universality: A theory of nursing* (pp. 147–178). New York: National League for Nursing.

Wenger, A. F. Z. (1991b). Culture-specific care and the Old Order Amish. *Imprint, 38*(2), 81–82, 84, 87, 93.

Wenger, A. F. Z. (1991c). The role of context in culture-specific care. In P. L. Chinn (Ed.), *Anthology of caring* (pp. 95–110). New York: National League for Nursing.

Wenger, A. F. Z. (1994). Health and health-care decision-making: The Old Order Amish. In J. R. Dow, W. Enninger, & J. Raith, (Eds.), *Internal and external perspectives on Amish and Mennonite life 4: Old and New World Anabaptists studies on the language, culture, society and health of the Amish and Mennonites* (pp. 88–110). Essen, Germany: University of Essen.

Wenger, A. F. Z. (1995). Cultural context, health and health-care decision making. *Journal of Transcultural Nursing, 7*(1), 3–14.

Wenger, M. R. (1970). *A Swiss German dialect study: Three linguistic islands in Midwestern USA.* Ann Arbor, MI: University Microfilms.

What is in a language? (1986, February). *Family Life,* p. 12.

Wolkomir, R., & Wolkomir, J. (1991, July). The doctor who conquered a killer. *Readers Digest, 139,* 161–166.

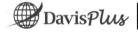 **DavisPlus** | For case studies, review questions and additional information, go to http://davisplus.fadavis.com.

Chapter 5

People of Appalachian Heritage

KATHLEEN W. HUTTLINGER and LARRY D. PURNELL

Overview, Inhabited Localities, and Topography

OVERVIEW

Appalachia consists of that large geographic expanse in the eastern United States that is associated with the Appalachian mountain system, a 200,000-square-mile region that extends from the northeastern United States in southern New York to northern Mississippi. It includes all of West Virginia and parts of Alabama, Georgia, Kentucky, Maryland, Mississippi, New York, North Carolina, Ohio, Pennsylvania, South Carolina, Tennessee, and Virginia. This very rural area is characterized by a rolling topography with very rugged ridges and hilltops, some extending over 4000 feet high, with remote valleys between them. The surrounding valleys are often 2000 feet or more in elevation and give one a sense of isolation, peacefulness, and separateness from the lower and more heavily traveled urban areas. This isolation and rough topography have contributed to the development of secluded communities in the hills and natural hollows or narrow valleys where people, over time, have developed a strong sense of independence and family cohesiveness. These same isolated valleys and rugged mountains present many transportation problems for those who do not have access to cars or trucks. Very limited public transportation is available only in the larger urbanized areas.

Even though the Appalachian region includes several large cities, many people live in small settlements and in inaccessible hollows or "hollers" (Huttlinger, Schaller-Ayers, & Lawson, 2004a). The rugged location of many communities in Appalachia results in a population that is often isolated from the mainstream of health-care services. In some areas of Appalachia, substandard secondary and tertiary roads, as well as limited public bus, rail, and airport facilities, prevent easy access to the area (Fig. 5–1). Difficulty in accessing the area is partially responsible for continued geographic and sociocultural isolation. The rugged terrain can significantly delay ambulance response time and is a deterrent to people who need health care when their health condition is severe. This is one area in which telehealth innovations can and often do provide needed services.

Many of the approximately 24 million people who live in Appalachia can trace their family roots back 150 or more years, and it is common to find whole communities comprising extended, related families. The cultural heritage of the region is rich and reflected in their distinctive music, art, and literature. Even though family roots are strong, many of the region's younger residents have left the area to pursue job opportunities in the larger urban cities of the north. The remaining, older population reflects a group that often has less than a high-school education, is frequently unemployed, may be on welfare and/or disability, and is regularly uninsured (20.4 percent) (Virginia Health Care Foundation, 2001). In fact, of the total current population in Appalachia, 12.4 percent are 65 years or older (Haaga, 2004).

The lack of education has often been associated with nonparticipation in health promotion activities (Graduate Medical Education Consortium [GMEC], 2001). Graduation rates from high school in the year 2000 vary widely from 60.7 to 91.4 percent, with the lowest number of graduates occurring in West Virginia, southwestern Virginia, eastern Kentucky, and northeastern Tennessee (Haaga, 2006).

95

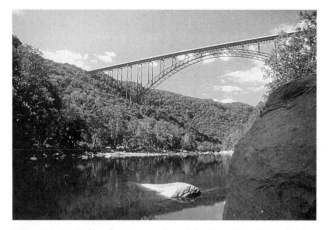

FIGURE 5–1 Before the construction of the New River Gorge bridge, many people were isolated from health care. (Courtesy of West Virginia Division of Tourism and Parks.)

HERITAGE AND RESIDENCE

Appalachians generally identify by family name and by their country of origin, such as German, Scotch-Irish, Welsh, French, or British, the primary groups who settled the region between the 17th and the 19th centuries. It is important to remember that migrating into the area does not make one an Appalachian. Historically, the population has been predominantly white, although many maintain a strong family identity with Native American groups who once populated the area (e.g., Cherokee, Choctaw) (Huttlinger, Schaller-Ayers, Kenney, & Ayers, 2004b).

Appalachians in general cannot be distinguished from other white cultural and ethnic groups by either dress or physical appearance. However, similarities in beliefs and practices, tempered by the primary and secondary characteristics of culture (see Chapter 1), give them a unique and rich ethnic identity. Like many disenfranchised groups, the people of Appalachia have been described in stereotypically negative terms (e.g., "poor white trash") that in no way represent the people or the culture as a whole. They have also been called "mountaineers," "hill-billies," "rednecks," and "Elizabethans." The media perpetuates these stereotypes with cartoon strips such as "Li'l Abner" and "Snuffy Smith," television programs such as the *Dukes of Hazzard*, and stories of the feuding Hatfields and McCoys and the Whites and Garrards. Interestingly, these feuds were among wealthy families over salt deposits and land and families who had high political profiles. Failure of the courts to intervene and a propensity of Appalachians to "handle things themselves" perpetuated the longevity of the feuds.

In reality, Appalachians value a deep-seated work ethic, a low cost of living, and a high quality of life. Appalachians see themselves as loyal, caring, family-oriented, religious, hardy, independent, honest, patriotic, and resourceful (Huttlinger et al., 2004a).

Other groups in the region who may identify with Appalachian culture include Native Americans, African Americans, and Melungeons, who are of mixed African American, Native American, Middle Eastern, Mediterranean, and white ethnic descent (Costello, 2000; Kennedy, 1997).

Although Melungeon heritage is often denied, there is, of late, a resurgence of identification of Melungeon ancestry. In fact, annual Melungeon get-togethers are now held once a year in Appalachia (Kennedy, 1997). With the increase in immigration to the United States since the 1970s, the Appalachian region is becoming more ethnically and culturally diverse, and it is now common to observe various southeast Asian, Chinese, and Hispanic groups.

REASONS FOR MIGRATION AND ASSOCIATED ECONOMIC FACTORS

Approximately 300 years ago, people came to Appalachia to seek religious freedom, land for themselves, and personal control over interactions with the outside world. Over the years, mining and timber resources became depleted, farmland eroded, and jobs became scarce, which resulted in an out-migration of people, especially those of working age, to larger urban areas of the North such as Cincinnati, Cleveland, and Louisville. This migration began after World War II and has remained constant ever since (Obermiller & Brown, 2002). Those who moved to urban areas often felt alone and sometimes became depressed as they were separated from family and friends. Many feared the large cities because of high crime and their unfamiliarity with how to get along in an urban environment. Those who remained in urban settings have become bicultural, adapting to the culture of urban life while retaining, as much as possible, their traditional Appalachian culture.

The limited opportunities for employment in Appalachia often require wage earners to leave their families to seek work elsewhere, returning home only to maintain close ties with their kinfolk as resources allow. Their migration pattern is regional, where individuals from one area primarily migrate to the same urban areas as their relatives and friends—a pattern that is common with many migrants. This practice helps decrease the occurrence of depression and feelings of isolation and provides a support network of family and friends so important for members of an Appalachian culture.

Appalachian migration patterns reflect the economic conditions found in the area as well as some of the cultural values of home, connection to the land, and importance of the family. Working-age individuals move from Appalachia to make their living but often return to the area to retire. Because of these patterns, Appalachia has one of the highest existing aging populations (Haaga, 2004). The pattern of returning home to retire has given rise to challenges for health-care delivery. In fact, older people were once able to rely on home care services, but severe budget cuts in 1977 left home care health service unreliable and ineffective. Therefore, older people and the chronically ill have to rely on options for short-term and expensive hospital care, nursing homes, or no care at all (Hurley & Turner, 2000).

For generations, the region has been a symbol of poverty in a land of wealth and opportunity. During the 1960s, the Appalachian Regional Commission (ARC) appropriated funds for building roads to attract industry and provided loans for residents to start their own businesses. In many areas of Central Appalachia, the unemployment rate and the number of people living in poverty have remained consistently above the national average, while the per capita income has remained below the national average. Eight of the 13 states in Appalachia have an unemployment rate higher than the national average of 4.8 percent, and the national poverty rate of 12.6 percent is exceeded by 10 of the 13 states in Appalachia. The average per capita income rate in Appalachia is $20,872. Not one Appalachian state achieves the national per capita income of $25,470. Of 410 counties in Appalachia, 77 are considered economically distressed, 81 are at risk, and 222 are transitional (ARC, 2006a). Even though the cost of living in much of the area is lower than that in many other parts of the United States, costs for transportation of food, basic living supplies, and transportation fuels rise, thus creating hardships for an area that is already economically stressed (ARC, 2006a).

EDUCATIONAL STATUS AND OCCUPATIONS

Although many of the original immigrants to this area were highly educated when they arrived, limited access to more formal education resulted in the isolation of later generations with fewer educational opportunities. Despite the value placed on education, a disparity in the number and placement of educational facilities exists throughout the region. Access to colleges and universities has improved, but there is still a lack of knowledge about life outside of Appalachia and the educational opportunities available. Examples of universities and colleges in Appalachia include, but are not limited to, West Virginia University, Appalachian State, University of Virginia's College at Wise, East Tenneesse State, Shawnee State, and the University of North Alabama. A dichotomy between those who are poorly educated and those who are extremely well educated still exists today (Huttlinger et al., 2004a).

Because isolationism results in a cultural lag, IQ scores of children from Appalachia are sometimes lower than those in the populations outside of Appalachia who have access to larger schools and live in urban settings. However, with television and the Internet now available throughout the area, this cultural lag has been slowly improving. In fact, U.S. Representatives from many of the districts that lie in Appalachia made it a priority to have broadband and Internet connections made accessible. Factors such as improved mobility, access to better schools with qualified teachers, increased employment opportunities in some regions, and greater use of technology are responsible for improving socioeconomic conditions and better performance on standard IQ tests (ARC, 2006a).

Although a value is placed on education, many see education beyond high school as not as important as earning a living to help support the family. Many Appalachian parents, and especially those who belong to more conservative and secular religious sects, do not want their children influenced by mainstream middle-class American behaviors and actions. However, fewer children drop out of school today than in previous decades. One interesting fact is that several states in Appalachia have

laws that grant permanent driving privileges only upon completion of high school, which has lowered dropout rates significantly.

Parents who value higher education encourage their children to seek quality education at the best institutions possible. Despite this value, the graduation rate from college has remained at 36 percent, compared with 45 percent for non-Appalachian counterparts (ARC, 2006a). Unfortunately, the highly educated, including health-care workers, who return to the area are often unable to secure financially lucrative employment.

Because educational levels of individuals within the Appalachian regions vary, it is essential for health-care providers to assess the health literacy and basic understanding of health and disease of individuals when providing any kind of intervention. Educational materials and explanations must be presented at literacy levels that are consistent with clients' understanding. If materials are presented at a level that is not understandable to clients, providers may be seen as being "stuck-up," "putting on airs," or "not understanding them and their ways" (Huttlinger et al., 2004b).

VIGNETTE 5.1

The Carter Family Fold lies deep in Appalachia at the base of Clinch Mountain in the Maces Springs or Poor Valley Community of southwestern Virginia. The Carter Family Fold is the home of the musical Carter family who provided the country with the rich legendary "Carter" family, a museum, a church, a cemetery, and a music center where lively concerts featuring local, national, and international musicians are featured. The concerts are family centered and, in keeping with a traditional style, feature only acoustic instruments (no electric instruments allowed!). Seating is in a barnlike structure with tiered platforms with seats made from discarded buses, cars, and tractors. The hospitality is contagious and as welcoming as the bluegrass and country musical tradition of the Appalachian culture. The "fold" includes the home sites of the family. Outsiders, young and old, are encouraged to dance, sing, and celebrate the rich musical heritage of the area.

Go to the Carter Family Fold website at http://www.carterfamilyfold.org/

1. What is the Center's objective?
2. For what are Maybelle, Sara, and A. P. Carter given historical credit?
3. How do the Fold and Center contribute to Appalachian culture?

Communication

DOMINANT LANGUAGE AND DIALECTS

The dominant language of the Appalachian region is English, with many words derived from 16th-century Saxon and Gaelic. Because the Appalachian dialect tends to be very concrete, continued exposure is necessary to avoid misunderstandings. Negative interpretations of Appalachian behaviors by non-Appalachian health-care workers can be detrimental to positive and facilitative working relationships.

Some of the more isolated groups in Appalachia speak an Elizabethan English, which has its own distinct vocabulary and syntax and can cause communication difficulties for those who are not familiar with it. Some examples of variations in pronunciation for words are *allus* for "always" and *fit* for "fight." Word meanings that may be different include *poke* or *sack* for "paper bag" and *sass* for "vegetables." The Appalachian region is also noted for its use of strong preterits such as *clum* for "climbed," *drug* for "dragged," and *swelled* for "swollen." Plural forms of monosyllabic words are formed like Chaucerian English, which adds *es* to the word, for example: "post" becomes *postes*, "beast" becomes *beastes*, "nest" becomes *nestes*, and "ghost" becomes *ghostes*. Many people, especially in the nonacademic environment, drop the *g* on words ending in *ing*. For example, "writing" becomes *writin'*, "reading" becomes *readin'*, and "spelling" becomes *spellin'*. In addition, vowels may be pronounced with a diphthong that can cause difficulty to one unfamiliar with this dialect; hence, *poosh* for "push," *boosh* for "bush," *warsh* for "wash," *hiegen* for "hygiene," *deef* for "deaf," *welks* for "welts," *whar* for "where," *hit* for "it," *hurd* for "heard," and *your'n* for "your." However, when the word is written, the meaning is apparent. Comparatives and superlatives are formed by adding a final *er* or *est*, making the word "bad" become *badder* and "preaching" become *preachin'est* (Wilson, 1989).

If health-care workers are unfamiliar with the exact meaning of a word, it is best to ask clients to explain. Otherwise, miscommunication can occur and will probably result in incorrect diagnoses and/or other poor health outcomes. The health-care worker may want to ask the person to write the words (if the person has writing skills) to help prevent errors in communication and to improve outcomes and following directions with health prescriptions and treatments.

CULTURAL COMMUNICATION PATTERNS

Appalachians practice the ethic of neutrality, which helps shape communication styles, their worldview, and other aspects of the Appalachian culture. Four dominant themes affect communication patterns in the Appalachian culture: (1) avoiding aggression and assertiveness, (2) not interfering with others' lives unless asked to do so, (3) avoiding dominance over others, and (4) avoiding arguments and seeking agreement (Smith & Tessaro, 2005).

Appalachians often tend to accept others and do not want to judge others. This value is reflected in written and oral communications in which fewer adjectives and adverbs are used. Thus, many Appalachians may be less precise in describing their emotions, may be more concrete in conversations, and will answer questions in a more direct manner. Accordingly, the health-care worker may need to use more open-ended questions when obtaining health information and eliciting opinions and beliefs about health-care practices. Otherwise, Appalachian clients are likely to give a yes or no answer without expanding or clarifying their answers.

In general, Appalachians are a very private people who do not want to offend others, nor do they easily trust or share their thoughts and feelings with *outsiders*. They are more likely to say what they think the listener wants to hear rather than what the listener needs to hear. In addition, because of past, and often unfavorable, experiences with large mining and timber companies, many Appalachians dislike authority figures and institutions that attempt to control their behavior. Individualism and self-reliant behavior are idealized; personalism and individualism are admired; and people are accepted on the basis of their personal achievements, qualities, and family lineage.

Appalachians' perceptions of themselves, their community, and their families influence many aspects of their communication styles. Families are more than genetic relationships and are described as including brothers, sisters, aunts, uncles, parents, grandparents, cousins, in-laws, and out-laws (those related by marriage). This perception of family and community transcends the concept of self as "I." The use of the pronoun "we" throughout speech patterns recognizes the concept of self. Thus, "we can make it," "we will survive," "we will be there" may refer to only the person speaking.

An example of a typical interaction in an Appalachian community may be illustrated by this statement from a key informant in the Counts and Boyle (1987) Genesis Project, which took place from 1985 to 1994. Miss Ruth, a 94-year-old native Appalachian, was interviewed in the house in which she was born. In fact, she had her appendix removed in the living room of this same house by a traveling nurse. After returning from a trip to Africa (she had a doctorate and liked to travel, but always returned home), Miss Ruth described the concept of "neighboring" as a double-edged sword. The positive side is that when you are sick, everyone comes around to take care of you; however, on the negative side, when you try to do something quietly, everyone knows about it.

Appalachians may be sensitive to direct questions about personal issues. Sensitive topics are best approached with indirect questions and suggestions and any critical innuendo. Appalachians are taught to deny anger and not complain. Information should be gathered in the context of broader relationships with respect for the ethic of equality, which implies more horizontal than hierarchical relationships, allowing cordiality to precede information sharing. Starting with sensitive issues may invite ineffectiveness; thus, the health-care worker may need to "sit a spell" and "chat" before getting down to the business of collecting health information. To establish trust, the health-care worker must show interest in the community, the client's family, and other personal matters, drop hints instead of give orders, and solicit the client's opinions and advice. These actions increase the client's self-worth and self-esteem and helps to establish the trust needed for an effective working relationship.

Traditional Appalachians value personal physical space, so they are more likely to stand at a distance when talking with people in both social and health-care situations. This physical distancing has its origins in religious persecution endured by this group in their history and has been perpetuated by a social isolationism that has encouraged family members to become the main social contact (Coyne, Demian-Popescu, & Friend, 2006). Therefore, many people may perceive direct eye contact, especially from strangers, as an aggressive or hostile act. Staring is considered bad manners.

To communicate effectively with Appalachian clients, nonverbal behavior must be assessed within the contextual framework of the culture. Many Appalachians are comfortable with silence, and when talking with health-care providers who are outsiders, they are likely to speak without emotion, facial expression, or gestures and avoid telling unpleasant news to avoid hurting someone's feelings. Health-care providers who are unfamiliar with the culture may interpret these nonverbal communication patterns as not caring. Within this context, the health-care provider needs to allow sufficient time to develop rapport by dropping hints instead of giving orders (Coyne et al., 2006).

VIGNETTE 5.2

Dr. Smythe has just finished his residency training and has moved to a small town in Appalachia to serve out his commitment of government service as payment for medical school. He is married and has three school-aged children. He is opening a general medical practice with another physician who has lived in the area for 30 years and is getting ready to retire. The community in which he will live is approximately 150 miles from any large metropolitan area. Although shopping areas are limited, the community does support several schools, churches, and community centers. In fact, the community boasts the prowess of their "boys" and "girls" basketball teams who generally finish high in the state rankings each year. Most of the families who live here can trace their heritage back 200 or more years. Once Dr. Smythe has moved in, he sends his children out of the area to boarding schools, and he and his wife travel to the larger city to attend church on Sundays. His wife is seldom observed shopping in local stores. He prefers to spend his "off-time" playing golf with fellow physicians from larger, neighboring communities and has, so far, not engaged in community service activities.

1. How do you think the community will respond to Dr. Smythe and his family? How might the local people perceive him?
2. What do you think Dr. Smythe and his family will need to do to be accepted into the community?
3. Identify potential communication problems that might arise in the clinical setting between Dr. Smythe and his patients.

TEMPORAL RELATIONSHIPS

The traditional Appalachian culture is "being"-oriented (i.e., living for today) as compared with "doing"-oriented (i.e., planning for the future). A being orientation not only opposes progress but also may mean ignoring expert advice and "accepting one's lot in life." With the potential for economic and cultural lag, other problems may be more pressing, and "just getting by" may be the most important activity. Health-care workers must realize that

the emphasis on illness prevention in our current society is still relatively new for many Appalachians (GMEC, 2001). For those living in poverty and isolation, the trend is to "live for today" and to rely on more traditional approaches for those things that cannot be controlled. This worldview is common with present-oriented societies, in which some higher power is in charge of life and its outcomes, but it is a deterrent to preventive health services. With a fatalistic view in which individuals have little or no control over nature and the time of death is "predetermined by God," one frequently hears expressions such as "I'll be there, God willing and if the crick [creek] don't rise." As communication systems such as televisions, satellite dishes, and the Internet become more commonplace, temporal relationships are becoming more future-oriented.

For the traditional Appalachian, life is unhurried and body rhythms, not the clock, control activities. One may come early or late for an appointment and still expect to be seen. If individuals are not seen because they are late for an appointment and are asked to reschedule, they are likely to not return because they may feel rejected. Many Appalachians are hesitant to make appointments because "somethin' better might come up."

Appalachians who live outside the area usually talk about, and sometimes even dwell upon, "home" in a nostalgic way. To some, this might seem like a glorification of a past temporal orientation. However, these authors believe that it is nostalgia for "the way things used to be" as, in reality, most people do not want to return to the harshness of the life experienced by past generations.

FORMAT FOR NAMES

Although the format for names in Appalachia follows the standard given name plus family name, individuals address nonfamily members by their last name. A common practice that denotes neighborliness with respect is to call a person by his or her first name with the title Mr. or Miss (pronounced "miz" similar to "Ms.," when referring to women, whether single or married); for example, Miss Lillian or Mr. Bill. Miss Lillian may or may not be married. There is also a need to provide a link with both families of origin. Many times Appalachians refer to a married woman as "she was [born] a . . . ," thus linking the families and enhancing the feeling of continuity.

To communicate effectively with traditional Appalachians, health-care workers must not ignore speech patterns; they must clarify any differences in word meanings, translate medical terminology into everyday language using concrete terms, explain not only what is to be done but also why, and ask clients to repeat or demonstrate instructions to ensure understanding. Adopting an attitude of respect and flexibility demonstrates interest and helps bridge barriers imposed by health-care workers' personal ideologies and cultural values. Throughout history, Appalachians have enjoyed storytelling, a practice that still continues; accordingly, some individuals may respond better to verbal instructions and education, with reinforcement from videos rather than printed communications.

Family Roles and Organization

HEAD OF HOUSEHOLD AND GENDER ROLES

In previous decades, gender roles for Appalachian men and women were more clearly defined. Men were supposed to do physical work, to support the family financially, and to provide transportation. Women took care of the house and assumed responsibility for child rearing. Self-made individuals and families, those who carried out their own subsistence and depended little on outsiders, were idealized.

The traditional Appalachian household continues to be patriarchal, although many families are becoming more egalitarian in their beliefs and practices. This is especially true if the woman makes more money than the man. Women are generally the providers of emotional strength, with older women having a lot of clout in health-care matters. Older women are usually responsible for preparing herbal remedies and folk medicines and are sought out by family members and neighbors for these preparations. Older women have a higher status in the community than older men, who in turn have a higher status than younger women. With the advent of better access to education and improved transportation throughout the Appalachian region, more women are working outside the home, thus creating an environment in which gender roles are becoming more egalitarian.

PRESCRIPTIVE, RESTRICTIVE, AND TABOO BEHAVIORS FOR CHILDREN AND ADOLESCENTS

Children are important to the Appalachian culture (Coyne et al., 2006). Large families are common and children are usually accepted regardless of whether the parents are married. Parents may impose strict social conformity for family members in fear of community censure and their own parental feelings of inferiority. Permissive behavior at home is unacceptable, and hands-on physical punishment, to a degree that some perceive as abuse, is common. For Appalachian children who have problems with school performance, the most effective approach to increase performance is to provide individualized attention rather than group support or attention, an approach that is congruent with the ethic of neutrality. To be effective in changing negative behavior, it is necessary to emphasize positive points.

As children progress into their teens, mischievous behavior is accepted but not condoned. Continuing formal education may not be stressed because many teens are expected to get a job to help support the family. Children are seen as being important, and to many, having a child, even at an early age (less than 18 years), means fulfillment. Motherhood increases the woman's status in the church and the community. In previous generations, it was not uncommon for teenagers to marry by the age of 15, and some as early as 13. Children, single or married, may return to their parents' home, where they are readily accepted, whenever the need arises.

Teens in Appalachia are often in a cultural dilemma upon exposure to other lifestyles outside the home and family. Health-care workers can assist adolescents and family members in working through these cultural differences by helping them resolve personal conflicts. One way is to promote a positive self-awareness that conveys a respect for their culture, by discussing personal parenting practices, and by providing information about health promotion and wellness; disease, illness, and injury prevention; and health restoration and maintenance in a culturally congruent way.

FAMILY GOALS AND PRIORITIES

Appalachian families take great pride in being independent and doing things for themselves. Even though economics may permit paying others to do some tasks, great pride is taken in being able to do for oneself. This is an area in which one of the authors can still strongly relate to Appalachian roots. Even though reaching a financial position at which he can pay someone to do chores on home and farm, he continues to take pride in doing them for himself. For many, family priorities include men getting a job and making a living and, for women, bearing children. Traditionally, nuclear and extended families are important in the Appalachian culture, so family members frequently live in close proximity. Relatives are sought for advice on child rearing and most other aspects of daily living.

Elders are respected and honored in the Appalachian family. Grandparents frequently care for grandchildren, especially if both parents work. This form of child care is readily accepted and is an expectation in large extended families. Elders usually live close to or with their children when they are no longer able to care for themselves. The physical structure of the home is designed to assist aging parents. Many adult children do not consider nursing home placement because it is the equivalent of a death sentence. Migration of children out of the home area may force many older people to relocate outside their home area to be with their children. A dilemma occurs because they have an equally strong Appalachian value of attachment to place and family. As a compromise, some practice "snow birding"—leaving their home in the winter and moving in with their children, then returning to their home in the summer. It is not unusual for adult children to drive 3 to 5 hours on days off work to spend time with and help maintain their aging parents at their homes in Appalachia.

One's obligation to extended family outweighs the obligations to school or work. The nuclear family feels a personal responsibility for nieces and nephews and readily takes in relatives when the need arises. This extended family is important regardless of the socioeconomic level. Upon migration to urban areas, the nuclear family becomes dominant because the extended family is usually left behind in Appalachia. This strong sense of family, in which the family distrusts outsiders and values privacy, can be a deterrent to getting involved in community activities or joining self-help group activities.

The Appalachian family network can be a rich resource for the health-care worker when health teaching and assistance with personalized care are needed. For programs with Appalachians to be effective, support must begin with the family, specifically the grandmothers, and immediate neighborhood activities. The health-care worker must respect each person as an individual and be nonbureaucratic in nature. The family, rather than the individual, must be considered as the basic treatment unit.

Social status is gained from having the respect of family and friends. Formal education and position do not gain one respect. Respect has to be earned by proving that one is a good person and "living right." Living right is based on the ethic of neutrality and on being a good "Christian person." Having a job, regardless of what the work might be, is as important as having a prestigious position. Families are very proud of their family members and let the entire community know about their accomplishments. In some instances, migration to the city may result in mixed views toward one's status. Monetary gain does not necessarily improve one's status in the family and community. Rather, skills and character traits that allow one to achieve financial comfort are given high status.

ALTERNATIVE LIFESTYLES

Alternative lifestyles including single and divorced parents are usually readily accepted in the Appalachian culture. Same-sex couples and families living together are accepted, but rarely discussed. Such acceptance is congruent with the ethic of neutrality, the Appalachian need for privacy, not interfering with other's lives unless asked to do so, avoiding arguments, and seeking agreement, even though agreement may be implied rather than spoken.

Workforce Issues

CULTURE IN THE WORKPLACE

As many Appalachians value family above all else, reporting to work may become less of a priority when a family member is ill or other family obligations are pressing. When family illnesses occur, many Appalachian individuals willingly quit their jobs to care for family members. For some, the preferred work pattern is to work for an extended period of time, take some time off, and then return to work. Although work patterns may change, a deep-seated work ethic exists. Liberal leave policies for funerals and family emergencies are seen as a necessary part of work environment.

Because personal space is important, many Appalachians use a greater distance when communicating in the workplace. Close, face-to-face encounters, hugs, and the like are rarely seen. A harmonious environment that fosters cooperation and agreement in decision making is valued and desired. Health-care workers who come from outside the area may have some difficulty establishing rapport in the workplace if they lack an understanding and appreciation for Appalachian workplace etiquette.

Appalachian individuals usually wish to maintain independent lifestyles and often frown upon or not engage in the latest fads of the larger, macroculture. Although most people want progress, they also wish to remain isolated from the mainstream. Thus, more tradi-

tional Appalachians may be slower to assimilate the values of middle-class society into their daily work habits.

ISSUES RELATED TO AUTONOMY

In general, a lack of leadership is not uncommon because ascribed status is more important than achieved status and because there is an attempt to keep hierarchal relationships to a minimum (Coyne et al., 2006). The Appalachian ethic of neutrality and the values of individualism and nonassertiveness, with a strong people orientation, may pose a dichotomous perception at work for outsiders who may not be familiar with the Appalachian way of life. However, when conflicts occur, mutual collaboration for seeking agreement is consistent with the ethic of neutrality. Because many Appalachians align themselves more closely with horizontal rather than hierarchical relationships, they are sometimes reluctant to take on management roles. When they do accept management roles, they take great pride in their work and in the organization as a whole.

Most middle-class Americans gain self-actualization through work and personal involvement with doing. Appalachians seek fulfillment through kinship and neighborhood activities of being. To foster positive and mutually satisfying working relationships, organizations should capitalize on individual strengths such as independence, sensitivity, and loyalty, which are recognized values in the Appalachian culture. Many Appalachians prefer to work at their own pace, devising their own work rules and methods for getting the job done. Some local factories, mines, lumber, and health-care facilities that hire managers and administrators from outside the region often provide educational seminars about the Appalachians' worldview, work culture, and way of life in order to foster cultural sensitivity and a general understanding of the people with whom they work.

Biocultural Ecology

SKIN COLOR AND OTHER BIOLOGICAL VARIATIONS

Since its first settlement, the Appalachian region has had a predominantly white population with little variation over time. Some individuals can trace their heritage to a mixture of white ancestry along with Cherokee, Apalachee, Choctaw, and other indigenous tribes of the region. A few blacks, a distinct minority of 3.2 percent, may identify themselves as Appalachian, and intermarriage with Native Americans and white settlers was not uncommon (ARC, 2006a). The influence of Native Americans and blacks can be seen in skin color along with pronounced epicanthic eye folds, high cheekbones characteristic for Native American ancestry, and darker skin tone and black, curly hair that is a characteristic in black people.

DISEASES AND HEALTH CONDITIONS

Those Appalachians who have migrated and live in the urban centers of the north are often exposed to poor housing conditions that include inadequate sewage and plumbing systems, lack of refrigeration, and various environmental problems stemming from industrial pollution (Obermiller & Brown, 2002). Even those who have remained and live in Appalachia are often exposed to substandard housing where there is a lack of safe potable water and sewage disposal (GMEC, 2000).

Although national safety programs implemented by the Occupational Safety and Health Administration have been implemented throughout Appalachia, many people are still exposed to the harmful by-products of the predominant occupations in the region—farming, textile manufacturing, mining, furniture making, and timbering (ARC, 2006a). Occupational hazards include respiratory diseases such as black lung, brown lung, emphysema, and tuberculosis. The incidence of other health conditions including hypochromic anemia, otitis media, cardiovascular diseases, female obesity, non–insulin-dependent diabetes mellitus, and parasitic infections is greater than the national norm (GMEC, 2001; Huttlinger et al., 2004a). White Appalachian residents may have a 20 percent greater chance of dying from heart disease between the ages of 35 and 64 than other white Americans. This rate may be due to limited access to healthy foods, a general lack and use of recreational facilities, and a lack of access to medical care (GMEC, 2001; Centers for Disease Control and Prevention [CDC], 2001). Appalachia is one of the areas in the United States with the highest rate of disability (Hurley & Turner, 2000).

Children are at greater risk for sudden infant death syndrome, congenital malformations, and infections. The infant mortality rate throughout the Appalachian region varies greatly, with an overall rate of 7.7 per 100 live births, which is lower than the national average of 7.9. However, the states of Alabama, Mississippi, and North Carolina have an infant mortality rate that exceeds the national rate (ARC, 2006a). Only 70 percent of children are immunized, compared with 90 percent for the nation as a whole. Childhood injuries due to burns, trauma, poisoning, child neglect, and abuse are also higher than the national average (*Voices of Appalachia*, 2001).

Cancer, suicide, and accident rates in some parts of Appalachia are significantly greater than the national average. The higher rate of cancer in Appalachia prompted the National Cancer Institute in 1999 to create the Appalachian Leadership Initiative on Cancer (ALIC) to help communities challenge cancer at the grassroots level. Through ALIC, significant progress has been made on screening for cervical and breast cancer among low-income older women (CDC, 2004).

Educational information presented in a nonjudgmental manner can have a significant impact on the health of Appalachian clients. Clients generally prefer verbal rather than printed material to obtain health-related information. In fact, an effective success strategy used by ALIC is storytelling, a strong tradition in Appalachia and one in which people can relate. Thus, the presentation of health and educational material needs to include the entire family and be linked with improvement in function in order to be taken seriously.

VARIATIONS IN DRUG METABOLISM

Current medical and research literature reports no studies specific to the pharmacodynamics of drug interactions among Appalachians. Given the diverse gene pool of many residents, the health-care worker needs to observe each individual for adverse drug interactions.

High-Risk Behaviors

Compared with non-Appalachians, Appalachians seem to be less concerned about their overall health and risks associated with smoking (Huttlinger et al., 2004a, 2004b). Their use of smokeless tobacco is the highest in the country, and deaths from tobacco-related uses are the highest in the nation (CDC, 2004). Underage use of tobacco and alcohol is widespread among teens.

The Appalachian definition of health encompasses three levels: body, mind, and spirit. This definition precludes viewing disease as a problem unless it interferes with one's functioning. Consequently, many conditions are denied or ignored until they progress to the point of decreasing function. (Nutrition practices are covered more extensively later in the chapter.)

OxyContin has become one of the most widely abused drugs in America. Dubbed "Hillbilly heroin," it has become the drug of choice for narcotic abusers in Appalachia. Although chronic pain sufferers are finding it increasingly difficult to obtain, elaborate OxyContin underground transportation systems have developed to sustain a lucrative drug trafficking business throughout many mountain communities (Hays, 2004; Lubell, 2006). There has been a tremendous response from lawmakers and law enforcement agencies throughout the region to curb the trafficking of OxyContin. The result is that many physicians have become increasingly unwilling to provide the drug, even to the cancer patients and chronic pain sufferers who need it (Lubell, 2006). One woman with cancer relates how she searched 7 months before she found a specialist near Cincinnati who would prescribe OxyContin for her (Hays, 2004).

Several states have tightened the control of Oxy-Contin. At least nine have limited Medicaid patients' access to the drug. Virginia adopted a resolution to study the use and abuse of OxyContin, whereas Kentucky has legislation pending that would restrict distribution of the drug. In Virginia, police have provided fingerprint kits to pharmacies for customers wanting OxyContin (ARC, 2006b; Lubell, 2006).

Another high-risk behavior involves the proliferation of methamphetamine laboratories throughout Appalachia. The seclusion of mountain hollows and the number of remote and available barns and sheds have contributed to the rise in methamphetamine production. This highly addictive drug is made using common ingredients such as over-the-counter (OTC) cold medications, acetone, and rock salt. Setting up a laboratory doesn't require a lot of room. Unfortunately, ingredients and recipes aren't hard to find. It is cooked up in homemade laboratories using items such as paint thinner, camping fuel, starter fluid, gasoline additives, mason jars, and coffee filters (U.S. Drug Enforcement Agency [DEA], 2006a).

Marijuana abuse and trafficking is a serious problem throughout the region and especially in the more remote areas. Tennessee is a major supplier of domestically grown marijuana. In fact, the DEA (2006b) reported that Tennessee, along with West Virginia and Kentucky, produces the majority of the U.S.'s supply of domestic marijuana. Prosecution of marijuana growers in the state has been extremely difficult owing to a lack of intelligence and because many of the domestic marijuana sites detected are so small that even if the owner/grower were identified, the U.S. Attorney would be reluctant to prosecute (DEA, 2006b).

HEALTH-CARE PRACTICES

A 10-step pattern of health-seeking behaviors has been identified among Appalachians.

1. At the onset of symptoms, Appalachians typically implement self-care practices that are usually learned from mothers.

2. When the symptoms persist, they call their mother, if she is available.

3. If the mother is unavailable, they call the female in their kin network who is perceived as knowledgeable regarding health. If a nurse is available, they may seek the nurse's advice.

4. If relief is not achieved, they use OTC medicine they have seen advertised on television for symptoms that most closely match their own.

5. If that is ineffective, they use some of "Mable's medicine" (she lives down the road, had similar symptoms, and did not finish her medicine).

6. Next, they ask the local pharmacist for a recommendation; this usually marks the first encounter with a professional health provider. (Of course, they usually do not tell the pharmacist that they tried Mable's medicine.) The pharmacist may strongly suggest that they see a health-care provider; however, on their insistence, the pharmacist may recommend another OTC medication.

7. When no relief is achieved, they seek a local health-care provider or utilize local emergency- and urgent-care centers.

8. If the condition does not resolve itself, the local health-care provider refers them to a specialist in the area or to a larger urban area (e.g., Lexington, Cincinnati).

9. The specialist treats the condition to the best of her or his ability.

10. If unsuccessful, the specialist refers him or her to the closest tertiary medical center.

These 10 steps may not always follow the sequence presented here; some steps may be skipped, and not all steps are always completed. Moreover, the time frame around these 10 steps may be several years. Often by the time typi-cal Appalachians are referred for definitive treatment, compensatory reserves have been depleted and they die at large medical centers. The story is then passed on in the "holler": "So-and-So went to [Hospital X] and died." This pattern leads to a significant mistrust of large medical centers and continued reluctance to use these facilities effectively.

Health-care workers can have a significant impact on improving a client's health-seeking behaviors by providing information early in this pattern. Nurses especially can help to reverse this pattern because they are viewed as knowledgeable, nonjudgmental, and respectful of Appalachian lifestyles.

VIGNETTE 5.3

A public health nurse is traveling to a remote area of Appalachia on a follow-up visit to check on a baby born 2 weeks ago at home with the assistance of a granny midwife. The granny midwife left a written description of the uncomplicated, term birth for the nurse so the nurse is making a service visit to talk with the new mother about well-baby care, immunization schedules, and nutrition and to answer any questions that the mother, aged 17, might have about the care of her new infant. Travel to the home is along unpaved and winding roads with no signage. Upon reaching her destination, the nurse notes that the family is living in a clearing in a mobile home. There is no sign of electricity, but she sees a gasoline-powered generator on one side of the dwelling and hears the sounds of a stream nearby. Three shedlike buildings are within 150 feet of the home. She tries to call into the public health department to tell them that she has arrived at her destination, as per protocol, but there is no reception for her cell phone. As she exits her car, she notes that one of the buildings has a small greenhouse behind it and another has a "chemical"-smelling smoke coming from a chimney. Several cooking pans, milk cartons, kerosene cans, and other debris are piled outside of the building with the smoke.

1. Given the location and description of this home, what activity do you believe might be taking place?
2. Discuss courses of action the nurse should take.
3. Should the nurse continue with her original assignment? Why? Why not?

Nutrition

MEANING OF FOOD

As with most ethnic and cultural groups, food has meaning beyond providing nutritional sustenance. To many Appalachians, wealth means having plenty of food for family, friends, and social gatherings. One should drink plenty of fluids and eat plenty to have a strong body. A strong body is a healthy body. Food and the sharing of food has broad social implications. Appalachians love to get together with family members, friends, and neighbors for meals. Weekend meals at a family member's home are common and serve as a mechanism to share information, community events and happenings, and gossip. Church suppers are also commonplace, with members contributing favorite dishes.

COMMON FOODS AND FOOD RITUALS

Many Appalachians, and especially those living in the more remote areas, include wild game in their diet. Muskrat, groundhog, rabbit, squirrel, duck, turkey, and venison commonly supplement "store-bought" meats. Wild game traditionally has a lower fat content than meat raised for commercial purposes. However, consistent with traditional practices from previous decades, most parts of both wild and domesticated animals are eaten. High-cholesterol organ meats such as tongue, liver, heart, lungs (called *lights*), and brains are considered delicacies. Bone marrow is used to make sauces, and stomach, intestines (chitlins or chitterlings), pigs' feet, tail, and ribs are also commonly eaten. Low-fat game meat is usually breaded and fried with lard or animal fat, negating the overall gains from these low-fat meat sources. Most diets include sweet prepackaged drinks, Kool-Aid with added sugar, very sweet iced tea, and soda.

Food preparation practices may increase dietary risk factors for cardiac disease because many recipes contain lard and meats are preserved with salt. Other common foods in particular regions of Appalachia that may be unfamiliar to non-native Appalachians are sweet potato pie; molasses candy; apple beer; gooseberry pie; pumpkin cake; and pickled beans, fruit, corn, beets, and cabbage, all of which are high in sodium. Frying foods with bacon grease or lard was once a common practice, but recent publicity on the dangers of lard have initiated a cut-back in its use in cooking (Huttlinger et al., 2004a). Fried green tomatoes, biscuits, and thick gravies are favorites.

Appalachians celebrate Thanksgiving, Christmas, other national and religious holidays, and many other occasions with food. In rural areas, people celebrate with food when game and livestock are slaughtered because this is usually an extended-family or community affair. The value of self-reliance is enhanced during the "cannin'" season when foodstuffs are preserved. Canning becomes a social or family occasion and is an excellent avenue for health teaching if the health-care provider is willing to participate and learn. Additional celebrations with food occur during times of death and grieving, when friends and participants bring dishes specifically prepared for the occasion.

DIETARY PRACTICES FOR HEALTH PROMOTION

Many Appalachians believe that good nutrition has an effect on one's health. In one study with rural Appalachians, young mothers were asked what it meant to eat well for good health. They referred to "taking fluids" and "eating right," but they were unable to describe healthy eating patterns any further (Gainor, Fitch, & Pollard, 2006). Because of health intervention programs, publicity though television, magazines, newspapers, and the internet, residents of most Appalachian communities are aware of "good foods" and "bad foods" in terms of general health. However, a lack of money and having a meager budget including Food Stamps may limit choices.

Many believe that the sooner a baby can take food other than milk, the healthier it will be. At one time, babies from the first month were fed grease, sugar, and coffee to promote hardiness, but the practice seems to have fallen by the wayside with the younger generations of mothers. One author fondly remembers being fed teaspoons of bacon grease as a child to be sure to growing up strong and healthy. Another example is a family who saved the skin from fried chicken for the author to eat to increase his body fat, because they believed that he was too thin. The Women, Infants, and Children program, commonly known as WIC, has done much to change some of these practices. Health-care workers have a rich opportunity to provide education in healthy eating practices. Factual information that describes health risks with early feeding of solid foods may help prevent later nutritional allergies in children.

An example of how a community intervention can work is illustrated by the decrease in the incidence of hypertension in one community. A local health-care worker participated in the cannin' of beans and showed the residents that the beans would remain crisp with a "tige (a pinch) of vinegar" rather than a "pile of salt." It is essential for health-care workers to assess specific food practices and food preparation practices in order to provide effective dietary counseling for health promotion and wellness. Health-care workers in clinics and school settings have an excellent opportunity to have a positive impact on the nutritional status of individuals and families. School breakfast and lunch programs, Meals on Wheels, and church-sponsored meal plans are some of the ways in which health-care workers can encourage and support families to attain better nutrition practices.

NUTRITIONAL DEFICIENCIES AND FOOD LIMITATIONS

A common practice for rural and urban Appalachian children is to replace meals with snacks. The most common snacks are candy, salty foods, desserts, and carbonated beverages. Many adolescents skip breakfast and lunch entirely, preferring to eat snack foods. This pattern of snacking can result in deficiencies in vitamin A, iron, and calcium.

No specific food limitations or enzyme deficiencies exist among Appalachians. With subsistence farming and commercial farms from nearby areas, all foods for a healthy diet are readily available during the growing season. Even though the climate is ideal for growing a large variety of vegetables, broccoli, cauliflower, or asparagus are rarely seen as vegetables of choice in the mountainous regions of Appalachia.

Pregnancy and Childbearing Practices

FERTILITY PRACTICES AND VIEWS TOWARD PREGNANCY

Birth outcomes among some regions of Appalachia are poorer than among middle-class white groups in rural, suburban, and urban populations. In one study comparing birth outcomes among rural, rural-adjacent, and urban women, rural women had the worst birth outcomes overall; rural-adjacent women had the best birth outcomes of the three groups, yet were the youngest, least educated, least likely to be married, and least likely to be privately insured (Gainor et al., 2006). Contraceptive practices of Appalachians follow the general pattern of the U.S. population. Methods include birth control pills, condoms, and tubal ligation; abortion is an individual choice. A popular belief among many is that taking laxatives facilitates an abortion. As a group, a disproportionate number of teenage pregnancies occur at a younger age compared with non-Appalachians.

Fertility practices and sexual activity, both sensitive topics for many teenagers, are areas in which outsiders unknown to the family may be more effective than health-care practitioners who are known to the family. To be effective, counseling by the health-care provider must be accomplished within the cultural belief patterns of this group and must be approached in a nonhierarchical manner, preferably with a health-care provider of the same gender.

PRESCRIPTIVE, RESTRICTIVE, AND TABOO PRACTICES IN THE CHILDBEARING FAMILY

Although the literature reports no specific research or studies related to prescriptive, restrictive, or taboo practices during pregnancy, the following are some of the current beliefs:

- Pregnant women subscribe to the belief that to have a healthy baby they need to eat well and take care of themselves.
- Boys are carried higher and the mother's belly appears pointy, whereas girls are carried low.
- The expectant mother should not have her picture taken because it can cause a stillbirth.
- Reaching over one's head can cause the cord to strangle the baby.
- Wearing an opal ring during pregnancy may harm the baby.
- Being frightened by a snake or eating strawberries or citrus fruit can cause birthmarks.
- If the mother experiences a tragedy, a congenital anomaly may occur.
- If the mother craves a particular food during her pregnancy, then she should eat that food or the baby will have a birthmark resembling the craved food.

Childbearing is a family affair. The birthing mother is expected to accept childbirth as a short, intense, natural process that will bring her closer to the earth and must be endured (Gainor et al., 2006).

The literature reports no specific studies on beliefs related to postpartum practices. When a new baby is born, relatives and extended family members gather to assist the new mother with household chores until she is able to complete them herself. Some newborns wear a band around the abdomen to prevent umbilical hernias and an asafetida bag around the neck to prevent or ward off contagious disease. The health-care professional pro-viding pregnancy counseling to the Appalachian family needs to demonstrate an openness to discuss cultural differences.

Death Rituals

DEATH RITUALS AND EXPECTATIONS

When a death is expected, family and friends may stay through the night and prepare food for the event. Because death is such an important occasion in Appalachia, many employers give workers 3 days of funeral leave for deaths of extended family members. After a death, extended family and friends may spend the night with the deceased's immediate family to prevent loneliness.

Deaths in Ohio, Michigan, and other adjoining states are frequently published in Appalachian newspapers with a notice that the individual will be returned to their mountain home for burial. Funeral services serve an important social function and are usually simple. This is a time when extended family and friends come together for services that can last for 3 hours or longer. The length of time for a service varies according to the age of the deceased. The service for an older person may be longer than that for a younger person. The body is displayed for hours, either in the home or at the church, so that all those who wish to view the body can do so. At the end of the service, all who wish to can view the body again, with the closest relative being the last. Many Appalachian families go to funeral homes that specialize in personal services to the Appalachian culture. Urban Appalachian areas have funeral homes that specialize in long-distance transport for burial and have become familiar with Appalachian customs to meet culturally specific requirements.

The deceased is usually buried in her or his best clothes. Some individuals have a custom-made set of clothes in which to be buried and may even design their own funeral services long before their death. A common practice is to bury the deceased with personal possessions. At the funeral home, the person's favorite chair, a picture of the deceased, or other personal items may be displayed. Flowers are more important than donations to a charity. Cremation is an acceptable practice, and disposition of the ashes is a personal decision. After the funeral services are completed, elaborate meals are served either in the home or at the church. Services are accompanied by singing before, during, and after the service. Cemeteries throughout Appalachia show frequent visitations and give a sense of place and relationship to the land. Plots are carefully tended with displays of flowers, wreaths, and flags. Other beliefs regarding burial practices include placing graveyards on hillsides for fear that graves may be flooded out in low-lying areas. If the body is exhumed and reburied, it is believed that the person may not go to heaven.

RESPONSES TO DEATH AND GRIEF

Clergy help families through the grieving process by providing counseling and support to family members. Family members, fellow church members, friends, and community leaders often assist the bereaved. Typically, family members get together and reminisce about their deceased loved one. Friends and neighbors bring food for about a week and share memories of the "one who passed on."

Spirituality

DOMINANT RELIGION AND USE OF PRAYER

The original inhabitants of Appalachia were mostly Protestant and Episcopalian. In the early settlement years, as central organization of churches was difficult to retain, people individualized their chosen church structure. Today, the predominant religions in the Appalachian region are Baptist, Methodist, Presbyterian, Holiness, Pentecostal, and Episcopalian. For most Appalachians, the church is the center for social and community activities. Some of the more religiously devout pray daily whether or not they formally attend church. Very often, religious beliefs are of a spiritual nature and not tied to the tenets of any singular faith and reflect the harmony of the mountains and being at one with life.

In addition to Protestant and Episcopalians, there are congregations of Roman Catholics and Jehovah's Witnesses as well as other groups who, although they call themselves Baptists, are not associated with the national church organization. These Baptist "sects" are quite diverse and have important central beliefs, including the belief in autonomy at the local level. As a result, many divisions have occurred within and among churches to accommodate more personal beliefs and philosophies. Regardless of the denomination, most churches in the region stress fundamentalism in religious practices and use the King James Version of the Bible.

Many small churches have lay preachers instead of trained ministers, and there is a belief that to be a preacher, a person must have a divine calling. Thus, a minister may or may not be ordained. Many of the Baptist faiths believe that baptism must be done in a river, pond, or lake so that the body can be submerged. Another practice, feet washing, is believed to demonstrate humility and occurs when men wash men's feet and women wash women's feet. Many of the more fundamentalist churches segregate women and children from men in the seating arrangement within the church—men and older boys sit on one side, and women and children sit on the opposite side. In some churches, men sit on the right side of the church to represent the "right hand of God," while women sit on the left (Huttlinger, personal communication, 2006).

Some denominations believe in divine healing, and the region is full of examples to testify to its effectiveness. Two or more weekly services are common, and revival meetings are customary. Revivals tend to be lively, allowing individuals to shout out when the spirit moves them. Some denominations speak in tongues and believe in visions. Stringed music is played in some churches.

Some freewill churches, for example, the Holiness Church, preach against attending movies, ball games, and social functions where dancing occurs. Other sects believe in handling poisonous snakes. Although the practice is rare, it is believed that the snake will not bite those who have faith. A few people do get bitten by snakes, and their usual course of action is to heal themselves rather than to go to a hospital even though deaths occur each year following snake-handling rituals.

Another practice, the ingestion of strychnine in small doses during religious services, is believed to increase sensory stimuli. Needless to say, this practice can precipitate convulsions if ingested in large enough amounts. Fire-handling is still practiced by some groups, again with the belief that the hot coals will not burn those who have faith.

Prayer for many Appalachians is a primary source of strength. Prayer is personally designed around specific church and religious beliefs and practices, which vary widely throughout the region and between and among churches of similar faith.

MEANING OF LIFE AND INDIVIDUAL SOURCES OF STRENGTH

Meaning in life comes from the family and "living right," which is defined by each person and usually means living right with God and in the beliefs of a chosen church. Religion tends to be less focused on institutional rituals and ceremonies and consists more of personalized beliefs in God, Christ, and church. Because life in the mountainous regions can often be harsh, religious beliefs and faith make life worth living in a grim situation. The church provides a way of coping with the hurts, pains, and disappointments of a sometimes hostile environment and becomes a source for celebration and a social outlet.

Common themes that give Appalachians strength are family, traditionalism, personalism, self-reliance, religiosity, a worldview of being, and not having undue concern about things that one cannot control, such as nature and the future. Appalachians believe that rewards come in another life, in which God repays one for kind deeds done on earth.

SPIRITUAL BELIEFS AND HEALTH-CARE PRACTICES

Within the context of **fatalism** comes the belief that what happens to the individual is largely a result of God's will. Many Appalachians may not seek health care until symptoms of illness are well advanced. This practice is described more thoroughly under "High-Risk Behaviors," earlier in this chapter. Forming partnerships between health-care workers and faith-related organizations for health promotion and illness and disease prevention has strong potential for improving the health status of Appalachians. Health-care workers who are aware of clients' religious practices and spirituality needs are in a better position to promote culturally competent health care and to incorporate nonharmful practices into clients' care plans. Practitioners must indicate an appreciation and respect for the dignity and spiritual beliefs of Appalachians without expressing negative comments about differing religious beliefs and practices.

Health-Care Practices

HEALTH-SEEKING BELIEFS AND BEHAVIORS

Beliefs that influence health-care practices for many Appalachians are derived from concepts such as family, fatalism, traditionalism, self-reliance, individualism, and the ethic of neutrality. Even though many Appalachians believe that health is God's will, the concept of self-reliance can foster good health practices through self-care. Many may not see formal biomedical health-care practitioners until self-medicating and folk remedies have been exhausted. At one time, Appalachians, compared with non-Appalachians, were less likely to use the emergency room or to have private physicians, but the trend has since changed and emergency rooms and urgent-care centers are communly used (GMEC, 2000; Obermiller & Brown, 2002).

Health information on the Appalachian client should be gathered in the context of broader family relationships and cordiality that precedes information sharing, as the family rather than the individual is the basic unit for treatment. Because direct approaches are frowned upon, health-care workers need to learn to approach sensitive topics, such as contraception and alcohol and drug use, indirectly. Many Appalachians expect the health-care worker to establish an advocacy role and to understand and accept their cultural differences; thus, it is best to involve professionals from the same backgrounds, if they are available.

Huttlinger et al. (2004a) surveyed a large sample of Appalachians from southwestern Virginia and northeastern Tennessee to determine access to health care. They also addressed factors related to "good health." Over 75 percent stated that their health was "God's will," and over half stated that their families, church, and community played a vital role in their overall health and well-being.

RESPONSIBILITY FOR HEALTH CARE

When entering the biomedical health-care arena, Appalachians might feel powerless to control their own health. They often abdicate responsibility for their own care and expect that the health-care worker will completely take over their care. Many have high expectations for their health-care worker and provider, with an unrealistic dependence on the system and an abandonment of more self-reliance activities (Coyne et al., 2006).

One major health concern for many Appalachians is the state of the blood, which is described as being thick or thin, good or bad, and high or low; these conditions can be regulated through diet (Huttlinger, personal communication, 2006; Obermiller & Brown, 2002). Venereal disease and Rh-negative blood fall into the category of bad blood. Sour foods can also cause bad blood. Appalachian men, in general, report a greater number of backaches, with women reporting a greater number of headaches, than the rest of society (Coyne et al., 2006).

Self-care is a primary focus of health. Self-care is primarily perceived as an individual responsibility, and care is focused within the family rather than within the community. Because many Appalachians value the ability to respond to, and cope with, events of daily life, home remedies, treatments, and active consultation with family members are sought before seeking outside help (Huttlinger et al., 2004a). Good health is feeling well and being able to meet one's obligations. Care within the medical system is used when the condition is perceived as serious, does not respond to self-care, or has a high potential for death. Furthermore, because self-reliance activities and nature predominate over people, many believe that it is best to let nature heal. Health-care workers need to keep this in mind when giving explanations and instructions to make them more acceptable to clients and their families.

When older Appalachians go to a physician or another health-care provider, they usually expect immediate help. Physicians who dispense medications in their offices are seen as helpful; providing prescriptions may be interpreted as rejection. The average Appalachian client does not understand the restrictions and limitations that are placed on physicians and nurse practitioners with respect to dispensing "sample" medications.

Health-care workers can assist Appalachian clients by reinforcing their preferred coping methods and strategies when they are ill. The five most frequently used coping methods are helping, thinking positively, worrying about the problem, trying to find out more about the problem, and trying to handle things one step at a time. Coping strategies include talking the problem over with friends, praying, thinking about the good things in life, trying to handle things one step at a time, and trying to see the good side of the situation (Hunsucker, Flannery, & Frank, 2000). When establishing rapport, a health-care worker can go a long way in achieving trust by using churches, grange halls, and other community places (e.g., libraries, schools) as meeting places for the entire family to work with Appalachian families at the community level.

FOLK AND TRADITIONAL PRACTICES

A strong belief in folk medicine is a traditional part of the Appalachian culture. Using herbal medicines, poultices, and teas is common practice among individuals of all socioeconomic levels. Table 5–1 presents a reference guide for the health-care practitioner with the major ingredients and conditions for which the folk treatments are used. These treatments can be adjusted to accommodate prescription therapies or education regarding folk treatments. Information in this table has been derived from the *Foxfire* series, the authors' backgrounds and experiences, and health-care workers who practice in the area. Note that specific amounts are not given, and in many cases, the amounts vary from person to person, according to the geographic region and local family practices. Local names are given rather than scientific names because this is how the residents identify them. Many folk and traditional practices were learned from the Cherokee and Apalachee Indians living in the region and have been passed down from generation to generation. Although many of these home remedies are not harmful, some may have a deleterious effect when used to the exclusion of, or in combination with, prescription medications. This

TABLE 5.1   *Health Conditions and Appalachian Folk Medicine Practices*

Health Condition	Folk Medicine Practices
Arthritis	Make tea from boiling the roots of ginseng. Drink the tea or rub it on the arthritic joint.
	Mix roots of ginseng and goldenseal in liquor and drink it. Ginseng is used heavily by many Koreans and was exported to Korea in the 18th and 19th centuries.
	Eat large amounts of raw fruits and vegetables.
	Carry a buckeye around in a pocket.
	Drink tea from the stems of the barbell plant.
	Drink a mixture of honey, vinegar, and moonshine (or other liquor).
	Drink tea made from alfalfa seeds or leaves.
	Drink tea made from rhubarb and whiskey.
	Place a magnet over the joint to draw the arthritis out of the joint.
Asthma	Drink tea from the bark of wild yellow plum trees, mullein leaves, and alum. Take every 12 hr.
	Combine gin and heartwood of a pine tree. Take twice a day.
	Suck salty water up the nose.
	Smoke or sniff rabbit tobacco.
	Swallow a handful of spiderwebs.
	Smoke strong tobacco until choking occurs.
	Drink a mixture of honey, lemon juice, and whiskey.
	Inhale smoke from ginseng leaves.
Bedbugs/chiggers	Apply kerosene liberally to all parts of the body. *Caution:* Kerosene can cause significant irritation to sensitive skin, especially when exposed to sunlight.
Bleeding	Place a spiderweb across the wound. This is also used in rural Scotland.
	Put kerosene oil on the cut.
	Place soot from the fireplace into a cut. Be sure to wash out the soot after bleeding is stopped or the area will scar.
	Apply a mixture of honey and turpentine on the bleeding wound.
	Apply a mixture of soot and lard on the wound.
	Place a cigarette paper over the wound.
	Put pine resin over the cut.
	Place kerosene oil on the wound. *Caution:* If used in large doses, kerosene will burn the skin.
Blood builders	Drink tea from the bark of a wild cherry tree.
	Combine cherry bark, yellowroot, and whiskey. Take twice each day.
	Eat fried pokeweed leaves.
Blood purifiers	Drink tea from burdock root.
	Drink tea from spice wood.
Blood tonic	Take a teaspoon of honey and a tiny amount of sulfur.
	Take a teaspoon of molasses and a tiny amount of sulfur.
	Drink tea made from bloodroot.
	Soak nails in a can of water until they become rusty. Drink the rusty water.
Boils or sores	Apply a poultice of walnut leaves or the green hulls with salt.
	Apply a poultice of the houseleek plant.
	Apply a poultice of rotten apples.
	Apply a poultice of beeswax, mutton tallow, sweet oil, oil of amber, oil of spike, and resin.
	Apply a poultice of kerosene, turpentine, Vaseline, and lye soap.
	Apply a poultice of heart leaves, lard, and turpentine.
	Apply a poultice of bread and milk.
	Apply a poultice of slippery elm and pork fat.
	Apply a poultice of flaxseed meal.
	Apply a poultice of beef tallow, brown sugar, salt, and turpentine.
Burns	Apply a poultice of baking soda and water.
	Place castor oil on the burn.
	Apply a poultice of egg white and castor oil.
	Place a potato on the burn.
	Wrap the burn in a gauze and keep moist with salt water.
	Place linseed oil on the burn.

TABLE 5.1	*Health Conditions and Appalachian Folk Medicine Practices (Continued)*
Health Condition	**Folk Medicine Practices**
	Apply a poultice of lard and flour.
	Put axle grease on the burn. This is also a practice with some Germans in Minnesota.
Chapped hands and lips	Apply lard, grease, or tallow from pork or mutton.
Chest congestion	Apply a poultice of kerosene, turpentine, and lard to the chest. Make sure the poultice is not applied directly to the chest but rather on top of a cloth.
	Apply mutton tallow directly to the chest.
	Apply a warm poultice of onions and grease.
	Rub pine tar on the chest.
	Chew leaves and stems of peppermint.
	Drink a combination of ginger and sugar in hot water.
	Make a mixture of rock candy and whiskey. Take several teaspoons several times each day.
	Drink tea made from ginger, honey, and whiskey.
	Drink tea made from pine needles.
	Put goose grease on the chest.
	Drink red pepper tea.
	Eat roasted onions.
	Drink brine from pickles or kraut.
	Make tea from boneset, rosemary, and goldenrod.
	Make tea from butterfly weed.
Colic	Make tea from calamus root and catnip. (Calamus is a suspected carcinogen.)
	Tie an asafetida bag around the neck.
	Drink baking soda and water.
	Chew and swallow the juice of camel root.
	Massage stomach with warm castor oil.
	Drink ginseng tea.
Constipation	Take two tablespoons of turpentine.
	Combine castor oil and mayapple roots.
	Take castor oil or Epsom salts.
Croup	Have child wear a bib containing pine pitch and tallow.
	Apply cloth to the chest saturated with groundhog fat, turpentine, and lamp oil.
	Drink juice from a roasted onion.
	Apply a poultice of mutton tallow and beeswax to the back.
	Eat a spoonful of sugar with a drop of turpentine.
	Eat honey with lemon or vinegar.
	Eat onion juice and honey.
Diarrhea	Drink tea from the ladyslipper plant.
	Place soot in a glass of water, let the soot settle to the bottom of the glass, and drink the water.
	Drink tea made from blackberry roots.
	Drink tea from red oak bark.
	Drink blackberry or strawberry juice.
	Drink tea made from strawberry or blackberry leaves.
	Drink tea made out of willow leaves.
	Drink the juice from the bark of a white oak or a persimmon tree.
Earache	Place lukewarm salt water in the ear.
	Put castor oil or sweet oil in the ear.
	Put sewing machine oil in the ear.
	Place a few drops of urine in the ear.
	Place cabbage juice in the ear.
	Blow smoke from tobacco in the ear.
	Place a Vicks-soaked cotton ball in the ear.
Eye ailments	Place a few drops of castor oil in the eye.
	Drop warm salty water in the eye.
	Drink tea made from rabbit tobacco or snakeroot.

(Continued on following page)

TABLE 5.1	*Health Conditions and Appalachian Folk Medicine Practices (Continued)*
Health Condition	**Folk Medicine Practices**
Fever	Drink tea made from butterfly weed, wild horsemint, or feverweed.
	Mash garlic bulbs and place in a bag tied around the pulse points.
	Drink water from wild ginger.
Headache	Drink tea made of ladyslipper plants.
	Tie warm fried potatoes around the head.
	Take Epsom salts.
	Tie ginseng roots around the head.
	Place crushed onions on the head.
	Rub camphor and whiskey on the head.
Heart trouble	Drink tea made from heartleaf leaves or bleeding heart.
	Eat garlic.
High blood pressure (not to be mistaken for high blood)	Drink sarsaparilla tea.
	Drink a half cup of vinegar.
Kidney trouble	Drink tea made from peach leaves or mullein roots.
	Drink tea made from corn silk or arbutus leaves.
Liver trouble	Drink tea made from lion's tongue leaves.
	Drink tea made from the roots of the spinet plant.
Poison ivy	Urinate on the affected area.
	Take a bath in salt water and then apply Vaseline.
	Wash the area with bleach.
	Wash the area with the juice of the milkweed plant.
	Apply a poultice of gunpowder and buttermilk.
	Apply baking soda to wet skin.
Sore throat	Gargle with sap from a red oak tree.
	Eat honey and molasses.
	Eat honey and onions.
	Drink honey and whiskey.
	Tie a poultice of lard of cream with turpentine and Vicks to the neck.
	Apply a poultice of cottonseed to the throat.
	Swab the throat with turpentine.

should be evident from the 10-step pattern health-seeking behaviors among Appalachians presented in the section on health-care practices.

Because ingredients in some of these herbal medicines can have serious side effects, especially if taken in large quantities, health-care providers must become familiar with folk medicines used by Appalachians as part of client assessments. Health-care workers must ascertain whether individuals intend to use folk medicines simultaneously with prescription medications and treatment regimens so that these remedies can be incorporated into the plan of care and that dialogue can be undertaken to prevent adverse effects. Health-care workers who integrate folk medicine into allopathic prescriptions have a greater chance of improving clients' compliance with health prescriptions and interventions. Health-care workers must remember that today's scientific medicine may be traditional or folk medicine to the next generation.

BARRIERS TO HEALTH CARE

Barriers to health care for Appalachians are numerous and center on accessibility, affordability, adaptability, accept-ability, appropriateness, and awareness. Bureaucratic, written forms foster fear and suspicion of health-care workers, which can lead to confusion, distrust, and negative stereotyping by both parties. Some individuals fear "being cut on" or "going under the knife" and feel that a hospital is a place where you go to give birth or die.

As noted earlier, the rugged terrain and distance to health-care facilities and service is a deterrent to accessing services. Even though ARC has sponsored road-building campaigns in the mountainous regions of Appalachia since 1965, transportation problems continue to exist in parts of the region (see Fig. 5–1). The high rate of unemployment in Appalachia means that many people cannot afford basic health care. A disproportionate number of Appalachians, especially those who are self-employed, unemployed, or underemployed, do not have health insurance. For some who do not believe in owing money, seeing a health-care provider may be postponed until the condition is severe or until they have the money. If services can be offered on a sliding scale, more people may be willing to access them.

Health-care facilities are closing in some areas of Appalachia. Most often, the closings are related to decreasing availability of health-care workers and the ability to pay competitive salaries, especially for registered nurses (Huttlinger, personal communication, 2006). These changes have resulted in the relocation of highly educated and trained professionals of all professions.

Recent studies have demonstrated that there is not a lack of primary-care providers in Appalachia (Huttlinger et al., 2004a). The shortage of primary-care providers resulted in a large portion of health-care being provided by nurses, which continues today in some areas. There is, however, an acute shortage of specialty providers in respiratory and pulmonary diseases, oncology, dental services, and ophthalmology. Those physicians who settle in the region quickly learn that flexible fee schedules, patience, and hands-on treatment approaches work best. Referral to "specialty" care in the larger urban centers must be made with consideration of travel and other expenses. For example, a referral to a pulmonologist in Charlottesville, Virginia, for a person who lives in Wise might require a 3-day trip: 1 full 8-hour day of travel each way, with the expense of gasoline, a relative taking off work to drive the person, and 2 nights in a motel. For some, this is an expense that simply cannot be incurred.

Preventive health services have not been stressed in the past and are not perceived as important by many (GMEC, 2001). Even when services are available, people may feel they are not delivered in an appropriate manner. Outsider health-care workers may be seen as disrespectful of Appalachian ways and self-care practices, and clients may see the health-care workers advice as criticism. If the health-care worker uses language that the patient does not understand, the health-care worker may be perceived as "stuck up." Many Appalachians do not like the impersonal care delivered in large clinics and, therefore, shop around and ask friends and family for suggestions for a private health-care provider. "Sittin' for a spell and engagin' in small talk" with the patient before an examination or treatment will help ensure return visits for follow-up care.

When health-care facilities have limited hours or are not adaptable, patients may not return for scheduled appointments. For example, a mother may bring her child in for an immunization. If the mother has a health problem and perhaps needs a Pap smear, she may be willing to have the test performed while having the child examined. However, if she is given an appointment to return at a later date, she may not keep the appointment because it is too far to travel for a problem she sees as nonurgent. If services are not available during evening hours, people may be afraid of taking time off during regular work hours for fear of losing their job.

CULTURAL RESPONSES TO HEALTH AND ILLNESSES

Appalachians take care of their own and accept a person as a "whole individual." Thus, those with mental impairments or physical handicaps are generally accepted into their communities and not turned away. The mentally handicapped are not crazy but are seen as having "bad nerves," "quite turned," or "odd turned." Appalachians may label certain behaviors as "lazy," "mean," "immoral," "criminal," or "psychic" and recommend punishment by

either the social group or the legal system or tolerance of these behaviors (Obermiller & Brown, 2002).

Traditional Appalachians believe that disability is a natural and inevitable part of the aging process. Their culture of being discourages the use of rehabilitation as an option. To establish trust and rapport when working with Appalachian clients with chronic diseases, health-care workers must avoid assumptions regarding health beliefs and provide health maintenance interventions within the scope of cultural customs and beliefs.

Individual responses to pain cannot be classified among Appalachians. The Appalachian background is too varied, and no studies regarding cultural beliefs about pain could be found in the literature. For many Appalachians, pain is something that is to be endured and accepted stoically. However, when a person becomes ill or has pain, personal space collapses inward, and the person expects to be waited on and to be cared for by others. A belief among many is that if one places a knife or axe under the bed or mattress of a person in pain, the knife will help cut the pain. This practice occurs with childbearing and other conditions that cause pain. The authors are aware of an Appalachian woman who requested to have a knife or axe placed under the bed or mattress postoperatively to help cut (or decrease) the pain associated with surgery. One of the authors offered a small pocketknife or butter knife to place under the bed. Both were unacceptable as the pocketknife was too small and the butter knife was too dull to be of use. A sharp meat-cutting knife from the kitchen was deemed appropriate because it was both large enough and sharp enough to help cut the pain.

BLOOD TRANSFUSIONS AND ORGAN DONATION

Appalachians generally do not have any specific rules or taboos about receiving blood, donating organs, or undergoing organ transplantation. These decisions are largely one's own, but advice is usually sought from family and friends.

Health-Care Practitioners

TRADITIONAL VERSUS BIOMEDICAL PRACTITIONERS

For decades, both lay and trained nurses have provided significant health-care services, including obstetrics. Grannies midwives and more formally trained midwives have provided obstetric services throughout the history of Appalachia. Although many practitioners and herbalists are older women, men may also become healers. Grannies and herb doctors are trusted and known to the individual and the community for giving more personalized care.

The entire Appalachian area has a shortage of health personnel even though recent years have evidenced a good supply of primary-care providers, thanks to government incentives for medical school loans. As a result and as mentioned before, nurses have delivered the bulk of health care to some areas of Appalachia (Huttlinger et al., 2004a, 2004b).

The Frontier Nursing Service, started by Mary Brecken-ridge, is one of the oldest and most well-known nurse-run clinics in the United States and is a notable example of nurses taking the initiative to provide health care in Appalachia. It was started in one of the most rural areas of Appalachia in response to a lack of physicians and the high birth and child mortality rates in the area (Dawley, 2003; Jesse & Blue, 2004). Many Appalachians prefer to go to *insider* health-care professionals, especially in the more rural areas, because the system of payment for services is accepted on a sliding scale, and in some communities, even an exchange of goods for health services exists. One nurse-practitioner in private practice states that the only time she locks her car is when the zucchini are "in." If she does not, when she gets in her car after a clinic session, she has no room to drive because of all the "presents" of the large vegetable.

Locally respected Appalachians are engaged to facilitate acceptance of outside programs and of the staff who participate at the grassroots level in planning and initiating programs. For Appalachian clients to become more accepting of biomedical care, it is important for health-care providers to approach individuals in an unhurried manner consistent with their relaxed lifestyle, to engage clients in decision making and care planning, and to use locally trained support staff whenever possible.

STATUS OF HEALTH-CARE PROVIDERS

Most herbal and folk practitioners are highly respected for their treatments, mostly because they are well known to their people and trusted by those who need health care. Physicians and other health-care professionals are frequently seen as outsiders to the Appalachian population and are, therefore, mistrusted. This initial mistrust is rooted in outsider behaviors that exploited the Appalachian people and took their land for timbering and coal mining in earlier generations. Trust for an outsider is gained slowly. Once the person gets to know and trust the health-care provider, the provider is given much respect. Trust and respect for health-care providers depend more on personal characteristics and personal behavior than on knowledge.

In terms of provider care, Appalachians seem to prefer home-based nurses, health-care workers, and social workers. To obtain full cooperation, the health-care provider needs to ask clients what they consider to be the problem before devising a plan of care. If the provider begins with an immediate diagnosis without considering the patient's explanation, there is a good chance that the provider's treatment or recommendation will be ignored. Lastly, it is important to decrease language barriers by decoding the jargon of the health-care environment.

REFERENCES

Appalachian Regional Commission (ARC). (2006a). Available at http://www.arc.gov Contains various articles on economics, populations statistics, health-care delivery, education, and general life in Appalachia.

Appalachian Regional Commission (ARC). (2006b). Twenty-six communities awarded seed grants to battle substance abuse in Appalachia. News Brief. http://arc.gov Viewed 01/03/07.

Centers for Disease Control and Prevention (CDC). (2001). http://www.cdc.gov

Centers for Disease Control and Prevention (CDC). (2004). CDC report shows cancer death rates in Appalachia higher than national. https://www.scienceblog.com/community

Costello, C. (2000, May 30). Beneath myth, Melungeons find roots of oppression: Appalachian descendants embrace heritage. *The Washington Post*, p. A4.

Counts, M. M., & Boyle, J. S. (1987). Nursing, health, and policy within a community context. *Advances in Nursing Science, 9*(3), 12–23.

Coyne, C., Demian-Popescu, C., & Friend, D. (2006). Social and cultural factors influencing health in southern West Virginia: A qualitative study. *Preventing Chronic Disease, 3*(4), A. 124.

Dawley, K. (2003). Origins of nurse-midwifery in the United States and its expansion in the 1940s. *Journal of Midwifery and Womens' Health, 48*(2), 86–95.

Gainor, R., Fitch, C., & Pollard, C. (2006). Maternal diabetes and perinatal outcomes in West Virginia Medicaid enrollees. *West Virginia Medical Journal, 102*(1), 314–316.

Graduate Medical Education Consortium (GMEC). (2001, August). Report to the board. Wise, VA: Graduate Medical Education Consortium.

Haaga, J. (2004). The aging of Appalachia: Demographic and socioeconomic change in Appalachia. Washington, DC: Appalachian Regional Commission.

Haaga, J. (2006). Educational attainment in Appalachia: Regional and national trrends. Washington, DC: Appalachian Regional Commission. http://www.arc.gov/index

Hays, J. (2004). A profile of oxycontin addiction. *Journal of Addictive Disorders, 23*(4), 1–9.

Hunsucker, S., Flannery, J., & Frank, D. (2000). Coping strategies of rural families of critically ill patients. *Journal of the American Academy of Nurse Practitioners, 12*(4), 123–127.

Hurley, J., & Turner, H. S. (2000). Development of a health service at a rural community college in Appalachia. *Journal of American College Health, 48*(4), 181–189.

Huttlinger, K., Schaller-Ayers, J., & Lawson, T. (2004a). Health care in Appalachia: A population-based approach. *Public Health Nursing, 21*(2), 103–110.

Huttlinger, K., Schaller-Ayers, J., Kenny, B., & Ayers, J. (2004b). Rural, community health nursing, research and collaboration. *Online Journal of Rural Nursing and Health Care, 4*(1), www.rno.org

Jesse, D., & Blue, C. (2004). Mary Breckinridge meets *Healthy People 2010*: A teaching strategy for visioning and building healthy communities. *Journal of Midwifery & Womens' Health, 49*(2), 126–131.

Kennedy, N. (1997). *Melungeons.* Macon, GA: Mercer University Press.

Lubell, J. (2006). Virginia doctors report controlled substances. Program targets substances with high potential for abuse. *Modern Healthcare, 36*(26), 32.

Obermiller, P., & Brown, M. (2002, February). *Appalachian health status in greater Cincinnati: A research overview.* Urban Council Working Paper No. 18. Cincinnati, OH: Urban Appalachian Council.

Smith, S., & Tessaro, I. (2005). Cultural perspectives on diabetes in an Appalachian population. *American Journal of Health Behavior, 29*(4), 291–301.

U.S. Drug Enforcement Agency (DEA). (2006a, September 9). DEA briefs and backgound drugs and drug abuse, drug descriptions. News Release. Washington, DC: Drug Enforcement Agency.

U.S. Drug Enforcement Agency (DEA). (2006b, November 29). National methamphetamine awareness day events represent largest single-day education effort in the dangers of methamphetamine. News Release. Washington, DC: Drug Enforcement Agency.

Virginia Health Care Foundation. (2001). *Results of Virginia's 2001 health access survey.* Joint Commission on Health Care. Richmond, VA: Virginia Health Care Foundation.

Voices of Appalachia Health Start Project. (2001). Whitley County Public Health Department. Available at http://www.wcphd.com.

Wilson, C. M. (1989). Elizabethan America. In W. K. Neil (Ed.), *Appalachian images in folk and popular cultures* (pp. 205–216). London: UMI Press.

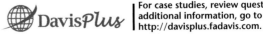

For case studies, review questions, and additional information, go to http://davisplus.fadavis.com.

Chapter 6

People of Arab Heritage

ANAHID DERVARTANIAN KULWICKI

Overview, Inhabited Localities, and Topography

OVERVIEW

Arabs trace their ancestry and traditions to the nomadic desert tribes of the Arabian Peninsula. They share a common language, **Arabic**, and most are united by **Islam**, a major world religion that originated in 7th-century Arabia. Despite these common bonds, even Arab residents of a single Arab country are characterized by diversity in thoughts, attitudes, and behaviors. Indeed, a poor tradition-bound farmer from rural Yemen may appear to have little in common with an educated professional from cosmopolitan Beirut. Additional factors such as refugee status, time since arrival, **ethnic identity**, disparity between cultures, economic status, employment status, social support, and English language skills influence the immigration experience and the Arab's adjustment to life in America.

The September 11, 2001, al Qaeda terrorist attack on the United States has increased negative comments about Arabs by some people. Health-care providers need to understand that few Arab Americans support the terrorist attacks, and they must not pigeonhole people by their cultural background.

The diversity among Arabs makes presenting a representative account of Arab Americans a formidable task because of the primary and secondary characteristics of culture (see Chapter 1) and the limited research literature on Arabs in the Americas. The earliest Arab immigrants arrived as part of the great wave of immigrants at the end of the 19th century and the beginning of the 20th century.

They were predominantly Christians from the region that is present-day Lebanon and Syria, and like most newcomers of the period, they valued assimilation and were rather easily absorbed into mainstream U.S. society. Arab Americans tend to disappear in national studies because they are counted as white in census data rather than as a separate ethnic group. Therefore, to portray Arab Americans as fully as possible, including the large numbers of new arrivals since 1965, literature that describes Arabs is used to supplement research completed by groups studying Arab Americans residing in Michigan and the San Francisco Bay area of California. An underlying assumption is that the attitudes and behaviors of first-generation immigrants are similar in some aspects to those of their counterparts in the Arab world.

Islamic doctrines and practices are included because most post-1965 Arab American immigrants are **Muslims**. Religion, whether official Islam, Christianity, or a local folk variant, is an integral part of everyday Arab life. Historically, Christians, Muslims, and Jews share a common religious background, and the three prophets are descendants from the same father, Abraham. Moses, the messenger of Judaism, and Jesus, the messenger of Christianity, are believed to be descendants of Isaac; whereas, Mohammed, the messenger of Islam, is believed to be a descendant of Abraham's eldest son, Ishmael. Moreover, because Arabism and Islam are so intrinsically interwoven and because Islam has some elements of Christianity, Arabs, whether Christian or Muslim, share some basic traditions and beliefs. Consequently, knowledge of religion is critical to understanding the Arab American client's cultural frame of reference and for providing care that considers specific religious beliefs and practices of devout Arab Muslim clients.

113

HERITAGE AND RESIDENCE

Arab Americans are defined as immigrants from the 22 Arab countries of North Africa and Southwest Asia: Algeria, Bahrain, Comoros, Djibouti, Egypt, Iraq, Jordan, Kuwait, Lebanon, Libya, Mauritania, Morocco, Oman, Palestine, Qatar, Saudi Arabia, Somalia, Sudan, Syria, Tunisia, United Arab Emirates, and Yemen. The Arab American Institute (2007) estimates 3.5 million Arab Americans live in the United States, with approximately 94 percent living in urban settings. The largest concentrations are in Los Angeles County, California; Wayne County, Michigan; and Kings, New York. However, Zogby International (2007) estimates the number of Arab American as three times greater than estimates from the Arab American Institute.

REASONS FOR MIGRATION AND ASSOCIATED ECONOMIC FACTORS

First-wave immigrants came to the United States between 1887 and 1913 seeking economic opportunity and perhaps the financial means to return home and buy land or set up shop in their ancestral villages. Most first-wave Arab Americans worked in unskilled jobs, were male and illiterate (44 percent), and were from mountain or rural areas (Naff, 1980). Today, 39 percent of Arab Americans are from Lebanon, and 12 percent come from Syria (Arab American Institute, 2007).

Second-wave immigrants entered the United States after World War II; the numbers increased dramatically after the Palestinian-Israeli conflict erupted and the passage of the Immigration Act of 1965 (Naff, 1980). Unlike the more economically motivated Lebanese-Syrian Christians, most second-wave immigrants are refugees from nations beset by war and political instability—chiefly, occupied Palestine, Jordan, Iraq, Yemen, Lebanon, and Syria. Included in this group are a large number of professionals and individuals seeking educational degrees who have subsequently remained in the United States. Of the current Arab American population, 57 percent are male, 25 percent are age 18 years or younger, and 9 percent are age 65 years or older; their median age is 33 years (Arab American Institute, 2007).

EDUCATIONAL STATUS AND OCCUPATIONS

Because Arabs favor professional occupations, education, as a prerequisite to white-collar work, is valued. Not surprisingly, both U.S.- and foreign-born Arab Americans are more educated than the average American. Over 84 percent of Arab Americans have a high school education, compared with all Americans at 81 percent, and 41 percent have a college education, compared with 24 percent of the total population (U.S. Bureau of the Census, 2005).

In comparison with Americans, Arab Americans are more likely to be self-employed and much more likely to be in managerial and professional specialty occupations (U.S. Bureau of the Census, 2005). Nearly 42 percent are employed in managerial and professional positions, 32 percent in sales, and 11.7 percent in retail trade. Few Arab Americans are employed in farming, forestry, fishing, precision production, crafts, or work as operators and fabricators (U.S. Bureau of the Census, 2005). Arab American households in the United States have a mean annual income of $47,000, compared with $42,000 for all households (Arab American Institute, 2007).

Communication

DOMINANT LANGUAGE AND DIALECTS

Arabic is the official language of the Arab world. Modern or classical Arabic is a universal form of Arabic used for all writing and formal situations ranging from radio newscasts to lectures. Dialectal or colloquial Arabic, of which each community has a variety, is used for everyday spoken communication. Arabs often mix Modern Standard Arabic and colloquial Arabic according to the complexity of the subject and the formality of the occasion. The presence of numerous dialects with differences in accent, inflection, and vocabulary may create difficulties in communication between Arab immigrants from Syria and Lebanon and Arab immigrants from Iraq and Yemen.

The Arab person's speech is likely to be characterized by repetition and gesturing, particularly when involved in serious discussions. Arabs may be loud and expressive when involved in serious discussions to stress their commitment and their sincerity in the subject matter. Observers witnessing such impassioned communication may assume that Arabs are argumentative, confrontational, or aggressive.

English is a common second language in Egypt, Jordan, Lebanon, Yemen, Bahrain, and Kuwait. In contrast, literacy rates among adults in the Arab world vary from 44 percent in Yemen to 88 percent in Lebanon and Jordan. Literacy rates among women also vary, ranging from 23.7 percent in Yemen to 84 percent in Lebanon, where women often earn university degrees (*Arab human development report*, 2000). More than half (65 percent) speak a language other than English at home, although 44 percent report a good command of the English language (U.S. Bureau of the Census, 2005). Despite this, ample evidence indicates that language and communication pose formidable problems in American health-care settings. For example, Kulwicki and Miller (1999) reported that 66 percent of respondents using a community-based health clinic spoke Arabic at home and only 30.2 percent spoke both English and Arabic. Even English-speaking Arab Americans report difficulty in expressing their needs and understanding health-care providers.

Health-care providers have cited numerous interpersonal and communication problems, including erroneous assessments of patient complaints, delayed or failed appointments, reluctance to disclose personal and family health information, and in some cases, noncompliance with medical treatments (Kulwicki, 1996; Kulwicki, Miller, & Schim, 2000), and a tendency to exaggerate when describing complaints (Sullivan, 1993).

CULTURAL COMMUNICATION PATTERNS

Arab communication has been described as highly nuanced, with more communication contained in the context of the situation than in the actual words spoken. Arabs value privacy and resist disclosure of personal information to strangers, especially when it relates to familial disease conditions. Conversely, among friends and relatives, Arabs express feelings freely. These patterns of communication become more comprehensible when interpreted within the Arab cultural frame of reference. Many personal needs may be anticipated without the individual having to verbalize them because of close family relationships. The family may rely more on unspoken expectations and nonverbal cues than overt verbal exchange.

Arabs need to develop personal relationships with a health-care provider before sharing personal information. Because meaning may be attached to both compliments and indifference, manner and tone are as important as what is said. Arabs are sensitive to the courtesy and respect they are accorded, and good manners are important in evaluating a person's character. Therefore, greetings, inquiries about well-being, pleasantries, and a cup of tea or coffee precede business. Conversants stand close to one another, maintain steady eye contact, and touch (only between members of the same sex) the other's hand or shoulder. Sitting and standing properly is critical; to do otherwise is taken as a lack of respect. Within the context of personal relationships, verbal agreements are considered more important than written contracts. Keeping promises is considered a matter of honor.

Substantial efforts are directed at maintaining pleasant relationships and preserving dignity and honor. Hostility in response to perceived wrongdoing is warded off by an attitude of **maalesh**, "never mind, it doesn't matter." Individuals are protected from bad news for as long as possible and are then informed as gently as possible. When disputes arise, Arabs hint at their disagreement or simply fail to follow through. Alternatively, an intermediary, someone with influence, may be used to intervene in disputes or present requests to the person in charge. Mediation saves face if a conflict is not settled in one's favor and reassures the petitioner that maximum influence has been employed (Nydell, 1987).

Guidelines for communicating with Arab Americans include

1. Employ an approach that combines expertise with warmth. Minimize status differences, as Arab Americans report feeling uncomfortable and self-conscious in the presence of authority figures. Pay special attention to the person's feelings. Arab Americans perceive themselves as sensitive, with the potential for being easily hurt, belittled, and slighted (Reizian & Meleis, 1987).

2. Take time to get acquainted before delving into business. If sincere interest in the person's home country and adjustment to American life is expressed, he or she is likely to enjoy relating such information, much of which is essential to assessing risk for traumatic immigration experience (see Barriers to Health Care, later in this chapter) and understanding the person's cultural frame of reference. Sharing a cup of tea does much to give an initial visit a positive beginning (Kulwicki, 1996).

3. Nurses may need to clarify role responsibilities regarding history taking, performing physical examinations, and providing health information for newer immigrants. Although recent Arab American immigrants may now recognize the higher status of nurses in the United States, they are still accustomed to nurses' functioning as medical assistants and housekeepers (see Status of Health-Care Providers, later in this chapter).

4. Perform a comprehensive assessment. Explain the relationship of the information needed for physical complaints.

5. Interpret family members' communication patterns within a cultural context. Recognize that a spokesperson may answer questions directed to the client, and that the family members may edit some information that they feel is inappropriate (Kulwicki, 1996). Family members can also be expected to act as the client's advocates; they may attempt to resolve problems by taking appeals "to the top" or by seeking the help of an influential intermediary.

6. Convey hope and optimism. The concept of "false hope" is not meaningful to Arabs because they regard God's power to cure as infinite. The amount and type of information given should be carefully considered.

7. Be mindful of the patient's modesty and dignity. Islamic teachings forbid unnecessary touch (including shaking hands) between unrelated adults of opposite sexes (al-Shahri, 2002). Observation of this teaching is expressed most commonly by female patients with male health-care professionals, and may cause the patient to be shy or hesitant in allowing the professional to do physical assessments. Health-care providers must make concerted efforts to understand the patient's feelings and to take them into consideration.

TEMPORAL RELATIONSHIPS

First-generation Arab immigrants may believe in predestination; that is, God has predetermined the events of one's life. Accordingly, individuals should work hard to make the best of life while acknowledging that God has ultimate control over all that happens. Consequently, plans and intentions are qualified with the phrase **inshallah**, "if God wills," and blessings and misfortunes are attributed to God rather than to the actions of individuals.

Throughout the Arab world, there is nonchalance about punctuality except in cases of business or professional meetings; otherwise, the pace of life is more leisurely than in the West. Social events and appointments tend not to have a fixed beginning or end. Although certain individuals may arrive on time for appointments, the tendency is to be somewhat late. However, for most Arab Americans who belong to professional occupations or who are in the business field, punctuality and respecting deadlines and appointments are considered important (Kulwicki, 2001).

FORMAT FOR NAMES

Etiquette requires shaking hands on arrival and departure. However, when an Arab man is introduced to an Arab woman, the man waits for the woman to extend her hand. Devout Muslim men may not shake hands with women.

Titles are important and are used in combination with the person's first name (e.g., Mr. Khalil or Dr. Ali). Some may prefer to be addressed as mother (*Um*) or father (*Abu*) of the eldest son (e.g., Abu Khalil, "father of Khalil").

Family Roles and Organization

VIGNETTE 6.1

Mrs. Nasser arrived at the urgent-care center with her 16-year-old daughter, who had been experiencing burning upon urination, itching around her genital area, and a high fever. Mrs. Nasser appeared very anxious, explaining to the nurse that her daughter had never had these symptoms before. The nurse tried to calm Mrs. Nasser and asked that her daughter, Samia, get undressed in preparation for a physical examination. Mrs. Nasser appeared concerned and requested that the nurse inform the doctor that she will not allow the doctor to perform a vaginal examination on her daughter.

The nurse explained to Mrs. Nasser that it will be necessary for the doctor to examine Samia so that she can determine the cause of Samia's discomfort. Mrs. Nasser became extremely agitated and explained to the nurse that in her culture, young girls are not allowed to have vaginal examination for fear that their virginity will be compromised. Mrs. Nasser insisted that she would not allow her daughter to be examined by the female doctor on duty. Mrs. Nasser requested that the nurse ask the doctor to write a prescription for her daughter's infection, or else she would leave the clinic immediately.

1. How should the nurse respond to Mrs. Nasser's request? Explain your rationale.
2. Identify culturally congruent strategies that may be most effective in addressing the needs of Mrs. Nasser.
3. How might the nurse ensure that Mrs. Nasser's concerns are addressed appropriately and that Samia has received the appropriate care?

HEAD OF HOUSEHOLD AND GENDER ROLES

Arab Muslim families are characterized by a strong patrilineal tradition (Aswad, 1999). Women are subordinate to men, and young people are subordinate to older people. Consequently, within his immediate family, the man is the head of the family and his influence is overt. In public, a wife's interactions with her husband are formal and respectful. However, behind the scenes, she typically wields tremendous influence, particularly in matters pertaining to the home and children. A wife may sometimes be required to hide her power from her husband and children to preserve the husband's view of himself as head of the family.

Within the larger extended family, the older male figure assumes the role of decision maker. Women attain power and status in advancing years, particularly when they have adult children. The bond between mothers and sons is typically strong, and most men make every effort to obey their mother's wishes, and even her whims (Nydell, 1987).

Gender roles are clearly defined and regarded as a complementary division of labor. Men are breadwinners, protectors, and decision makers, whereas women are responsible for the care and education of children and for maintenance of a successful marriage by tending to their husbands' needs.

Although women in more urbanized Arab countries such as Lebanon, Syria, Jordan, and Egypt often have professional careers, with some women advocating for women's liberation, the family and marriage remain primary commitments for the majority. Most educated women still consider caring for their children as their primary role after marriage. Arab women value modesty, especially among devout Muslim Arabs—modesty is expressed with their attire. For example, many Muslim women view the **hijab**, "covering the body except for one's face and hands," as offering them protection in situations in which the sexes mix, because it is a recognized symbol of Muslim identity and good moral character.

Ironically, many Americans associate the *hijab* with oppression rather than protection. Similarly, the authority structure and division of labor within Arab families are often misinterpreted, fueling common stereotypes of the overtly dominant Arab male and the passive and oppressed Arab woman. Thus, by extension, conservative Arab Americans perceive the stereotypical understanding of the submissive role of women as a criticism to the Arab culture and family values (Kulwicki, 2000).

PRESCRIPTIVE, RESTRICTIVE, AND TABOO BEHAVIORS FOR CHILDREN AND ADOLESCENTS

In the traditional Arab family, the roles of the father and mother as they relate to the children are quite distinct. Typically, the father is the disciplinarian, whereas the mother is an ally and mediator, an unfailing source of love and kindness. Although some fathers feel that it is advantageous to maintain a degree of fear, family relationships are usually characterized by affection and sentimentality. Children are dearly loved, indulged, and included in all family activities.

Among Arabs, raising children so they reflect well on the family is an extremely important responsibility. A child's character and successes (or failures) in life are attributed to upbringing and parental influence. Because of the emphasis on familialism rather than individualism within the Arab culture, conformity to adult rules is favored. Correspondingly, child-rearing methods are oriented toward accommodation and cooperation. Family reputation is important; children are expected to behave in an honorable manner and not bring shame to the family. Child-rearing patterns also include great respect toward parents and elders. Children are raised to not question elders and to be obedient to older brothers and sisters (Kulwicki, 1996). Methods of discipline include physical punishment and shaming. Children are made to feel ashamed because others have seen them misbehave, rather than to experience guilt arising from self-criticism and inward regret.

Whereas adolescence in the West is centered on acquiring a personal identity and completing the separation process from family, Arab adolescents are expected to remain enmeshed in the family system. Family interests and opinions often influence career and marriage decisions. Arab adolescents are pressed to succeed academically, in part because of the connections between professional careers and social status. Conversely, behaviors that would bring family dishonor, such as academic failure, sexual activity, illicit drug use, and juvenile delinquency, are avoided. For girls in particular, chastity and decency are required. Adolescence in North America may provide more opportunities for academic success and more freedom in making career choices than can be accessed by their counterparts in the Arab countries. Cultural conflicts between American values and Arab values often cause significant conflicts for Arab American families. Arab American parents cite a variety of concerns related to conflicting values regarding dating, after-school activities, drinking, and drug use (Zogby, 2002).

FAMILY GOALS AND PRIORITIES

The family is the central socioeconomic unit in Arab society. Family members cooperate to secure livelihood, rear children, and maintain standing and influence within the community. Family members live nearby, sometimes intermarry (first cousins), and expect a great deal from one another regardless of practicality or ability to help. Loyalty to one's family takes precedence over personal needs. Maintenance of family honor is paramount.

Within the hierarchical family structure, older family members are accorded great respect. Children, sons in particular, are held responsible for supporting elderly parents. Therefore, regardless of the sacrifices involved, the elderly parents are almost always cared for within the home, typically until death.

Responsibility for family members rests with the older men of the family. In the absence of the father, brothers are responsible for unmarried sisters. In the event of a husband's death, his family provides for his widow and children. In general, family leaders are expected to use influence and render special services and favors to kinsmen.

Although educational accomplishments (doctoral degrees), certain occupations (medicine, engineering, law), and acquired wealth contribute to social status, family origin is the primary determinant. Certain character traits such as piety, generosity, hospitality, and good manners may also enhance social standing.

ALTERNATIVE LIFESTYLES

Most adults marry. Although the Islamic right to marry up to four wives is sometimes exercised, particularly if the first wife is chronically ill or infertile, most marriages are monogamous and for life. Recent studies have reported that 2 to 5 percent of Arab Muslim marriages are polygamous (Kulwicki, 2000). Whereas homosexuality occurs in all cultures to some extent, it is stigmatized among Arab cultures. In some Arab countries, it is considered a crime; fearing family disgrace and ostracism, gays and lesbians remain closeted (Global Gayz, 2006). However, in recent years, Arab American gays and lesbians have been active in gay and lesbian organizations, and some have been outspoken and publicly active in raising community awareness about gay and lesbian rights in Arab American communities.

Workforce Issues

CULTURE IN THE WORKPLACE

Cultural differences that may have an impact on work life include beliefs regarding family, gender roles, one's ability to control life events, maintaining pleasant personal relationships, guarding dignity and honor, and the importance placed on maintaining one's reputation. Arabs and Americans may also differ in attitudes toward time, instructional methods, patterns of thinking, and the amount of emphasis placed on objectivity. However, because many second-wave professionals were educated in the United States, and thereby socialized to some extent, differences are probably more characteristic of less-educated, first-generation Arab Americans.

Stress is a common denominator in recent studies of first-generation immigrants. Sources of stress include separation from family members, difficulty adjusting to American life, marital tension, and intergenerational conflict, specifically coping with adolescents socialized in American values through school activities (Seikaly, 1999). Issues related to discrimination have been reported as a major source of stress among Arab Americans in their work environment. In a recent study exploring the perceptions and experiences of Arab American nurses in the aftermath of 9/11, the majority of nurses did not experience major episodes of discrimination at work such as termination and physical assaults; however, some did experience other types of discrimination such as intimidation, being treated suspiciously, negative comments about their religious practices, and patient refusal to be treated by them (Kulwicki & Khalifa, 2007). Arab Americans are keenly aware of the misperceptions Americans hold about Arabs, such as notions that Arabs are inferior, backward, sinister, and violent. In addition, the American public's ignorance of mainstream Islam and the stereotyping of Muslims as fanatics, extremist, and confrontational burden Arab American Muslims.

Muslim Arab Americans face a variety of challenges as they practice their faith in a secular American society. For example, Islamic and American civil law differ on matters such as marriage, divorce, banking, and inheritance. Individuals who wish to attend Friday prayer services and observe religious holidays frequently encounter job-related conflicts. Children are often torn between fulfilling Islamic obligations regarding prayer, dietary restrictions, and dress and hiding their religious identity in order to fit into the American public school culture.

ISSUES RELATED TO AUTONOMY

Whereas American workplaces tend to be dominated by deadlines, profit margins, and maintaining one's competitive edge, a more relaxed, cordial, and relationship-oriented atmosphere prevails in the Arab world. Friendship and business are mixed over cups of sweet tea to the extent that it is unclear where socializing ends and work begins. Managers promote optimal performance by using personal influence and persuasion, and performance evaluations are based on personality and social behavior as well as job skills.

Significant differences also exist in workplace norms. In the United States, position is usually earned, laws are applied equally, work takes precedence over family, honesty is an absolute value, facts and logic prevail, and direct and critical appraisal is regarded as valuable feedback. In the Arab world, position is often attained through one's family and connections, rules are bent, family obligations take precedence over the demands of the job, subjective perceptions often dictate actions, and criticism is often taken personally as an affront to dignity and family honor (Nydell, 1987). In Arab offices, supervisors and managers are expected to praise their employees to assure them that their work is noticed and appreciated. Whereas such direct praise may be somewhat embarrassing for Americans, Arabs expect and want praise when they feel they have earned it (Nydell, 1987).

Biocultural Ecology

SKIN COLOR AND OTHER BIOLOGICAL VARIATIONS

Although Arabs are uniformly perceived as swarthy, and whereas many do, in fact, have dark or olive skin, they may also have blonde or auburn hair, blue eyes, and fair complexions. Because color changes are more difficult to assess in dark-skinned people, pallor and cyanosis are best detected by examination of the oral mucosa and conjunctiva.

DISEASES AND HEALTH CONDITIONS

The major public health concerns in the Arab world include trauma related to motor vehicle accidents, maternal-child health, and control of communicable diseases. The incidence of infectious diseases such as tuberculosis, malaria, trachoma, typhus, hepatitis, typhoid fever, dysentery, and parasitic infestations varies between urban and rural areas and from country to country. For example, disease risks are relatively low in modern urban centers of the Arab world, but are quite high in the countryside where animals such as goats and sheep virtually share living quarters, open toilets are commonplace, and running water is not available. Schistosomiasis (also called bilharzia), infecting about one-fifth of Egyptians, has been called Egypt's number-one health problem. Its prevalence is related to an entrenched social habit of using the Nile River for washing, drinking, and urinating. Similarly, outbreaks of cholera and meningitis are continuous concerns in Saudi Arabia during the Muslim pilgrimage season. In Jordan, where contagious diseases have declined sharply, emphasis has shifted to preventing accidental death and controlling noncommunicable diseases such as cancer and heart disease. Correspondingly, seatbelt use, smoking habits, and pesticide residues in locally grown produce are major issues. Campaigns directed at improving children's health include hepatitis B vaccinations and dental health programs.

Glucose-6-phosphate dehydrogenase (G-6-PD) deficiency, sickle cell anemia, and the thalassemias are extremely common in the eastern Mediterranean region, probably because carriers enjoy an increased resistance to malaria (Hamamy & Alwan, 1994). High consanguinity rates—roughly 30 percent of marriages in Iraq, Jordan, Kuwait, and Saudi Arabia are between first cousins—and the trend of bearing children up to menopause also contribute to the prevalence of genetically determined disorders in Arab countries (Hamamy & Alwan, 1994).

With modernization and increased life expectancy, multifactorial disorders—hypertension, diabetes, and coronary heart disease—have also emerged as major problems in eastern Mediterranean countries (Kulwicki, 2001). In many countries, cardiovascular disease is a major cause of death. In Lebanon, the increased frequency of familial hypercholesterolemia is a contributing factor. Individuals of Arabic ancestry are also more likely to inherit familial Mediterranean fever, a disorder characterized by recurrent episodes of fever, peritonitis, or pleurisies, either alone or in some combination.

The extent to which these conditions affect the health of Arab Americans is limited. However, a Wayne County Health Department (1994) project, a telephone survey including Arabs residing in the Detroit, Michigan, area, identified cardiovascular disease as one of two specific risks, based on the high prevalence of cigarette smoking, high-cholesterol diets, obesity, and sedentary lifestyles. Although the prevalence of hypertension was lower in the Arab community than in the rest of Wayne County, Arab respondents were less likely to report having their blood pressure checked. In fact, lower rates for appropriate testing and screening, such as cholesterol testing, cholorectal cancer screening, and uterine cancer screening, were considered a major risk for this group of Arab Americans. In recent years, the rate of mammography has increased dramatically. The Institute of Medicine's report *Unequal Treatment: Confronting Racial and Ethnic Disparities in Health Care* (2002) indicated that death rates for Arab females, compared with those of other white groups, was higher from heart disease and cancer but lower from strokes. However, the death rate for Arab males from coronary heart disease is higher when compared with that of white males. Lung and colorectal cancer are the two leading causes of death among Arab Americans. For Arab American men, lung cancer is the leading cause of death, and breast cancer is the leading cause of death in Arab American women (Schwartz, Darwish-Yassine, & Wing, 2005).

The rate of infant mortality in the Arab world is very high, ranging from 24 per 1000 births in Syria to 108 per 1000 births in Iraq. In Bahrain, the infant mortality is low: 8.5 per 1000 births (World Health Organization [WHO], 2006). Although overall infant mortality rates for Arab Americans are the same as for white infants, figures for Michigan show a lower infant mortality rate for Arab Americans (6.2 per 1000 births) than for white infants (7.8 per 1000).

VARIATIONS IN DRUG METABOLISM

Information describing drug disposition and sensitivity in Arabs is limited. Between 1 and 1.4 percent of Arabs are known to have difficulty metabolizing debrisoquine and substances that are metabolized similarly: antiarrhythmics, antidepressants, beta-blockers, neuroleptics, and opioid agents. Consequently, a small number of Arab Americans may experience elevated blood levels and adverse effects when customary dosages of antidepressants are prescribed. Conversely, typical codeine dosages may prove inadequate because some individuals cannot metabolize codeine to morphine to promote an optimal analgesic effect (Levy, 1993).

High-Risk Behaviors

Despite Islamic beliefs discouraging tobacco use, smoking remains deeply ingrained in Arab culture. For many Arabs, offering cigarettes is a sign of hospitality. Consistent with their cultural heritage, Arab Americans are characterized by higher smoking rates and lower quitting rates than European Americans (Darwish-Yassine & Wang, 2005; Rice & Kulwicki, 1992).

According to the *2001–2002 Special Cancer Behavioral Risk Factor Survey*, Arab Americans who are 50 years and older have the highest smoking rates compared with other populations in Michigan. Smoking rates for Arab women in the same age group are considerably lower (39.9 versus 10.9 percent) (Michigan Department of Community Health and Michigan Department of Public Health Institute, 2003). Preliminary research results related to tobacco use among Arab Americans suggests that the rates of tobacco smoking among Arab American youth are considerably lower than those among non-Arab youth in Michigan, with only 16 percent of Arab youths smoking versus 34 percent of non-Arabs (Templin, Rice, Gadelrab, Weglicki, Hammad, & Kulwicki, 2003).

Limited information is available on alcohol use among Arab Americans. However, Islamic prohibitions do appear to influence patterns of alcohol consumption and attitudes toward drug use (Wayne County Health Department, 1994). Ninety percent of the Arab respondents in the survey reported that they abstain from drinking alcohol. None reported heavy drinking, with a limited number reporting binge drinking (2.2 percent) and driving under the influence of alcohol (1.4 percent). All respondents believed that occasional use of cocaine entails "great" risk, with most saying the same about occasional use of marijuana.

The actual risk for, and incidence of, HIV infection and AIDS in Arab countries and among Arab Americans is low. However, an increase in the rate of infection has been noticed among many Arab countries and among Arab Americans (Centers for Disease Contral and Prevention [CDC], 2006). The reported number of individuals having AIDS in the Arab countries varies and may not be an accurate reflection of the real incidence owing to restrictions placed on HIV/AIDS research by some Arab countries. The largest number of AIDS cases is seen in Djibouti (214); the lowest numbers of individuals reported as having AIDS are found in Palestine (1), Kuwait (11), Syria (18), Lebanon (24), Yemen (45), and Egypt (63) (WHO, 2004).

Despite the reported low rate of HIV/AIDS among Arab Americans, 4 percent of the Arab American respondents surveyed by Kulwicki and Cass (1994) reported that they were at high risk for AIDS. In addition, the sample demonstrated less knowledge of primary routes of transmission and more misconceptions regarding unlikely modes of transmission than other populations surveyed.

Cultural norms of modesty for Arab women are also a significant risk related to reproductive health among Arab Americans. For example, the rate of breast cancer screening among Arab women was 50.8 percent, compared with 71.2 percent for other women in Michigan. The rate of cervical Pap smears was 59.9 percent, and the rate of mammogram screenings was 51.2 percent (Kulwicki, 2000). Arab American women, especially new immigrants, may be at a higher risk for domestic violence because of the higher rates of stress, poverty, poor spiritual and social support, and isolation from family members owing to immigration (Kulwicki, 2001).

Sedentary lifestyle and high fat intake among Arab Americans place them at higher risk for cardiovascular diseases. For instance, 43 percent of the participants surveyed by Wayne County Health Department indicated that they had been told that their cholesterol level was high (Office of Minority Health [OMH], 2001). Studies in Arab countries and in Michigan have also reported higher rates of cardiovascular disease and diabetes among Arabs and Arab Americans.

Many Arab Americans are refugees fleeing war and political and religious conflicts, placing them at greater risk for psychological distress, depression, and other psychiatric illnesses (Hikmet, Hakim-Larson, Farrag, & Jamil, 2002; Kinzie, Boehnlein, Riley, & Sparr, 2002). Psychological distress was also documented among immigrants who themselves were not victims of war and conflict but who worried over family members that were in areas of conflict. Studies conducted with Iraqi refugees and victims of torture in the United States identified higher prevalence of post-traumatic stress disorder and depression (Kinzie et al., 2002).

HEALTH-CARE PRACTICES

According to the Wayne County Health Department (1994), Arab Americans' risk in terms of safety is mixed. Factors enhancing safety include low rates of gun ownership and high recognition of the risks associated with having guns in the house. Conversely, lower rates of fire escape planning and seatbelt usage for adults and older children (car seats are generally used for younger children), as well as higher rates of physical assaults, threaten their safety.

In most health areas surveyed in Michigan, education and income were important determinants of risk for people of Arab descent. Socioeconomic status was also a strong indicator in accessing health-care services. The Wayne County Health Department (1994) indicated that 37.2 percent of the adult Arab respondents were not covered by health insurance. Use of health-care services for prenatal care was, however, higher among Arab American females than other ethnic groups in Michigan (Michigan Department of Public Health, 1995). Physical or mental disability among Arab Americans in Michigan was almost equal to that of white Americans.

Nutrition

MEANING OF FOOD

Sharing meals with family and friends is a favorite pastime. Offering food is also a way of expressing love and friendship, hospitality, and generosity. For the Arab woman, whose primary role is caring for her husband and children, the preparation and presentation of an elaborate midday meal is taken as an indication of her love and caring. Similarly, in entertaining friends, the types and quantity of food served, often several entrees, is a measure of one's hospitality and esteem for one's guests. Honor and reputation are based on the manner in which guests are received. In return, family members and guests express appreciation by eating heartily.

COMMON FOODS AND FOOD RITUALS

Although cooking and national dishes vary from country to country and seasoning from family to family, Arabic cooking shares many general characteristics. Familiar spices and herbs such as cinnamon, allspice, cloves, ginger, cumin, mint, parsley, bay leaves, garlic, and onions are used frequently. Skewer cooking and slow simmering are typical modes of preparation. All countries have rice and wheat dishes, stuffed vegetables, nut-filled pastries, and fritters soaked in syrup. Dishes are garnished with raisins, pine nuts, pistachios, and almonds.

Favorite fruits and vegetables include dates, figs, apricots, guavas, mangos, melons, papayas, bananas, citrus fruits, carrots, tomatoes, cucumbers, parsley, mint, spinach, and grape leaves. Lamb and chicken are the most popular meats. Muslims are prohibited from eating pork and pork products (e.g., lard). For Arab Christians, pork is not prohibited; however, pork consumption by Arab Christians is low. Similarly, because the consumption of blood is forbidden, Muslims are required to cook meats and poultry until well done. Bread accompanies every meal and is viewed as a gift from God. In many respects, the traditional Arab diet is representative of the U.S. Department of Agriculture's food pyramid. Bread is a mainstay, grains and legumes are often substituted for meats, fresh fruit and juices are especially popular, and olive oil is widely used. In addition, because foods are prepared "from scratch," consumption of preservatives and additives is limited.

Lunch is the main meal in Arab households. Encouraging guests to eat is the host's duty. Guests often begin with a ritual refusal and then succumb to the host's insistence. Food is eaten with the right hand because it is regarded as clean. Beverages may not be served until after the meal because some Arabs consider it unhealthy to eat and drink at the same time. Similar concerns may exist regarding mixing hot and cold foods.

Health-care providers should also understand **Ramadan**, the Muslim month of fasting. The fast, which is meant to remind Muslims of their dependence on God and the poor who experience involuntary fasting, involves abstinence from eating, drinking (including water), smoking, and marital intercourse during daylight hours. Although the sick are not required to fast, many pious Muslims insist on fasting while hospitalized, necessitating adjustments in meal times and medications, including medications given by nonoral routes. In outpatient settings, health-care providers need to be alert to potential "noncompliance." Patients may omit or adjust the timing of medications. Of particular concern are medications requiring constant blood levels, adequate hydration, or both (e.g., antibiotics that may crystallize in the kidneys). Health-care providers may need to provide appointment times after sunset during Ramadan for individuals requiring injections (e.g., allergy shots).

DIETARY PRACTICES FOR HEALTH PROMOTION

Arabs associate good health with eating properly, consuming nutritious foods, and fasting to cure disease. For some, concerns about amounts and balance among food types (hot, cold, dry, moist) may be traced to the Prophet Mohammed, who taught that "the stomach is the house of every disease, and abstinence is the head of every remedy" (Al-Akili, 1993, p. 7). Within this framework, illness is related to excessive eating, eating before a previously eaten meal is digested, eating nutritionally deficient food, mixing opposing types of foods, and consuming elaborately prepared foods. Conversely, abstinence allows the body to expel disease.

The condition of the alimentary tract has priority over all other body systems in the Arab perception of health (Meleis, 2005). Gastrointestinal complaints are often the reason Arab Americans seek care (Meleis, 2005). Obesity is a problem for second-generation Arab American women and children, most of whom report eating American snacks that are high in fat and calories. Most women try to lose weight by reducing caloric intake (Wayne County Health Department, 1994).

NUTRITIONAL DEFICIENCIES AND FOOD LIMITATIONS

In Arab countries, diet is influenced by income, government subsidies for certain foods (e.g., bread, sugar, oil), and seasonal availability. Arab Americans most at risk for nutritional deficiencies include newly arrived immigrants from Yemen and Iraq (Ahmad, 2004) and Arab American households below the poverty level. Lactose intolerance sometimes occurs in this population. However, the practice of eating yogurt and cheese, rather than drinking milk, probably limits symptoms in sensitive people.

Many of the most common foods are available in American markets. Some Muslims may refuse to eat meat that is not **halal**, "slaughtered in an Islamic manner." *Halal* meat can be obtained in Arabic grocery stores and through Islamic centers or **mosques**.

Islamic prohibitions against the consumption of alcohol and pork have implications for American health-care providers. Conscientious Muslims are often wary of eating outside the home and may ask many questions about ingredients used in meal preparation: Are the beans vegetarian? Was wine used in the meat sauce or lard in the pastry crust? Muslims are equally concerned about the ingredients and origins of mouthwashes, toothpastes, and medicines (e.g., alcohol-based syrups and elixirs), as well as insulins and capsules (gelatin coating) derived from pigs. However, if no substitutes are available, Muslims are permitted to use these preparations.

Pregnancy and Childbearing Practices

FERTILITY PRACTICES AND VIEWS TOWARD PREGNANCY

Fertility rates in the countries from which most Arab Americans emigrate range from 1.9 in Tunisia and 2.2 in Lebanon to 5.9 in Yemen (UNICEF, 2005). Fertility practices of Arabs are influenced by traditional Bedouin values supporting tribal dominance, popular beliefs that "God decides family size," and "God provides," and Islamic rulings regarding birth control, treatment of infertility, and abortion.

High fertility rates are favored. Procreation is regarded as the purpose of marriage and the means of enhancing family strength. Accordingly, Islamic jurists have ruled that the use of "reversible" forms of birth control is "undesirable but not forbidden." These should be employed only in certain situations, listed in decreasing order of legitimacy, such as threat to the mother's life, too frequent childbearing, risk of transmitting genetic disease, and financial hardship. Moreover, irreversible forms of birth control such as vasectomy and tubal ligation are **haram**, "absolutely unlawful." Muslims regard abortion as *haram* except when the mother's health is compromised by pregnancy-induced disease or her life is threatened (Ebrahim, 1989). Therefore, unwanted pregnancies are dealt with by hoping one miscarries "by an act of God" or by covertly arranging for an abortion. Recently, great decline in fertility rates has occurred in Arab countries and among Arab Americans. According to Michigan's birth registration data, fertility rates among Arab Americans are highest (approximately 4) when compared with those of the total population (OMH, 2001).

Among Jordanian husbands, religion and the fatalistic belief that "God decides family size" were most often given as reasons why contraceptives were not used. Contraceptives were used by 27 percent of the husbands, typically urbanites of high socioeconomic status. Although the intrauterine device (IUD) and the pill were most widely favored, 4.9 percent of females used sterilization despite religious prohibitions (Hashemite Kingdom of Jordan, 1985). A survey of a random sample of 295 Arab American women in Michigan indicated that 29.1 percent of the surveyed women did not use any birth control methods because of their desire to have children, 4.3 percent did not use any form of contraceptives because of their husband's disapproval, and 6 percent did not use contraceptive methods because of religious reasons. The use of birth control pills was the highest

(33.2 percent) among the users of contraceptive methods, followed by tubal ligation (12.9 percent) and IUD (10.7 percent) (Kulwicki, 2000).

Indeed, among Arab women, in particular, fertility may be more of a concern than contraception because sterility in a woman could lead to rejection and divorce. Islam condones treatment for infertility, as **Allah** provides progeny as well as a cure for every disease. However, approved methods for treating infertility are limited to artificial insemination using the husband's sperm and in vitro fertilization involving the fertilization of the wife's ovum by the husband's sperm.

PRESCRIPTIVE, RESTRICTIVE, AND TABOO PRACTICES IN THE CHILDBEARING FAMILY

Because of the emphasis on fertility and the bearing of sons, pregnancy traditionally occurred at a younger age and the fertility rate among Arab women was higher in the Arab world. However, as the educational and economic conditions for Arab women have improved both in the Arab world and in the United States, fertility patterns have also changed accordingly.

The pregnant woman is indulged and her cravings satisfied, lest she develop a birthmark in the shape of the particular food she craves. Because of the preference for male offspring, the sex of the child can be a stressor for mothers without sons. Friends and family often note how the mother is "carrying" the baby as an indicator of the baby's sex (i.e., high for a girl and low for a boy). Although pregnant women are excused from fasting during Ramadan, some Muslim women may be determined to fast and thus suffer potential consequences for glucose metabolism and hydration.

Labor and delivery are women's affairs. In Arab countries, home delivery, with the assistance of **dayahs** ("midwives") or neighbors was common because of limited access to hospitals, "shyness," and financial constraints. However, recently, the practice of home delivery has decreased dramatically in Arab countries, and hospital deliveries have become common. During labor, women openly express pain through facial expressions, verbalizations, and body movements. Nurses and medical staff may mistakenly diagnose Arab women as needing medical intervention and administer pain medications more liberally to alleviate the pain.

Care for the infant includes wrapping the stomach at birth, or as soon thereafter as possible, to prevent cold or wind from entering the baby's body (Luna, 1994). The call to prayer is recited in the Muslim newborn's ear. Male circumcision is almost a universal practice, and for Muslims, it is a religious requirement.

Folk beliefs influence bathing and breastfeeding. Arab mothers may be reluctant to bathe postpartum because of beliefs that air gets into the mother and causes illness (Luna, 1994) and washing the breasts "thins the milk" (Cline, Abuirmeileh, & Roberts, 1986).

Breastfeeding is often delayed until the 2nd or 3rd day after birth because of beliefs that the mother requires rest, that nursing at birth causes "colic" pain for the mother, and that "colostrum makes the baby dumb" (Cline et al., 1986). Postpartum care also includes special foods such as lentil soup to increase milk production and tea to flush and cleanse the body.

Statistics describing the pregnancy and birth experiences of Michigan mothers, including 2755 Arab Americans, depict the experiences of Arab American mothers and infants as fairly comparable with their white counterparts with regard to adequacy of prenatal care, maternal complications, infant mortality, and birth complications. In addition, fewer Arab American mothers smoke, drink alcohol, or gain too little weight (Kulwicki, Smiley, & Devine, 2007).

Although these statewide statistics are quite favorable, it is important to mention that earlier studies revealed an alarming rate of infant mortality among Arab American mothers in Dearborn, Michigan, a particularly disadvantaged community of new immigrants with high rates of unemployment. Factors contributing to poor pregnancy outcomes include poverty; lower levels of education; inability to communicate in English; personal, family, and cultural stressors; cigarette smoking; and early or closely spaced pregnancies. Fear of being ridiculed by American health-care providers and a limited number of bilingual providers limit access to health-care information.

Death Rituals

DEATH RITUALS AND EXPECTATIONS

Although Arabs insist on maintaining hope regardless of prognosis, death is accepted as God's will. According to Muslim beliefs, death is foreordained and worldly life is but a preparation for eternal life. Hence, from the Qur'an, Surrah III, v. 185:

> Every soul will taste of death. And ye will be paid on the Day of Resurrection only that which ye have fairly earned. Whoso is removed from the Fire and is made to enter Paradise, he indeed is triumphant. The life of this world is but comfort of illusion (Pickthall, 1977, p. 70).

Muslim death rituals include turning the patient's bed to face the holy city of Mecca and reading from the Qur'an, particularly verses stressing hope and acceptance. After death, the deceased is washed three times by a Muslim of the same sex. The body is then wrapped, preferably in white material, and buried as soon as possible in a brick- or cement-lined grave facing Mecca. Prayers for the deceased are recited at home, at the mosque, or at the cemetery. Women do not ordinarily attend the burial unless the deceased is a close relative or husband. Instead, they gather at the deceased's home and read the Qur'an. Cremation is not practiced.

Family members do not generally approve of autopsy because of respect for the dead and feelings that the body should not be mutilated. Islam allows forensic autopsy and autopsy for the sake of medical research and instruction.

Death rituals for Arab Christians are similar to Christian practices in the rest of the world. Arab American Christians may have a Bible next to the patient, expect a visit from the priest, and expect medical means to prolong life if possible. Organ donations and autopsies are acceptable. Wearing black during the mourning period is also common. For both Christians and Muslims, patients, especially children, are not told about terminal illness. The family spokesperson is usually the person who should be informed about death. The spokesperson will then communicate news to family members.

RESPONSES TO DEATH AND GRIEF

Mourning periods and practices may vary among Muslims and Christians emigrating from different Arab countries. Extended mourning periods may be practiced if the deceased is a young man, a woman, or a child. However, in some cases, Muslims may perceive extended periods of mourning as defiance of the will of God. Family members are asked to endure with patience and good faith in Allah what befalls them, including death. Whereas friends and relatives are to restrict mourning to 3 days, a wife may mourn for 4 months, and in some special cases, mourning can extend to 1 year. Although weeping is allowed, beating the cheeks or tearing garments is prohibited. For women, wearing black is considered appropriate for the entire period of mourning.

Spirituality

RELIGIOUS PRACTICES AND USE OF PRAYER

Not all Arab Americans are Muslims. Prominent Christian groups include the Copts in Egypt, the Chaldeans in Iraq, and the Maronites in Lebanon (Kulwicki & Kridli, 2001). Despite their distinctive practices and liturgies, Christians and Muslims share certain beliefs because of Islam's origin in Judaism and Christianity. Muslims and Christians believe in the same God and many of the same prophets, the Day of Judgment, Satan, heaven, hell, and an afterlife. One major difference is that Islam has no priesthood. Islamic scholars or religious **sheikhs**, the most learned individuals in an Islamic community, assume the role of **imam**, or "leader of the prayer." The imam also performs marriage ceremonies and funeral prayers and acts as a spiritual counselor or reference on Islamic teachings. Obtaining the opinion of the local imam may be a helpful intervention for Arab American Muslims struggling with health-care decisions.

As with any religion, observance of religious practices varies among Muslims; some nominally practice their religion whereas others are devout. However, because Islam is the state religion of most Arab countries, and in Islam, there is no separation of church and state, a certain degree of religious participation is obligatory.

To illustrate, consider a few examples of Islam's impact on Jordanian life. Because of Islamic law, abortion is investigated as a crime, and foster parenting is encouraged, whereas adoption is forbidden. The infertility treatments available are those approved by Islamic jurists. **Shariah**, Islamic law courts, rule on matters such as marriage, divorce, guardianship, and inheritance. Public schools have classes on Islam and prayer rooms. School and work schedules revolve around Islamic holidays and the weekly prayer. During Ramadan, restaurants remain closed during daylight hours and workdays are shortened to facilitate fasting. Because Muslims gather for communal prayer on Friday afternoons, the workweek runs from Saturday through Thursday. Finally, because of Islamic tradition that adherents of other monotheistic religions be accorded tolerance and protection, Jordan's Christians have separate religious courts and schools, and non-Muslims attending public schools are not required to participate in religious activities.

For Arab American Christians, church is an important part of everyday life. Most celebrate Catholic and Orthodox Christian holidays with fasting and ceremonial church services. They may display or wear Christian symbols such as a cross or a picture of the Virgin Mary.

VIGNETTE 6.2

Bilal, the terminally ill son of Mr. and Mrs. Khoury, has been on an inpatient unit for 3 weeks. Mrs. Khoury had been extremely critical of the nurses and the care they had been giving her son. Bilal has died. Upon being informed of their son's death, Mrs. Khoury appeared shocked and started sobbing loudly. The nurse tried to comfort her without success. Mrs. Khoury blamed herself for not bringing their son to the hospital sooner. Mr. Knoury appeared upset about the death but still tried to comfort his wife, also without success. He seemed reserved, and despite all efforts to calm his wife, she continued crying and beating on her chest. Patients from nearby rooms gathered in the hallway and inquired about the incident.

1. Based on your readings about the Arab culture, what measures should the nurse have taken prior to informing Mr. and Mrs. Khoury about their son's death?
2. Explain Mrs. Khoury's behavior, the critical behavior of the nurses, and the care they provided her son.
3. What is the role of Mr. Khoury in caring for his wife? How can a nurse ensure that Mr. Khoury's emotional needs are being met?

MEANING OF LIFE AND INDIVIDUAL SOURCES OF STRENGTH

For Muslims, adherents of the world's second largest religion, Islam means "submission to Allah." Life centers on worshipping Allah and preparing for one's afterlife by fulfilling religious duties as described in the Qur'an and the **hadith**. The five major pillars, or duties, of Islam are (1) declaration of faith, (2) prayer five times daily, (3) alms-giving, (4) fasting during Ramadan, and (5) completion of a pilgrimage to Mecca.

Despite the dominance of familialism in Arab life, religious faith is often regarded as more important. Whether Muslim or Christian, Arabs identify strongly with their respective religious groups, and religious affiliation is as much a part of their identity as family name. God and his power are acknowledged in everyday life.

SPIRITUAL BELIEFS AND HEALTH-CARE PRACTICES

Many Muslims believe in combining spiritual medicine, performance of daily prayers, and reading or listening to the Qur'an with conventional medical treatment. The devout patient may request that her or his chair or bed be turned to face Mecca and that a basin of water be provided for ritual washing or ablution before praying. Providing for cleanliness is particularly important because the Muslim's prayer is not acceptable unless the body, clothing, and place of prayer are clean.

Islamic teachings urge Muslims to eat wholesome food; abstain from pork, alcohol, and illicit drugs; practice moderation in all activities; be conscious of hygiene; and face adversity with faith in Allah's mercy and compassion, hope, and acceptance. Muslims are also advised to care for the needs of the community by visiting and assisting the sick and providing for needy Muslims.

Sometimes, illness is considered punishment for one's sins. Correspondingly, by providing cures, Allah manifests mercy and compassion and supplies a vehicle for repentance and gratitude (Al-Akili, 1993). Some emphasize that sickness should not be viewed as punishment, but as a trial or ordeal that brings about expiation of sins and that may strengthen character (Ebrahim, 1989). Common responses to illness include patience and endurance of suffering because it has a purpose known only to Allah, unfailing hope that even "irreversible" conditions might be cured "if it be Allah's will," and acceptance of one's fate. Suffering by some devout Muslims may be viewed as a means for greater reward in the afterlife (Lovering, 2006). Because of the belief in the sanctity of life, euthanasia and assisted suicide are forbidden (Lawrence, & Rozmus, 2001).

Spiritual beliefs and health-care practices for Arab American Christians are similar to those of Orthodox or Catholics. Caring for the body and burial practices are similar. A priest is always expected to visit the patient; if the patient is Catholic, a priest administers the sacrament of the sick.

Health-Care Practices

HEALTH-SEEKING BELIEFS AND BEHAVIORS

Good health is seen as the ability to fulfill one's roles. Diseases are attributed to a variety of factors such as inadequate diet, hot and cold shifts, exposure of one's stomach during sleep, emotional or spiritual distress, and envy or the evil eye. Arabs are expected to express and acknowledge their ailments when ill. Muslims often mention that the Prophet urged physicians to perform research and the ill to seek treatment because "Allah has not created a disease without providing a cure for it," except for the problem of old age (Ebrahim, 1989, p. 5).

Despite beliefs that one should care for health and seek treatment when ill, Arab women are often reluctant to seek care. Because of the cultural emphasis placed on modesty, some women express shyness about disrobing for examination. Similarly, some families object to female family members being examined by male physicians. Because of the fear that a diagnosed illness, such as cancer or psychiatric illness, may bring shame and influence the marriageability of the woman and her female relatives, delays in seeking medical care may be common.

Evidence also suggests that the cultural preference for male offspring influences the health care that low-income parents provide for female children. In poor communities in Jordan, boys were better nourished, more likely to be immunized, and more apt to receive prompt medical attention for illnesses (West, 1987). Delay in seeking treatment was noted by a local health-care provider who diagnosed "failure to thrive" in a young Iraqi female infant when her refugee parents sought medical attention for a feverish male sibling.

Whereas Arab Americans readily seek care for actual symptoms, preventive care is not generally sought (Kulwicki, 1996; Kulwicki et al., 2000). Similarly, pediatric clinics are used primarily for illness and injury rather than for well-child visits (Lipson, Reizian, & Meleis, 1987). Laffrey, Meleis, Lipson, Solomon, and Omidian (1989) attributed these patterns to Arabs' present orientation and reluctance to plan and to the meaning Arab Americans attach to preventive care. Whereas American health-care providers focus on screening and managing risks and complications, Arab Americans value information that aids in coping with stress, illness, or treatment protocols. Arab Americans' failure to use preventive care services may be related to other factors such as insurance coverage, the availability of female physicians who accept Medicaid patients, and the novelty of the concept of preventive care for immigrants from developing countries.

RESPONSIBILITY FOR HEALTH CARE

Dichotomous views regarding individual responsibility and one's control over life's events often cause misunderstanding between Arab Americans and health-care providers (Abu Gharbieh, 1993). For example, individualism and an activist approach to life are the underpinnings of the American health-care system. Accordingly, practices such as informed consent, self-care, advance directives, risk management, and preventive care are valued. Patients are expected to use information seeking and problem solving in preference to faith in God, patience, and acceptance of one's fate as primary coping mechanisms. Similarly, American health-care providers expect that the patient's hope be "realistic" in accordance with medical science.

However, in Arab culture, quite the opposite values—familialism and fatalism—influence health care and responses to illness. For Arabs, the family is the context within which health care is delivered (Lipson et al., 1987). Rather than engage in self-care and decision making, clients often allow family members to oversee care. Family members indulge the individual and assume the ill person's responsibilities. Although the patient may seem overly dependent and the family overly protective by American standards, family members' vigilance and "demanding behavior" should be interpreted as a measure of concern. For Muslims, care is a religious obligation associated with individual and collective meanings of honor (Luna, 1994). Individuals are seen as expressing care through the performance of gender-specific role responsibilities, as delineated in the Qur'an.

Although most American health-care professionals consider full disclosure an ethical obligation, most Arab physicians do not believe that it is necessary for a client to know a serious diagnosis or full details of a surgical procedure. In fact, communicating a grave diagnosis is often viewed as cruel and tactless because it deprives clients of hope. Similarly, preoperative instructions are believed to cause needless anxiety, hypochondriasis, and complications. Apart from the educated, most clients are not interested in actively participating in decision making (Abu Gharbieh, 1993). Most Arabs expect physicians, because of their expertise, to select treatments. The client's role is to cooperate. The authority of physicians is seldom challenged or questioned. When treatment is successful, the physician's skill is recognized; adverse outcomes are attributed to God's will unless there is evidence of blatant malpractice (Sullivan, 1993).

Not all Arabs may be familiar with the American concept of health insurance. Traditionally, the family unit, through its communal resources, provides insurance. Certain Arab countries, such as Saudi Arabia and Kuwait, provide free medical care, whereas in other countries, many citizens are government employees and are entitled to low-cost care in government-sector facilities. Private physicians and hospitals are preferred because of the belief that the private sector offers the best care.

Because many medications requiring a prescription in the United States are available over the counter in Arab countries, Arabs are accustomed to seeking medical advice from pharmacists. In comparison with other Americans in Wayne County, Arab Americans were less likely to take prescription medications, but when they did, they were more likely to use medications as directed (Wayne County Health Department, 1994).

FOLK PRACTICES

Although Islam disapproves of superstition, witchcraft, and magic, concerns about the powers of jealous people, the evil eye, and certain supernatural agents such as the devil and **jinn** are part of the folk beliefs. Those who envy the wealth, success, or beauty of others are believed to cause adversity by a gaze, which brings misfortune to the victim. Beautiful women, healthy-looking babies, and the rich are believed to be particularly susceptible to the evil eye, and expressions of congratulations may be interpreted as envy. Protection from the evil eye is afforded by wearing amulets, such as blue beads or figures involving the number 5, reciting the Qur'an, or invoking the name of Allah (Kulwicki, 1996). Barren women, the poor, and the unfortunate are usually suspects for casting the evil eye.

Mental or emotional illnesses may be attributed to possession by evil jinn. Some believe that insanity, or **jinaan** ("possessed by the jinn"), may also be caused by the evil wishes of jealous individuals.

Traditional Islamic medicine is based on the theory of four humors and the spiritual and physical remedies prescribed by the Prophet. Because illness is viewed as an imbalance between the humors—black bile, blood, phlegm, and yellow bile—and the primary attributes of dryness, heat, cold, and moisture, therapy involves treating with the disease's opposite: hot disease, cold remedy. Although methods such as cupping, cautery, and phlebotomy may be employed, treating with special prayers or simple foods such as dates, honey, salt, and olive oil is preferred (Al-Akili, 1993). Yemeni or Saudi Arabian patients may apply heat (cupping, moxibustion) or use cautery in combination with modern medical technology.

BARRIERS TO HEALTH CARE

Newly arrived and unskilled refugees from poorer parts of the Arab world are at particular risk for both increased exposure to ill health and inadequate access to health care. Factors such as refugee status, recency of arrival, differences in cultural values and norms, inability to pay for health-care services, and inability to speak English add to the stresses of immigration (Kulwicki, 2000; Kulwicki et al., 2000), affecting both health status and responses to health problems. Moreover, these immigrants are less likely to receive adequate health care because of cultural and language barriers, lack of transportation, limited health insurance, poverty, a lack of awareness of existing services, and poor coordination of services (Kulwicki, 1996, 2000).

Although a lack of insurance coverage affects a significant number of Wayne County Health Department respondents (Wayne County Health Department, 1994), other studies suggest that Arab Americans regard other barriers and services as more significant. For instance, language and communication remain serious barriers for recent Arab American immigrants (Kulwicki, 2000). Transportation to health-care facilities and culturally competent service providers also adds to the problems of accessing health-care services.

VIGNETTE 6.3

Amal is a 22-year-old pregnant woman who has just immigrated from Lebanon. She is 6 months' pregnant and has not seen a doctor because she does not have health insurance. She is visiting the health department for the first time, hoping to be seen by a doctor and enroll in the Women, Infants, and Children (WIC) program. She, her husband, and her 4-year-old son fled Lebanon 1 year ago owing to the political unrest in their home country. Amal is hesitant to fill out the necessary paperwork or answer questions about her residency status for fear of being deported. She states that her son constantly coughs and has breathing problems, especially when her husband smokes. Her husband works in a local restaurant as a dishwasher but was recently laid off because of his frequent absences from work owing to his constant coughing and breathing difficulties. Amal does not smoke, but her husband has smoked two packs a day since he was 18 years old. Amal speaks only limited English.

1. What additional information is needed to complete an assessment for Amal and her family? Given Amal's limited English proficiency, how would you obtain the necessary information?
2. Explain the cultural barriers Amal is experiencing in accessing prenatal care.
3. What type of intervention can the nurse provide to Amal regarding her husband's smoking?

CULTURAL RESPONSES TO HEALTH AND ILLNESS

Arabs regard pain as unpleasant and something to be controlled (Reizian & Meleis, 1986). Because of their confidence in medical science, Arabs anticipate immediate postoperative relief from their symptoms. This expectation, in combination with a belief in conserving energy for recovery, often contributes to a reluctance to comply with typical postoperative routines such as frequent ambulation. Although expressive, emotional, and vocal responses to pain are usually reserved for the immediate family, under certain circumstances, such as childbirth and illnesses accompanied by spasms, Arabs express pain more freely (Reizian & Meleis, 1986). The tendency of Arabs to be more expressive with their family and more restrained in the presence of health professionals may lead to conflicting perceptions regarding the adequacy of pain relief. Whereas the nurse may assess pain relief as adequate, family members may demand that their relative receive additional analgesia.

The attitude that mental illness is a major social stigma is particularly pervasive. Psychiatric symptoms may be denied, attributed to "bad nerves" (Hattar-Pollara, Meleis, & Nagib, 2001) or evil spirits (Kulwicki, 1996). Underrecognition of signs and symptoms may occur because of the somatic orientation of Arab patients and physicians, patients' tolerance of emotional suffering, and relatives' tolerance of behavioral disturbances (El-Islam, 1994). Indeed, home management with standard but crucial adjustments within the family may abort or control symptoms until remission occurs. For example, female family members manage postpartum depression by assuming care of the newborn and/or by telling the mother she needs more help or more rest. Islamic legal prohibitions further confound attempts to estimate the incidence of problems such as alcoholism and suicide, resulting in underreporting of these conditions because of a potential for severe social stigma.

When individuals suffering from mental distress seek medical care, they are likely to present with a variety of vague complaints, such as abdominal pain, lassitude, anorexia, and shortness of breath. Patients often expect and may insist on somatic treatment, at least "vitamins and tonics" (El-Islam, 1994). When mental illness is accepted as a diagnosis, treatment by medications rather than by counseling is preferred. Hospitalization is resisted because such placement is viewed as abandonment (Budman, Lipson, & Meleis, 1992). Although Arab Americans report family and marital stress as well as various mental health symptoms, they often seek family counseling or social services rather than a psychiatrist (Aswad & Gray, 1996).

Yousef (1993) described the Arab public's attitude toward the disabled as generally negative, with low expectations for education and rehabilitation. Yousef also related misconceptions about mental retardation to the dearth of Arab literature about disability and the public's lack of experience with the disabled. Because of social stigma, the disabled are often kept from public view. Similarly, although there is a trend toward educating some children with mild mental retardation in regular schools, special education programs are generally institutionally based.

Reiter, Mar'i, and Rosenberg (1986) found that parents who were most intimately involved with the developmentally disabled held rather positive attitudes. More tolerant views were expressed among Israeli Arab parents, Muslims, the less educated, and residents of smaller villages than among Christians, the educated, and residents of larger villages with mixed populations. Reiter et al. (1986) linked the less positive attitudes of the latter groups to the process of modernization, which affects a drive toward status and a weakening of family structures and traditions. Traditions include regarding the handicapped as coming from God, accepting the disabled person's dependency, and providing care within the home.

Dependency is accepted. Family members assume the ill person's responsibilities. The ill person is cared for and indulged. From an American frame of reference, the patient may seem overly dependent and the family overly protective.

BLOOD TRANSFUSIONS AND ORGAN DONATION

Although blood transfusions and organ transplants are widely accepted, organ donation is a controversial issue among Arabs and Arab Americans. Practices of organ donation may vary among Arab Muslims and non-Muslims based on their religious beliefs about death and dying, reincarnation, or their personal feelings about helping others by donating their organs to others or for scientific purposes (Kulwicki, 2001). Health-care professionals should be sensitive to personal, family, or religious practices toward organ donation among Arab Americans and should not make any assumptions about organ donation unless family members are asked.

Health-Care Practitioners

TRADITIONAL VERSUS BIOMEDICAL PRACTITIONERS

Although Arab Americans combine traditional and biomedical care practices, they are very cognizant of the effective medical treatments in the West and consider themselves privileged to be able to use the American health-care system, which would not have been accessible to them in their country of origin (Kulwicki, 1996). Because of their profound respect for medicine, Arab Americans seek treatments for physical disorders or ailments. Medical treatments that require surgery, removal of causative agents, or eradicating by intravenous treatments are valued more than therapies aimed at health promotion or disease prevention. Although most Arab Americans have high regard for medicine related to physical disorders, many do not have the same respect or trust for mental or psychological treatment. A pervasive feeling among many Arab Americans is that psychiatric services or therapies related to mental disorders are not effective and are required only for individuals who have severe mental disorders or who are considered "crazy." Psychiatric services are, therefore, underutilized among Arab Americans despite greater need for such services among distressed immigrant populations.

Gender and, to a lesser extent, age are considerations in matching Arab patients and health-care providers. In Arab societies, unrelated males and females are not accustomed to interacting. Shyness in women is appreciated, and Muslim men may ignore women out of politeness. Health-care settings, client units, and sometimes waiting rooms are segregated by sex. Male nurses never care for female patients.

Given this background, many Arab Americans may find interacting with a health-care professional of the opposite sex quite embarrassing and stressful. Discomfort may be expressed by refusal to discuss personal information and a reluctance to disrobe for physical assessments and hygiene. Arab American women may refuse to be seen by male American health-care providers, excluding or denying men the opportunity to interact or appropriately diagnose health conditions for high-risk Arab American females.

STATUS OF HEALTH-CARE PROVIDERS

Arab Americans have great respect for science and medicine. Most Arab Americans are aware of the historical contributions of Arabs in the field of medicine and are proud of their accomplishments. Knowledge held by a doctor is believed to convey authority and power. When ill, most Arab American clients who lack English communication skills prefer to see Arabic-speaking doctors because of their feelings of cultural and linguistic affinity toward Arab American doctors. Many Arabic-speaking clients also feel that Arab American doctors understand them better, and they feel more at ease speaking with someone from their own culture. However, clients who are able to communicate in English do not usually show preferences for seeing Arab doctors rather than American doctors. In some cases, these clients prefer to be seen by American doctors because they view American doctors as more professional and more respectful to clients than their Arab American counterparts.

Although medicine is perhaps the most respected profession in Arab society, nursing is viewed as a menial profession that conflicts with societal norms proscribing certain female behavior. In this conservative culture, in which contact between unrelated males and females is often discouraged, nursing is considered particularly undesirable as an occupation because it requires close contact between the sexes and work during evening and night hours (Abu Gharbieh, 1993). American nurses are regarded more favorably because of their education, expertise, and performance of roles ascribed solely to Arab physicians (e.g., performing physical examinations). However, younger immigrants, and especially immigrants who come from Lebanon, Iraq, and Jordan, have more favorable perceptions about nursing as a profession than the older generation of Arab American immigrants (Kulwicki & Kridli, 2001).

Perhaps because Arab physicians tend to be older males and Arab nurses are typically young females, the status and roles of physicians and nurses mirror the hierarchical family structure of Arab society. Physicians require that nurses "know their place" and leave the interpretation of data, decision making, and disclosure of information to them. Nurses conform to the role expectations of physicians and the public and function as medical assistants and housekeepers rather than as critical thinkers and health educators.

REFERENCES

Abu Gharbieh, P. (1993). Culture shock. Cultural norms influencing nursing in Jordan. *Nursing and Health Care, 14*(10), 534–540.

Ahmad, N. M. (2004). Arab-American culture and health care. Retrieved January 15, 2007, from http://www.case.edu/med/epidbio/mphp439/Arab-Americans.html

Al-Akili, M. (1993). *Natural healing with the medicine of the prophet.* Philadelphia, PA: Pearl Publishing House.

Al-Shahri, M. Z. (2002). Culturally sensitive caring for Saudi patients, *Journal of Transcultural Nursing, 13*(2), 133–138.

Arab American Institute. (2007). *Demographics.* Retrieved January 14, 2007, from http://www.aaiusa.org/arab-americans/22/demographics

Arab human development report. (2000). Retrieved October 30, 2002, from http://www.UNESCO.org/education

Aswad, B. (1999). Arabs in America: Building a new future. In M. W. Suleiman (Ed.), *Attitudes of Arab immigrants toward welfare* (pp. 177–191). Philadelphia: Temple University Press.

Aswad, B. C., & Gray, N. (1996). Challenges to the Arab-American family and ACCESS (Arab Community Center for Economic and Social Services). In B. C. Aswad & B. Bilgé (Eds.), *Family and gender among American Muslims: Issues facing Middle Eastern immigrants and their descendants* (pp. 223–240). Philadelphia: Temple University Press.

Budman, C., Lipson, J., & Meleis, A. (1992). The cultural consultant in mental health care: The case of an Arab adolescent. *American Journal of Orthopsychiatry, 62*(3), 359–370.

Centers for Disease Control and Prevention (CDC). (2006). *Complete HIV/AIDS resource.* Retrieved January 15, 2007, from http://thebody.com/cdc/cdcpage.html

Cline, S., Abuirmeileh, N., & Roberts, A. (1986). *Woman's life cycle. Fundamentals of health education* (pp. 48–77). Yarmouk, Jordan: Yarmouk University.

Darwish-Yassine, M., & Wang, D. (2005). Cancer epidemiology in Arab Americans and Arabs outside the Middle East. *Ethnicity and Disease, 15*, S1–S8.

Ebrahim, A. (1989). *Abortion, birth control and surrogate parenting. An Islamic perspective.* Indianapolis, IN: American Trust Publications.

El-Islam, M. (1994). Cultural aspects of morbid fears in Qatari women. *Social Psychiatry Psychiatric Epidemiology, 29*, 137–140.

Global Gayz: Muslims. (2006). Retrieved January 15, 2007, from http://www.globalgayz.com/art-index.html#middleeast

Hamamy, H., & Alwan, A. (1994). Hereditary disorders in the Eastern Mediterranean region. *Bulletin of the World Health Organization, 72*(1), 145–154.

Hashemite Kingdom of Jordan, Department of Statistics. (1985). *Jordan's husbands' fertility survey.* Amman, Jordan: Author, in collaboration with Division of Reproductive Health, Centers for Disease Control and Prevention, Atlanta, GA.

Hattar-Pollara, M., Meleis, A. I., & Nagib, H. (2001). A study of spousal role of Egyptian women in clerical jobs. *Health Care for Women International, 21*(4), 305–517.

Hikmet, J., Hakim-Larson, J., Farrag, M., & Jamil, L. (2002). A retrospective study of Arab American mental health clients: Trauma and the Iraqi refugees. *American Journal of Orthopsychiatry, 72*, 355–361.

Institute of Medicine (2002). *Unequal treatment: Confronting racial and ethnic disparities in health care.* Retrieved January 15, 2007, from http://www.iom.edu/?id=4475

Kinzie, J., Boehnlein J. K., Riley, C., & Sparr, L. (2002) The effects of September 11 on traumatized refugees: Reactivation of posttraumatic stress disorder. *Journal of Nervous and Mental Disease, 190*, 437–441.

Kulwicki, A. (1996). Health issues among Arab Muslim families. In B. C. Aswad & B. Bilgé (Eds.), *Family and gender among American Muslims: Issues facing Middle Eastern immigrants and their descendants* (pp. 187–207). Philadelphia: Temple University Press.

Kulwicki, A. (2000). Arab women. In M. Julia (Ed.), *Constructing gender: Multicultural perspectives in working with women* (pp. 89–98). Nelson, BC, Canada: Brooks/Cole.

Kulwicki, A. (Ed.). (2001). *Ethnic resource guide.* Dearborn, MI: Henry Ford Hospital.

Kulwicki, A., & Cass, P. (1994). An assessment of Arab-American knowledge, attitudes, and beliefs about AIDS. *IMAGE: Journal of Nursing Scholarship, 26*(1), 13–17.

Kulwicki, A., & Khalifa, R. (2007). *The impact of September 11th, 2001, on Arab American nurses in Michigan.* Manuscript submitted for publication.

Kulwicki, A., & Kridli, S. (2001). *Health-care perceptions and experiences of Chaldean, Arab Muslim, Arab Christian, and Armenian women in the metropolitan area of Detroit.* Unpublished manuscript.

Kulwicki, A., & Miller, J. (1999). Domestic violence in the Arab American population: Transforming environmental conditions through community education. *Issues in Mental Health Nursing 20*(3) 199–215.

Kulwicki, A., Miller, J., & Schim, S. (2000). Collaborative partnership for culture care: Enhancing health services for the Arab community. *Journal of Transcultural Nursing, 11*(1), 31–39.

Kulwicki, A., Smiley, K., & Devine, S. (2007, in press). Smoking behavior in pregnant Arab Americans. *The American Journal of Maternal/Child Nursing.*

Laffrey, S., Meleis, A., Lipson, J., Solomon, M., & Omidian, P. (1989). Assessing Arab-American health care needs. *Social Science and Medicine, 29*(7), 877–883.

Lawrence, P., & Rozmus, C. (2001). Culturally sensitive care of the Muslim patient. *Journal of Transcultural Nursing, 12*, 228–233.

Levy, R. (1993). Ethnic and racial differences in response to medicines: Preserving individualized therapy in managed pharmaceutical programmes. *Pharmaceutical Medicine, 7*, 139–165.

Lipson, J., Reizian, A., & Meleis, A. (1987). Arab-American patients: A medical record review. *Social Science and Medicine, 24*(2), 101–107.

Lovering, S. (2006). Cultural attitudes and beliefs about pain. *Journal of Transcultural Nursing, 17*(4), 389–395.

Luna, L. (1994). Care and cultural context of Lebanese Muslim immigrants: Using Leininger's theory. *Journal of Transcultural Nursing, 5*(2), 12–20.

Meleis, A. (2005). Arabs. In J. Lipson, & S. Dibble (Eds.), *Culture and clinical care* (pp. 42-57). San Francisco, CA: The Regents, University of California.

Michigan Department of Public Health. (1993). *Health profiles of Michigan populations.* Lansing, MI: Author.

Michigan Department of Community Health and Michigan Public Health Institute. (2003). *2001–2002 special cancer behavioral risk factor survey.* Lansing, MI: Author.

Naff, A. (1980). *Arabs in America: A historical overview* (pp. 128–136), Boston: Harvard Encyclopedia of American Ethnic Groups.

Nydell, M. (1987). *Understanding Arabs. A guide for Westerners.* Yarmouth, ME: Intercultural Press.

Office of Minority Health (OMH). (2001). *Health facts.* Retrieved October 21, 2001, from http://www.mdch.state.mi.us/pha/omh/ aram-ch.htm

Pickthall, M. (1977). *The meaning of the glorious Qur'an.* Mecca, Saudi Arabia: Muslim World League.

Reiter, S., Mar'i, S., & Rosenberg, Y. (1986). Parental attitudes toward the developmentally disabled among Arab communities in Israel: A cross-cultural study. *International Journal of Rehabilitation Research, 9*(4), 335–362.

Reizian, A., & Meleis, A. (1986). Arab-Americans' perceptions of and responses to pain. *Critical Care Nurse, 6*(6), 30–37.

Reizian, A., & Meleis, A. (1987). Symptoms reported by Arab-American patients on the Cornell Medical Index (CMI). *Western Journal of Nursing Research, 9*(3), 368–384.

Rice, V., & Kulwicki, A. (1992). Cigarette use among Arab Americans in the Detroit metropolitan area. *Public Health Reports, 107*(5), 589–594.

Schwartz, S., Darwish-Yassine, M., & Wing, D. (2005). Cancer diagnosis in Arab Americans and Arabs outside the United States. *Ethnicity and Disease, 15*, 1–8.

Seikaly, M. (1999). Arabs in America: Building a new future. In M. W. Suleiman (Ed.), *Attachment and identity: The Palestinian community of Detroit* (pp. 25–38). Philadelphia: Temple University Press.

Sullivan, S. (1993). The patient behind the veil: Medical culture shock in Saudi Arabia. *Canadian Medical Association Journal, 148*(3), 444–446.

Templin, T., Rice, H., Gadelrab, H., Weglicki, L., Hammad, A., & Kulwicki, A. (2003). Michigan Trends in tobacco use among Arab/Arab American adolescents: Preliminary findings. *Ethnicity and Disease, 15*(1), S-65–S-69.

UNICEF. (2005). United Nations Population Division. Retreived January 2, 2007, from http://www.unicef.org/infobycountry/index.html

U.S. Bureau of the Census. (2005). Special Report. We the People of Arab Ancestry in the United States. Retrieved January 14, 2007, from http://www.census.gov/prod/2005pubs/censr-21.pdf

Wayne County Health Department. (1994). *Arab community in Wayne County, Michigan: Behavior risk factor survey (BRFS).* East Lansing, MI: Michigan State University, Institute for Public Policy and Social Research.

West, M. (1987, April 29). Surveys indicate girls face discrimination in provision of nutrition and health care. *Jordan Times.*

World Health Organization (WHO). (2006). *Country and selection for infant deaths.* Retrieved August 22, 2007, from http://www.int/whosis/ database/mortable.2cfm

World Health Organization (WHO). (2004). *Regional database on HIV/AIDS,* WHO Regional Office for the Eastern Mediterranean. Retrieved January 2, 2007, from http://www.emro.who.int/ASD/Facts-regional-profile.html

Yousef, J. (1993). Education of children with mental retardation in Arab countries. *Mental Retardation, 31*(2), 117–121.

Zogby, J. (1990). *Arab America today. A demographic profile of Arab Americans.* Washington, DC: Arab American Institute.

Zogby, J. (2002). *What Arabs think: Values, beliefs and concerns.* Retrieved January 15, 2007, from http://www.zogby.com/News/ReadNews. dbm?ID=629

Zogby International. (2007). Retrieved January 14, 2007, from http://www. zogby.com/features/zogbytables3.cfm

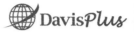 Davis*Plus*

For case studies, review questions and additional information, go to
http://davisplus.fadavis.com

Chapter 7

People of Chinese Heritage

YAN WANG and LARRY D. PURNELL

Overview, Inhabited Localities, and Topography

OVERVIEW

Although some Western health-care providers categorize all Asians into one group, each nationality is very different. Cultural values differ even among Chinese according to their geographic location within China—north, south, east, west; rural versus urban; interior versus port city—as well as other primary and secondary characteristics of culture (see Chapter 1). Chinese immigrants to Western countries are even more diverse, with a mixture of traditional and Western values and beliefs. These differences must be acknowledged and appreciated.

Han Chinese are the principal ethnic group of China, constituting about 92 percent of the population of mainland China, especially as distinguished from Manchus, Mongols, Huis, and other minority nationalities. The remaining 8 percent are a mixture of 56 different nationalities, religions, and ethnic groups. Substantial genetic, linguistic, cultural, and social differences exist among these subgroups. Because of the complexity of their values, it is impossible to develop specific cultural interventions appropriate for all Chinese clients. Therefore, the information included in this chapter should serve simply as a beginning point for understanding Chinese people, not as a definitive profile.

Children born to Chinese parents in Western countries tend to adopt the Western culture easily, whereas their parents and grandparents tend to maintain their traditional Chinese culture in varying degrees. Chinese who live in the "Chinatowns" of North America and other places outside of China, maintain many of their cultural and social beliefs and values and insist that health-care providers respect these values and beliefs with their prescribed interventions.

HERITAGE AND RESIDENCE

The Chinese culture is one of the oldest in recorded human history, beginning with the Xia dynasty, dating from 2200 B.C., to the present-day People's Republic of China (PRC). The Chinese name for their country is *Zhong guo,* which means "middle kingdom" or "center of the earth." Many of the current values and beliefs of the Chinese remain grounded in their history; many believe that the Chinese culture is superior to other Asian cultures. Ideals based on the teachings of Confucius (551–479 B.C.) continue to play an important part in the values and beliefs of the Chinese. These ideals emphasize the importance of accountability to family and neighbors and reinforce the idea that all relationships embody power and rule.

During early Communist rule, an attempt was made to break down the values grounded in Confucianism and substitute values consistent with equal social responsibility. This was initially achieved, and rank in society was no longer seen as important. During the People's Revolution, feudal rank frequently meant loss of social importance, physical punishment, imprisonment, and even death. Later, during the Cultural Revolution, the young were held responsible for the deaths of many previously esteemed elderly and educated Chinese. Today, many of the Confucian values have reasserted themselves. Families, the elderly, and highly educated individuals are again considered important. Research completed by the Chinese Culture Connection, a group of Chinese sociologists, lists 40 important values in modern China, including filial piety, industry, patriotism, paying deference to those in hierarchal status positions, tolerance of others, loyalty to superiors, respect for rites and social rituals, knowledge, benevolent authority, thrift, patience, courtesy, and respect for tradition (Hu & Grove, 1991).

The population of China is 1.31 billion people (China Population Information and Research Center, 2007), with 80 percent living in rural communities. The country is over 9.6 million square kilometers (3.7 million square miles), with 23 provinces; 5 regions including Tibet, Hong Kong, and Taiwan; and 3 municipalities. Each province, region, and municipality functions independently and in many different ways. The Chinese consider each region as part of greater China and predict that the day will come when all of China is reunited. Tibet has already been reassimilated, Hong Kong returned to Chinese control in 1997, and Macau in 1999.

Chinese Americans compose the largest subgroup among Asians/Pacific Islanders (APIs), exceeding 2.8 million people (Yu, Huang, & Singh, 2004). Every year since 1996, the quota for Chinese immigration to the United States has been filled, with more than 625,000 immigrants obtaining permanent legal status from mainland China, Taiwan, and Hong Kong (U.S. Department of Homeland Security, 2005). In the United States, the largest communities of Chinese Americans are in California, New York, Florida, and Texas.

REASONS FOR MIGRATION AND ASSOCIATED ECONOMIC FACTORS

Chinese immigrated to the United States in three different waves: in the 1800s, in the 1950s, and in more recent years. Chinese immigration was initially fueled by economic needs. Over 100,000 male peasants from Guangdong and Fujian came to the United States without their families in the early 1830s to make their fortune on the transcontinental railroad. This immigration continued through the Gold Rush of 1849. Many believed that they could make money in the United States to help their families and later return to China. Unfortunately, most found that opportunities were limited to hard labor and other vocations not desired by European Americans. Their culture and physical features made them readily identifiable in the predominantly white American society. They could not simply change their names and blend in with other, primarily European immigrant populations. The Chinese had few rights and were barred from becoming U.S. citizens. Racial violence and prejudice against them were common, and the courts did not punish the violators. Compared with other ethnic groups, their immigration numbers were small until 1952, when the McCarran-Walters Bill relaxed immigration laws and permitted more Chinese to enter the country.

The most recent immigrants from Taiwan, Hong Kong, and mainland China are strikingly different from earlier Chinese immigrants in that they are more diverse. In addition, whereas many emigrated to reunite with families, students, scholars, and professionals flocked to the United States to pursue higher education or research. For their safety and the maintenance of their cultural values, most Chinese settled in closed communities.

EDUCATIONAL STATUS AND OCCUPATIONS

Education is compulsory in China, and most children receive the equivalent of a ninth-grade education. Middle school students must complete a state examination to determine their eligibility to enter a general high school, to go to a preparatory high school before entering technical school or college, or to begin their lives as workers. Those who complete either the general or the preparatory high school experience compete academically to continue their education at college and university levels. The Chinese educational system is complex and is not presented here in its entirety; further study is encouraged.

A university education is highly valued; however, few have the opportunity to achieve this life goal because enrollments in better educational institutions are limited. Because competition for top universities is keen, many families select less valued universities to ensure that their child is accepted into a university rather than slated for a technical school education. After their undergraduate or graduate programs, many young adults come to Western countries to attend universities to seek more advanced education or research. A foreign education is considered prestigious in China.

In the West, initially the Chinese tend to be either highly or poorly educated. This dichotomy may result in healthcare providers categorizing clients in a similar manner. Many people believe that Chinese occupations are limited to restaurant work, service employment, and the garment industry. However, this phenomenon has changed since the 1980s. A significant number of Chinese students and scholars from the PRC and Taiwan come to the United States to study every year. Because of the competitive educational system in mainland China and Taiwan, where only the brightest students go to a university, Chinese immigrants with a college education are often very well educated. Student immigrants are expected to return to China or Taiwan when their education and research are completed. However, many do not return but elect to remain in Western countries, having obtained graduate degrees in the United States, and many find employment in high-technology companies or educational and research institutes.

Another group of Chinese immigrants are professionals from Hong Kong who moved to North America and other Western countries to avoid the repatriation in 1997. These immigrants usually have family connections or close friends in Western countries who are highly educated and skilled. A third group of immigrants consists of uneducated individuals with diverse manual labor skills. Finding employment opportunities for these Chinese people may be more difficult. They often settle with family members who are not skilled or highly educated. This arrangement drains family resources for many years until they obtain financial security, learn the language, and become acculturated in other ways.

Communication

VIGNETTE 7.1

Mrs. Yu, a 48-year-old from Beijing, immigrated to the United States 5 years ago to live with her daughter. She speaks and reads very little English, but most of the time she seems to understand what physicians and nurses tell her. Today, she walked 12 blocks to the clinic for her monthly check-up regarding arthritis problems and chronic bronchitis from smoking when she lived in China. The physician on duty is a male and prescribes several new medicines. The nurse needs to give instructions on how to take her new medication three times a day with meals.

1. Does the gender of the physician have any implications for Mrs. Yu's visit?
2. Provide written instructions for Mrs. Yu to take her medications.
3. Given limited English language ability, how might the nurse ensure that Mrs. Yu understands how to take her medication?
4. Where might the nurse find someone to translate the English instructions into Chinese?
5. Does it make any difference which dialect Mrs. Yu speaks for the written instructions? Explain.

The official language of China is *Mandarin* (**pu tong hua**), which is spoken by about 70 percent of the population, primarily in northern China, but there are 10 major, distinct dialects, including Cantonese, Fujianese, Shanghainese, Toishanese, and Hunanese. For example, *pu tong hua* is spoken in Beijing, the capital of China in the north, and Shanghainese is spoken in Shanghai. The two cities are only 1462 kilometers (about 665 miles)

apart, but because the dialects are so different, the two groups cannot understand one another verbally. Even though people from one part of China cannot understand those from other regions, the written language is the same throughout the country and consists of over 50,000 characters (about 5000 common ones); thus, most children are at least 10 to 12 years old before they can read the newspaper.

Although many times Chinese sound loud when talking with other Chinese, they generally speak in a moderate to low voice. Americans are considered loud to most Chinese, and health-care providers must be cautious about their voice volume when interacting with Chinese in English so that intentions are not misinterpreted.

When possible, health-care providers should use the Chinese language to communicate (see Table 7–1 for some common phrases), being careful to avoid jargon and use the simplest terms. Many times, verbs can be omitted because the Chinese language has only a limited number of verbs. The Chinese appreciate any attempt to use their language. They do not mind mistakes and will correct speakers when they believe it will not cause embarrassment. When asked whether they understand what was just said, the Chinese invariably answer yes, even when they do not understand. Such an admission causes loss of face; thus, it is better to have clients repeat the instructions they have been given.

Negative queries are difficult for Chinese people to understand. For example, do not say, "You know how to

TABLE 7.1 *Frequently Used Words and Phrases*

English Word or Phrase	Chinese Pinyin	Phonetic Pronunciation
Hello	Nǐ hǎo	Nee how (note tones to be used*)
Goodbye	Zài jiàn	Dzai jee en
How are you?	Nǐ hǎo mā	Nee how mah
Please	Qǐng	Ching
Thank you	Xīe xie	Shee eh shee eh
I don't understand	Wǒ bù dǒng	Wah boo doong
Yes	Shì de or dui	Shur da or doee (no real yes or no comparable saying—this means I agree or okay)
No	Bú shì de or bu hǎo	Boo shur or boo how
My name is	Wǒ jiào	Wah djeeow
Very good	Hěn hǎo	Hun hao
Hurt	Téng	Tung
I, you, he/she/it	Wo, nǐ, tā	Wah, nee, tah
Hot	Rè	Ruh
Cold	Lěng	Lung
Happy	Gāo xi ngu	Gow shing
Where	Nǎ li	Na lee
Not have	MéiYǒu	May yo
Doctor	Yī shēng	Yee shung
Nurse	Hù s hi	Who shur

*Note: Each *pu tong hua* Chinese word is pronounced with five different tones:
1. First tone is high and even across the word (–).
2. Second tone starts low and goes high (–`).
3. Third tone starts neutral, goes low, and then goes high (ˇ).
4. Fourth tone is curt and goes low (·`).
5. Fifth tone is neutral and pronounced very lightly.

do that, don't you?" Instead say, "Do you know how to do that?" Also, it is easier for them to understand instructions placed in a specific order, such as:

1. At 9 o'clock every morning, get the medicine bottle.
2. Take two tablets out of the bottle.
3. Get your hot water.
4. Swallow the pills with the water.

Do not use complex sentences with *ands* and *buts*. The Chinese have difficulty deciding what to respond to first when the speaker uses compound or complex sentences.

CULTURAL COMMUNICATION PATTERNS

Chinese have a reputation for not openly displaying emotion. Although this may be true among strangers, among family and friends they are open and demonstrative. The Chinese share information freely with health-care providers once a trusting relationship has developed. This is not always easy because Western health-care providers may not have the patience or time to develop such relationships. In situations in which Chinese people perceive that health-care practitioners or other people of authority may lose face or be embarrassed, they may choose not to be totally truthful.

Touching between health-care providers and Chinese clients should be kept to a minimum. Most Chinese maintain a formal distance with each other, which is a form of respect. Some are uncomfortable with face-to-face communications, especially when there is direct eye contact. Because they prefer to sit next to others, the health-care practitioner may need to rearrange seating to promote positive communication. When touching is necessary, the practitioner should provide explanations to Chinese clients.

Facial expressions are used extensively among family and friends. The Chinese love to joke and laugh. They use and appreciate smiles when talking with others. However, if the situation is formal, smiles may be limited. In most greeting and communication situations, shaking hands is common; hugs are limited. The health-care provider should watch for cues from their Chinese clients.

FORMAT FOR NAMES

Among the Chinese, introductions, either by name card or verbally, are different from those in Western countries. For example, the family name is stated first and then the given name. Calling individuals by any name except their family name is impolite unless they are close friends or relatives. If a person's family name is Li and the given name is Ruiming, then the proper form of address is Li Ruiming. Men are addressed by their family name, such as *Ma*, and a title such as *Ma xian sheng* ("Mister Ma"), *lao Ma* ("respected older Ma"), or *xiao Ma* ("young Ma"). Titles are important to Chinese people, so when possible, identify the person's title and use it.

Women in China do not use their husband's last name after they get married and retain their own family last name. Therefore, unless the woman is from Hong Kong or Taiwan, or has lived in a Western country for a long time, do not assume that her last name is the same as her husband's. Her family name comes first, followed by her given names, and finally, by her title. Many Chinese living in Western counties take an English name as an additional given name because their name is difficult for Westerners to pronounce. Their English name can be used in many settings. Addressing them as "Miss Millie" or "Mr. Jonathan" rather than simply by their English name is better. Even though they have adopted an English name, some Chinese may give permission to use only the English name. In addition, some Chinese switch the order of their names to be the same as Westerners, with their family name last. This practice can be confusing; therefore, health-care providers should address Chinese clients by their whole name or by their family name and title, and then ask them how they wish to be addressed.

Family Roles and Organization

HEAD OF HOUSEHOLD AND GENDER ROLES

Kinship traditionally has been organized around the male lineage. Fathers, sons, and uncles are the important, recognized relationships between and among families in politics and in business. Each family maintains a recognized head who has great authority and assumes all major responsibilities for the family. A common and desirable domestic traditional structure is to have four generations under one roof. However, with the improvement in the standards of living and other changes, families have gradually gotten smaller. The first generation of one-child families appeared in the 1970s when China introduced a policy of family planning. This phenomenon led to the nuclear family of three (parents and one child) gradually becoming the mainstream family structure in cities. By the end of 2001, of the 351,234 million households in China, the average number of people in each household was 3.46 (Women of China, 2006c).

Family life takes on various faces and follows new trends. Because young people face greater and greater pressure from work and want a higher standard of living and spiritual life, the traditional concept of raising children has faded and more couples are choosing the "double income, no kids" (DINK) way of life.

Because increasing numbers of young people leave home to work in other parts of the country or to study abroad, the number of households consisting of older couples is also rising. Improvements in housing conditions make it possible for the younger generations to move out of the house and live apart from senior members of the family. Longer life spans have resulted in more seniors living alone and those who have lost their spouse living by themselves in one-person households. "Empty nests" will become the norm for seniors as parents of the first generation of single-child families get older. That, in turn, means a switch from an old system in which children looked after their parents to one in which seniors are cared for by society in general through benefits.

Another traditional practice in many rural Chinese families is the submissive role of the daughter-in-law to the mother-in-law. Many times, the mother-in-law is demanding and hostile to the daughter-in-law and may treat her worse than the servants. This relationship has changed significantly since modern culture was introduced to Chinese society. However, such relationships may continue to influence some Chinese families today to some extent, or mothers-in-law and daughters-in-law may simply not get along with each other. Overseas, Chinese are quite different. The involvement of parents, especially the husband's parents, in the new family's life may have a great impact on families (Women of China, 2007).

The Chinese view of women is perpetuated to ensure male dominance in a society that has existed for centuries. Men still remain in control of the country, largely because of stereotypical roles of men and women. However, since the founding of the PRC, this has been changing somewhat. In 1949, the Communist Party stated that "women hold up half the sky" and are legally equal to men.

In 2001, almost half of the workforce were women. Favored professions are education, culture and arts, broadcasting, television and film, finance and insurance, public health, welfare, sports, and social services. In those trades requiring higher technical skills and knowledge, such as computer science, telecommunications, environmental protection, aviation, engineering design, real-estate development, finance and insurance, and the law. In 2001, the number of women employed increased from to 5 to 10 times what they were before China's reform (Women of China, 2006a).

The traditional gender roles of women are changing, but a sense remains that a woman's responsibility is to maintain a happy and efficient home life, especially in rural China. In recent times, some Chinese men include housework, cooking, and cleaning as their responsibilities when their spouses work. Most Chinese believe that the family is most important, and thus, each family member assumes changes in roles to achieve this harmony.

PRESCRIPTIVE, RESTRICTIVE, AND TABOO BEHAVIORS FOR CHILDREN AND ADOLESCENTS

Children are highly valued among the Chinese. China's one-child rule is still in effect (China Turns One Child Policy into Law, 2002). Because of overpopulation in China, the government has mandated that each married couple may have only one child; however, in some rural areas if the first-born child is female, the couple may get permission to have a second child. Families often wait many years, until they are financially secure, to have a child. After the child is born, many family resources are lavished on the child. Families may be able to afford only to live with relatives in a two-room apartment, but if the family believes that the child will benefit by having a piano, then the resources will be found to provide a piano. Children are well dressed and kept clean and well fed.

In China, the child is protected from birth and independence is not fostered. The entire family makes decisions for the child even into young adulthood. Children usually depend on the family for everything. Few teens earn money because they are expected to study hard and to help the family with daily chores rather than to seek employment. Children are pressured to succeed and improve the future of the family and the country. Their common goal is to score well on the national examinations when they reach age 18 years. Most Chinese children and adolescents value studying over playing and peer relationships. They recognize that they are constantly evaluated on having healthy bodies and minds and achieving excellent marks in school.

In rural communities, male children are more valued than female children because they continue the family lineage and provide labor. In urban areas, female children are valued as highly as male children. Children in China are taught to curb their expression of feelings because individuals who do not stand out are successful. However, this is changing. The young in China today frequently think that their parents are too cautious. The children are becoming even more outspoken as they read more and watch more television and movies.

From elementary school to university, students take courses in Marxist politics and learn not to question the doctrine of the country. If they do, they may be interrogated and ridiculed for their radical thoughts. Nationalism is important to Chinese children, and they want to help their country continue to be the center of the world. Children are also expected to help their parents in the home. Many times in the cities when children get home from school before their parents, they are expected to do their homework immediately and then do their household chores. They exhibit their independence not so much by expressing their individual views but by performing chores on their own. However, because of China's one-child rule and high competition for enrollment to colleges, parents and grandparents spoil most children. The children are expected to earn good grades and household chores are not encouraged; this is exhibited in overseas Chinese families as well. Lin and Fu (1990) studied 138 children: 44 Chinese, 46 Chinese Americans, and 48 white Americans in kindergarten through second grade and found that both Chinese and Chinese American parents expected increased achievement and parental control over their children. One surprising finding was the high expectation for independence in Chinese and Chinese American children.

Boys and girls play together when they are young, but as they get older, they do not because their roles and the corresponding expectations are predetermined by Chinese society. Girls and boys both study hard. Boys are more active and take pride in physical fitness. Girls are not nearly as interested in fitness as boys, preferring reading, art, and music.

Adolescents are expected to determine who they are and what they want to do with their lives. Adolescents maintain their respect for older people even when they disagree with them. Although they may argue with their parents and teachers, they have learned that it seldom does any good. Teens value a strong and happy family life and seldom do things that jeopardize that unanimity. Adolescents question affairs of life and make great efforts to see at least two sides of every issue. They enjoy exploring different views with their peers and try to explore them with their parents.

Teenage pregnancy is not common among the Chinese, but it is increasing among Chinese Americans. Young men and women enter the workforce immediately after high school if they are unable to continue their education. Many continue to live with their parents and contribute to the family, even after marriage, into their 20s, and with the birth of a child, in their 30s.

FAMILY GOALS AND PRIORITIES

The Chinese perception of family is through the concept of relationships. Each person identifies himself or herself in relation to others in the family. The individual is not lost, just defined differently from individuals in Western cultures. Personal independence is not valued; rather, Confucian teachings state that true value is in the relationships a person has with others, especially the family.

Older children who experienced the Cultural Revolution may feel some discomfort with their traditional parents. During the Cultural Revolution, the young were encouraged to inform on older people and peers who did not espouse the doctrine of the time. Most of those who were reported were sent to "reeducation camps" where they did hard labor and were "taught the correct way to think." As a result, many families have been permanently separated.

Extended families are important to the Chinese and function by providing ways to get ahead. Often, children live with their grandparents or aunts and uncles so individual family members can obtain a better education or reduce financial burdens. Relatives are expected to help each other through connections (**guan xi**), which are used by Chinese society in a manner similar to the use of money in other cultures. Such connections are perceived as obligations and are placed in a mental bank with deposits and withdrawals. These commitments may remain in the "bank" for years or generations until they are used to get jobs, housing, business contacts, gifts, medical care, or anything that demands a payback.

Filial loyalty to the family is extended to other Chinese. When Chinese immigrants need additional assistance, health-care providers may be able to call on local Chinese organizations to obtain help for clients.

Older people in China are venerated just as they were in earlier years. Chinese government leaders are often older and remain in power until they are in their 70s, 80s, and beyond. Traditional Chinese people view older people as very wise, a view that communism has not changed. Chinese children are expected to care for their parents, and in China, this is mandated by law.

Younger Chinese who adopt Western ideas and values may find that the expectations of older people are too demanding. Even though younger Chinese Americans do not live with their older relatives, they maintain respect and visit them frequently. Older Chinese mothers are viewed as central to family feelings, and older fathers retain their roles as leaders. As generations live in areas removed from China and families become more Westernized, family relationships need to be assessed on an individual basis. An extended-family pattern is common and has existed for over 2000 years. The traditional marriage still remains nuclear. Historically in China, marriage was used to strengthen positions of families in society.

Kinship relationships are based on the concept of loyalty, and the young experience pressure to improve the family's standing. Many parents give up items of daily living to provide more for their children, thereby increasing opportunities for them to get ahead.

Maintaining reputation is very important to the Chinese and is accomplished by adhering to the rules of society. Because power and control are important to Chinese society, rank is very important. True equality does not exist in the Chinese mind; their history has demonstrated that equality cannot exist. If more than one person is in power, then consensus is important. If the person in power is not present at decision-making meetings, barriers are raised and any decisions made are negated unless the person in power agrees. Even after negotiations have been concluded and contracts signed, the Chinese continue to negotiate.

The Chinese concept of privacy is even more important than recognized social status, corresponding values, and beliefs. The Chinese word for "privacy" has a negative connotation and means something underhanded, secret, and furtive. People grow up in crowded conditions, they live and work in small areas, and their value of group support does not place a high value on privacy. The Chinese may ask many personal questions about salary, life at home, age, and children. Refusal to answer personal questions is accepted as long as it is done with care and feeling. The one subject that is taboo is sex and anything related to sex. This may create a barrier for a Western health-care provider who is trying to assess a Chinese client with sexual concerns. The client may feel uncomfortable discussing or answering questions about sex with honesty. Privacy is also limited by territorial boundaries. Some Chinese may enter rooms without knocking or invade privacy by not allowing a person to be alone. The need to be alone is viewed as "not good" to some Chinese, and they may not understand when a Westerner wants to be alone. A mutual understanding of these beliefs is necessary for harmonious working relationships.

ALTERNATIVE LIFESTYLES

The Chinese do not condone same-sex relationships. In many provinces, these are illegal and punishable by death. Divorce is legal, but not encouraged; although it is evident that divorce is a growing trend in China (Women of China, 2006d). Xu Anqi, an analyst at the Shanghai Social Science Academy and standing director of the China Research Association for Women and Family, said the reason for the growing number of divorces in China is multifaceted. First, society is going through a transitional period, which is greatly affecting the stability of marriages. Second, as living standards improve, people have higher expectations toward marriage and love. Third, the simplification of marriage and divorce procedures has made getting a divorce much easier (Women of China, 2006d).

For reasons such as tradition, consideration of children's feelings, and difficulty in remarrying, many

Chinese families would rather stay in an unhealthy marriage than divorce. Remarriage is encouraged, but some difficult relationships may occur in the blended family, especially remarriage with children from previous marriages.

Workforce Issues

CULTURE IN THE WORKPLACE

China is becoming more Westernized with high technology and increased knowledge. The Communist Party is responsible for establishing the **dan wei**, local Chinese work units, that are responsible for jobs, homes, health, enforcement of governmental regulations, and problem solving for families. Although recent immigrants know that the culture in the workplace is different in the United States, they adapt to it quickly. The Chinese acculturate by learning as much as possible about their new culture in the workplace. They observe people from the culture and listen closely for nuances in language and interpersonal connections. They frequently call on other Chinese people to teach them and to discuss how to fit into the new culture more quickly. Chinese Americans support one another in new cultures and help each other find resources and learn to live effectively and efficiently in the new culture. They also watch television, listen to music, and go to movies to learn about Western ways of life. They read about the new culture in magazines, books, and newspapers. They love to travel, and when an opportunity arises to see different aspects of the new culture, they do not hesitate to do so.

The Chinese are accustomed to giving coworkers small gifts of appreciation for helping them acculturate and adapt to the American workforce. Often, Americans seek opportunities to reciprocate with a gift, such as at a birthday party, farewell party, or other occasion. Whereas a wide variety of gifts is appropriate, some gifts are not. For example, giving an umbrella means that one wishes to have the recipient's family dispersed; giving a gift that is white in color or wrapped in white could be interpreted as meaning the giver wishes the recipient dead; and giving a clock could be interpreted as never wanting to see the person again or wishing the person's life to end (Smith, 2002).

On the surface, Chinese Americans form classic external networks, including groupings by (1) family surname, (2) locality of origin in China, (3) dialect or subdialect spoken, (4) craft practiced, and (5) trust from prior experience or recommendation. Therefore, Chinese Americans approximate external networks with some characteristic of internal networks (Haley, Tan, & Haley, 1998).

Guanxi is a Mandarin term with no exact English translation. This term includes the concept of trust and presenting uprightness to build close relationships and connections. It definitely helps to build networks. This *Guanxi* network can be used in the work-related, decision-making process and is also used with family, friends, and community-related issues in the Chinese American community.

ISSUES RELATED TO AUTONOMY

Historically, the Chinese have been autonomous. They had to exhibit this characteristic to survive through difficult times. However, their autonomy is limited and is based on functioning for the good of the group. When a new situation arises that requires independent decision making, many times the Chinese know what should be done but do not take action until the leader or superior gives permission. However, the Western workforce expects independence, and some Chinese may need to be taught that true autonomy is necessary to advance. Health-care providers should be aware, however, that the training might not be successful because it is foreign to Chinese cultural values. A demonstration is the best alternative, leaving it up to the individuals to determine whether assertiveness can be a part of their lives. After acculturation takes place, Chinese Americans do not differ significantly in assertiveness.

Language may be a barrier for Chinese immigrants seeking assimilation into the Western workforce. Western languages and Chinese have many differences, among them sentence structure and the use of intonation. The Chinese language does not have verbs that denote tense, as in Western languages. Whereas the ordering of the words in a sentence is basically the same, with the subject first and then the verb, the Chinese language places descriptive adjectives in different orders. Intonation in Chinese is in the words themselves, rather than in the sentence. Chinese people who have taken English lessons can usually read and write English competently, but they may have difficulty in understanding and speaking it.

Biocultural Ecology

SKIN COLOR AND OTHER BIOLOGICAL VARIATIONS

The skin color of Chinese is varied. Many have skin color similar to that of Westerners with pink undertones. Some have a yellow tone, whereas others are very dark. Mongolian spots, dark bluish spots over the lower back and buttocks, are present in about 80 percent of infants. Bilirubin levels are usually higher in Chinese newborns, with the highest levels occurring on the 5th or 6th day after birth.

Although Chinese are distinctly Mongolian, their Asian characteristics have many variations. China is very large and includes people from many different backgrounds, including Mongols and Tibetans. Generally, men and women are shorter than Westerners, but some Chinese are over 6 feet tall. Differences in bone structure are evidenced in the ulna, which is longer than the radius. Hip measurements are significantly smaller: Females are 4.14 cm smaller, and males 7.6 cm smaller than Westerners (Seidel, Ball, Dains, & Benedict, 1994). Not only is overall bone length shorter, but bone density is also less. Chinese have a high hard palate, which may cause them problems with Western dentures. Their hair is generally black and straight, but some have naturally curly hair. Most Chinese men do not have much facial or chest hair. The Rh-negative blood group is rare, and twins are not common in

Chinese families, but are greatly valued, especially since the emergence of China's one-child law.

DISEASES AND HEALTH CONDITIONS

Many Chinese who come to the United States settle in large cities like San Francisco and New York, so they are at risk for the same problems and diseases experienced by other inner-city populations. For example, crowding in large cities often results in poor sanitation and increases the incidence of infectious diseases, air pollution, and violence.

The three leading causes of death were, among men, malignant neoplasms, heart diseases, cerebrovascular disease, accidents, and infectious diseases, and among women, heart diseases, cerebrovascular disease, and malignant neoplasms (He, Gu, Wu, Reynolds, & Cao, 2005).

The average life expectancy in China is 72.58 years (CIA, 2007), thanks to improved living conditions and medical facilities, as well as a nationwide fitness campaign. In 1949, the average life expectancy was only 35 years (People's Daily, 2002). Disease incidence has decreased as well, but major problems still exist in rural China, where perinatal deaths and deaths from infectious diseases remain high. Tobacco use is a major problem and results in an increased incidence of lung disease. Healthcare providers must screen newer immigrants from China for these health-related conditions and provide interventions in a culturally congruent manner.

Many Chinese immigrants have an increased incidence of hepatitis B and tuberculosis. Poor living conditions and overcrowding in some areas of China enhance the development of these diseases, which persist after immigrants settle in other countries.

According to the Office of Minority Health (2007), Chinese American women have a 20 percent higher rate of pancreatic cancer and higher rates of suicide after the age of 45 years, and all Chinese have higher death rates owing to diabetes. The incidence of different types of cancer, including cervical, liver, lung, stomach, multiple myeloma, esophageal, pancreatic, and nasopharyngeal cancers, is higher among Chinese Americans (Office of Minority Health, 2007). Overall, the incidence of disease in this population has not been studied sufficiently, and continuing research is desperately needed.

VARIATIONS IN DRUG METABOLISM

Multiple studies outlining problems with drug metabolism and sensitivity have been conducted among the Chinese. Results suggest a poor metabolism of mephenytoin (e.g., diazepam) in 15 to 20 percent of Chinese; sensitivity to beta-blockers, such as propranolol, as evidenced by a decrease in the overall blood levels accompanied by a seemingly more profound response; atropine sensitivity, as evidenced by an increased heart rate; and increased responses to antidepressants and neuroleptics given at lower doses. Analgesics have been found to cause increased gastrointestinal side effects, despite a decreased sensitivity to them. In addition, the Chinese have an increased sensitivity to the effects of alcohol (Levy, 1993).

Delineating specific variations in drug metabolism among the Chinese is difficult because various studies tend to group them in aggregate as Asians. Much more research needs to be completed to determine variations between Westerners and Asians as well as among Asians.

High-Risk Behaviors

High-risk behaviors are difficult to determine with accuracy among Chinese in the United States because most of the data on Chinese are included in the aggregate called *Asian Americans*. Smoking is a high-risk behavior for many Chinese men and teenagers. A study by Yu, Edwin, Chen, Kim, and Sawsan (2002) indicated that the male prevalence of smoking in Chicago is higher than that reported in California, the National Health Inventory Survey (NHIS), and the Behavioral Risk Factor Surveillance System (BRFSS); exceeds the rate for African Americans aged 18 years and older; is comparable with the rate for African American males aged 45 to 64 years; and is far above the *Healthy People 2010* target goal of less than 12 percent (Healthy People 2010, 2000). Most Chinese women do not smoke, but recently, the numbers for women are increasing, especially after immigration to the United States. Travelers in China see more cigarette vendors than any other type in the streets. The decrease in smoking in the United States resulted in cigarette manufacturers' identifying China as a good market in which to sell their product.

Even though alcohol consumption among Chinese has been high at times, the level is currently low (Weatherspoon, Danko, & Johnson, 1994). Despite these findings, the use of alcohol contributes to a high incidence of vehicle accidents and related trauma. HIV, AIDS, and sexually transmitted diseases are lower among Chinese and other Asian Americans compared with other groups in the United States (Centers for Disease Control [CDC], 2001).

Nutrition

MEANING OF FOOD

Food habits are important to the Chinese, who offer food to their guests at any time of the day or night. Most celebrations with family and business events focus on food. Foods served at Chinese meals have a specific order, with the focus on a balance for a healthy body. The importance of food is demonstrated daily in its use to promote good health and to combat disease and injury. Traditional Chinese medicine frequently uses food and food derivatives to prevent and cure diseases and illnesses and increase the strength of weak and older people.

COMMON FOODS AND FOOD RITUALS

The typical Chinese diet is difficult to describe because each region in China has its own traditional foods. Peanuts and soybeans are popular. Common grains include wheat, sorghum, and maize. Rice is usually steamed but can be fried with eggs, vegetables, and meats. Many Chinese eat beans or noodles instead of rice. The Chinese eat steamed and fried rice noodles, which are usually prepared with a broth base and include vegetables and meats. Meat choices include pork (the most common), chicken, beef, duck, shrimp, fish, scallops, and mussels. Tofu, an excellent source of protein, is a staple of the Chinese diet and can be fried or boiled or eaten cold like ice cream. Bean products are another source of protein, and many of the desserts or sweets in Chinese diets are prepared with red beans.

At celebrations, before-dinner toasts are usually made to family and business colleagues. The toasts may be interspersed with speeches, or the speeches may be incorporated in the toasts. Cold appetizers often include peanuts and seasonal fruits. Chopsticks, a chopstick holder, a small plate, and a glass are part of the table setting. If the foods are messy, like Beijing duck, then a finger towel may be available. The Chinese use ceramic or porcelain spoons for soup. Knives are unnecessary because the food is usually served in bite-sized pieces. Eating with chopsticks may be difficult for some at first, but the Chinese are good-natured and are pleased by any attempt to use them. Chopsticks should never be stuck in the food upright because that is considered bad luck (Smith, 2002). Westerners soon learn that slurping, burping, and other noises are not considered offensive, but are appreciated. The Chinese are very relaxed at meals and commonly rest their elbows on the table.

Fruits and vegetables may be peeled or eaten raw. Some vegetables commonly eaten raw by Westerners are usually cooked by the Chinese. Unpeeled raw fruits and vegetables are sources of contamination owing to unsanitary conditions in China. The Chinese enjoy their vegetables lightly stir-fried in oil with salt and spice. Salt, oil, and oil products are important parts of the Chinese diet.

Drinks with dinner include tea, soft drinks, juice, and beer. Foreign-born Chinese and older Chinese may not like ice in their drinks. They may just not like cold while eating or may believe that it is damaging to their body and shocks the body systems out of balance. Conversely, hot drinks are enjoyed and believed to be safe for the body. This "goodness" of hot drinks may stem from tradition in which the only safe drinks were made from boiled water. All food is put in the center of the table, arriving all at one time, but usually multiple courses are served. The host either serves the most important guests first or signals everyone to start.

DIETARY PRACTICES FOR HEALTH PROMOTION

For the Chinese, food is important in maintaining their health. Foods that are considered **yin** and **yang** prevent sudden imbalances and indigestion. A balanced diet is considered essential for physical and emotional harmony. Health-care providers need to provide special instructions regarding risk factors associated with diets that are high in fats and salt. For example, the Chinese may need education regarding the use of salty fish and condiments, which increase the risk for nasopharyngeal, esophageal, and stomach cancers.

NUTRITIONAL DEFICIENCIES AND FOOD LIMITATIONS

Little information is available about dietary deficiencies in the Chinese diet. The life span of the Chinese is long enough to suggest that severe dietary deficiencies are not common as long as food is available. Periodically, some deficiencies, such as rickets and goiters, have occurred. The Chinese government added iodine to water supplies, and fish, which is rich in iron, is encouraged to enhance the diets of people with goiters. Native Chinese generally do not drink milk or eat milk products because of a genetic tendency for lactose intolerance. Their healthy selection of green vegetables limits the incidence of calcium deficiencies. Health-care providers may need to screen newer Chinese immigrants for these deficiencies and assist them in planning an adequate diet.

Most Chinese do not eat desserts with a high sugar content. Their desserts are usually peeled or sliced fruits or desserts made of bean and bean curd. The higher death rate from diabetes in Western countries mentioned earlier in this chapter may be due to a change from the typical Chinese diet with few sweets to a Western diet with many sweets.

Pregnancy and Childbearing Practices

FERTILITY PRACTICES AND VIEWS TOWARD PREGNANCY

China continues to make efforts to slow the rate of population growth by enforcing a one-child law. The most popular form of birth control is the intrauterine device. Sterilization is common even though oral contraception is available. Contraception is free in China. Abortion is fairly common, but statistics are hard to find.

Most Chinese families see pregnancy as positive and important in the immediate and extended family. Many couples wait a long time to have their first and only child. If a woman does become pregnant before the couple is ready to start a family, she may have an abortion. When the pregnancy is desired, the nuclear and extended family rejoice in the new family member. Overall, pregnancy is seen as a woman's business, although the Chinese man is beginning to demonstrate an active interest in pregnancy and the welfare of the mother and baby.

China has 80 million one-child families. The gender imbalance has become a serious issue in recent years because many families, especially those in rural areas, prefer boys to girls. China has 119 boys born for every 100 girls, whereas the global ratio is 103 to 107 boys for every 100 girls. In China, the "Care for Girls" program was initiated in 2003 to promote the social status of women, and attempts are being made to decrease gender identification abortions without a medical purpose and the abandonment of newborn girls (XinHua News Agency, 2006)

PRESCRIPTIVE, RESTRICTIVE, AND TABOO PRACTICES IN THE CHILDBEARING FAMILY

Because Chinese women are very modest, many women insist on a female midwife or obstetrician. Some agree to use a male physician only when an emergency arises.

Pregnant women usually add more meat to their diets because their blood needs to be stronger for the fetus. Many women increase the amount of organ meat in their diet, and even during times of severe food shortages, the Chinese government has tried to ensure that pregnant women receive adequate nutrition. These traditions are also reflected in Chinese families living in the West.

Other dietary restrictions and prescriptions may be practiced by pregnant women, such as avoiding shellfish during the first trimester because it causes allergies. Some mothers may be unwilling to take iron because they believe that it makes the delivery more difficult.

The Chinese government is proud of the fact that since the People's Revolution in 1949, infant mortality has been significantly reduced. In 2001, the mortality rates for infants and children under age 5 years were reduced to 30 per 1000 and 35.9 per 1000 (Women of China, 2006e). This has been accomplished by providing a three-level system of care for pregnant women in rural and urban populations. Over 90 percent of childbirths take place under sterile conditions by a qualified personnel. This has reduced the maternal mortality rate significantly to 50.2 in 100,000 (Women of China, 2006e). Therefore, most Chinese who have immigrated to Western countries are familiar with modern sterile deliveries.

In China, a woman stays in the hospital for a few days after delivery to recover her strength and body balance. Traditional postpartum care includes 1 month of recovery, with the mother eating cooked and warm foods that decrease the *yin* (cold) energy. The Chinese government supports this 1-month recuperation period through labor laws that entitle the mother from 56 days to 6 months of maternity leave with full pay (Ministry of Public Health, 1992). Women who return to work are allowed time off for breastfeeding, and in many cases, factories provide a special lounge for the women to breastfeed. Families who come to Western societies expect the same importance to be placed on motherhood and may be surprised to find that many Western countries do not provide similar benefits.

Traditional prescriptive and restrictive practices continue among many Chinese women during the postpartum period. Drinking and touching cold water are taboo for women in the postpartum period. Raw fruits and vegetables are avoided because they are considered "cold" foods. They must be cooked and be warm. Mothers eat five to six meals a day with high nutritional ingredients including rice, soups, and seven to eight eggs. Brown sugar is commonly used because it helps rebuild blood loss. Drinking rice wine is encouraged to increase the mother's breast milk production. But mothers need to be cautioned that it may also prolong the bleeding time. Many mothers do not expose themselves to the cold air and do not go outside or bathe for the first month postpartum because the cold air can enter the body and cause health problems, especially for older women. Some women wear many layers of clothes and are covered from head to toe, even in the summer, to keep the air away from their bodies. However, this practice has changed among some young women who live in Western cultures for a long period of time and when there are no older Chinese parents around during the postpartum period.

Adopted Chinese children display a similar pattern of growth and developmental delays and medical problems as seen in other groups of internationally adopted children. An exception is the increased incidence of elevated lead levels (overall 14 percent). Although serious medical and developmental issues were found among Chinese children, overall their health was better than expected based on recent publicity about conditions in the Chinese orphanages. The long-term outcome of these children remains unknown (Miller, 2000). Many children adopted from China have antibody titers that do not correlate with those expected from their medical records. These children, unlike children adopted from other countries, have documented evidence of adequate vaccinations. However, they should be tested for antibody concentrations and reimmunized as necessary (Schulpen, 2001).

Death Rituals

DEATH RITUALS AND EXPECTATIONS

Chinese death and bereavement traditions are centered on ancestor worship. Ancestor worship is frequently misunderstood; it is not a religion, but rather a form of paying respect. Many Chinese believe that their spirits can never rest unless living descendants provide care for the grave and worship the memory of the deceased. These practices were so important to early Chinese that Chinese pioneers to the West had statements written into their work contract that their ashes or bones be returned to China (Halporn, 1992).

The belief that the Chinese greet death with stoicism and fatalism is a myth. In fact, most Chinese fear death, avoid references to it, and teach their children this avoidance. The number 4 is considered unlucky by many Chinese because it is pronounced like the Chinese word for death; this is similar to the bad luck associated with the number 13 in many Western societies. Huang (1992) wrote:

> At a very young age, a child is taught to be very careful with words that are remotely associated with the "misfortune" of death. The word "death" and its synonyms are strictly forbidden on happy occasions, especially during holidays. People's uneasiness about death often is reflected in their emphasis on longevity and everlasting life. . . . In daily life, the character "Long Life" appears on almost everything: jewelry, clothing, furniture, and so forth. It would be a terrible mistake to give a clock as a gift, simply because the pronunciation of the word "clock" is the same as that of the word "ending." Recently, many people in Taiwan decided to avoid using the number "four" because the number has a similar pronunciation to the word "death." (p. 1)

Many Chinese are hesitant to purchase life insurance because of their fear that it is inviting death. The color white is associated with death and is considered bad luck. Black is also a bad-luck color.

Many Chinese believe in ghosts, and the fear of death is extended to the fear of ghosts. Some ghosts are good and some are bad, but all have great power. Communism discourages this thinking and sees it as a hindrance to future growth and development of the society, but the ever-pragmatic Chinese believe it is better not to invite trouble with ghosts just in case they might exist.

The dead may be viewed in the hospital or in the family home. Extended family members and friends come together to mourn. The dead are honored by placing objects around the coffin that signify the life of the dead: food, money designated for the dead person's spirit, and other articles made of paper. In China, cremation is preferred by the state because of a lack of wood for coffins and a limited space for burial. The ashes are placed in an urn and then in a vault. As cities grow, even the space for vaults is limited. In rural areas, many families prefer traditional burial and have family burial plots. It is preferable to burying an intact body in a coffin.

RESPONSES TO DEATH AND GRIEF

The Chinese react to death in various ways. Death is viewed as a part of the natural cycle of life, and some believe that something good happens to them after they die. These beliefs foster the impression that Chinese are stoic. In fact, they feel similar emotions to Westerners but do not overtly express those emotions to strangers. During bereavement, a person does not have to go to work, but instead can use this mourning time for remembering the dead and planning for the future. Bereavement time in the larger cities is 1 day to 1 week, depending on the policy of the government agency and the relationship of family members to the deceased. Mourners are recognized by black armbands on their left arm and white strips of cloth tied around their heads.

Spirituality

DOMINANT RELIGION AND USE OF PRAYER

In mainland China, the practice of formal religious services is minimal. The ideals and values of the different religions are practiced alone rather than with people coming together to participate in a formal religious service. In recent years, in some parts of China, religion is becoming more popular. The main formal religions in China are Buddhism, Catholicism, Protestantism, Taoism, and Islam.

As immigration from China increases, Chinese people who practice Christian religions have become more visible on the American landscape. Chinese immigrants from the PRC may express perspectives on religious beliefs different from those of the Chinese from other countries, or from Hong Kong and Taiwan, where they have been permitted to practice Christianity. At first, they may go to a church attended by other Chinese people; eventually some are baptized, and others continue to attend Bible studies. In cities in the United States, churches are playing a very important role in the local Chinese community in terms of providing support and services to Chinese immigrants, students, scholars, and their families. An understanding of this concept is essential when the health-care provider attempts to obtain religious counseling services for Chinese clients.

Prayer is generally a source of comfort. Some Chinese do not acknowledge a religion such as Buddhism, but if they go to a shrine, they burn incense and offer prayers.

MEANING OF LIFE AND INDIVIDUAL SOURCES OF STRENGTH

The Chinese view life in terms of cycles and interrelationships, believing that life gets meaning from the context in which it is lived. Life cannot be broken into simple parts and examined because the parts are interrelated. When the Chinese attempt to explain life and what it means, they speak about what happened to them, what happened to others, and the importance and interrelatedness of those events. They speak not only of the importance of the current phenomena but also about the importance of what occurred many years, maybe even centuries, before their lives. They live and believe in a true systems framework.

"Life forces" are sources of strength to the Chinese. These forces come from within the individual, the environment, the past and future of the individual, and society. Chinese use these forces when they need strength. If one usual source of strength is unsuccessful, they try another. The individual may use many different techniques such as meditation, exercise, massage, and prayer. Drugs, herbs, food, good air, and artistic expression may also be used. Good-luck charms are cherished, and traditional and nontraditional medicines are used.

The family is usually one source of strength. Individuals draw on family resources and are expected to return resources to strengthen the family. Resources may be financial, emotional, physical, mental, or spiritual. Calling on ancestors to provide strength as a resource requires giving back to the ancestors when necessary. The interconnectedness of life provides a source of strength for individuals from before birth to death and beyond.

Health-care providers need to understand this multidimensional manner of thinking and believing. Assessments, goal setting, interventions, and evaluations may be different for Chinese clients than for American clients. The context of client problems is the emphasis, and the physical, mental, and spiritual aspects of the person's life are the focal points.

Health-Care Practices

HEALTH-SEEKING BELIEFS AND BEHAVIORS

Health care in China is provided for most citizens. Every work unit and neighborhood has its own clinic and hospital. Traditional Chinese medicine shops abound (Fig. 7–1). Even department stores and supermarkets have Western medicines and traditional Chinese medicines and herbs.

The focus of health has not changed over the centuries, and includes having a healthy body, a healthy mind, and a healthy spirit. Preventive health-care practices are a major focus in China today. An additional focus is placed on infectious diseases such as schistosomiasis, tuberculosis, childhood diseases, and malaria; cancer; heart diseases; and maternal-infant care. Chinese Ministry of Health statistics indicate China had 840,000 HIV-infected people in 2004 (Chinese Ministry of Health, 2004). That means that China had the 14th highest number of HIV-infected people in the world and the second highest in Asia. Between 2000 and 2005, the percentage

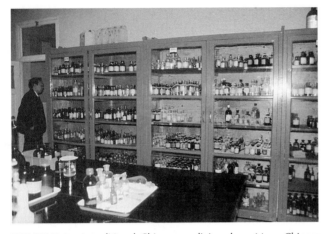

FIGURE 7–1 A traditional Chinese medicine shop. Many Chinese practice traditional Chinese medicine, either alone or in conjunction with Western medicine.

of people infected with HIV rose from 19.4 percent to 28.1 percent (Women of China, 2006b). China now faces a critical period in the fight to curb the spread of, and ultimately cure, HIV and AIDS. The World Health Organization (WHO) has predicted that China, if it fails to control the disease's spread, will have 10 million AIDS sufferers by 2010 (Gu, 2006). A new regulation on AIDS prevention and control (effective January 1, 2007) spells out the plan to administer the free test in areas of the province where the AIDS situation is "grave." HIV carriers and AIDS patients will be asked to inform their spouses or sex partners of the results, or the local disease prevention authorities will do so (Women of China, 2006b).

Whereas many Chinese have made the transition to Western medicine, others maintain their roots in traditional Chinese medicine, and still others practice both types. The Chinese are similar to other nationalities in seeking the most effective cure available. Younger Chinese people usually do not hesitate to seek health-care providers when necessary. They generally practice Western medicine unless they feel that it does not work for them; then they use traditional Chinese medicine. Conversely, older people may try traditional Chinese medicine first, and only seek Western medicine when traditional medicine does not seem to work.

Among Chinese Americans, these health-seeking beliefs, practices, and patterns remain the same as the ones in China. This results in sicker older people seeking care from Western health-care providers. Even after seeking Western medical care, many older Chinese continue to practice traditional Chinese medicine in some form. However, some Chinese clients may not tell health-care providers about other forms of treatment they have been using because they are conscious of saving face. Health-care providers need to understand this practice and include it in their care. Members of the health-care team need to develop a trusting relationship with Chinese clients so that all information can be disclosed. Health-care providers must impress upon clients the importance of disclosing all treatments because some may have antagonistic effects.

RESPONSIBILITY FOR HEALTH CARE

Chinese people often self-medicate when they think that they know what is wrong or if they have been successfully treated by their traditional medicine or herbs in the past. They share their knowledge about treatments and their medicines with friends and family members. This often happens among Chinese Americans as well because of the belief that occasional illness can be ameliorated through the use of nonprescription drugs. Many consider seeing Western health-care providers as a waste of time and money. Health-care providers need to recognize that self-medication and sharing medications are accepted practices among the Chinese. Thus, health-care providers should inquire about this practice when making assessments, setting goals, and evaluating the results of treatments. A trusting relationship between members of the health-care team and the client and family is necessary to enhance the disclosure of all treatments.

TRADITIONAL CHINESE MEDICINE PRACTICES

Traditional Chinese medicine is practiced widely, with concrete reasons for the preparation of medications, taking medicine, and the expected outcomes. Western medicine needs to be explained to Chinese people in equally concrete terms.

Traditional Chinese medicine has many facets, including the five basic substances (**qi**, energy; **xue**, blood; **jing**, essence; **shen**, spirit; and **jing ye**, body fluids); the pulses and vessels for the flow of energetic forces (**mai**); the energy pathways (**jing**); the channels and collaterals, including the 14 meridians for acupuncture, moxibustion, and massage (**jing luo**); the organ systems (**zang fu**); and the tissues of the bones, tendons, flesh, blood vessels, and skin. The scope of traditional Chinese medicine is vast and should be studied carefully by professionals who provide health care to Chinese clients.

Acupuncture and moxibustion are used in many of the treatments. Acupuncture is the insertion of needles into precise points along the channel system of flow of the *qi* called the 14 meridians. (The system has over 400 points.) Many of the same points can be used in applying pressure and massage to achieve relief from imbalances in the system. The same systems approach is used to produce localized anesthesia.

Moxibustion is the application of heat from different sources to various points. For example, one source, such as garlic, is placed on the distal end of the needle after it is inserted through the skin, and the garlic is set on fire. Sometimes, the substance is burned directly over the point without a needle insertion. Localized erythema occurs with the heat from the burning substance, and the medicine is absorbed through the skin. Cupping is another common practice. A heated cup or glass jar is put on the skin, creating a vacuum, which causes the skin to be drawn into the cup. The heat generated is used to treat joint pain.

The Chinese believe that health and a happy life can be maintained if the two forces, the *yang* and the *yin*, are balanced. This balance is called the **dao**. Heaven is *yang*, and Earth is *yin*; man is *yang*, and woman is *yin*; the sun is *yang*, and the moon is *yin*; the hollow organs (bladder, intestines, stomach, gallbladder), head, face, back, and lateral parts of the body are *yang*, and the solid viscera (heart, lung, liver, spleen, kidney, and pericardium), abdomen, chest, and the inner parts of the body are *yin*. The *yang* is hot, and the *yin* is cold. Health-care providers need to be aware that the functions of life and the interplay of these functions, rather than the structures, are important to Chinese people.

Central to traditional medicine is the concept of the *qi*. It is considered the vital force of life; includes air, breath, or wind; and is present in all living organisms. Some of the *qi* is inherited, and other parts come from the environment, such as in food. The *qi* circulates through the 14 meridians and organs of the body to give the body nourishment. The channels of flow are also responsible for eliminating the bad *qi*. All channels, the meridians and organs, are interconnected. The results resemble a system in which a change in one part of the system results in a change in other parts, and one part of the system can assist other parts in their total functioning.

Diagnosis is made through close inspection of the outward appearance of the body, the vitality of the person, the color of the person, the appearance of the tongue, and the person's senses. The practitioner uses listening, smelling, and questioning techniques in the assessment. Palpation is used by feeling the 12 pulses and different parts of the body. Treatments are based on the imbalances that occur. Many are directly related to the obvious problem, but many more are related through the interconnectedness of the body systems. Many of the treatments not only "cure" the problem but are also used to "strengthen" the entire human being. Traditional Chinese medicine cannot be learned quickly because of the interplay of symptoms and diagnoses. Practitioners take many years to become adept in all phases of diagnosis and treatment.

T'ai chi, practiced by many Chinese, has its roots in the 12th century. This type of exercise is suitable for all age groups, even the very old. *T'ai chi* involves different forms of exercise, some of which can be used for self-defense. The major focus of the movements is mind and body control. The concepts of *yin* and *yang* are included in the movements, with a *yin* movement following a *yang* movement. Total concentration and controlled breathing are necessary to enable the smoothness and rhythmic quality of movement. The movements resemble a slow-motion battle, with the participant both attacking and retreating. Movements are practiced at least twice a day to bring the internal body, the external body, and the environment into balance (T'ai Chi Chen Homepage, 2007). A recent survey in China indicated that 41.3 percent respondents believe that "Yoga" is the most fashionable kind of exercise among women (Women of China, 2006c). Yoga incorporates meditation, relaxation, imagery, controlled breathing, stretching, and other physical movements. Yoga has become increasingly popular in Western cultures as a means of exercise and fitness training. Yoga needs to be better recognized by the health-care community as a complement to conventional medical care.

Herbal therapy is integral to traditional Chinese medicine and is even more difficult to learn than acupuncture and moxibustion. Herbs fall into four categories of energy (cold, hot, warm, and cool), five categories of taste (sour, bitter, sweet, pungent, and salty), and a neutral category. Different methods are used to administer the herbs, including drinking and eating, applying topically, and wearing on the body. Each treatment is specific to the underlying problem or a desire to increase strength and resistance.

BARRIERS TO HEALTH CARE

VIGNETTE 7.2

The Chiang family brings their 6-year-old daughter, Yan, to the Emergency Department (ED) on 2 consecutive days. Yesterday, when they first brought her to the ED, the nurse found six quarter-sized round ecchymotic areas on the child's back from traditional Chinese medicine. Yan was discharged on liquid antibiotics for a pulmonary infection. The parents bring Yan to the ED again today because she does not seem to be improving and has diarrhea. Mrs. Chiang has the medicine in a plastic bag with a tablespoon. After much discussion and calling the language interpretation line, the nurse determined that Mrs. Chiang was using a tablespoon instead of a teaspoon of the liquid antibiotic.

1. What type of traditional Chinese medicine leaves round ecchymotic areas?
2. For what type of conditions is this treatment used?
3. Why does Yan have diarrhea?
4. What could the nurse have done initially to ensure that a teaspoon would have been used instead of a tablespoon?
5. What Chinese beliefs regarding Western health care are perpetrated by Yan's reaction to the antibiotic?

In China, the government is primarily responsible for providing basic health care within a multilevel system. Native Chinese are accustomed to the neighborhood work units called **dan wei**, where they get answers to their questions and health-care services are provided. After transition to the United States, Chinese clients face many of the same barriers to health care faced by Westerners, yet they have other special concerns and difficulties that prevent them from accessing health-care services. Ma (2000) summarized these barriers as the following:

1. *Language barriers:* This is one of the major reasons that Chinese Americans do not want to see Western health-care providers. They feel uncomfortable and frustrated with not being able to communicate with them freely and not being able to adequately express their pains, concerns, or health problems. Even highly educated Chinese Americans, who have limited knowledge in the medical field and are unfamiliar with medical terminology, have difficulty complying with recommended procedures and health prescriptions.

2. *Cultural barriers:* Lack of culturally appropriate and competent health-care services is another key obstacle to health-care service utilization. Many Chinese Americans have different cultural

responses to health and illness. Although they respect and accept the Western health-care provider's prescription drugs, they tend to alternate between Western and traditional Chinese physicians.

3. *Socioeconomic barriers:* Being unable to afford medical expenses is another barrier to accessing health-care services for some Chinese Americans. However, having health insurance does not always assure the utilization of the health-care system or the benefits of health insurance. There may be a sense of distrust between patients and health-care providers or between patients and insurance companies. In addition, many do not know the cost of the service when they enter a clinic or hospital. They are frustrated with being caught in the battle between health insurance companies and the clinic or hospital.

4. *Systemic barriers:* Not understanding the Western health-care system and feeling inconvenienced by managed-care regulations deters many from seeking Western health-care providers unless they are seriously ill. The complexity of the rules and regulations of public agencies and medical assistance programs such as Medicaid and Medicare blocks their effective use.

Tan (1992), in a different perspective, summarized barriers for Chinese immigrants seeking health care:

1. Many Chinese Americans have great difficulty facing a diagnosis of cancer because families are the main source of support for patients, and many family members are still in China.

2. Because many Chinese Americans do not have medical insurance, any serious illness will lead to heavy financial burdens on the family.

3. Once the client responds to initial treatment, the family tends to stop treatment and the client does not receive follow-up care or becomes non-compliant.

4. Chinese American families may be reluctant to allow autopsies because of their fear of being "cut up."

5. The most difficult barrier is frequently the reluctance to disclose the diagnosis to the patient or the family.

In recent years, clinics of Chinese medicine and health-care providers who are originally from China have been significantly visible in the United States, especially in the larger cities. These provide opportunity or options for those Chinese Americans who prefer to seek traditional Chinese treatment for certain illness.

CULTURAL RESPONSES TO HEALTH AND ILLNESS

VIGNETTE 7.3

Mr. and Mrs. Lin, first-generation Chinese Americans, bring Mrs. Lin's 75-year-old father, Mr. Xu, who does not speak English, to the neighborhood clinic because he has not been eating well or socializing with the family. This morning, he is complaining of fire in his chest and stomach. Mr. Lin admits finding several empty alcohol bottles in the trash, which they said were put there by neighbors. Mr. Lin is adamant that his father is not drinking the alcohol. When the physician suggests family counseling, Mr. and Mrs. Lin leave with Mr. Xu, replying that this was not necessary.

1. Mr. and Mrs. Lin have the same surname. How does this compare with traditional Chinese when they marry?
2. What was Mrs. Lin's family name before she married Mr. Lin?
3. How does Mr. Xu's description of pain vary from what a European American might describe?
4. What might the complaint of "fire in the chest and stomach" signify?
5. What drug metabolism issues are relevant to the assessment?
6. Identify a more appropriate approach for the physician to use when prescribing medication and conducting family counseling.
7. What cultural concerns might a social worker have to consider to effectively assist this family?
8. How are Mr. and Mrs. Lin showing respect for Mrs. Lin's father?

Chinese people express their pain in ways similar to those of Americans, but their description of pain differs. A study by Moore (1990) included not only the expression of pain but also common treatments used by Chinese. The Chinese tend to describe their pain in terms of more diverse body symptoms, whereas Westerners tend to describe pain locally. The Western description includes words like "stabbing" and "localized," whereas the Chinese describe pain as "dull" and more "diffuse." They tend to use explanations of pain from the traditional Chinese influence of imbalances in the *yang* and *yin* combined with location and cause. The study determined that the Chinese cope with pain by using externally applied methods, such as oils and massage. They also use warmth, sleeping on the area of pain, relaxation, and aspirin.

The balance between *yin* and *yang* is used to explain mental as well as physical health. This belief, coupled with the influence of Russian theorists such as Pavlov, influence the Chinese view of mental illness. Mental illness results more from metabolic imbalances and organic problems. The effect of social situations, such as stress and crises, on a person's mental well-being is considered inconsequential, but physical imbalances from genetics are the important factors. Because a stigma is associated with having a family member who is mentally ill, many families initially seek the help of a folk healer. Many use a combination of traditional and Western medicine. Many mentally ill clients are treated as outpatients and remain in the home.

Although Chinese do not readily seek assistance for emotional and nervous disorders, a study of 143 Chinese Americans found that younger, lower socioeconomic, and married Chinese with better language ability seek help more frequently (Ying & Miller, 1992). The researchers recommended that new immigrants be taught that help is available when needed for mental disorders within the mental health-care system.

Chinese people in larger cities are becoming more supportive of the disabled, but for the most part, support services are popular. Because the focus has been on improving the overall economic growth of the country, the needs of the disabled have not had priority. The son of Deng Xiaoping was crippled in the Cultural Revolution and has been active in making the country more aware of the needs of the disabled. The Beijing Paralympic Games will be held September 6 to 17, 2008, and will open 12 days after the 29th Olympic Games. A successful Paralympics in Beijing will promote the cause of disabled persons in Beijing as well as throughout China. The Games will urge the whole of society to pay more attention to this special segment of our population and will reinforce the importance of building accessible facilities for the disabled and thus enhance efforts to construct a harmonious society in China (Nan, 2006). Overall, the Chinese still view mental and physical disabilities as a part of life that should be hidden.

The expression of the sick role depends on the level of education of the client. Educated Chinese people who have been exposed to Western ideas and culture are more likely to assume a sick role similar to that of Westerners. However, the highly educated and acculturated may exhibit some of the traditional roles associated with illness. Each client needs to be assessed individually for responses to illness and for expectations of care. Traditionally, the Chinese ill person is viewed to be passive and accepting of illness. To the Chinese, illness is expected as a part of the life cycle. However, they do try to avoid danger and to live as healthy a life as possible. To the Chinese, all of life is interconnected; therefore, they seek explanations and connections for illness and injury in all aspects of life. Their explanations to health-care providers may not make sense, but the health-care provider should try to determine those connections so the connections can be incorporated into treatment regimens. The Chinese believe that because the illness or injury is caused from an imbalance, there should be a medicine or treatment that can restore the balance. If the medicine or treatment does not seem to do this, they may refuse to use it.

Native Chinese and Chinese Americans like treatments that are comfortable and do not hurt. Treatments that hurt are physically stressful and drain their energy. Health-care providers who have been ill themselves can appreciate this way of thinking, because sometimes the cure seems worse than the illness. Treatments will be more successful if they are explained in ways that are consistent with the Chinese way of thinking. The Chinese depend on their families and sometimes on their friends to help them while they are sick. These people provide much of the direct care; health-care providers are expected to manage the care. The family may seem to take over the life of the sick person, and the sick person is very passive in allowing them the control. One or two primary people assume this responsibility, usually a spouse. Health-care providers need to include the family mem-

bers in the plan of care and, in many instances, in the actual delivery of care.

BLOOD TRANSFUSIONS AND ORGAN DONATION

Modern-day Chinese accept blood transfusions, organ donations, and organ transplants when absolutely essential, as long as they are safe and effective. Chinese Americans have the same concerns as Americans about blood transfusion because of the perceived high incidence of HIV and hepatitis B. No overall ethnic or religious practices prohibit the use of blood transfusions, organ donations, or organ transplants. Of course, some individuals may have religious or personal reasons for denying their use.

Health-Care Practitioners

TRADITIONAL VERSUS BIOMEDICAL PRACTITIONERS

China uses two health-care systems. One is grounded in Western medical care, and the other is anchored in traditional Chinese medicine. The educational preparation of physicians, nurses, and pharmacists is similar to Western health-care education. Ancillary workers have responsibility in the health-care system, and the practice of midwifery is widely accepted by the Chinese. Physicians in Chinese medicine are trained in universities, and traditional Chinese pharmacies remain an integral part of health care.

STATUS OF HEALTH-CARE PROVIDERS

Traditional Chinese medicine practitioners are shown great respect by the Chinese. In many instances, they are shown equal, if not more, respect than Western practitioners. The Chinese may distrust Western practitioners because of the pain and invasiveness of their treatments. The hierarchy among Chinese health-care providers is similar to that of Chinese society. Older health-care providers receive respect from the younger providers. Men usually receive more respect than women, but that is beginning to change. Physicians receive the highest respect, followed closely by nurses with a university education. Other nurses with limited education are next in the hierarchy, followed by ancillary personnel.

Health-care practitioners are usually given the same respect as older people in the family. Chinese children recognize them as authority figures. Physicians and nurses are viewed as individuals who can be trusted with the health of a family member. Nurses are generally perceived as caring individuals who perform treatments and procedures as ordered by the physician. Nursing assistants provide basic care to patients. Adult Chinese respond to practitioners with respect, but if they disagree with the health-care provider, they may not follow instructions. They may not verbally confront the health-care provider because they fear that either they or the provider will suffer a loss of face.

The Chinese respect their bodies and are very modest when it comes to touch. Most Chinese women feel uncomfortable being touched by male health-care providers, and most seek female health-care providers.

REFERENCES

Centers for Disease Control and Prevention (CDC). (2001). Retrieved March 28, 2007, from http://www.cdc.gov

China Population Information and Research Center. (2007). Retrieved March 28, 2007, from http://www.cpirc.org

China turns one child policy into law. (2002). Center for Reproductive Rights. Retrieved February 17, 2007, from http://www.crlp.org/ww_asia_1child.html

Chinese Ministry of Health. (2004). *An about face on AIDS prevention.* Retrieved August 29, 2007, from http://www.highbeam.com/doc/pi-103213525.htm

CIA. (2007). *World FactBook: China.* Retrieved February 17, 2007, from https://www.cia.gov/cia/publications/factbook/geos/ch.html

Gu, W. (2006). *Women of China, The human face of HIV/AIDS.* Retrieved February 17, 2007, from http://www.womenofchina.cn

Haley, G., Tan, C., & Haley, U. (1998). *New Asian emperors: The overseas Chinese, their strategies and competitive advantages.* Woburn, MA: Butterworth-Heinemann.

Halporn, R. (1992). Introduction. In C. L. Chen, W. C. Lowe, D. Ryan, A. H. Kutscher, R. Halporn, & H. Wang (Eds.), *Chinese Americans in loss and separation* (pp. v–xii). New York: Foundation of Thanatology.

He, J. Gu, D., Wu, X., Reynolds, L., Duan, X., & Cao, C. (2005). Major causes of death among men and women in China. *New England Journal of Medicine, 353,* 1124–1134.

Healthy People 2010. (2000). http://www.healthypeople.gov

Hu, W., & Grove, C. L. (1991). *Encountering the Chinese.* Yarmouth, MA: Intercultural Press.

Huang, W. (1992). Attitudes toward death: Chinese perspectives from the past. In C. L. Chen, W. C. Lowe, D. Ryan, A. H. Kutscher, R. Halporn, & H. Wang (Eds.), *Chinese Americans in loss and separation* (pp. 1–5). New York: Foundation of Thanatology.

Levy, R. A. (1993). Ethnic and racial differences in response to medicines: Preserving individualized therapy in managed pharmaceutical programmes. *Pharmaceutical Medicine, 7,* 139–165.

Lin, C. C., & Fu, V. R. (1990). A comparison of child-rearing practices among Chinese, immigrant Chinese, and Caucasian-American parents. *Child Development, 61,* 429–433.

Ma, G. X. (2000). Barriers to the use of health services by Chinese Americans. *Journal of Allied Health, 29*(2), 64–70.

Miller, L. C. (2000). Health of children adopted from China. *Pediatrics, 105*(6), 76.

Ministry of Public Health. (1992). *A brief introduction to China's medical and health services.* Beijing, People's Republic of China: Author.

Moore, R. (1990). Ethnographic assessment of pain coping perceptions. *Psychosomatic Medicine, 52,* 171–181.

Nan, C. (2006). *Beijing gears up for 2008 Paralympic Games.* Retrieved February 17, 2007, from http://www.btmbeijing.com

Office of Minority Health. (2007). *Asian American profiles.* Retrieved February 17, 2007, from http://www.omhrc.gov/templates/browse.aspx?lvl=2&lvlID=32

People's Daily. (2002). *China's life expectancy averaged 71.8 year.* Retrieved February 17, 2007, from http://english.peopledaily.com.cn

Schulpen, T. (2001). Immunization status of children adopted from China. *The Lancet, 358,* 2131–2132.

Seidel, H., Ball, J., Dains, J., & Benedict, W. (1994). *Quick reference to cultural assessment.* St. Louis, MO: Mosby.

Smith, C. S. (2002, April 30). Beware of cross-cultural faux pas in China. *New York Times.* Retrieved April 30, 2002, from http://www.nytimes.com

Tai Chi Chen Homepage. (2007). Retrieved August 29, 2007, from http://thetaichisite.htm

Tan, C. M. (1992). Treating life-threatening illness in children. In C. L. Chen, W. C. Lowe, D. Ryan, A. H. Kutscher, R. Halporn, & H. Wang (Eds.), *Chinese Americans in loss and separation* (pp. 26–33). New York: Foundation of Thanatology.

U.S. Department of Homeland Security. (2005). *Yearbook of immigration statistics.* Author. Retrieved February 17, 2007, from http://www.hsdl.org/hslog/?q=node/3281

Weatherspoon, A. J., Danko, G. P., & Johnson, R. C. (1994). Alcohol consumption and use norms among Chinese Americans and Korean Americans. *Journal of Studies on Alcohol, 55*(2), 203–206.

Women of China. (2006a). *Employment status of women.* Retrieved February 17, 2007, from http://www.womenofchina.cn

Women of China. (2006b). *HIV test mandatory.* Retrieved February 17, 2007, from http://www.womenofchina.cn

Women of China. (2006c). *Marriage and family.* Retrieved February 17, 2007, from http://www.womenofchina.cn

Women of China. (2006d). *Survey of divorce rates in different countries.* Retrieved February 17, 2007, from http://www.womenofchina.cn

Women of China. (2006e). *Women and children's health care services.* Retrieved February 17, 2007, from http://www.womenofchina.cn

Women of China. (2007). *Mother and daughter-in-law.* Retrieved February 17, 2007, from http://www.womenofchina.cn

XinHua News Agency. (2006). *Official calls for more efforts to curb gender imbalance.* Retrieved February 17, 2007 from http://english.peopledaily.com.cn

Ying, Y., & Miller, L. S. (1992). Help-seeking behavior and attitude of Chinese Americans regarding psychological problems. *American Journal of Community Psychology 20*(4), 549–556.

Yu, E. S., Edwin, H., Chen, K., Kim, K., & Sawsan, A. (2002). *Smoking among Chinese Americans: Behavior, knowledge, and beliefs.* Retrieved February 17, 2007, from http://www.pubmedcentral.nih.gov

Yu, S. M., Huang, S. J., & Singh, G. K. (2004). Health status and health services utilization among US Chinese, Asian Indian, Filipino, and Other Asian/Pacific Islander Children. *Pediatrics, 113*(1), 101–107.

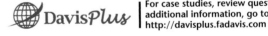

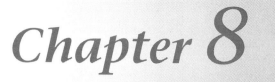

Chapter 8

People of Guatemalan Heritage

TINA A. ELLIS and LARRY D. PURNELL

Overview, Inhabited Localities, and Topography

OVERVIEW

People of Guatemalan heritage compose a growing number of Hispanic/Latino populations in the United States. Whereas Guatemalans may share a common Spanish language with other Hispanic ethnic groups, they are, nonetheless, a unique cultural group. Health-care providers must be knowledgeable regarding distinct Hispanic cultural characteristics to provide culturally competent care for patients of Guatemalan heritage.

HERITAGE AND RESIDENCE

Guatemala is a Central American country characterized by beautiful landscapes and peoples. This land, referred to as "eternal spring," has an estimated population of over 12.3 million (CIA, 2007). The northernmost of the Central American nations, Guatemala has 41,700 square miles and is the size of the state of Tennessee in the United States. Its neighbors are Mexico on the north and west, and Belize, Honduras, and El Salvador on the south and east. The country consists of three main regions—the cool highlands with the heaviest population, the tropical area along the Pacific and Caribbean coasts, and the tropical jungle in the northern lowlands, known as the *Petén* (Information Please Almanac, 2007). Guatemala is inhabited by Mestizo (mixed Amerindian Spanish—in local Spanish called *Ladino*) and European 59.4 percent, K'iche 9.1 percent, Kaqchikel 8.4 percent, Mam 7.9 percent, Q'eqchi 6.3 percent, other Mayan 8.6 percent, indigenous non-Mayan 0.2 percent, other 0.1 percent. More than half of Guatemala's rural population resides in the highlands,

the most populated region of the country. The capital, Guatemala City with a population of 1.1 million, is located within the highland area. Soil in the Pacific lowlands is the most fertile within the country owing to the ash deposited by active volcanoes. Ladinos compose the majority population in this region of Guatemala (Information Please Almanac, 2007).

Guatemala was inhabited for approximately 3000 years by Mayan Indians who lived a simple life based on the culture, customs, and religion of their ancestors. Farming was the primary occupation, although the Maya excelled in architecture, weaving, pottery, and hieroglyphics. Whereas a few cities (*pueblos*) were established during Mayan times, the majority of Guatemalans now live in small villages (*aldeas*).

In the 15th century, the Spaniards came to Guatemala seeking a route to the East Indies. Many remained, establishing a formal government, economy, and way of life based on Spanish culture, traditions, and the Catholic religion (Information Please Almanac, 2007).

REASONS FOR MIGRATION AND ASSOCIATED ECONOMIC FACTORS

Civil war during the 1960s, 1970s, and 1980s created widespread death, loss of land rights, economic instability, and disruption of the way of life for most Guatemalans. The indigenous population was most adversely affected. As a result, huge numbers fled to Mexico and the United States seeking safety and political asylum. A peace accord signed in 1996 formally ended 36 years of violence in Guatemala. The country continues to be plagued by "abject" poverty. With 56 percent of the population living below the poverty level (CIA, 2007), families with one member earning as little as 14 *quetzales* a day (equivalent to 2 U.S. dollars) can survive (Walsh, 2006).

Two distinct types of migration, internal and external, occur among people of Guatemalan heritage. The first occurs within the country of Guatemala. Large company-owned farms (*fincas*) along the Pacific lowlands grow coffee beans, cotton, cardamom, and sugar. During the harvest season, indigenous people from the highlands migrate to the Pacific lowlands to harvest the crops grown there. Migrants may remain in the *fincas* for months prior to returning home. Although for many only the male head of household and mature boys migrate, in some cases, the entire family migrates. Another in-country migration is the relocation of indigenous people to Guatemala City. Owing to economic necessity, young women leave their families to work as housekeepers for wealthy Ladino families. Their earnings are sent home to supplement the family income. In some cases, whole families relocate to Guatemala City. Some are able to secure adequate income for their needs; however, many cannot and resort to living within the Guatemala City dump.

The second type of migration occurs primarily to the United States. Over 700,000 Guatemalans currently reside in the United States, of whom an estimated 150,000 are undocumented (U.S. Bureau of the Census, 2005).

Approximately 85 percent of America's farm workers are Hispanic, some of whom are Guatemalan. The average farm worker in the United States averages less than $10,000 a year (National Center for Farmworker Health [NCFH], 2005). These wages provide Guatemalans with sufficient income to send money back home to help support their families. When the opportunity presents itself, many move into nonagricultural jobs, as these generally offer increased stability and higher wages.

EDUCATIONAL STATUS AND OCCUPATIONS

Prior to the Spanish conquest, education in Guatemala was informal. The Mayan languages and cultures were passed down orally from generation to generation. There was no written Mayan language. Children learned language and culture from their parents, extended family, and community. Ladinos established the first public education system within the country. Higher education was developed as well. The education system teaches the official language of the country, Spanish, along with Spanish culture and traditions. High school and university graduates are primarily Ladinos (Shea, 2001).

Within the Mayan culture, boys are permitted to attend school. Parents believe that developing skills in the Spanish language prepares them for additional economic opportunities. Female children traditionally have not been permitted to attend school. They spent as much time as possible with their mothers to learn homemaking skills. This, however, is changing. More female children are encouraged to attend school. The literacy rate for men is 78 percent, and for women, it is 63 percent (CIA, 2007).

Most Guatemalans are involved in occupations related to farming. Rural families may own a small plot of land passed on by their ancestors; however, many of these plots were confiscated by the government during the civil war. Often, the plot is just large enough for a small adobe brick home with a tin roof and an area to grow corn (*maize*), beans, and a few other vegetables for family consumption.

Children miss school when needed to help with farming or household duties. Rather than completing high school, many children around the age of 12 years begin working as soon as they are able to do so in order to supplement the family income.

Women in rural areas may earn money by selling, at the local marketplace, woven clothing, handmade items, or small animals they have raised. Weavings using a traditional back strap loom contain colors and designs related to the specific indigenous group, village, and family by whom they are made.

Communication

VIGNETTE 8.1

Francisco Salvador Siantz, a 42-year-old Ladino from the Guatemalan Highlands, fell from a ladder and broke his femur while picking apples. Working through an interpreter during his health assessment, he admitted to having a 6-month history of generalized musculoskeletal pain, dizziness, and intermittent fevers that he has not revealed to anyone. His laboratory reports return with an elevated blood glucose level. His physician plans to complete a further work-up for diabetes mellitus.

1. This Ladino gentleman has three names. What is the surname of his father? Of his mother? If he were to sign his first and last name, what would they be?
2. What language interpreter was used if he speaks the language of the Ladino Guatemalan population?
3. Identify three possible reasons he did not notify anyone about his history of generalized musculoskeletal pain, dizziness, and intermittent fevers?
4. Besides his diabetes, what might other diagnoses be?
5. If the nutritionist provides him with a diabetic diet, what "typical" Ladino foods should be included?

DOMINANT LANGUAGE AND DIALECTS

The major languages in Guatemala include the official language, Spanish, which is spoken by 60 percent of the population, and Amerindian languages, which are spoken by the remaining 40 percent. Officially, 23 Amerindian languages are recognized, including Quiche, Cakchiquel, Kekchi, Mam, Garifuna, and Xinca. Ladinos speak Spanish as their primary language. In addition, there are various unofficial Mayan languages (Shea, 2001). Each Mayan ethnic group speaks one dialect as their primary language. If Mayans attend school in Guatemala, they learn Spanish.

Some Mayan men do not have a formal education but are able to speak Spanish because of frequent interactions with Spanish speakers. This occurs most often through business relationships. Mayan men, therefore, may be bilingual, speaking their Mayan dialect and Spanish.

Spanish is the primary language of blacks who attend school in Guatemala. If a black individual immigrated to Guatemala, then her or his primary language is most likely the language of their home country. Most black immigrants to Guatemala speak French as their primary language and learn Spanish after arriving in Guatemala.

TEMPORAL RELATIONSHIPS

Guatemalan people tend to value the past and live in the present, being more concerned with today than the future because the future is uncertain for many. Some of life's uncertainties for Guatemalans are related to the daily challenges they face securing adequate employment, housing, food, and other basic necessities such as health care for themselves and their families.

For those in poverty, there is usually not enough money to save for the future and send their children for higher education. Social Security or retirement benefits are not available to the average citizen in Guatemala. Medicare or Medicaid insurance is not available. Most Guatemalans hope that they can work until the time of their death. When an individual is unable to work, it is customary for him or her to be taken care of by the family.

Because work is such a priority in the life of many Guatemalans, they seek health care only when their illness has progressed to the point of preventing them from working or carrying out their duties or roles within the family. Taking time to go to the doctor means time lost from work and loss of pay.

Most Guatemalans live in poverty in rural areas and may not own a watch or clock and may not be able to tell time. Time is related to the natural environment, such as sunrise, sunset, and the rainy season. Businesses in Guatemala are much more relaxed about time. Punctuality is difficult for many because of limited transportation and unexpected family needs.

Future orientation and punctuality are highly valued in the United States. Because these are in direct contrast to Guatemalan values, patient/health-care provider relationships often result in conflict. Guatemalans may be late for appointments or not show up at all. Health-care providers may interpret this behavior as immature or disrespectful, whereas the reason may actually have to do with a family emergency, lack of transportation, inability to get time off from work, limited finances, or fear of losing one's job. Moreover, health-care providers may expect Guatemalan patients to participate in preventive health screenings and adopt behaviors to reduce their risk of long-term complications of disease. These behaviors require a future orientation that conflicts with the present orientation of many Guatemalans.

FORMAT FOR NAMES

Guatemalans who have a Hispanic heritage use the Spanish format for names. At birth, a child is given a first name (Ovidio) followed by the surname of his father (Garcia), and then the surname of his mother (Salvador), resulting in Ovidio Garcia Salvador. Men's names remain the same through their lifetime. However, when a woman named Jovita Garcia Salvador marries Francisco Vasquez Gutierrez, she then becomes Jovita Garcia de Vasquez or simply Jovita Garcia Vasquez.

Sometimes, health-care providers incorrectly assume Guatemalan couples are not married because of the format of their names. Guatemalan couples use this format when married in either the church or a civil ceremony.

Couples who live together (*unidos*) may use this format or choose for the woman to retain her unmarried name.

To convey respect, the health-care providers should address the Guatemalan in a formal manner unless otherwise requested by the patient. Male children and adults are referred to as Mr. (*señor*). Females are referred to as Ms. (*señorita*) or Mrs. (*señora*). Guatemalans are customarily greeted with a handshake. In rural areas, people shake hands softly. To give a firm handshake indicates aggressive behavior. In the cities, however, the handshake tends to be more firm. Guatemalans avoid direct eye contact with others, including health-care providers, which is a way of demonstrating respect and should not be misinterpreted as avoidance, low self-esteem, or disinterest. They speak softly in public. Speaking loud is considered rude.

Family Roles and Organization

HEAD OF HOUSEHOLD AND GENDER ROLES

Many Guatemala families follow traditional roles for husbands, wives, and children, although this is changing for some. Traditionally, the man has been the head of household and is the primary "breadwinner" and provider for the family. This usually requires men to work outside of the home. Ultimate decision-making power resides with the man of the house.

Women's roles have traditionally involved raising the children and caring for the home. In rural areas, the wife usually rises around 5:00 a.m. or even earlier. She carries water for drinking and firewood from the nearest sources available. Then she returns home, builds a fire, and begins cooking for the family on a wood-burning stove. Once the family has eaten breakfast, she cleans house by sweeping the dirt floors, grinds corn to make *tortillas*, washes clothes, cares for the young children, breastfeeds as needed, sews, weaves, cares for chickens and other small animals, and prepares for market day (Shea, 2001). Little girls begin fetching water at the age of 3 to 4 years. At age 7 years, they are washing clothes, gathering wood, and caring for younger siblings. At age 9 years, young girls learn to weave and embroider (Glittenberg, 1994).

Guatemalans place a high value on the family and the extended family. Most families are nuclear—comprising a father, mother, and children. Extended family is important to Guatemalans and may include grandparents, aunts, uncles, and cousins.

A young woman's 15th birthday (*quinceñera*) is celebrated as her passage to womanhood. Coming of age for a young man is at 18 years. A young man asks the young woman's father for her hand in marriage. Engagements may last several years. In the indigenous population, a young man's father may seek out a matchmaker to find a suitable bride under age 16. Once an arrangement is reached, the young man offers a dowry. A wedding feast celebrates the marriage.

More Guatemalan women are entering the workforce outside of the home, resulting in more egalitarian male/female roles. Husbands and wives share more of the child rearing and household responsibilities.

PRESCRIPTIVE, RESTRICTIVE, AND TABOO PRACTICES FOR CHILDREN AND ADOLESCENTS

Guatemalans place a high value on the institution of family, which includes nuclear and extended family members who most often live together or very close. They are involved in each other's lives on a daily basis. Family is structured as a patrilineal system. Males are the only family members who receive an inheritance (Glittenberg, 1994).

Children are a gift from God and are highly valued in Guatemalan society. Sons are more valued than daughters (Glittenberg, 1994). Children are taught to be obedient and demonstrate respect for older people. In Mayan communities, family members and other adults take an active part in raising a child. They believe it takes a village to raise a child to become a productive member of the community and to continue their culture (Menchu, 1984). Values include being humble, content, and respectful of others; working hard; avoiding arguments; and placing the needs of the family before one's own individual needs. In Ladino families, individualism and competition are more highly valued (Glittenberg, 1994).

Disobedience among children in Guatemala may be handled with physical punishment (Menchu, 1984). Health-care providers in the United States need to use care in assessing evidence of this to avoid misdiagnosing it as child abuse.

FAMILY GOALS AND PRIORITIES

The Guatemalan family demonstrates a desire to provide for the needs of each member. Parents provide for their children in hopes that they will grow up, marry, work, and have children. When family members are unable to take care of themselves, the expectation is that their family will take care of them. Life is hard in Guatemala. Families work much of their lives without luxuries such as days off or vacations. Most know poverty will likely prevail in their lives regardless of how hard they work. Parents feel they must prepare their children for the same hard life they have lived because very little changes from generation to generation (Menchu, 1984).

Guatemalans expect to work hard and believe that their hard work will result in an increased quality of life. Guatemalan families who migrate to the United States do so with the hope of a better life for themselves and their children. More opportunities are available in the United States, which is why Guatemalans often risk everything to migrate.

ALTERNATIVE LIFESTYLES

When "family" falls outside of defined norms, there is a lack of understanding and acceptance toward those involved. Religious beliefs and tradition often dictate the attitude one holds about what does and does not constitute family in Guatemala.

Catholic, Protestant, and Evangelical Guatemalans do not believe in homosexuality, sexual activity among the unmarried, or infidelity. Persons involved in these activities must do so in secrecy. Even today, indigenous women dress conservatively with a woven long skirt (*corte*), blouse (*huipil*), a scarf (*tzute*), and shawl (*rebozo*) that promote modesty. A single woman is believed to be a prostitute if she is out in public alone.

Despite a prevailing "macho" attitude with a deep-rooted homophobia, some inroads have been made for gays, lesbian, and transgendered populations in Guatemala with *Lesbiradas*, an organization for lesbians and bisexual women, and an annual Gay Pride March in Guatemala City since 2000 (Gay Guatemala, 2007). Larger cities in the United States offer organizations such as *Ellas*, a support group for Latina lesbians; El Hotline of Hola Gay, an organization with information and referrals in Spanish; and Dignity, a gay Catholic support organization. Health-care providers need to be sensitive toward and knowledgeable regarding the resources in their community for Guatemalans who present with an alternative lifestyle.

Workforce Issues

CULTURE IN THE WORKPLACE

During the civil war in Guatemala, residents were permitted to migrate to the United States and apply for political asylum. If granted, this allowed Guatemalans to stay permanently in the United States, but they were not permitted to ever return to Guatemala. Many who chose this route had no family left in their home country; their lives were at risk should they return. In 1986, the Immigration Reform and Control Act allowed many Guatemalan agricultural workers to bypass the process involved in political asylum and simply obtain residency as farm laborers. This promoted an increase in emigration (Wellmeier, 1998). Guatemalans who migrate to the United States today often find employment in the agricultural industry, including hand-harvesting crops and working on egg or chicken farms, citrus processing plants, and plant and flower nurseries.

Wellmeier (1998) found that Guatemalans in Indiantown, Florida, acquired a reputation for hard work, complained little, and paid close attention to detailed work in agriculture. However, Mayans were not often hired for picking oranges or cutting sugar cane because of their small stature. Agricultural employers preferred Mexican or Haitian workers for these jobs.

When possible, Mayan farm workers in the United States secure nonagricultural employment that offers less migration and more economic stability. Some find positions in housekeeping or maintenance in businesses or schools. Those with skills in English and Spanish may qualify for interpreter positions. If they speak a Mayan dialect as well, their services are even more highly sought by agencies that serve that particular population (Wellmeier, 1998).

Guatemalan women may work in agriculture or housekeeping in the United States or cook instead for Guatemalan men who are single or working in the United States without their families. This provides men with a connection to home, convenience, and the enjoyment of consuming foods prepared according to cultural traditions. Prices for the meals are generally affordable.

Undocumented Guatemalans have difficulty securing a bank account or driver's license. Many carry the cash they earn with them. This habit and their small stature have resulted in Guatemalans being victims of robbery. Some Mayan agencies in the United States have developed co-ops that offer simple banking services to reduce the incidence of robbery among Guatemalans (Wellmeier, 1998).

Guatemalans may purchase a vehicle in order to secure employment far from home while in the United States. Most have never had formal driver's training or a driver's license or driven a vehicle prior to arrival in the United States. Moreover, they may be unaware of driving rules and regulations in the United States owing to unfamiliarity with the English language. Driving under these circumstances places the Guatemalan and other drivers at risk for serious accidents. In addition, Guatemalans may be ticketed or arrested for driving violations owing to their lack of understanding regarding laws in the United States, such as seatbelt laws.

Because family is highly valued among Guatemalans, needs of the family take priority over obligations in the employment setting. Guatemalans may miss work owing to an illness of a loved one, a need for transportation to an appointment, or a lack of child care. When Guatemalans living in the United States learn that a loved one in Guatemala is ill or has passed away, they feel compelled to return to Guatemala for an extended period of time, risking loss of their job if a leave of absence is not possible.

Because punctuality is not valued in Guatemala, the Guatemalan employee in the United States may arrive for work late. They may not wear a timepiece, be able to tell time, or understand the importance of punctuality in the United States. This misunderstanding also occurs in health-care settings. The Guatemalan patient may be late for an appointment owing to circumstances related to family, work, or transportation and find the appointment has been cancelled or rescheduled when she or he arrives. To achieve a positive relationship, health-care providers need to demonstrate respect for the Guatemalan patient's need for flexibility and help her or him to understand the expectations within the health-care setting.

ISSUES RELATED TO AUTONOMY

Guatemalans tend to respect persons in positions of authority. Those of lower socioeconomic status and/or with formal education and English language skills usually acquire positions with responsibility but little authority. They prefer to get along well with others and not criticize or voice complaints when treated poorly. Moreover, the Guatemalan is likely to remain in a position equal to his or her peers rather than seek a promotion.

Biocultural Ecology

SKIN COLOR AND OTHER BIOLOGICAL VARIATIONS

Most Guatemalans are a mixture of Spanish and Mayan Indian heritage. There is a small population of black Guatemalans with ancestry from the Caribbean and Africa. This accounts for variations in skin color, facial features, hair, body structure, and other biological variations. Intermarriage among the racial groups in Guatemala has produced variations in their appearance. No one appearance is "typical" for a Guatemalan individual.

Guatemalans who are predominantly Spanish have the appearance of Caucasians. They may have blonde or brown hair, fair (white) complexion, and blue eyes and be of average or taller height with a medium to large build. Guatemalans with predominantly Mayan Indian ancestry tend to have black hair, brown skin, and dark eye color and are of short height with a petite build. Black Guatemalans tend to have black hair, black skin, and dark eyes and be of average or taller height with a medium to large build.

Cyanosis and anemia are assessed differently in dark-skinned people than in white-skinned people. Instead of being bluish in color, the skin color of a cyanotic patient of Indian or black ancestry may appear more ashen. Physical assessment of these individuals should include examination of the sclera, conjunctiva, buccal mucosa, tongue, lips, nailbeds, and palms of hands and soles of feet. In addition, jaundice is more difficult to detect among dark-skinned Guatemalans. Examination of the sclera and buccal mucosa for evidence of bilirubin is important for accurate assessment.

DISEASES AND HEALTH CONDITIONS

Health literature regarding Guatemalans is limited. The primary literature is related to public health statistics compiled by Pan American Health Organization (PAHO) and direct observations by North American health-care professionals who provide primary care through their volunteer efforts in Guatemala (*jornadas*). Even data compiled by the NCFH do not differentiate Guatemalan farm workers from other groups within the designation of Hispanic farm workers when discussing health.

The leading causes of mortality in Guatemala are pneumonia, diarrhea, communicable diseases, diseases of the circulatory system, perinatal conditions, and tumors (PAHO, 2004). These may be directly linked to environmental factors, lifestyle, and lack of adequate medical care. Chickering (2006) compiled data of the most frequent complaints of Guatemalans to North American health-care practitioners during *jornadas*. These are described in order of highest to lowest frequency:

1. *Musculoskeletal pain:* This is not really surprising, considering the lifestyle of many Guatemalans. They are exposed to difficulties in life, including violence, malnutrition, disease, and high child-bearing rates, all of which take their toll on one's health and well-being.

    Much of the work involved in the daily lives of Guatemalans is difficult. For example, young girls start fetching water, which they carry on their heads, and caring for siblings, whom they carry on their backs, at very young ages.

    Boys begin farm work with their fathers as soon as they are physically able. Farming continues much as it traditionally has with primitive tools, requiring lifting, bending, climbing steep mountains, and carrying heavy loads without the use of modern machinery.

Adulthood brings requirements for more work, along with an increased need for physical stamina to maintain economic stability, the family, and the home. Guatemalans often believe that life is hard and pain is expected; instead of complaining about pain, they usually learn to endure the pain and continue their duties until the pain is unbearable or they physically are unable to function as desired.

Other causes for musculoskeletal pain in Guatemalans are diseases such as malaria or dengue fever. ". . . Whole body pain with a history of fever should be considered malaria until proven otherwise" (Chickering, 2006). Guatemalans with dengue are not as likely to be seen by a health-care provider because they are usually too ill to even leave their home (Chickering, 2006).

2. *Abdominal pain:* These complaints are divided into epigastric and non-epigastric pain. Most commonly, epigastric pain is due to gastritis (*gastritis*), intestinal worms, or chronic giardia. Guatemalans may hold traditional beliefs about the symptoms caused by intestinal worms. These include thunder (*trueño*) noise in the stomach, swelling (*hinchazón*) in the stomach (especially in the afternoon following the largest meal of the day), chronic abdominal swelling (*panzudo*) in children, a ball-like mass (*bola*) in the stomach, gas moving back and forth in the upper abdomen, itchy nose, pica (especially for eating dirt, ashes, and paper), loss of appetite, and sleeping prone (*embrocado*) (Chickering, 2006).

3. *Cough and upper respiratory symptoms:* A complaint of chronic coughing or a cough that persists can be a symptom of pulmonary tuberculosis (TB). This may be accompanied by fever, night sweats, or weight loss. Typhoid can also have symptoms of a mild, dry cough, although typhoid is not a very common disease in Guatemala (Chickering, 2006).

A factor increasing the Guatemalan's risk for acute upper respiratory infections is related to poverty and living conditions. Many Guatemalans of low socioeconomic status are malnourished, so their immune function is compromised. They often live in one- or two-room homes, placing them in close quarters with other family members and enabling germs to spread easily from one person to another.

In addition to acute upper respiratory infections, chronic lung disease is seen among Guatemalans. Some areas of Guatemala have very poor air quality, exposing people to high levels of toxic inhalants. Regulations for air quality are few and poorly monitored. Another source of exposure for many Guatemalans is from cooking on wood-burning stoves. Cooking remains primitive for many, and dependence on wood for fuel is high. Exposure to carbon monoxide presents a risk in itself, but the danger becomes even higher because the cooking area is often enclosed in the home or a building adjacent to the home, with little, if any, ventilation to the outside. Chronic lung disease may result from years of one or both of these exposures.

Health-care providers may misinterpret signs and symptoms of chronic lung disease in Guatemalans as related to cigarette smoking when, in reality, far more people are exposed to environmental factors than smoke cigarettes. In cases in which the Guatemalan patient does smoke, the risk is obviously higher than that of nonsmokers.

4. *Headaches:* Headaches can be due to a number of factors. Malnutrition and anemia are common and some headaches are attributed to these. In addition, cooking on the wood-burning stove causes women, especially, to be exposed to high levels of carbon monoxide, which can produce headaches.

Although men usually carry heavy loads on their backs, women carry them on their heads, which leads some women to experience headaches. Finally, worms can cause headaches. Guatemalans themselves often relate the cause of headaches to be from anger or exposure to sun. Relationships that do not involve conflict are highly valued among Guatemalans. Unresolved issues in relationships may increase one's stress, thereby creating headaches. There is no literature to suggest sun exposure may cause headaches among Guatemalans, but perhaps the belief is related to the hot/cold paradigm. Health-care providers should also assess blood pressure and neurological function in Guatemalans complaining of headaches (Chickering, 2006).

5. *Weakness:* Weakness (*debilidad*), fatigue (*cansancio*), and dizziness (*mareos, baidos,* or *tarantamiento*) are common complaints. Anemia is the most common cause for these symptoms. Health-care providers must note that weakness can also be used to describe a health problem involving one body organ. For example, weakness of the stomach (*debilidad del estomago*) can refer to a Guatemalan patient's self-report of poor nutrition, and weakness of the heart (*debilidad del corazon*) can imply being upset emotionally (Chickering, 2006).

When Guatemalan patients complain of dizziness with or without the weakness and fatigue, dehydration should be considered. Guatemalans consume very little water on a daily basis because of the scarcity and poor quality of the accessible drinking water. Adults are more likely to drink coffee than water, which can lead to dehydration.

6. *Skin lesions and/or itching:* The most common skin lesions are skin spots (*manchas*) known scientifically as the yeast *Malassezia furfur*. Pruritus may result from dry skin, fungi, scabies, worms, or AIDS, known in Spanish as SIDA. In Guatemala,

HIV, known in Spanish as VIH, is most often transmitted by heterosexual intercourse. Men may contract it through sexual activity with women they meet at bars; wives then contract it from their infected husbands (Chickering, 2006).

Health-care providers should suspect HIV/AIDS when the Guatemalan patient offers the next most common presenting complaints of anorexia and weight loss and their history includes diarrhea, cough, pruritus, painful swallowing, persistent unexplained fever, weakness, or night sweats. The health-care provider should not hesitate to ask about risky sexual behaviors with which the patient may have been involved to further determine if HIV/AIDS may be the most likely diagnosis; testing/counseling should follow (Chickering, 2006).

7. *Diarrhea* (asientos, chorrio): Causes for diarrhea primarily include shigella, amoebas, and giardia, although it may accompany HIV/AIDS as well (Chickering, 2006). Exposure to these pathogens is high in Guatemala, especially in the rural areas. The infrastructure of the communities simply cannot provide water and sewage services necessary for promoting healthy lifestyles because these are nonexistent for most Guatemalans.

   Drinking water is obtained from polluted waterways, so it is nonpotable. Either bottled water must be purchased, which is cost prohibitive for most Guatemalans, or contaminated water must be boiled for at least 20 minutes to ensure pathogenic organisms are eradicated. Factors such as depending on wood for cooking to boil drinking water and the time required for this option lead to low levels of compliance.

   Dehydration, obviously, is the most serious side effect of diarrhea. This is especially true for children and is the second leading cause of death for children under 5 years of age in Guatemala (PAHO, 2004). Severe dehydration needs to be treated promptly with IV fluids when possible. When IV fluids are not available to administer, oral rehydration solutions should be used. They are available in prepared packets or can be made with ingredients readily available at low cost. Whereas the pathogens mentioned are the most common causes of diarrhea in Guatemala, health-care providers who treat immigrant populations in North America should consider these causes when patients have a history of traveling to and from Guatemala.

8. *Eye disorders:* Wind, dust, sunlight, and cooking smoke contribute to eye pain in Guatemala through conjunctiva irritation or by the stimulation of ptergia (*carnosidades*). Relief from discomfort and pain can be accomplished through the use of cool, moist compresses over the eyes. Moistening the compresses with chamomile tea (*té de manzanilla*) is ideal (Chickering, 2006).

   Other painful eye disorders among Guatemalan patients include dacrocytosis and tracoma.

Cataracts (even in children), congenital toxoplasmosis, toxic optic neuropathy (usually related to TB treatment), vitamin A deficiency, and actinic allergy are examples of nonpainful eye conditions common to Guatemalans. Vitamin A deficiency, however, is decreasing because sugar has been fortified with vitamin A (Chickering, 2006).

Chickering (2006) identified additional presenting complaints of Guatemalan patients as falling into categories related to menstrual/vaginal, psychiatric, urinary tract infection, pregnancy, pure fever and chills, ear and hearing, chest pain, and male genitourinary issues.

VARIATIONS IN DRUG METABOLISM

Although some studies have identified differences in drug metabolism related to racial/ethnic groups, it is difficult to use these for Guatemalans owing to the mixed heritage of many. These variations, however, can influence the determination of a therapeutic dose and affect absorption, distribution, metabolism, and excretion of drugs. A few studies using one subgroup of Hispanics noted that they required lower doses of antidepressants and experienced more side effects than non-Hispanic whites.

High-Risk Behaviors

Although Guatemala as a country struggles to maintain traditional and faith-based values, the reality is that increasing numbers of residents seek relief from the hardships of life through abuse of substances. The prevalence of substance abuse is highest among men. Alcohol is the most readily available substance and the most widely abused. In Guatemala, it is not uncommon to see men staggering in public owing to drunkenness and unconscious on sidewalks and roads from excessive intoxication. Accidents are more prone to occur in these settings. Injuries and even death occur from falls, confrontations, and collisions with vehicles.

Men who immigrate to the United States from Guatemala for work may find themselves drinking alcohol excessively, even if they did not prior to migration. This may be due to such factors as (1) the stress of living in another country illegally, (2) being away from the family, friends, and support systems, (3) fears of inadequate work and deportation, and (4) illness and being victims of violence and injury. They may work and live closely with other men they hardly know and yet develop a camaraderie based on their shared lifestyle. Their role changes from being actively involved in family to that of a long-distance economic provider, which leads to loneliness, emptiness, and unstructured time when the work day is done. Alcohol can become the antidote (NCFH, 2005).

HEALTH-CARE PRACTICES

Guatemalans of low socioeconomic status receive little health education, have limited access to health care, and often believe illness is punishment from God. These factors result in their poor participation in illness prevention practices. In addition, health care in rural areas is mostly provided by government health promoters who focus on episodic illness care rather than preventive measures such as sanitary housing, potable water, balanced diets, and family planning (Icu, 2000).

Guatemalan families readily participate in immunization programs for their children yet do not participate themselves. Adult immunizations such as tetanus, flu, and pneumonia are underutilized by Guatemalans. Moreover, women do not participate in routine screening for breast and cervical cancer. Guatemalan men do not participate in routine screening for testicular or colon cancer.

Lack of routine health-care screenings place Guatemalans at high risk for communicable diseases and cancers at advanced stages of disease, severely compromising positive outcomes. Health-care professionals should educate Guatemalans in a family context for disease, illness, and injury prevention; assist with low-cost referrals; and respect their cultural beliefs.

Nutrition

VIGNETTE 8.2

Pablo Salvador, a Ladino Guatemalan political refugee, has been in the United States for 15 years. Señor Salvador has worked in the same poultry processing plant since his arrival. Over the last 10 years, he has sent almost half of his salary to his parents in Guatemala. His parents were able to afford the trip to the United States and moved in with him 4 months ago. He told his supervisor that he is happy that his mother is cooking his childhood Guatemalan foods, especially tortillas treated with limestone, which he has missed since his arrival in the United States.

1. What are the implications of being a political refugee and a political asylee? What is the difference?
2. What foods might be included in a Ladino Guatemalan diet? How might they be prepared?
3. What health problem can occur with eating tortillas cooked with limestone?
4. What evidence of the value of familism is in this vignette?

MEANING OF FOOD

Food to Guatemalans signifies physical, spiritual, and cultural wellness. Foods vary among Guatemalans based on cultural traditions and accessibility.

COMMON FOODS AND FOOD RITUALS

Gari'funa cuisine reflects the Caribbean coast and includes recipes from African ancestors. Common foods include sea bass, flounder, red snapper, tarpon, shrimp, seviche, coconut milk, tomato, onion, garlic, lime, and lemon (Shea, 2001).

Their ancestors taught that the Maya come from the corn. As a result, corn is highly valued in the Mayan culture. Corn is the chief crop and the basis for many food products and meals. Foods bring strength, good health,

and a spiritual connection to the past. The Mayan diet primarily consists of maize, black beans, rice, chicken, squash, tomatoes, carrots, chilies, beets, cauliflower, lettuce, cabbage, chard, leek, onion, and garlic. These foods are used to make tortillas, *atole* (liquid corn drink), *pinol* (chicken-flavored corn gruel), *pepi'an* (chicken stew with squash seeds, hot chilies, tomatoes, and tomatillos [small green tomato]), and *caldos* (soups made of chicken stock and vegetables) (Shea, 2001). Preferred beverages are Hibiscus tea and coffee. Coffee is brewed weaker than that in North America.

Ladino foods reflect their Spanish ancestry and include maize, rice, beans, beef, chicken, pork, milk, cheese, plantains, carrots, peppers, tomatoes, squash, avocado, cilantro, chilies, onion, garlic, lemon, lime, and chocolate. Common dishes include *arroz con pollo* (chicken with rice), *chile rellenos* (peppers stuffed with pork or beef with carrot, onion, and tomato and fried in egg batter), and *tamales* (chicken or pork in a corn paste steamed in banana leaves or corn husks) (Shea, 2001). Foods are seasoned with toasted squash seeds ground to a powder. Guatemalan food is not served spicy. A spicy hot sauce may be served alongside a meal for individuals who prefer to add it.

DIETARY PRACTICES FOR HEALTH PROMOTION

Guatemalans value corn because it brings good health. Corn is eaten at every meal, most often in the form of tortillas. Tortillas are made by soaking corn kernels in lime, creating dough by adding animal fat, flattening the dough, and cooking it over an open fire or wood-burning stove. The lime used is limestone rather than the fruit lime and is believed to strengthen bones. Consuming foods with limestone, however, has also been associated with dental problems and gallstones (Glittenberg, 1994).

NUTRITIONAL DEFICIENCIES AND FOOD LIMITATIONS

The diet of many Guatemalans is low in protein (Steltzer, 1983), iron, and vitamin C (Chickering, 2006). Lactose intolerance is especially prevalent among indigenous populations (National Digestive Diseases Information Clearinghouse, 2007). Some families encourage their children to drink coffee with sugar when they refuse the poor-tasting drinking water. This practice leads to gastritis, dehydration, and dental caries.

Pregnancy and Childbearing Practices

VIGNETTE 8.3

A 15-year-old "typical" Mayan, Angelica speaks Mam, which is not a written language. She is 8 months' pregnant and was sent by her family with a group of migrant Guatemalan and Mexican workers to prepare their meals. Her family sent her because they did not want to face the stigma of her unwed pregnancy, even though she was a victim of rape. The public health worker has witnessed her walking through the fields in the late afternoon looking at her abdomen and talking to her fetus. Initially, the public health nurse thought Angelica was 11 or 12 years old.

1. Identify Mayan beliefs regarding pregnancy and virginity.
2. Why is Angelica talking to her fetus?
3. Describe the physical attributes of "typical Mayans." Why did the public health worker initially think Angelica was only 11 or 12 years of age?
4. Identify Mayan foods that Angelica might eat to ensure a healthy baby.

FERTILITY PRACTICES AND VIEWS TOWARD PREGNANCY

Guatemalans value life beginning from conception; a baby is a gift from God. For religious reasons, most do not believe in contraception or abortion. A Guatemalan woman may bear 10 or more children in her lifetime. Of these, many die before the age of 5 years (PAHO, 2004). Women who desire contraception will not actually seek it because of lack of support from their spouse, family, and church. Access to modern birth control methods is difficult, if not impossible, for many Guatemalan women who may consider alternatives to pregnancy.

In Guatemala, Mayan midwives (*comadronas*) deliver 80 percent of all children in the home. The other 20 percent are delivered by medical professionals in the hospital setting. *Comadronas* are "wise" women who are trusted in their community. They feel midwifery is a sacred "calling" by God or a saint who requires special knowledge and rituals. The Ministry of Health has permitted midwives to practice since 1935 (Lang & Elkin, 1997). Many midwives do not have formal training. They may have learned the practice from their mother (*mama*) or grandmother (*abuela*) or through "dreams or visions." Prior to delivery, the midwife prays at her own home and then again at the home of the pregnant mother. Some use candles, incense, or religious icons during prayer. The delivery is followed by additional prayers. If the baby dies during delivery, the midwife and family accept it as God's will (Walsh, 2006).

Health-care providers must ask the Guatemalan woman whether she is interested in family planning instead of directing the question as "which form of birth control do you prefer?" The latter clearly arises from the health-care provider's own values, which may be in direct conflict with those of the patient. Moreover, when the patient does express a desire to learn more about family planning, she may request the session include her husband. Arrangements should be made to accommodate the patient's request.

PRESCRIPTIVE, RESTRICTIVE, AND TABOO PRACTICES IN THE CHILDBEARING FAMILY

On the day a Guatemalan woman becomes pregnant, she and her husband share the news with respected elders of the village. The community becomes the grandparents (*abuelos*) of the unborn child. Godparents are also selected at this time (Menchu, 1984).

In the seventh month of pregnancy, the woman introduces her fetus to the environment. She walks the fields and hills and goes through her daily activities, showing and telling her fetus about the life she leads. The mother tells the fetus to be honest and never abuse nature. If someone eats in front of the pregnant woman without offering her food, she believes she will have a miscarriage. Children are permitted at the delivery. The woman's husband, village leaders, and parents of the couple may be present. A single woman must not observe the birth of the baby (Menchu, 1984). A midwife and a witch (*brujo*) may both attend the birth. The midwife helps with delivery, while the *brujo* prays for long life, good health, and protection from the evil eye (*mal ojo*). A breech delivery or one in which the baby's cord is around the neck is considered good luck.

Mayan women do not believe in lying down to give birth or delivering in a hospital. Following delivery, the placenta has to be burned, not buried, because it is disrespectful to the earth to do so. The placenta can be burned on a log and then the ashes used for a steam bath, *temascal* (Menchu, 1984).

To celebrate the birth of a baby, the villagers slaughter a sheep. The mother and baby are kept separated from others for 8 days. When the baby is born, its hands and feet are bound for 8 days. This signifies that they are meant for hard work, not for stealing, and they are not meant to have things the rest of the community does not have (Menchu, 1984). Guatemalan women may continue breastfeeding until the child reaches the age of 5 years. Moreover, they may be breastfeeding a new baby while continuing to breastfeed a toddler.

During the first 8 postpartum days, friends and extended family bring food, clothing, small animals, or wood as gifts for the newborn's family. They also offer their services, like carrying water or chopping wood. The family of the newborn does nothing for these 8 days. All their needs are taken care of by others (Menchu, 1984).

After 8 days, the newborn's hands and feet are untied. While the newborn is in bed with mom, all community members visit to officially welcome him or her. The baby is told he or she is made of corn. A bag with garlic, lime, salt, and tobacco is hung around the baby's neck and a red thread is used to tie the umbilical cord to protect the baby, provide strength, and denote respect for the ancestors. If the baby is a female, the midwife pierces her ears at birth (Menchu, 1984).

Death Rituals

DEATH RITUALS AND EXPECTATIONS

Death rituals among Guatemalans vary depending on traditional and/or religious beliefs. Guatemalans grow up experiencing far more death than most North Americans. They see babies and children die of malnutrition and disease, parents and grandparents die from violence, and loved ones die because the health care they needed was too far away or was too expensive. The family may decide the cost for treatment of one family member is too much and decide against it because of the financial strain on the entire family.

When a person is seriously ill, she or he is usually cared for at home. Family members and the community provide assistance and support. When family must take a seriously ill family member to a hospital, extended family and the community help care for members left at home. Often, hospitals are such a great distance that the ill person dies before she or he arrives or during the hospitalization. Prayers are offered for the sick. Rituals and ceremonies are offered to prepare the body and spirit of the dying for death.

RESPONSES TO DEATH AND GRIEF

When death occurs in Guatemala, it is customary to place the deceased in a simple wooden coffin/casket and conduct a funeral. In small villages, the entire community is present. The casket may be carried by key family members through town from the church to the cemetery while onlookers show their respect, mourn, and offer flowers. Graves are decorated with flowers on All Saint's Day in memory of the deceased. Some Guatemalans relate their illness to "punishment" or impending death to "God's will" and refuse an intervention or heroic measures to reverse the outcome.

When a Guatemalan dies in the United States, the family may request repatriation, because it is important for the final resting place to be the home country. Often, immediate and extended family and social service agencies pool their resources to send the body home.

Guatemalans believe in burial; they do not practice cremation. At Indian funerals, the Mayan priest may spin the coffin at the grave to fool the devil and point the spirit of the deceased toward heaven. Yellow is the color of mourning. Yellow flowers are placed at the grave. Food is placed at the head for the spirit of the departed. Church bells are rung to gain favor with the gods. Ladinos mourn the dead by wearing black. Maya do not believe in this practice.

Spirituality

DOMINANT RELIGION AND USE OF PRAYER

Approximately 65 to 80 percent of Guatemalans are Roman Catholic. Regular church attendance is not possible for many, as there is a shortage of priests. Most priests in Guatemala are foreigners (Gall, 1998).

Prior to the Spanish conquest, the Maya practiced a religion based on gods associated with the sun, moon, and other natural phenomena. The causes of natural disasters were related to punishments from heavenly beings. They believed animal spirits (*nahuales*) inhabited the human spirit (Shea, 2001). *Maximon* is a Mayan saint popular among Maya and Ladinos. He is believed to represent ordinary Guatemalans, has supernatural powers, and produces witches (*brujos*) and shaman (*zajorines*) (Sexton, 1999).

When the Spanish brought Roman Catholicism to Guatemala, some Maya converted to Christianity. Others continued to practice their Mayan religion. Still other Guatemalans combined beliefs and practices of the two. In some cases, Guatemalans integrated aspects of Catholicism

into their lives while continuing to believe in the spirituality of their ancestors in private (Shea, 2001).

Two practices influenced by the Spanish are *guachibal* and *cofradia*. *Guachibal* involves the practice of keeping an image of a Christian saint in the home and celebrating on the particular saint's day. *Cofradia* refers to a "religious brotherhood" that serves to maintain the "cult" of a particular saint. *Cofradias* consist of dues-paying members and elected leaders. In addition to religious activities, they often serve needy persons in the community by visiting the sick and paying for funerals (Shea, 2001).

Protestantism arrived in Guatemala in the 19th century. Today, there are an increasing number of evangelical Christian religions in Guatemala. The Christian holidays of Holy Week, All Saint's Day, and Christmas are celebrated by Catholic and Protestant Guatemalans (Shea, 2001). Health-care providers must determine whether the Guatemalan patient has a religious preference and demonstrate respect and sensitivity for his or her beliefs.

MEANING OF LIFE AND INDIVIDUAL SOURCES OF STRENGTH

Family provides Guatemalans with meaning in their lives. Life revolves around the nuclear and extended family. Spirituality helps to explain life and the circumstances faced by Guatemalans. For example, whether Catholic, Protestant, or traditional Maya, many believe that life's events happen for a reason. The reason may be attributed to favor from God or gods when positive experiences occur and to punishment or disfavor from God or gods when negative events occur. Some feel nothing can be done to change the outcome of these experiences. This belief is referred to as *fatalism*.

SPIRITUAL BELIEFS AND HEALTH-CARE PRACTICES

When illness occurs, many Guatemalans turn to their faith for strength, wisdom, and hope. Health-care providers may be uncomfortable with patients who have a statue of a patron saint, picture of a saint, or candles burning while prayers are being said. The family may pray together; they need time and space to do so. They may even ask the health-care professional to join prayer, which is acceptable if the provider wishes. Praying with the family promotes confidence in the relationship. The patient and family feel the compassion and respect such actions demonstrate. The health-care provider may also help arrange for spiritual care services for the patient and family through their church or hospital resources.

Health-Care Practices

HEALTH-SEEKING BELIEFS AND BEHAVIORS

Transculturation is continually occurring in Guatemala. Characteristics between Ladinos and Indians used to vary greatly. Ladinos were Spanish speakers, wore Western style clothing, practiced Catholicism, were better educated, worked in nonagricultural occupations, were economically better off, lived in superior housing with sanitation, had a better diet, and were healthier. Indians more often than not spoke a Mayan dialect; wore traditional woven clothing (*traje*); worked in agriculture; used primitive technology; and maintained social, political, and religious life through *cofradias* (Woods & Graves, 1973).

Today, the distinction between the Ladino and the Indian in Guatemala is less clear. For example, more Indian men speak Spanish, wear Western clothing, and receive an education.

The preferred mode of treatment among Ladinos is medication administered by hypodermic injection. For example, if an infant has a cold, Ladinos believe an injection is necessary to treat it effectively. If someone has the flu, an IV infusion is preferred. Intramuscular medications are preferred to those taken orally (Kunkel, 1985).

Health-care seeking among Guatemalans generally occurs by first seeking advice from a mother, grandmother, or other respected elder. If this approach is unsuccessful, then the family usually seeks health care from folk healers. Modern medical care may be the last resort. Many are fearful of hospitals. In Guatemala, when hospital care is necessary, patients are often seriously ill, resulting in death, which perpetuates the belief that "hospitals are places where patients go to die."

RESPONSIBILITY FOR HEALTH CARE

Guatemalans often delay seeking health care until they are incapacitated by illness, disease, or injury. Many times, they are unaware of the dangers associated with working in agriculture in the United States. They may be exposed to pesticides and dangerous equipment without proper training. Although the government has specific laws in place to protect farm workers, enforcement is limited. Companies may not tell the workers the dangers or the workers may not understand owing to language differences. Health-care providers caring for Guatemalan patients who are farm workers must be aware of the chemical exposures, laws, and resources available in order to adequately advocate for the patient.

BARRIERS TO HEALTH CARE

Only 33 percent of Guatemalans have regular access to health services (Gall, 1998). Guatemalans experience barriers to health care, whether in Guatemala or in the United States, that include

1. *Availability:* The hours many health services are offered are inconvenient for Guatemalan patients who cannot afford to take time off work.

2. *Accessibility/reliability:* Transportation is not available to access health-care services.

3. *Affordability:* Most Guatemalans do not have health insurance and are limited to health-service agencies offering low-cost care.

4. *Appropriateness:* Low-cost health care offers limited services; dental, women's, or pediatric care may not be available.

5. *Accountability:* Health-care providers lack education regarding Guatemalan cultures, languages, and lifestyles required to offer culturally competent care.

6. *Adaptability:* Many health-care settings do not offer one-stop shopping in which the patient may be seen for dental care and a mammogram the same day in the same location.

7. *Acceptability:* Many health-care settings do not offer patient education materials in the languages or literacy levels common to Guatemalan patients.

8. *Awareness:* Many times, Guatemalan patients are unaware of the services available in the area in which they live.

9. *Attitudes:* Sometimes health-care providers convey negative attitudes toward the Guatemalan patient, making it unlikely she or he will return for care.

10. *Approachability:* Guatemalan patients may not feel welcome in the health-care setting because they interpret verbal and nonverbal communication from providers as lacking in care and compassion.

11. *Alternative practices and practitioners:* Guatemalan patients may prefer to integrate modern medicine with traditional therapies; yet, the health-care provider may be resistant to this.

12. *Additional services:* The health-care setting may lack child care; the Guatemalan family that does not have extended family members in the United States to assist is required to bring children and older family members with them to the visit, which is disruptive.

CULTURAL RESPONSES TO HEALTH AND ILLNESS

Guatemalans tend to view health and illness in relation to their ability to perform duties associated with their roles. As long as women are functioning in their role of caring for the home and family, and men are functioning in their job, then they feel "healthy." Aches, pains, and minor illnesses that do not prevent functioning are tolerated. When an illness prevents normal functioning required for their roles, then Guatemalans view it seriously.

The cause of debilitating illness or disease may be viewed as punishment from God rather than lack of prevention or early detection. Sometimes, early warning signs of illness or disease are ignored in hopes they will go away on their own. When symptoms persist, fear may keep the Guatemalan patient from seeking medical attention.

When a member of a Guatemalan family needs to be cared for, others gladly comply. This occurs for reasons of advanced age, illness, and mental or physical disability, among others. Residential homes for persons with these conditions are not readily available in Guatemala and are usually cost prohibitive for families living in the United States. Family members would rather care for their loved one at home if at all possible.

Health-care providers may demonstrate respect for the cultural values of Guatemalan patients by providing community resources that enable them to adequately care for a family member at home if they so desire.

BLOOD TRANSFUSIONS AND ORGAN DONATION

Blood transfusions and organ donation are not common in Guatemala, and with many living outside of the realm of modern medicine, residents may be uneducated regarding the medical situations in which they are indicated, benefits, and risks. Questions related to organ donation will be puzzling and elicit fear and anxiety. The Guatemalan patient may think the health-care provider is asking his or her to consent to organ donation because he or she is going to die rather than understanding the context to which the question applies.

Some Guatemalans fear venipuncture because taking blood leaves the body without enough blood to keep them strong and healthy. Health-care providers need to carefully assess the level of education and understanding of the Guatemalan patient regarding these issues and use an interpreter who is competent in the language and culture of the patient in order to promote successful communication.

Health-Care Practitioners

TRADITIONAL VERSUS BIOMEDICAL PRACTITIONERS

Three distinct health care systems exist in Guatemala: modern medicine, Ladino folk medicine, and Indian folk medicine. *Modern medicine* refers to health care provided by educated physicians and nurses. *Ladino folk medicine* is provided by Ladino pharmacists, spiritualists, and lay healers (*curanderos*). *Mayan Indians* seek medical care from Mayan *shaman, herbalists,* and *comadronas.* When Ladinos and Mayan Indians have access to modern medicine, the utilization increases.

STATUS OF HEALTH-CARE PROVIDERS

Guatemalans have great respect and admiration for health-care providers, who are viewed as authority figures with clinical expertise. Guatemalans expect their health-care provider to have the appearance and manners of a professional (Purnell, 2001). When this is not the case, Guatemalans lose confidence in the provider.

Guatemalans are very private and are not accustomed to discussing issues and concerns openly. It may take a while to develop the trust and rapport with the provider necessary for them to share. They fear disclosure may result in deportation or rejection. Patients also fear confidentiality will not be maintained in the health-care setting.

Health-care providers who are most successful in caring for Guatemalan patients practice *personalismo*, respect, and genuine compassion in their approach to care.

Moreover, Purnell (2001) found the following behaviors and comments by health-care providers best conveyed respect to their Guatemalan patients:

1. Greets me when I come in.
2. The way the doctor/nurse talks to me (denotes respect).
3. Asks questions about what bothers me.
4. Says things to make me feel better.
5. Explains things to me.

Guatemalan women are usually very modest. They may refuse to discuss personal issues or receive an examination by a male health-care provider. Likewise, a male Guatemalan patient may refuse a female health-care provider. Because Guatemalans dislike conflict, they may not actually refuse care; yet they withhold personal information owing to discomfort with the health-care provider. Incorporating these preferences into the encounter with Guatemalan patients enhances the development of relationships that result in effective and meaningful care.

REFERENCES

Chickering, W. H. (2006). A guide for visiting clinicians to Guatemala: Common presenting symptoms and treatment. *Journal of Transcultural Nursing, 17*(2), 190–197.

CIA. (2007). *World FactBook: Guatemala.* Retrieved March 16, 2007, from https://www.cia.gov/cia/publications/factbook/geos/gt.html#People

Gall, T. L. (Ed.). (1998). *Worldmark encyclopedia of cultures and daily life: Vol. 2, Americas.* Detroit, MI: Gale Research.

Gay Guatemala. (2007). Retrieved March 17, 2007, from www.zoomvacations.com/guatemala.htm

Glittenberg, J. (1994). *To the mountain and back: The mysteries of Guatemalan highland family life.* Lake Zurich, IL: Waveland Press, Inc.

Icu, H. (2000). *Health care reform in Guatemala.* Retrieved March 17, 2007, from http://phmovement.org/pha2000/stories/icu.html

Information Please Almanac. (2007). *Guatemala.* Retrieved March 16, 2007, from http://www.infoplease.com/encyclopedia/

Kunkel, P. (1985). Paul Kunkel: Guatemala journal part 2. *The Washington Nurse, 15*(4), 34–35.

Lang, J. B., & Elkin, E. D. (1997). International exchange: A study of the beliefs and birthing practices of traditional midwives in Guatemala. *Journal of Nurse Midwifery, 42*(1), 25–31.

Menchu, R. (1984). *I, Rigoberta Menchu: An Indian woman in Guatemala.* London: Verso.

National Center for Farmworker Health (NCFH). (2005). *Facts about farmworkers.* Retrieved November 22, 2006, at http://www.ncfh.org

National Digestive Diseases Information Clearinghouse. (2007). *Lactose intolerance.* Retrieved February 3, 2007, at http://digestive.niddk.nih.gov

Pan American Health Organization (PAHO). (2004). *Country profile: Guatemala.* Retrieved January 6, 2007, at http://www.paho.org

Purnell, L. (2001). Guatemalan's practices for health promotion and the meaning of respect afforded them by health care providers. *Journal of Transcultural Nursing, 12*(1), 40–47.

Sexton, J. D. (1999). *Heart of heaven, heart of earth and other Mayan folktales.* Washington, DC: Smithsonian Institution Press.

Shea, M. E. (2001). *Culture and customs of Guatemala.* Westport, CT: Greenwood Press.

Steltzer, V. (1983). Health in the Guatemalan highlands. *Anthropological Quarterly, 57*(3), 141–142.

U.S. Bureau of the Census. (2005). *Census 2000 demographic profiles.* Retrieved January 6, 2007, at http://www.census.gov

Walsh, L. V. (2006). Beliefs and rituals in traditional birth attendant practices in Guatemala. *Journal of Transcultural Nursing, 17*(2), 148–154.

Wellmeier, N. (1998). *Ritual, identity, and the Mayan diaspora.* New York: Garland Publishing, Inc.

Woods, C. M., & Graves, T. D. (1973). *The process of medical change in a highland Guatemalan town.* Los Angeles: University of California.

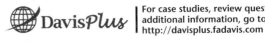

Chapter 9

People of Egyptian Heritage

AFAF IBRAHIM MELEIS and
MAHMOUD HANAFI MELEIS

Overview, Inhabited Localities, and Topography

OVERVIEW

Egypt, the country of origin of Egyptian Americans, has a landmass of 386,900 square miles (about 1½ times the size of Texas) and a population of over 78 million people, giving it a population density of 177 per square mile. More than 95 percent of the land is barren desert, resulting in 90 percent of the population's living on 3 percent of the total land area, in the Nile Valley and Delta (CIA, 2007). The Nile has been and still is significant in shaping life and living patterns in Egypt. The average annual rate of population increase is 1.75 percent, with a birth rate of 22.94 per 1000 and an infant mortality rate of 31.3 per 1000 (CIA, 2007). The capital, Cairo, has over 11 million people, followed in population by Alexandria with 3.5 million people. The population of Egypt continues to grow by about 1.4 million per year (Zohry & Harrell-Bond, 2003).

Egypt is bordered by Libya on the west, Sudan on the south, the Mediterranean Sea on the north, and the Red Sea and Israel on the east. The eastern region, across the Suez Canal, is Sinai. Egypt's climate is hot and dry most of the year. The average daily temperature on the Mediterranean coast is 68°F with a maximum of 88°F, and in Aswan, average temperatures are 80°F but can reach 120°F with little or no humidity. The Mediterranean region receives most of the country's annual rainfall (7.5 in.). The northern summers are balmy with moderate temperatures and 80 percent humidity. Between March and April, *khamsi* winds blow in from the Western Desert at up to 93 miles per hour. Except for a few hills outside Cairo, Egypt has a flat terrain on both sides of the southern Nile valley and the Sinai Peninsula. The Nile River, a main artery for Egypt and an orientation point for its terrain, runs through the center of the country from south to north to the Mediterranean Sea. The Nile—considered to be Egypt's lifeline—provides water and supports agriculture.

Egypt is considered by many politicians, historians, and social scientists to be part of 22 Arabic-speaking countries in North Africa. Egyptians are among the 255 million Arab people of the world, as well as part of the 1 billion persons who are Muslim. Others write about Egypt as a Middle Eastern country and count its population as Middle Eastern. A review of scholarly literature about Egyptian Americans is embedded in writing that aggregates them with Arab Americans, African Americans, and Middle Eastern Americans, as well as separates them out as Egyptian Americans. Scholarly literature about Egyptians in the United States is limited; therefore, the reader will find citations that reflect a broader geographic territory, which in turn reflects how Egyptians are often connected to or embedded in many Arab, Middle Eastern, African, and Muslim cultures.

This chapter is also based on the authors' own experiences. Both authors are Egyptian Americans who came to the United States in the early 1960s and observed many Egyptian Americans as they defined themselves within the multiple identities generated by the different groupings, such as generation and length of time away from the country of origin. Both authors have been insiders as well as outsiders to Middle Eastern communities in the United States and globally. They have participated in different community celebrations, experienced immigrants' grief over the impending or actual death of a family member, provided social and emotional support during times of crisis, and counseled many immigrants. One of the authors has been professionally involved with health care for this population for over 30 years as part of a project that was designed to provide health-care services to Middle Eastern immigrants in California. Therefore, data in this chaper are from our lived experiences in the two worlds Egyptian Americans claim as their own—Egypt and the United States.

Arab Americans are estimated to number 3 million (Salari, 2002), although census data estimate that population at only 1.1 million (U.S. Bureau of Census, 2002). The variation is an artifact of census survey problems. Among these estimates is around 1 million Arab Americans who reside in the United States as permanent residents, citizens, or residents in the process of becoming permanent residents. Egyptians reside in most states in the United States; 66 percent of Arab Americans are concentrated in 16 states (Zogby, 2001). Heavily populated states are New Jersey, California, Michigan, Illinois, and New York. Egyptian Americans' religious affiliations resemble those of others from the rest of the Arab countries. The majority are Christians, and among the Christians are Orthodox (Greek and Copts), Catholics, and Protestants. Egyptian American Muslims who are Sunni are increasing in numbers and represent the fastest growing religious group among Egyptian immigrants (Salari, 2002). Ninety percent of Egyptians are Muslims, and the overwhelming majority of these are Sunni Muslims.

Egyptian Americans are diverse in other ways. They come from urban and rural communities, upper and lower Egypt, and diverse educational backgrounds, and they possess a wide range of cultural characteristics influenced by colonialization, occupations, and a variety of immigration experiences that shaped their responses. However, only the most common patterns of responses and experiences of Egyptian Americans with regard to heath and illness are presented in this chapter. Diversity among Egyptians is not well depicted, and this description does not represent a universal profile either. By defining the similarities among Egyptian Americans, we hope to stimulate interest in more systematic scholarhip about this unique community and their lifestyles, health, and health-care practices.

HERITAGE AND RESIDENCE

In spite of the many attributions of geographic belonging to Egypt, the Egyptian people have a strong sense of identity with their country and demonstrate pride in coming from such an old civilization. Egyptian history is inextricably connected to the Nile River and dates back to about 4000 B.C., when the kingdoms of upper and lower Egypt were united by King Menes, who presented himself as a god. The ancient Egyptians were the first to believe in life after death, mummify bodies, and build elaborate tombs to preserve and protect these bodies for the afterlife. Egyptians also developed the plow, a system of writing, and medical skills such as surgical operations.

The Arab conquest of Egypt around A.D. 641, which spread the Islamic and Arabic culture among the Egyptians, has lasted to this day. The minority (Christian) Copts, who preserved the African-Asiatic language of ancient Egypt, now use the Arabic language and have been assimilated into the Arabic culture. The Ottoman Turks invaded Egypt in 1517, adding it to their vast empire. While living under Turkish rule, Egypt enjoyed religious and cultural stability because the Turks shared the Islamic and Arabic cultures. In the last 2 centuries, Egypt experienced invasions by the French, followed by the British in 1882, who remained in the country until 1954. In 1952, an Egyptian army group led by Lieutenant Colonel Gamal Abdel Nasser took control of the government and removed King Farouk from power. Since then, Egypt has been an independent state called the *Arab Republic of Egypt* (CIA, 2007).

An influential part of modern Egyptian history is the Arab-Israeli conflict. The conflict between Egypt, as part of the Arab League, and Israel ended in 1979 when the two countries signed the Camp David Accords. Anwar Sadat was the president of Egypt at the time. Egypt continues to be involved in diplomatic efforts to arrive at peace between Israel and its neighboring Arab countries. This long history and the diversity of populations have influenced the value systems, beliefs, and explanatory frameworks Egyptians use in their daily lives and have contributed to the diverse thinking processes they use to resolve issues and conflict.

REASONS FOR MIGRATION AND ASSOCIATED ECONOMIC FACTORS

Many Egyptians immigrated to the United States in an attempt to escape economic stagnation during President Nasser's regime and his failed economic policies that nationalized all privately owned companies and enterprises. The United States offered educational opportunities, career options, and economic incentives that rewarded hard-working individuals. After the 1952 military revolution, Egyptians immigrated in three main waves. The first wave, in the 1950s, consisted of graduate students who came to the United States to obtain advanced degrees. After the defeat of the Egyptian army by the Israelis in 1967, many of these students, believing the totalitarian military regime of Egypt did not offer hope for economic recovery, changed their status to immigrant. For most, this ensured a promising future for their children, even though they would have been assured decent positions in Egypt because of their American education.

The second wave of immigration resulted from the heightened mass dissatisfaction, hopelessness, and anger toward the government of the educated and professional community after the 1967 war. A lenient government policy made it easy and safe for anyone who wanted to leave the country, resulting in the largest exodus from Egypt in modern history. Included in this wave were many Coptic and other Egyptian Christians (Shaw, 2000).

The third wave, in the 1980s and beyond, had many more risk takers. They came to seek better lives and forsake the security of government jobs for unknown adventures. They sought new opportunities such as cab driving and working at food outlets in large cities (Meleis, 2002). It is important to note here that the terrorist attacks in New York, Pennsylvania, and Washington, DC, and the tragic consequences of September 11, 2001, have rendered many newly immigrated Egyptian Americans vulnerable to profiling and stereotyping in their newly adopted country, the United States of America. Therefore, a newly acquired sense of stigma tends to influence their patterns of responses in ways that were not manifested previously. Long-term effects of this situation on their patterns of behaviors have yet to be studied and understood.

EDUCATIONAL STATUS AND OCCUPATIONS

Most of the first-wave Egyptian immigrants were highly educated individuals with graduate and postgraduate degrees earned in the United States. Members of this group were able to obtain teaching and research positions in universities or work in industries. Some joined companies or started their own businesses in the high-technology industries.

Egyptians in the second and third waves were more diverse in their educational backgrounds, although most of them were college graduates. Second-wave immigrants worked as engineers, physicians, dentists, accountants, and technicians; however, some with college degrees initially accepted employment as gas station attendants, cab drivers, security guards, and other blue collar positions to ensure employment. After improving their language skills and obtaining degrees from American universities, many obtained professional positions. A small minority never achieved an occupational status equivalent to their original training. Many from this group returned to their home country or plan for such a return.

Communication

DOMINANT LANGUAGE AND DIALECTS

The dominant language of Egyptians is **Arabic**, a Semitic language understood by all Arab nationals, who hear it in popular Egyptian movies, songs, and television programs. The written Arabic language is the same in all Arab countries, but spoken Arabic is dialectal and does not necessarily follow proper Arabic grammar. A number of Arabic dialects are spoken in Egypt. The *Saiidis* (Egyptians south of Cairo) have a different dialect from the northerners. The *Nubians* (who live around and south of Aswan) have another unique dialect, as do the *Bedouins*, who live in the desert. Despite these different dialects and their distinct vocabularies, neither Egyptians nor Egyptian Americans have any noticeable communication barriers among themselves.

For Egyptian immigrants in the United States, English is the language of communication in business and contact with American society. Within their own gatherings, they speak a mixture of Arabic and English, switch with great ease from one language to another, and sometimes speak a mixture of Arabic, English, and French. Egyptian social gatherings usually involve large numbers of people, with multiple conversations occurring simultaneously. When they are discussing subjects such as politics or religious issues, the level of excitement heightens and the tone of the speech is sharpened, so an outside observer may mistakenly characterize the exchanges as chaotic or angry.

CULTURAL COMMUNICATION PATTERNS

⬤— VIGNETTE 9.1

Rania Selim is a 37-year-old Egyptian American teacher who is married to 45-year-old engineer Abdel Samih Adeeb, who works for a moderate-sized construction company. They have one daughter, Salwa, who is 8 years old. Mrs. Selim went to her gynecologist on a routine visit, and her doctor discovered a lump in her breast. This led to a diagnosis of inflammatory carcinoma.

1. Identify cultural beliefs and values that may frame the assessment and intervention plan for this family.
2. What problems should the health-care provider anticipate related to communication between family members about the diagnosis?
3. Identify three problems and three strengths during the process of decision making and care.
4. What culturally congruent strategies should be used to support family decision making for the different treatment options?
5. Name two interventions that are immediately needed.

Several values govern interaction patterns among Egyptians. The first is respect (*ihteram*), which is expected when speaking with those who are older and those in higher social positions. Respect is demonstrated in the Arabic language by differentiation in the words used to address those who are equal in age or position and those who are older in age or higher in position (see Format for Names). A second important value, politeness (*adab*) is related to what is appropriate, expected, and socially sanctioned. Truth and reality may be sacrificed for what is appropriate and polite. Politeness results in a preference for more indirect modes of communication. Sharing negative news directly or asking for things directly is not polite. Therefore, a poor prognosis of an illness is not immediately shared; calamities should be slowly and deliberately introduced and shared in stages. It is more appropriate and expected that such news will be shared first with other family members who will provide a buffer that helps those coping with and responding to such news.

Significant value is related to the status of insiders and outsiders, the private and public spheres. Private spheres are reserved for immediate family, some members of the extended family, and friends who are elevated to the status of family. The public sphere includes acquaintances, public officials, and the rest of the world. Those who occupy a public sphere may get completely different communications and versions of the same events or incidents.

Because Egyptian Americans tend to be externally driven, they are concerned about what others think of their behaviors, which are considered a direct reflection on their entire family. Therefore, parents tend to be overzealous and anxious about the good or bad behaviors of children and adult sons and daughters. These behaviors reflect a measure of how well or how badly parents have raised their children.

Egyptian Americans tend to be in touch with their inner feelings and are highly expressive of them; however, this expression is governed by external orientation, spontaneity, and the differences between private and public spheres. Egyptians in America tend to share problems and the most minute details about their lives with their trusted circle of insiders. However, because they are externally oriented, they tend to look outside for explanations of their feelings, rather than to focus on their own actions. Egyptians tend to be comfortable and generous in sharing ideas and giving advice to others who might be family members or friends. This behavior stems from close family ties and trust that ensures the family will always be there to provide help. Advice is offered (even when not requested), out of love, care, and a sense of loyalty to friends or relatives. They do not shy away from becoming involved in the problems, trials, and tribulations of those in their private sphere. The extent and depth of involvement is less for those in the public sphere. Although these behavior patterns are a part of the lifestyle of first-generation immigrants, second-generation immigrants may not necessarily maintain them.

Egyptian Americans' nonverbal communication patterns are expressive. Because their personal space boundaries tend to be small, they stand and sit very close to each other. In spite of their preference for closeness, women and men use personal space boundaries differently during interactions. Women tend to keep male friends as far away as male strangers. Egyptian Americans speak with expressive words and facial expressions, gesticulating with hands and using body movements. They communicate with their entire body as much as with verbal language. Their facial expressions are mirrors of their internal processes and reflections of their inner evaluations of their situations. They tend to touch each other frequently and easily, and touch is both reflexive and deliberative. For example, they tend to touch others while speaking to solicit attention, concentration, and emphasis. To demonstrate trust, increase trust, or emphasize a point, they tend to touch each other on the hands, arms, legs, and shoulders. Men, whether strangers or acquaintances, touch each other. Similarly, it is acceptable for women to touch. Family members and friends of the same gender always hug and kiss on both cheeks. Friends of different sexes normally shake hands. However, traditionally, it is unacceptable for women and men to touch each other. Touch between the sexes is accepted in private and only between husbands and wives, parents and children, and adult brothers and sisters. Levels of religiosity govern the protocols about touching between males and females. The more religious the individuals, the more prohibitions about touching between males and females.

Devout Muslim men and women do not touch each other; even a handshake is not practiced. In these situations, a head nod substitutes for a physical greeting. Among devout Muslims, only *mahrams*, those individuals who are not permitted to marry (e.g., sisters and brothers), are permitted to greet each other with hugs. Among Christians and Westernized Egyptians and Egyptian Americans, greetings usually include formal courteous hugs and kisses on the cheeks. In Egypt, it is very common to see Egyptian men or women walking in public places

holding hands or embracing each other. In the United States, Egyptians are more self-conscious about touching members of the same sex, touching non-Egyptians only on the arm or shoulder as an expression of caring, assuring them that one is a friend. Some Westerners may be uncomfortable with these gestures.

Egyptians have their own nonverbal facial expressions. A momentary wide-eyed gaze to a child means "stop it now." A wink to an adult means "watch what you are saying" or "change the subject because you are treading on dangerous ground." Dissatisfaction is demonstrated by intentionally looking through the person or by avoiding eye contact. Egyptians think of those who do not maintain eye contact or have shifty eye contact as people who should not be trusted. Because Egyptians tend to stand in close proximity to each other, eye contact is automatic for them. However, among those who are more traditional, women and men who are strangers may avoid eye contact out of modesty and respect for religious rules. The situation is different if the communication is between men and women related by marriage or by blood. Children are taught not to *tebarrak* (stare), which denotes disrespect for those who are older or higher in status.

Egyptians tend to be congenial and personable, injecting humor to lighten stressful encounters or business meetings. They may exaggerate and overly assert judgments of events and situations for the sake of emphasizing a particular point of view.

An Egyptian greeting involves every person in a room standing and shaking hands within gender norms. Not standing can be considered an insult. A greeting may be just a nod or a few words. Similar greetings are practiced in the United States among immigrants.

TEMPORAL RELATIONSHIPS

Older Egyptians cherish the past, remembering the days when life was simple and easy. Reminiscing is a cultural pattern that becomes more prominent with age. Younger Egyptians live in the present, with its decreased availability of options, and in the future, with its potential, realizing that acquisition of goods comes with a high price tag. Thus, this generation is preoccupied with maximizing their incomes, often working two or three jobs to afford luxuries. For professional Egyptian immigrants, working hard has been their ticket to upward mobility and living the good life.

In Egypt, social time takes a high priority, and engagements are not concluded because of other scheduled appointments; therefore, guests are expected to arrive late. If a friend drops by as another is getting ready to leave for an appointment, the appointment is missed and the friend is not told about the prior engagement. Arrival at a social gathering, such as a lunch or dinner, as much as 1 or 2 hours late and to be late for business appointments because of heavy traffic and unanticipated and uncontrolled delays is common. A social custom is to offer coffee, tea, or a soft drink to business visitors. Therefore, a planned 10-minute office visit usually takes more time. Egyptian Americans' perception of time is in the context of the nationality of the group. Therefore, they follow "American time" and are punctual for business engagements and meetings with non–Egyptian Americans but prefer to use Egyptian time for Egyptian American gatherings.

FORMAT FOR NAMES

In all Arab countries, both male and female children are given a first name, and the father's first name is used as the middle name; the last name is the family name. In the Middle East, a person is called formally by the first name, such as Mr. William.

Respect for individuals is demonstrated in the use of certain titles. *Inta* (you) is saved for those in equal or lower positions, and *hadretak* (you) is reserved for those in higher-ranking positions or for older people. More flowery and more exaggerated variations of both of these appellations are used, such as *seyadtak*, which is reserved for the highest-level officials. *Inta*, used in place of *hadretak*, is an insult to older people and, more important, a reflection of bad manners and the poor upbringing of the young. Older people should never be called by their first names without an adjective or title attached to the name. The accepted custom in the United States of addressing clients by their first name may be insulting to people from other countries. An adjective, such as aunt, uncle, *ostaz* (Mr., Madame, Mrs.), or an adjective that denotes a profession, such as *bashmohandes* (engineer, doctor, physician) or a doctoral degree, may be used with the name. Family friends are addressed by both younger and adult children as uncle and aunt. Parental relatives are called either aunt or uncle or a special designation such as *ammeti* (sister of father), *ammy* (brother of father), *khalty* (sister of mother), or *khali* (brother of mother). Some Egyptian Americans, particularly those from rural Egypt, are addressed by the first name of their son, preceded by "*Abu*," which means "father of." This is more of an Arab custom adapted by Egyptians (Haddad & Hoeman, 2000).

Family Roles and Organization

VIGNETTE 9.2

The Fayez family came to the United States from Cairo, Egypt, in 1976. After spending 6 months with distant relatives in Daly City, California, Anwar and his wife, Fatma, moved into an apartment of their own. Anwar continued the job his Uncle Hussain had helped him get in the construction business. Fatma has never worked outside the home. In 1979, Mr. and Mrs. Fayez had their first child, a son named Moustafa. In 1980, they had their second child, a daughter named Somaya. Two years ago, Fatma miscarried in her 4th month of pregnancy and lost a male child. At present, Fatma is 6 months' pregnant, and Anwar owns and operates his own small construction and roofing company in the Richmond area of San Francisco. Moustafa is a healthy-looking boy who does well in school, and Somaya is in the first grade.

The public health nurse—a family nurse practitioner assigned to the Fayez family for their well-child and prenatal care—has made two visits to the family's home. On both occasions, the nurse noticed that Mrs. Fayez looked very fatigued and short of breath. Both Moustafa and Somaya were very quiet during the visits. Anwar boasted often of his son's achievements in school and said little about Somaya. Fatma was showing some slight edema in both feet, and the nurse noticed during these visits (both in the evening) that Fatma was frequently getting up to serve the family tea and food. Mr. Fayez described how Moustafa's teachers complain about his "aggressive behaviors in school." Mrs. Fayez was concerned about her daughter's "finicky" eating habits. During both visits, the nurse noticed an older, conservatively dressed woman who sat quietly during the early part of the visit and communicated with family members in Arabic. She always left the room soon after the nurse arrived, and the nurse sensed that the family acknowledged her with a great deal of respect. The house was nicely furnished, and no educational toys or books were visible.

1. Identify the strengths in the Fayez family that may support and enhance their health.
2. What problems are inherent in the situation?
3. What assessments are needed?
4. What might some goals be?
5. Identify priorities for health care and give rationales for these priorities.
6. Identify three cultural factors that influence the health of the Fayez family.
7. Describe two strategies the nurse might use to help the Fayez family deal with their son's "aggressive behaviors."
8. Describe two strategies the nurse might use to help the parents deal with their daughter's "finicky" eating habits.
9. Identify a culturally competent approach to assessing and intervening with the health-care concerns of the Fayez family.
10. Identify three culturally congruent intervention plans for Mrs. Fayez's pregnancy.
11. Describe three areas of at-risk behaviors that you might want to explore preventively with the Fayez family.
12. Compare and contrast first-wave and second-wave Egyptian immigrants in America according to their reasons for immigration.
13. Identify potential communication concerns in the American workforce with newer Egyptian American immigrants.
14. Identify infectious conditions that may be common among newer Egyptian American immigrants.
15. Identify culturally congruent bereavement patterns for Egyptian Americans.
16. Identify counseling strategies for Egyptian Americans in regard to self-medicating practices.

HEAD OF HOUSEHOLD AND GENDER ROLES

The man is formally considered the head of the household. The demands of life on immigrants and nuclear families drive couples to share responsibilities and decision making. Many Egyptian American men, however, tend to control family budgets, which gives them more power in the family and causes many interpersonal conflicts and much distress for Egyptian American women.

Egyptian American family roles change considerably after immigration. The fast pace and complexity of life in America, the many demands of child rearing, and the absence of an extended family to preserve traditional roles contribute to a more egalitarian family organization. Husbands and wives experience greater fluidity in their roles, substitute for each other when needed, and participate fully in all family matters. Egyptian American women tend to work both in temporary occupations and in career positions. Many who do not work outside the home consider their situation temporary, are between jobs, or are retooling their skills to become congruent with American job opportunities. Women who are not working outside the home tend to be more stressed than those who are employed. Unemployment brings with it economic limitations, social limitations in terms of developing a support network, or both. In the absence of extended families, lack of this support network increases vulnerability, isolation, and stress. Although couples may share daily household chores, the norm is similar to that of other educated middle-class families in America. The woman is responsible for the daily management of family affairs. The man is the major breadwinner for the family. Husbands, however, participate in shopping, cleaning, and activities related to entertaining with their wives. Fathers also participate proactively in activities and education with their children.

PRESCRIPTIVE, RESTRICTIVE, AND TABOO BEHAVIORS FOR CHILDREN AND ADOLESCENTS

Children are central to Egyptian families; they are treasured in the present and viewed as security for their parents' future. During their early years, they are expected to be studious and goal oriented, respectful, and loyal to the family. When they become adults, they are expected to take care of their older parents. However, second-generation Egyptians tend to blend with other Americans. Their sense of responsibility toward their parents is a topic of major concern among Egyptian Americans. Egyptian children are not permitted to use foul language or swear in the home or in front of parents, although this is true to a lesser degree in the United States. Answering back to parents is not condoned and is seen as rude and disrespectful. Some families adjust better than others to the Western style of child rearing, which permits and encourages the children's rights to question their parents' instructions. Families that allow their children more freedom to express their opinions and ask questions often end up with better-adjusted children and better-preserved family unity as their children grow into adulthood. Religious beliefs and teachings forbid premarital sex and adultery for both Egyptian Muslims and Christians.

As girls reach puberty and questions of dating, courting, and prom night arrive, some parents cannot cope with the freedom allowed within American society. They worry more about the consequences of dating and their daughters' getting pregnant and fleeing the home than about raising a healthy and well-adjusted young woman. In the extreme, a few families send their daughters with their mothers back to Egypt to complete their education through college under more restrictive conditions or to get married. Some families opt to return for good rather than raise their daughters in the American culture. Egyptian Muslim and Christian families usually have a hard time giving their young daughters enough space to grow (Meleis, 2002).

Hattar-Pollara, Meleis, and Nagib (2000) found that Egyptian American parents fear their daughters' losing their virginity, representing a major stress in their daily lives. The greatest calamity that may happen in a Christian or Muslim Egyptian American household is to have a daughter lose her virginity prematurely. This fear stems from a potential lack of marriageability of the daughter, loss of face for the father, and gossip within the Egyptian American community. Therefore, parents tend to be restrictive about their daughters' movements and to monitor their whereabouts carefully. Similar restrictions are placed on teenage sons, although they are allowed more freedom and more autonomy in decision making. Most parents prefer that their sons not date and discourage sexual activities. However, if sons disobey the rules of the household, the incident is not regarded as gravely as when daughters do.

Second-generation Egyptian Americans are rather philosophical about these restrictions. The open communication in the family allows children to see restrictions as temporary or to devise ways to do what they want without their parents' knowledge. Whereas similar situations may occur in their original country, the difference is that an extended family in the homeland may help mediate when confrontations between parents and children become inevitable. Without extended families, Egyptian Americans are at a loss for help in resolving family issues. The option of going to counselors or health-care professionals for advice is rarely exercised. Preserving family secrets and honor is more important than external support. Just as families have a strong need for virginity to be preserved, teen pregnancy is not openly discussed in the community. Because of the many restrictions placed on daughters' movements and the limited opportunities for teenage daughters to go out without chaperons, such pregnancies rarely occur. Birth control is not usually discussed in families until marriage, and Pap smears are not sought or accepted until after marriage. Egyptian American children are expected to marry Egyptian Americans. However, because many second-generation Americans do not reside in areas with other Egyptian Americans, cross-cultural marriages are becoming a trend. Many first-generation Egyptian Americans return to their home country to get married. Intermarriages among second-generation Americans are increasing.

FAMILY GOALS AND PRIORITIES

The family is the most sacred institution to Egyptian Americans. Although Egyptians in their own country have extended families, Egyptian American families tend to be more nuclear. Compared with other Arabs in the United States, most Egyptian Americans immigrated individually, were joined later by a bride, or immigrated as nuclear families. In some families, brothers, sisters, nephews, and nieces may arrive later. Even when extended families arrive later, they tend to live apart.

Job opportunities dictate living choices and patterns of living among Egyptian Americans. Egyptians in their own country view the relocation of sons or daughters for education or an occupation with trepidation and concern. However, once children move, though not bound by their extended family's geographic location, they remain connected with them. In their home country, Egyptians tend to include the extended family in social activities and consult them for advice in all matters pertaining to health, employment, and family. In the absence of such a family in the United States, they either resort to close Egyptian American friends or seek counseling from extended families in their home country. Christian families may resort to religious leaders in their church or community for assistance. Imams, who are Muslim religious leaders and therefore devout Muslims, who belong to a mosque may choose to consult with other Imams regarding marital, family, or mental health problems (Ali, Milstein, & Marzuk, 2005).

The most important goal for Egyptian American families is to raise children who are well educated, employable, and able to secure occupations that allow career mobility, financial security, and an acceptable social status. To that end, many other goals are subordinated. Because of this goal, parents may move to areas with better school systems and are willing to withstand financial or other hardships for the sake of their children.

Another goal of Egyptian American families is to keep children geographically close, if not living at home, until they get married to the right partner. Parents consider it their responsibility to assist their children, especially daughters, to find a suitable marriage partner, and they support children financially through wedding preparations. Raising children who are considered *moaddabeen* by Egyptian standards is important. A child who is *moaddab* is one who respects parents, defers to them for decisions, is mindful of older people, does not drink or indulge in immoral acts, listens to parents' advice, and does not answer back during conflict. One final goal of Egyptian families is to maintain a good face in public. This goal is achieved when children do not bring shame by engaging in activities forbidden by their parents, such as drinking, smoking, or going somewhere without their parents' permission.

As Egyptians grow older, they are considered richer in experiences and wiser and command more respect. They are treated with gentleness and never made to believe that their usefulness is limited just because of aging or retirement. Their children and extended family are expected to care for them. Older people prefer to do less management of their own affairs and expect more services, respect, and reverence from family members and subordinates. Women gain status with age and with childbearing. Young women know that inequities they may suffer as young brides are more than compensated for when they get older. Older women, however, are expected to care for older men in the family.

Because most of the Egyptian American community immigrated as young adults, as they advance in age they are the first generation to experience growing old in the United States. Many parents have a morbid fear that they may be forced to move into a nursing home. Many consider returning to their home country to avoid the humiliation of aging in America, with the potential loss of home, family care, and respect. Egyptian Americans do not believe that they can expect or hold their children responsible for becoming their caregivers during old age (Durrani, 2000). Growing old in America is surrounded by many images of abandonment, humiliation, loss of respect, and above all, loneliness. Those who adapt to a life without extended family and create an extended family will likely establish a new means to deal with their old age. Health-care professionals may consider alternative ways to support this community and enhance their self-care activities to help them avoid feelings of loneliness and a sense of abandonment in old age.

Many Egyptian Americans are part of a network of friends with whom they share their celebrations and calamities. Where mosques or Middle Eastern Orthodox churches exist, these organizations are used to promote social gatherings, maintain cultural norms, reinforce culturally driven restrictions on children's behavior, and promote historical continuity. In the absence of such organizations, Egyptian cultural clubs promote meetings, discussions, and sharing news from the homeland. Comparative analyses of life in Egypt and the United States often dominate these gatherings. During social gatherings, Egyptians are recognized by their elegant clothes, the hustle and bustle of children playing, adults chattering, and fine Egyptian food.

Egyptian Americans prefer family gatherings to adult gatherings for celebrations such as **Ramadan** (the month of fasting), the **Eid** feast celebrations, Christmas, and New Year's. Most often, they include extended family and their new networks of friends. Social networks are connected by their heritage rather than by their occupations. Without these large gatherings, loneliness and a sense of deprivation are exaggerated at times of crises or during normal developmental events such as the birth of a baby or the death of a family member.

In Egypt, extended family members play a strong role in the life of a family. It is an important goal of family members to live in the same city. Extended family members provide backup and support for working women by providing child care and for nonworking women with multiple children as they need tangible support. Families raise children, not mothers or fathers. All family members freely give advice on child rearing. In the United States, Egyptian immigrants do not usually have extended family members living with them, but they continue to consider the extended family living abroad as their support network. For those who have extended family members and professional careers, the relationship tends to be more limited by time, responsibilities, and other demands.

Social status is gained through professional accomplishments, financial success, and involvement in Egyptian community affairs. Respect is given to community leaders who give of themselves and share life experiences. No caste system exists based on color, familial lineage, or ancestry among Egyptians or Egyptian Americans. In some communities, Egyptian Americans are divided by religion (Muslims and Copts) and by professional status, with clubs for professionals, blue-collar workers, and other white-collar workers.

ALTERNATIVE LIFESTYLES

The divorce rate among Egyptian immigrants is low, a pattern similar to that in Egypt. In cases of divorce in which one parent raises the children, the Egyptian community supports the single parent, including his or her own children. Divorce is not seen as a stigma, but an unfortunate situation in which the children pay the greatest price. In second marriages, partners work hard to make a new life together and are committed to raising their stepchildren.

Communal and same-sex families are concepts that do not exist in Egyptian societies. Although a community of gays exists, homosexuality is rarely disclosed. They do have meeting places that are frequently ignored, intentionally overlooked, and more recently, raided, with jail as a result for those suspected of same-sex activities. The Web site GayEgypt.com includes stories of gay men who have been imprisoned, facing hard labor and torture. To be gay or lesbian is considered immoral and is not accepted by any Arab or Middle Eastern religion. To discover a gay son or lesbian daughter is akin to a catastrophic event for Egyptians and Egyptian Americans.

Workforce Issues

CULTURE IN THE WORKPLACE

Egyptian American nurses, who usually hold a minimum of a bachelor's degree, cope well with the demands inherent in providing nursing care in the United States. In the beginning of their careers in the United States, however, they encounter three challenges. First, Egyptian American nurses frequently expect detailed and careful communication of all steps and aspects of nursing care. This expectation is inherent in both their cultural patterns and their educational preparation. Although interactions and communications come naturally to Egyptian Americans, this naturalness is usually reserved for family and close acquaintances. In addition, their professional preparation does not emphasize communication skills for interacting with clients. Because Egyptian clients do not expect detailed information from physicians and nurses, the routine of informing clients about the rationale for interventions may challenge Egyptian American nurses.

The second challenge relates to the systematic and careful recording and documentation of nursing care. Egyptians are inclined to an oral tradition; therefore, the need to document in writing what can be shared verbally seems foreign to Egyptian American nurses.

The third challenge involves the work environment itself. For Egyptians, the work environment is also their social environment in which friendships are built and life experiences and personal issues are shared with a select few. The emphasis on privacy and separating work and social life expected in American work settings seems artificial to Egyptian Americans. Therefore, they tend to view American work relationships as superficial and often experience a sense of loss in terms of close,

meaningful work relationships and a supportive collegial network. This feeling is similar to how women in other professions view satisfying and stressful aspects of their work situation.

Many Egyptian communities in the United States form Egyptian cultural clubs to which a small percentage of these immigrant nurses belong. Such clubs help to decrease their sense of marginality. Activities usually include parties, dinners, picnics, and dances. Some of these clubs offer Arab language classes for the children. The more religious socialize around their local mosques and churches, which are good and safe forums for their teenage sons and daughters to meet prospective marital partners.

Egyptian immigrants to the United States work hard at becoming integrated into the Western work environment. They thrive on professional satisfaction, defining success in terms of advancement. They tend to be team players and effective contributors to the society at large. They are usually punctual and follow work rules and procedures. Being well assimilated, they create a close network of colleagues.

ISSUES RELATED TO AUTONOMY

Most Egyptians prefer to work in a job setting in which they are employees of an organization. They do not experience difficulty in reporting to a superior and following instructions. These cultural patterns do not preclude their being professionally motivated to work hard and advance their careers within respective organizations. As managers, leaders, or supervisors, they bring a personal touch and demonstrate human interest in their dealings with subordinates and coworkers. They demand loyalty and respect. On the whole, their religious affiliations do not pose problems for them when dealing with coworkers outside their own religions. However, the long history of Egyptian and Arab Israeli animosity causes some of them to approach their dealings with Jewish coworkers cautiously. Egyptian immigrants tend to be respectful of female coworkers, and often, their protective responses may be interpreted as patronizing by some women. They treat women as sisters or daughters.

Few Egyptians are entrepreneurial by nature. Those who opt to start their own businesses struggle to make them work. Egyptian Americans in general value job and economic security over the risk-taking inherent in operating a business. Therefore, they join established organizations with long-term goals.

Egyptians learn British English in schools and universities. On immigrating to the United States, they are confronted with unfamiliar slang and idioms. When viewed from an immigrant's point of view and with only basic knowledge of British English, some of these expressions are hard to interpret and could be construed as insults. An example of this type of misunderstanding happened to one of the authors (MHM). As he narrates it:

> When I arrived in the United States (over 30 years ago) as a graduate student in engineering, I had an occasion to be studying at a University of California Los Angeles library on a weekend day with my wife, a graduate student in nursing. When we decided to go to the local school cafeteria for a cup of tea, we noticed one of her psychology

professors in the library whom we knew very well inside and outside of the school. I approached him, greeted him, and asked if he would like to join us for a cup of tea. He responded by saying, "No, I don't care to have a cup of tea now." This, of course, is a very simple and totally acceptable American response. For me, a recent Egyptian immigrant (less than a year), this was a personal insult. The words "I do not care" meant to me that he did not care about *me*, not the process of having tea. We discussed this conversation a year later as he and I became close friends and laughed about it. He obviously meant no insult, and I just did not know enough about the idioms and commonly used expressions to "get it."

With increasing exposure to the media and life in the United States, it does not take long for a new immigrant to understand and accurately interpret idioms and commonly used expressions. The media is also a useful tool that helps Egyptian Americans and others to learn the English language and idiomatic and slang expressions.

Biocultural Ecology

SKIN COLOR AND OTHER BIOLOGICAL VARIATIONS

Most Egyptians have olive skin tones, some are fair-skinned, and others dark-skinned. Northern Egyptians exhibit a fairer complexion than most other Egyptians. Southern Egyptians (Nubians) are generally black, with very fine facial features. Upper Egyptians have a darker complexion. The average height of Egyptian men is about 5 ft 10 in., whereas women average 5 ft 4 in.

DISEASES AND HEALTH CONDITIONS

Several risk factors are peculiar to life along the banks of the Nile. Egyptians suffer from a host of parasitic diseases; the most common is schistosomiasis, known as *bilharzia* in Egypt. Schistosomiasis has been endemic in Egypt throughout history and has been found in mummified bodies from the pharaonic era. A high percentage of the Egyptian rural population is infected with *Schistosoma mansoni* or *S. haematobium*. The life cycle of schistosomiasis includes snails and human beings as hosts. Microscopic cercariae leave the snail in the warmth of the midday sun and penetrate the skin of humans who enter the shallow canals to irrigate crops, wash dishes or clothes, or swim. The cercariae migrate to areas near the liver, in the case of infection with *S. mansoni*, or near the bladder, in the case of infection with *S. haematobium*. The parasitic worms mature, mate, reproduce, and are expelled with urine or stools. If urine or stools are deposited in or near freshwater canals or rivers where snails live, the eggs seek out a snail to begin the cycle again.

In human hosts, as the female worm expels the eggs, some of them flow with the blood and become lodged in the liver or around the urinary tract. The body, treating the eggs as foreign irritants, surrounds them with granular tissue, leading to cirrhosis, liver failure, portal hypertension, esophageal varices, bladder cancer, and renal failure. Filariasis is another challenging parasitic disease endemic to Egyptians.

Rates of blindness in Egypt are among the highest in the world. Trachoma and other acute eye infections affect both rural and urban populations. Trachoma, a chronic infection of the lining of the eyelids caused by infection with *Chlamydia trachomatis*, is most common among children and can have severe disabling consequences in adulthood. Gel-like lymphoid follicles that subside over time, leaving residual scarring of the inner eyelids, characterize the active inflammatory stage. In the most severe cases, trichiasis, an end-stage complication of chronic trachoma, occurs when scarring shrinks the lid lining and turns the eyelashes inward, scratching the cornea. This painful condition often leads to corneal ulceration, opacity, and eventual blindness. Injuries and corneal ulcers secondary to other infections are also common causes of blindness in Egypt.

Other infectious diseases include typhoid and paratyphoid fevers, which are more frequent in urban than in rural areas. Streptococcal disease and rheumatic fevers are frequent among children, and tuberculosis continues to be a major problem in Egypt. Egyptian Americans who have positive tuberculin tests should be questioned about a history of Bacille Calmette-Guérin (BCG) vaccination.

Diarrheal diseases result from environmental conditions and family lifestyles. Heat contributes to the development of bacterial diseases, and dehydration results from diarrhea and vomiting caused by bacterial infections. Programs and campaigns using rehydration packets with water, salt, and sugar have drastically decreased mortality rates caused by diarrheal diseases. These endemic diseases are more common in rural areas than in urban areas. Egyptian immigrants come mainly from urban areas and, therefore, do not usually suffer from these diseases. However, some may have family members who come to the United States for treatment with complications caused by one of these diseases. Kidney diseases, lack of proper hydration, and eating habits may contribute to kidney failure and the subsequent need for kidney transplantation. Clinicians in the Middle East suspect that fasting during Ramadan increases the potential for dehydration, contributing to kidney problems.

The people of Egypt also suffer from diseases common to developing countries, such as undernutrition and malnutrition, and diseases resulting from overindulging in foods with high-fat and high-sugar contents. Modern diseases such as obesity, hypertension, and lower back pain affect a high percentage of Egyptians. Similarly, cardiovascular diseases resulting from stress, obesity, lack of exercise, and hypertension are on the rise. Egyptians who immigrate to the United States are more likely to become victims of these diseases of modernization than of rural diseases. Whereas breast cancer does not appear to be a uniformly manifest pattern among immigrant populations in an Australian study, rates were somewhat higher among the Egyptian born (McCredie, Coates, & Grulich, 1994). Type 2 diabetes is of concern to Egyptians and is further complicated by obesity. In addition, Egyptians are at a genetic risk for thalassemias, which can be detected from a molecular genetic standpoint through carrier screening and prenatal diagnosis.

VARIATIONS IN DRUG METABOLISM

The literature reports few studies related to variations in drug metabolism and specific drug interactions among Egyptian Americans. Some evidence indicates that Egyptians are poor metabolizers of beta-blockers (Levy, 1993). More research is needed in this area to provide better health care to Egyptian Americans.

High-Risk Behaviors

Certain behaviors may increase the risk of illness for Egyptians in America. One of these is a sedentary lifestyle and lack of regular exercise (Salari, 2002). Information about exercise has just begun to appear in the media in Egypt, and health clubs and gyms have begun to spring up in Cairo and Alexandria. This new phenomenon began after many Egyptians immigrated to America. Although exercise and fitness are regularly included in the curricula of schools and colleges, exercise is not part of the daily lives of adult Egyptians and, even less so, among Egyptian Americans.

Overeating food delicacies high in fat, sodium, and sugar; sedentary lifestyles; and an entertainment style based on eating contribute to obesity and immobility. Although no data exist on health risk factors for Egyptian Americans, the authors suspect that if such data were obtained, they would demonstrate an increased risk for coronary artery diseases, diabetes, and esophageal hernias. The premature deaths in Egyptian American communities are due to massive heart failure. There are also indications of an increase in risk factors for different types of cardiovascular diseases. Hassoun (1999) demonstrated that Arab Americans suffer from hypertension, high cholesterol levels, and diabetes more than other immigrants. These findings suggest that a similar pattern may exist among Egyptian Americans (Hatahet, Khosla, & Fungwe, 2002). Many Egyptians came to the United States as young adults; as the community of Egyptian Americans ages, questions related to sedentary lifestyles, overindulgence in food, and genetic makeup should be of interest.

Egyptian Americans are at risk for stomach and intestinal problems that include heartburn, flatulence, constipation, hemorrhoids, and fecal impaction. These conditions result from limited roughage, lack of fluids, and rapid consumption of food. Another factor contributing to constipation may be their expectations and the meaning they attach to regularity, which prompts them to push and strain to force a bowel movement prematurely. Egyptian Americans are also at risk for diabetes. Jaber, Brown, Hammad, Zhu, and Herman (2003) found that a decrease in acculturation to the United States is an important element in the increase in risk factors for Arab immigrants.

Like many less-developed countries, Egypt responded with zeal to campaigns launched by the cigarette industry. Cigarette smoking is on the rise in Egypt, mostly among men, but it is also increasing among women. Those who smoke, smoke heavily and are unwilling to quit. Rice, Templin, and Kulwcki (2003) reported that 17 percent of the adolescent Arab Americans in their study smoked, and 34 percent said they had never

smoked. Predictors for tobacco use were poor grades, peer or family smoking, passive smoking, receiving free samples of cigarettes, advertising, and believing that smoking helps in networking and stress. Smoking cessation programs, therefore, should reflect cultural gender norms and religious messages (Islam & Johnson, 2003).

One of the most dangerous risk factors among Egyptians in Egypt is their driving behavior. Most drive recklessly and aggressively, do not wear seatbelts, and drive without respect for speed limits. However, the extreme traffic congestion in Egypt provides a safety cushion. It takes Egyptian immigrants a number of years in America to learn to respect traffic rules, wear seatbelts, and drive cautiously.

The terrorist attacks on the United States on September 11, 2001, have resulted in harsh treatment of Arab Americans, including Egyptian Americans. Perceptions of scapegoating, discrimination, racism, and stigmatization increase their experience of stress. Outcomes of stress and marginalization will most probably be the subject of future research studies (Nieves, 2001; Salari, 2002; Zogby, 2001).

HEALTH-CARE PRACTICES

Two conditions increase the utilization of preventive health care by Egyptian Americans: having health insurance and having a health-care provider with whom they can develop a trusting and responsive relationship. Egyptian Americans like prompt and personal attention; they are usually among the most compliant clients if these conditions are met.

One reason for Egyptian Americans' seeking health care is a perception that they are experiencing high blood pressure. They believe it is important to have frequent readings but prefer to treat hypertension with medications rather than with changes in diet or lifestyle. Hypertension, the silent killer of many Americans, may not be so silent for Egyptians. Whether they can detect fluctuations in their blood pressure remains to be carefully studied. However, this behavior of reading one's own body cues should be encouraged and promptly addressed by health-care professionals.

Pap smears and mammograms tend to be new preventive health practices for Egyptian Americans. Education about the importance of these tests promotes compliance with regular checkups. As mentioned earlier, Pap smears for unmarried women are discouraged and considered totally unacceptable because of the expectations for preserving virginity until marriage. Gynecological examinations are given only to married women, usually during the checkup for a first pregnancy.

A study about health concerns among 99 Egyptian women and 135 American women aged 19 to 27 years reported that the top 10 health concerns among Egyptian women were halitosis/body odor, colds, cancer, poor teeth, population explosion, excess weight, birth control, water pollution, headaches, and heart disease. Among American women, the top 10 health concerns were birth problems, what the future would be like in 10 years, auto accidents, excess weight, cancer, use of contraceptives, death, nuclear war, childbirth, and air pollution (Engs &

Badr, 2001). The differences in health concerns of these two groups are probably due to cultural values and the degree of societal differences between the United States and Egypt. These results reinforce the need for community health education programs that address the specific needs of individuals.

Nutrition

MEANING OF FOOD

Food is an important component of Egyptian social life. Egyptians entertain lavishly and enjoy good food, which represents nurturing. The more food one provides, the more love is portrayed. Egyptians develop trust in each other by having a meal together. The saying *Akalt eish wa malh maa baad* literally means "eating bread and salt together" and symbolically signifies trust, care, and truthfulness.

In addition to being part of Egyptian social life, food is associated with health. The more food a person eats, the greater the potential expectation for health. Thus, children tend to be overfed. Food is also associated with the ability of the head of the family to provide for family members. Therefore, parents take pride in the amount and the quality of food they bring to their families. Because food is associated with caring and nurturing, mothers and wives spend much time and effort shopping and cooking family meals. Finally, food is associated with generosity and giving. To offer food and to accept food are indications of friendship. Mealtime is for eating and for socializing but not for conducting business or discussing issues.

Some beliefs surrounding meals may increase health risks. For example, Egyptians prefer not to drink water or fluids with meals because they believe that fluid displaces the volume that could be used for food, decreasing their appetite for solid nutrients. Some believe that fluids dilute the stomach "juices," make digestion difficult, and cause indigestion. Another potential risk factor to explore is the amount of salt added to food while cooking or at the table.

COMMON FOODS AND FOOD RITUALS

Egyptian food is tasty, well done, and well seasoned. Egyptian Americans take pride in the food they serve and the way they present it. Although in Egypt vegetable dishes are considered main dishes to be complemented by meat and rice dishes, this conception has changed for most Egyptian Americans. Preferred meats are lamb, chicken, beef, and veal. Favorite vegetables are peas, green beans, cauliflower, and molokhia, a green vegetable cooked like soup. Most consider meat dishes as main dishes, complemented by vegetables and rice. Rice, a main staple, adorns dinner or lunch tables on a daily basis even when potatoes are served. Tomato-based red sauces are popular, and some pasta and vegetable dishes are dressed with rich white sauces such as bechamel. Egyptians use lentils, fava beans, and bulgur in their cooking. Whole-wheat is the preferred bread.

Egyptians acquired a taste for tea from their years under British rule and drink strong tea with hot milk several times a day. Those who prefer tea without milk drink it with mint leaves. They tend to use several teaspoons of sugar to sweeten their tea. Although it is not easy for them to decrease their sugar intake, Egyptians do so if they understand its relationship to caloric intake, insulin requirements for those who are diabetic, or for other health considerations. Egyptians also drink coffee, a habit acquired from Turkish rule. The coffee is thick, strong, and served in small demitasse cups, with or without sugar. Egyptians also consume a large quantity of soft drinks.

Hostesses insist on giving guests excessive amounts of food and act insulted if guests refuse the food. Those who understand the ritual may insist on refusal or may take the food and not eat it. Leaving some food on the plate is more polite than refusing it. Completely emptying the plate may be seen as an indication that the guest did not have enough to eat. Egyptian Americans use modified versions of this ritual, depending on the guests and their length of time in the United States.

In Egypt, three main meals a day are served with a late afternoon or early evening snack of sweets with tea. The main meal is lunch, usually consumed at the end of the working day between 2 and 3 p.m., generally followed by a period of rest when many take an afternoon nap. Working men and women in the current economic climate of Egypt either return to work in the early evening between 5 and 6 p.m. or have a second job or business for the remaining part of the evening. Supper, usually a lighter meal, is eaten after 9 p.m.

On religious holidays, certain foods are prepared and shared with family and friends. An example is baking a variety of cookies at the end of the holy month of Ramadan, a time when Muslims fast daily from sunrise to sunset, and during the **Small Eid** feast (also called the *El Eid Alsagheer* or *Small Barrium*). During the **Great Eid** feast (also called the *El Eid Alkabeer* or *Big Barrium*), a sheep is sacrificed; the meat is given to needy families, and the family keeps some for consumption during that feast. Most of these rituals are modified in the United States. For example, Egyptian immigrants follow American eating habits of a small meal for lunch and then dinner at home after work between 6 and 7 p.m. Some immigrant families still make cookies at the end of Ramadan, but very few have a sheep slaughtered. Whether in Egypt or in America, the most devout Muslims do not consume pork or drink alcohol. Egyptian Copts may consume both in moderation.

For Egyptian American Muslims, many rituals are revived during the month of Ramadan, the ninth of 12 Islamic months that follow the lunar calendar. Therefore, Ramadan does not coincide with a particular month in the Christian calendar; instead it rotates and can fall on any of the Christian calendar months. Ramadan rituals are based on the teaching of the **Qur'an** (Koran) that calls for a month of fasting to experience the plight of the poor and the underprivileged. Fasting precludes taking anything by mouth or intravenously and abstaining from sexual activities. Muslims are expected to donate food for those in need, and they may eat modestly from sunset to sunrise. Egyptian American Christians fast for a varied number of days for several major religious celebrations. For them, fasting constitutes not eating any animal products.

Ramadan is a month of prayers and family festivities with many food rituals. At sunset, families gather to eat lavish meals consisting of several kinds of meat and poultry, rice, dried fruits, and desserts such as *konafa* (shredded phyllo dough stuffed with nuts and raisins and soaked in honey) and *kataif* (pancake-like dough dressed with nuts, raisins, and sugar and smothered in honey). The meals are usually high in protein, fat, sugar, salt, and calories. Just before sunrise, families consume a lighter meal in preparation for a day of fasting. Some Egyptian American Muslims follow these rituals in the United States. Even Egyptian Americans who do not follow and abide by the teachings of Islam during the year consider this month holy, and they become more devout Muslims during Ramadan. Some Egyptian Americans join others in social clubs and plan weekly potluck "sundown Ramadan breakfasts." During these gatherings, Egyptian Americans, their friends, and children exchange stories related to Ramadan, read from the Qur'an, and indulge in eating delicacies specific to Ramadan.

DIETARY PRACTICES FOR HEALTH PROMOTION

Egyptian Americans do not mix hot and cold nor sweet and sour foods at the same meal. For example, the accepted habit in America of eating ice cream as dessert with coffee was a foreign concept for Egyptians during the early stages of their immigration. However, they easily accommodate to this food habit. Some Egyptian Americans grew up believing that mixing fish and milk may cause digestive problems or create behavioral problems. Therefore, dairy products and fish are generally avoided in combination. Some may have practiced drinking milk with yeast to increase their intake of vitamin B complex, a popular custom in Egypt.

Most Egyptian Muslims do not eat pork, as proscribed by the Qur'an. They eat only well-cooked meat and do not touch rare meat. Recent Egyptian immigrants find it strange to eat cooked corn, which is only barbecued in their country. Most are partial to their own cooking, preferring not to eat in restaurants. They prefer kosher meat, trusting the dietary restrictions and food preparation practices of the Jewish population. In the absence of kosher meat, they shop at regular supermarkets.

NUTRITIONAL DEFICIENCIES AND FOOD LIMITATIONS

Egyptians, particularly those who live in rural and poor communities, experience fat-soluble vitamin and iron deficiency anemia. They eat more fresh vegetables, fresh fruits, and enriched or whole-wheat grain breads. Egyptians in the United States, like other Arab Americans, may resort to eating more processed foods and high-protein diets in the form of red meats because of increased availability (Hassoun, 1999). They also tend to eat more junk foods, preferring sweets. Therefore, Egyptian Americans may have a greater tendency to have diets higher in fat and consume fewer fresh fruits and vegetables. No literature exists about the changes in dietary habits and the effects on vitamin and mineral deficiencies among Egyptian Americans.

Pregnancy and Childbearing Practices

FERTILITY PRACTICES AND VIEWS TOWARD PREGNANCY

An Egyptian couple is not complete until they have a child and are usually under stress, fearing marriage instability caused by a lack of childbearing, until they conceive their first baby (Hattar-Pollara et al., 2000). Even if the husband is the cause of delayed or permanent infertility, women are threatened by the potential of divorce and are expected to conceive within their first year of marriage. Egyptian American families are under less stress and pressure to conceive because of the absence of extended family, although extended families continue to pressure their daughters and sons through letters and telephone calls. Pregnancies cement marriages, ensure a more lasting relationship, and are a way of getting men and women to mature in their relationship. Pregnancy brings women a sense of security and their husbands' and in-laws' respect. Giving birth, particularly to a son, considerably strengthens the status and power of women. Pregnancy gives women permission to decrease their responsibilities.

Systematic and concerted efforts have been initiated to develop and implement birth control practices in Egypt, with birth control being far more apparent in urban Egypt. Whereas Egyptian Americans may practice family planning and birth control, these are never advocated before conceiving the first child. Family planning is practiced through a variety of methods, including birth control pills, condoms, and early withdrawal. Abortion is used in Egypt, as in other countries, as a method of birth control. Desirable family size in urban Egypt is three or four children, whereas desirable family size in the United States among Egyptian Americans is two or three children. Women take an active role in limiting pregnancies; they are willing to use any method of birth control to achieve and maintain a small family size. Infertility is shrouded in secrecy and is attributed first and foremost to women. Among poor urban and rural families in Egypt *Kabsa* is considered to be the cause of infertility (Inhorn, 1994). *Kabsa* happens when vulnerable women come in contact with "polluted" individuals. *Kabsa* causes a threat to reproductive organs, a concept close to the way in which the "evil eye" affects an individual. It is unlikely that Egyptians who immigrate hold such a concept about infertility; however, assessing individuals who may be suffering from infertility nonetheless requires communication skills to uncover explanatory frameworks. This will lead to more compliance. It is also important to note that just like other underserved populations, Arab Americans tend to experience difficulties in accessing and receiving care in general, but infertility care in particular because of social marginalization especially after 9/11 (Inhorn & Fakih, 2006).

PRESCRIPTIVE, RESTRICTIVE, AND TABOO PRACTICES IN THE CHILDBEARING FAMILY

Women are expected and advised to curtail physical activities during pregnancy for fear of miscarriage (Meleis, 2002). Women are also advised to eat more because they are feeding two. Some Egyptian American women have strong cravings (*waham*) for certain foods that may extend to such scarce items as out-of-season strawberries. If these foods are not consumed, babies may be marked with the shape of foods that were craved. Therefore, every effort is made to provide the pregnant woman with the needed foods.

Providing support during labor and delivery is reserved for the woman's relatives, particularly her mother. Egyptian Americans invariably request that a female family member accompany the birthing mother. If an Egyptian American woman goes into labor with only her husband in attendance, it is considered an emergency. Acculturated Egyptian American men want to be included in the birthing experience, which may offend Egyptian newcomers. In Egypt, men are excluded from the birthing process because it is believed that men lack the ability to witness this highly emotional and painful process and lack the experience to support their wives.

The cold-and-hot theory for health and illness prevents women from bathing during the postpartum period. Bathing or washing hair could expose them to colds and chills. Egyptian Americans respond well to a sound rationale for bathing in a hot tub or taking a shower that dispels beliefs about the potential for infection. Chicken and chicken broth are expected to help women during their postpartum transition. The postpartum period lasts 40 days, during which new mothers are expected to rest, eat well, be confined to the house with their babies, and not engage in any sexual activities. They are usually cared for by family members and are not expected to have any demands put on them. This practice is eroding, however, because of increasing demands on women and the migration of families. Information related to birth control is always welcomed after the first pregnancy, although it may not be sought during the postpartum period.

Death Rituals

DEATH RITUALS AND EXPECTATIONS

Among Muslims in Egypt, Islam calls for burial of the deceased as soon as possible. The burial ritual includes cleaning the body and wrapping it in a white cotton wrap. Verses from the Qur'an are read and a special prayer is recited at the mosque before the body is buried underground in a simple tomb. Islam prohibits fancy tombstones; only a simple stone with the name of the deceased is placed above ground. The simple stone suggests that individuals are equal in death when meeting their creator. On the night of the burial, friends and family gather in a large tent outside the deceased's home to give their condolences and respect to the grieving family. No food is served, but Turkish coffee is usually offered. Forty days after the burial, another mourning ritual takes place in the home of the deceased's family. Family members listen while passages from the Qur'an are read by a religious man to console the family. Thereafter, a similar ritual takes place on the anniversary of the death. Egyptian Christian death rituals in Egypt and the United States are similar to American Christian death rituals.

For Egyptian immigrants, some cultural rituals are followed. For instance, the Islamic burial rituals are carried out in designated cemeteries. The evening before the burial, the Qur'an is recited, and occasionally, the mourning ritual is observed for 40 days after burial. The annual death observance ritual is rarely carried out. Some Muslim families insist on having the deceased buried in Egypt, which is a very costly process involving approval from both countries and transporting the deceased in a special casket. Abdel-Khalek and Ahmed (1986) found that Egyptian Americans have slightly higher anxiety about death than Americans. Health-care providers may be involved in and bewildered by the decision-making processes that Egyptian families go through on the death of family members. Plans for death are rarely made ahead of time, though a burial site is invariably selected in advance to protect families against being buried in non-Muslim burial places. Similar practices are observed among Christian Egyptian Americans.

RESPONSES TO DEATH AND GRIEF

Egyptians in Egypt and the United States react vigorously and dramatically to the loss of a family member, expressing their grief outwardly. Wailing and public crying occur when first learning of death. This public reaction is an expected demonstration of their grief; otherwise, the community may regard them as lacking affection for the deceased. Death is seen as inevitable, although any loss brings shock and despair. Older people speak calmly about their own impending death. Egyptian Americans with a strong religious foundation do not fear the nearness of death but rather view it as a journey to the other world, which is believed to be better. Egyptian Muslims and Christians believe in an afterlife and expect rewards for good deeds accomplished in their first life. They anticipate reuniting with those who preceded them.

Spirituality

DOMINANT RELIGION AND USE OF PRAYER

Religious practices for Egyptian Americans are performed during marriage, death, and religious holidays. Egyptian Americans participate in two wedding ceremonies: One is a religious and civil ceremony performed by the mosque's **Imam** (usually in place of Maazoon, who performs these rituals in Egypt), and the other a social ceremony in which friends and family gather for a gala evening. Both could be performed on the same day or days, months, or years apart. A separation after the religious ceremony is considered a divorce, but it is customary for brides and grooms to live together only after the social celebration has taken place. Egyptian American Christians have one religious marriage ceremony.

Prayers, even for the nondevout Muslim or Christian, are significant during times of illness. Egyptian Americans may bring the Qur'an or the Bible to their hospital beds and usually put it under the pillow or on the bedside table. Prayers may be recited by the individual, in groups for Muslims, or in religious settings such as mosques or churches. Families and friends pray for each other, invoking good health, cure of illness, and peace. Prayers during holidays are enjoyed particularly in groups and in religious settings.

MEANING OF LIFE AND INDIVIDUAL SOURCES OF STRENGTH

Religious Egyptians achieve inner peace through practicing their respective religious rituals, including individual or collective prayers, reading from the Qur'an or Bible, and other religious texts written by religious scholars. Muslims who can afford the expense and are in good health make the pilgrimage to Mecca sometime during their lifetime. The journey is believed to provide Muslims with a source of inner fulfillment. Similar patterns of fulfillment through participation in religious activities are common in the United States.

SPIRITUAL BELIEFS AND HEALTH-CARE PRACTICES

Most Egyptian Americans talk about their religious teachings during episodes of illness. They derive comfort, strength, and meaning from verses in the Qur'an and of prophets. Family members use these verses to remind them that they are at the mercy and under the control of God and that God may have a particular reason for their suffering. To lose hope may mean they are losing faith in God and His abilities.

Health-Care Practices

HEALTH-SEEKING BELIEFS AND BEHAVIORS

The health-care practices of Egyptian Americans can best be understood by looking at the historical roots and the meanings of health and health care for Egyptians. The pharaohs are credited with introducing medicine to the world, as evidenced by the writings on papyri from 4000 B.C. The practice of mummification, perfected to ensure that the pharaohs' bodies were preserved to wait for the return of the departed spirit, may have helped the pharaohs to understand the intricate anatomy of the body. Papyri writings have been found describing body organs, gynecological conditions, surgery, and signs and symptoms of illnesses. There are indications that the early Egyptians also had dental knowledge and had developed treatments for dental problems. Pharaonic writings introduced the idea of body parts and segmentation.

Egyptian health care is also influenced by Greek, or *unani*, medicine. The most famous medical library in the world was built in Alexandria during the reign of Alexander the Great, housing almost all the medical knowledge of the ancient world. The books contained in this library, which was later burned, chronicled numerous diseases and treatments. The Greeks combined medicine and philosophy and expanded the understanding of anatomy. Their texts influenced the entire region. As early as the 10th century B.C., medical schools based on *unani* medicine were established by the Arabs. These texts, known as the laws of medicine, were written by early Arab scholars and embodied the teachings of preventive and curative health care.

Egyptian beliefs about health care are also influenced by humoral systems described in Greek documents. The principles behind the humoral system are based on dividing many aspects of life into four: the year into four seasons; matter into fire, air, earth, and water; the body into black phlegm, black bile, yellow bile, and blood; and the environment into hot, cold, moist, and dry. Diseases follow these humors with treatments based on opposite humors. The pharaohs introduced the principle of balance and imbalance as the cause of illness. Egyptians believe that cold and moist environments cause illnesses, by changes from cold to hot or vice versa. The opposite humor is used for treating the illness.

Other influences on the Egyptian health belief system came from the colonization of Egypt by the Turks, French, and British. In addition to illnesses being caused by humoral imbalances, Egyptians believe them to be caused by being presented suddenly with bad news (*itkhad*, "startled/surprised by unexpected calamity") or by a fight. Whereas a person's mental and physical health are intricately interwoven, treatment sought from the health-care system is focused on physical or biomedical treatment. Family or religious people usually handle mental health problems outside the health-care system. Egyptians tend to manifest symptoms of mental health problems somatically. Therefore, they seek medical care to deal with the physical manifestations of mental illnesses.

Whereas Egyptian Americans are usually well educated, their views are colored by beliefs about the influence of imbalances, the evil eye, and Islamic beliefs about the role God plays in their illness. However, they are firm believers in Western medicine's miraculous ability to treat and cure illnesses. None of their beliefs prevents them from seeking or complying with the prescriptions of Western medicine. If they practice the belief of balancing or of warding off the evil eye, it is done in conjunction with Western medicine. Levels of acculturation and biculturalism play an important role in how Arab Americans respond and deal with health-care issues. For example, the level of acculturation was determined to be a risk factor for a number of health problems, such as dysglycemia (Jaber et al., 2003) and coronary artery disease (Hatahet et al., 2002). They are also at higher risk because limited research studies use them as research participants (Sayed, 2003). Finally, they are also at risk because of stereotyping (Soliman et al., 2001).

RESPONSIBILITY FOR HEALTH CARE

The Qur'an and the sayings of Mohammed, the Prophet of Islam, have made a major contribution to Muslim health care. In particular, preventive health care is embodied in many of Mohammed's prophetic sayings.

Cleanliness and hygiene are integral to practicing Muslims. A number of elaborate prayer rituals are also related to health care and prevention of illness. For example, before praying, Muslims must engage in a purification ritual, which consists of washing every exposed body part. Prayer, required five times daily, consists of elaborate bending and kneeling movements in systematic ways, increasing a person's range of movements, limbering stretches, and meditative poses. Religion and prayers are believed to provide protection from illnesses.

In Egypt, a government health insurance policy allows every citizen to receive free care, treatments, and medications. However, Egyptians believe that to receive better quality health care, they must shop, bargain, and negotiate. In the process, they learn that quality care means fees. If they can afford it, they prefer quality care. Most Egyptian Americans join a Health Maintenance Organization (HMO) or have private medical insurance. Whereas they may refuse to have life insurance (Islam does not condone insurance), they realize the importance of quality health care. Newcomers, however, may wait to develop financial security before they join a health insurance plan. Typically, Egyptian Americans experiencing a health problem consult family members and friends before visiting a trusted health-care professional. Once in the health-care system, they prefer immediate, personalized attention. They value tests and prescriptions for their illnesses and follow medical regimens and prescriptions carefully, particularly if they consist of oral medications, injections, or both. However, they tend to be skeptical of treatments such as weight reduction, exercise, and diet restrictions.

The family of a client expects and prefers to be involved in all health-care decisions. Their focus on human relations and interpersonal contact make it difficult for Egyptian Americans who encounter changing staff and assignments during treatments. They believe they have a better chance of receiving quality care if trusting relationships are formed. Thus, constancy and consistency of contacts decrease potential conflicts in their relationship with the health-care system.

Egyptian Americans may practice self-medication. They tend to share medications freely and use Western medications and home remedies such as herbs, hot compresses, and hot fluids and foods. Many Egyptians keep a very active medicine cabinet filled with antibiotics, tranquilizers, sleeping pills, and pain medications. They also believe that vitamins given intramuscularly and intravenously are more effective than vitamins taken in pills. In Egypt, vitamin B complex injections and iron supplements are common self-medicating activities. Some common herbal and home remedies are boiled mint leaves for a stomach ache; boiled cumin for gas; boiled caraway for coughs; and hot pads for aches, pains, and boils. Regulation of prescription drugs in the United States restricts the use of prescriptions, prompting some Egyptian Americans to get their supply of medications from their home country or friends. Use of illegal drugs is minimal in this community. Although some Egyptian Americans may overindulge in alcohol, the teachings of Islam prohibit its use. Many who drink alcohol tend to do so socially and in limited quantities.

FOLK AND TRADITIONAL PRACTICES

According to Islam, illnesses are caused by lack of hygiene, exposure to diseases, or environmental conditions, although it is up to God who gets sick and who does not. People are expected to care for themselves and work at preventing illnesses when possible. In addition, beliefs related to the healing powers of shrines and holy men or saints and the counterpowers of the devil (**Jenn**) and evil spirits (**arwah**) influence health care. Thus, ceremonies are designed to eliminate the devastating powers of the *Jenn*; among them is the famous **zar** ceremony and the *hegab*. The *zar* ceremony includes gathering friends and relatives around a sick person, with loud music playing and drums beating to increase the frenzy of dance and movement. The energy of the group and their solidarity help eliminate the bad spirits from the body, taking with them the illness or the handicapping condition. *Zar* is rarely practiced among Egyptian Americans. A person who is trying to get rid of an illness wears the *hegab*, an amulet with sayings from the Qur'an. Some also use the **amal**, which is designed to bring bad luck or illness to an unloved person.

Egyptians believe the evil eye is responsible for personal calamities. The evil eye is cast by those who have blue eyes, by those who tend to speak of an admired person or object in a boastful manner, or by the mere description of beauty, wealth, or health without saying some verses from the Qur'an or Bible. These verses protect the person from losing whatever good they possess. Some Egyptian Americans use blue beads or religious verses inscribed on charms to protect them or their children from the evil eye. Children are particularly at risk for the evil eye and need more protection than adults.

BARRIERS TO HEALTH CARE

VIGNETTE 9.3

Mr. Sauri went to the emergency room concerned about his blood pressure. He was having family problems that made him feel rather agitated (*asabi*) and he felt "he has high blood pressure." Sauri is a cab driver in an urban city, is married with one daughter, and speaks English moderately well. He is obese, and is fast to suggest all the tests that should be performed. He is impatient with the "many questions" that he perceives to be unrelated to his primary complaint. Furthermore, he believes that all he needs are "medications to lower his blood pressure."

1. What are the best strategies to begin the health assessment process?
2. Knowing the barriers to health care for underserved minorities, the schedules and work patterns of cab drivers, the meaning of Western medicine for Egyptian Americans, and their narrative style in recounting their illness stories, describe your assessment and intervention strategies.
3. Critically discuss a model of care that incorporates patterns of responses and explanatory frameworks of presenting problems and intervention plans.

Barriers to health care among Egyptian Americans are related to economics, work demands, and full schedules. Fitting appointments into their schedules proves to be somewhat difficult, particularly in families in which a spouse is working long hours and the family owns only one car. When the family has two working members, access to the health-care system at designated times is even more challenging. Another barrier is the difference in explaining health problems. The degree of specificity required in the U.S. health-care system, the narrative storytelling nature of Egyptians, and the contextual way in which Egyptians view a situation all contribute to a frustrating experience for both the immigrant and the health-care professional.

CULTURAL RESPONSES TO HEALTH AND ILLNESS

VIGNETTE 9.4

Salwa and Ahmed Sarhan recently moved from New York to New Jersey, where Ahmed is a cab driver. Salwa has a BA in Egyptology and Ahmed has a BS in Economics. They have three teenaged children—Maha, Saura, and Hazem. Over the past few weeks, Ahmed has been complaining of stomach pains. One night, the pain becomes more severe and feels like "he is being stabbed with a sharp knife." His brother brings him to the emergency room of a small community hospital. After a series of diagnostic tests, it is discovered that he has first-degree cancer. It is recommended that he undergo surgery to remove part of his stomach. He is given two different treatment options: surgery and no chemotherapy, and surgery followed by chemotherapy. He chooses to have the surgery and no chemotherapy, which is successful. The family indicates that they would like to send his diagnosis, x-rays, and all pertinent tests to Egypt. They receive many calls from various concerned family members. His wife does not want the staff to recount to them all the problems he is having or will have during his recovery. Ahmed becomes highly agitated and has been described as demanding and high maintenance. He is engaged with the staff at the hospital, but he wants his wife to attend to his wound changes. He does not want his teenaged children to know his diagnosis or prognosis. His daughter appears to be very quiet and withdrawn; one of his sons seems to be in charge. His wife is weepy and appears to be bewildered and concerned about her husband. He seems to expect her presence and does not want her to leave the room.

1. Identify three nursing problems and plan interventions in a cultural context.
2. What questions should the nurse ask in the initial family interviews to determine their needs?
3. How should the nurse plan care for Mr. and Mrs. Sarhan's state of mind?
4. Describe how Egyptian Americans respond to a serious diagnosis.
5. What should a health-care provider keep in mind in caring for Egyptian Americans with a terminal diagnosis?

Egyptians avoid pain at all costs by seeking prompt interventions. They tend to be verbally and nonverbally expressive about pain; moaning, groaning, sighing, and holding the painful body part tightly are common expressions of pain. As Reizian and Meleis (1987) demonstrated, Arab Americans tend to respond to an episode of pain depending on the intensity, severity, and their audience. Although they tend to be more constrained in front of health-care professionals or other "strangers," they are quite expressive in front of family members, using grunting, pushing, screaming, using guttural sounds, or gasping for air. These conflicting behaviors are confusing to health-care professionals when family members insist that the client needs pain relief. The absence of these responses in front of health-care professionals makes verification of the intensity of pain difficult.

Egyptian descriptions of pain may not be as specific as the Western health-care system prefers. Egyptians present a more generalized description of pain, regardless of whether it is localized. They usually describe general weakness, dizziness, or overall tension and stress associated with pain (Reizian & Meleis, 1987). They also use metaphors reflecting humoral medicine such as earth, rocks, fire, heat, and cold to describe their pain.

Age and birth order correlate significantly with individual responses and descriptions of pain. Younger children and first-born children are often more expressive about pain. Higher intensities of pain are also associated with increased behavioral responses in children. Egyptian children tend to describe their pain with sensory descriptors such as *sikkeenah*, or "it's like a knife" (Essaway, 1987). Giving birth is associated with severe pain, and it is not to be endured alone. Therefore, birthing mothers tend to be highly expressive of the intensity of their pain. Having a close family member present during the pain episode may be helpful for Egyptian Americans. Children prefer their mothers (Essaway, 1987), whereas adult women and men prefer female family members who are more nurturing, caring, and capable of comforting a person in pain (Meleis & Sorrell, 1981).

Although mental illness has been considered a stigma that should not be disclosed, more tolerance of emotional problems is the norm in modern Egypt. Rural Egyptians explain mental health problems within supernatural frameworks, including the *amal* (a curse) or *Jenn* (the devil). Urban Egyptians explain emotional problems in terms of grief, losses, and wrongdoing by others or by blaming the victims for not being able to control and snap out of their distress. Mental and emotional issues tend to be expressed somatically, and therefore, psychosomatic interventions are more effective than psychologically based interventions. Although Egyptians may seek therapy and counseling, they prefer to seek the advice of family members or trusted friends rather than go to strangers. They also do not like to call treatments psychotherapy or analysis. Egyptians tend to place the blame externally, looking for external actions or events to explain the situation. Because Egyptians are more community oriented, they tend to seek the approval and sanction of others; therefore, shame rather than guilt tends to explain their actions and their reactions.

Assessing and treating mental health problems among Egyptian Americans requires careful attention to gender relations, the history of how mental health is viewed in their country of origin, the individual's and family's level of acculturation, and their explanatory framework (Al-Krenawi & Graham, 2000). Integrating modern, Western, and cultural approaches will make the intervention more successful.

Disabilities are not hidden from public view. Whereas there is public sympathy and acceptance of people with disabilities, families still tend to be protective and shield them from public display. Families assume responsibility for the care of their disabled members, not expecting help or services from society. Egyptian Americans, however, tend to hide their disabled family members from other Egyptian Americans for fear of evoking reactions of pity. They are open, however, with health-care professionals in the hope of receiving better health care.

Egyptian Americans have a general belief that chronic illnesses can be controlled by the scientific sophistication of Western medicine. Therefore, health-care professionals and clients have a general pattern of cooperation on long-term treatments. Less regard is held for complementary therapies, and the demand is greater for scientifically supported remedies, regardless of their intrusiveness. Egyptian Americans tend to be hopeful, persistent, and optimistic about their prognoses. Therefore, they may shop around for health care that promises a better prognosis. Rehabilitation programs that include drastic changes in lifestyles are less appealing if the programs are not scientifically supported.

Egyptian families take care of their sick members. Promotion of self-care is viewed with suspicion by Egyptian Americans, just as by other Arab Americans, and sick people are not expected to participate in programs to enhance their self-care capabilities. Rather, they are expected to preserve their energy for healing. Attempts to engage Egyptian clients in self-care by promoting responsibility for daily care, for example, by keeping a colostomy incision clean, are resisted and perceived as a request to decrease the work of the nurse and the other staff. Sick people are also relieved from making major health-care decisions. Their families make all health-care decisions for them.

BLOOD TRANSFUSIONS AND ORGAN DONATION

Egyptian Americans have no taboos against blood transfusions or organ transplants. All measures needed to heal, cure, or prolong life are welcomed. Their trust and respect for the health-care system and health-care professionals facilitate their decision making, and they support recommendations offered by the health-care provider. They are hesitant, however, to pledge their own organs to others or to permit an autopsy. Because of their belief in the afterlife, they favor being buried whole.

Health-Care Practitioners

TRADITIONAL VERSUS BIOMEDICAL PRACTITIONERS

Although Egyptian Americans may consult family members and friends about their health and illnesses, they do not consult traditional or folk practitioners. In fact, they may be reluctant to seek health care from anyone but physicians. Using the services of acupuncturists, podiatrists, chiropractors, and physical therapists is foreign to those not integrated into the American culture. In general, members of the Egyptian American community have a positive perception of the American health-care system. They believe that physicians and nurses are experts and are caring and responsive to the needs of their community. Egyptian Americans are in awe of Western medicine, its scientific basis, and its vast resources. One of their most common responses is, "We were lucky to be in the United States when the illness occurred."

For some Egyptian Americans, however, the meticulous diagnostic approaches practiced by American physicians may be misinterpreted. Accustomed to Egyptian physicians whose clinical judgments and skills have been developed within a system that lacks adequate resources for meticulous diagnoses, some may misperceive an American physician's thoroughness as a lack of experience or appropriate knowledge. Therefore, they may shop for physicians whose clinical judgments are congruent with their cultural expectations of a prompt and firm diagnosis. Others may view the laborious and involved diagnostic process, which uses many resources and tests, as an indication of the gravity of the diagnosis.

A recent trend in Egypt is to consider gender as an important variable in the selection of health-care professionals. Although rural and less-educated urbanites have always valued this, religious influences have prompted a renewed preference for health-care providers of the same gender. Many Egyptian Americans immigrated before the wave of Islamic fundamentalism and its influence on life patterns and expressions. Therefore, first- and second-wave Egyptian Americans may not consider gender as an important criterion in the selection of their health-care providers. Third-wave immigrants may prefer gender-congruent health-care providers, although this preference may be mitigated by their respect for Western medicine. In addition to religious fundamentalism, modesty may influence the desire for gender-congruent health care. For some Egyptian Americans, sharing the intimate details of their health history is enhanced if the health-care provider is the same gender. Egyptian Americans may also view older female physicians as more experienced and, therefore, more trustworthy than younger female physicians.

STATUS OF HEALTH-CARE PROVIDERS

Physicians are highly respected by Egyptians and Egyptian Americans. As in most health-care systems throughout the world, Egyptian physicians expect to be the head of the health-care team and the primary decision makers for all aspects of clinical care. Egyptian Americans prefer physicians affiliated with large, respected organizations because they believe them to be more experienced. For some, the physician's age, years of experience, and position in the organization may indicate better qualifications.

As in the United States, nurses in Egypt are educated at many different degree levels and have similar patterns of practice. Most graduate from high school programs developed to meet the nursing shortage. Limited resources, an overabundance of physicians, limited educational preparation of the majority of nurses, low pay scales, and long work hours contribute to poor nursing care in Egypt. Consequently, nursing care in Egyptian hospitals is left to family members, who usually surround the client every waking moment. They are expected to carry out most of the care and act as advocates for the clients. Hence, they appear to us in the United States as more intrusive to Western routines, when in fact, they have been conditioned to be vigilant advocates for their family members.

Egyptians' contacts in the homeland with nurses who are knowledgeable and expert in their fields have been minimal. Consequently, their expectations of nurses are usually far below their experiences in the U.S. health-care system. They view American nurses as well educated and well qualified and are grateful for their expertise and for their attention.

Egyptian American physicians tend to be impressed with American nursing. Their limited views and expectations of nurses based on Egyptian experiences are drastically altered after short contact with American nursing practices. They consider nurses in the United States to be well educated and view their expertise as enhanced by years of experience and availability of resources. The emphasis on higher levels of education for American nurses is congruent with the high value Egyptians place on education. Egyptian physicians also believe that the better pay for American nurses is congruent with better education and better expertise.

REFERENCES

Abdel-Khalek, A., & Ahmed, M. (1986). Death anxiety in Egyptian samples. *Personality and Individual Differences, 7*(4), 479–483.

Al-Krenawi, A., & Graham, J. R. (2000). Culturally sensitive social work practice with Arab clients in mental health settings. *Health & Social Work, 25*(1), 9–22.

Ali, O. M., Milstein, G., & Marzuk, P. M. (2005). The imam's role in meeting the counseling needs of Muslim communities in the United States. *Psychiatric Services, 56*(2), 202–205.

CIA. (2007). *World Factbook: Egypt.* Retrieved February 22, 2007, from https://www.cia.gov/cia/publications/factbook/geos/eg.html

Durrani, A. (2000). Arab mothers like no other. *Arabia Online Ltd.* Retrieved February 22, 2007, from http://www.arabia.com

Engs, R., & Badr, L. (2001). The health concerns of young American and Egyptian women: A cross-cultural study. *Quarterly of Community Health Education, 4*(1), 1983–1984.

Essaway, M. A. H. (1987). The relationship of certain factors on the expression of pain among hospitalized surgical school age children. Unpublished doctoral dissertation, Alexandria University, Alexandria, Egypt.

Haddad, L. G., & Hoeman, S. P. (2000). Home healthcare and the Arab-American client. *Home Healthcare Nurse, 18*(3), 189–197.

Hassoun, R. (1999). Arab-American health and the process of coming to America: Lessons from the metropolitan Detroit area. In M. W. Suleiman (Ed.), *Arabs in America: Building a new future* (pp. 157–176). Philadelphia: Temple University Press.

Hatahet, W., Khosla, P., & Fungwe, T. V. (2002). Prevalence of risk factors to coronary heart disease in an Arab-American population in Southeast Michigan. *International Journal of Food Sciences and Nutrition, 53*(4), 325–335.

Hattar-Pollara, M., Meleis, A. I., & Hagib, H. (2000). A study of the spousal role of Egyptian women in clerical jobs. *Health-care for Women International, 21*(4), 305–317.

Inhorn, M. C. (1994). Kabsa (a.k.a. mushahara) and threatened fertility in Egypt. *Social Science and Medicine, 39*(4), 487–505.

Inhorn, M. C., & Fakih, M. H. (2006). Arab Americans, African Americans, and infertility: Barriers to reproduction and medical care. *Fertility and Sterility, 85*(4), 844–852.

Islam, S. M., & Johnson, C. A. (2003). Correlates of smoking behavior among Muslim Arab-American adolescents. *Ethnicity and Health, 8*(4), 319–337.

Jaber, L. A., Brown, M. B., Hammad, A., Zhu, Q., & Herman, W. H. (2003). Lack of acculturation is a risk factor of diabetes in Arab immigrants in the U.S. *Diabetes Care, 26*(7), 2010–2014.

Levy, R. (1993). Ethnic and racial differences in response to medicines: Preserving individualized therapy in managed programmes. *Pharmaceutical Medicine, 7*, 139–165.

McCredie, M., Coates, M., & Grulich, A. (1994). Cancer incidence in migrants to New South Wales (Australia) from the Middle East, 1972–91. *Cancer Causes and Control, 5*(5), 414–421.

Meleis, A. I. (2002). Egyptians. In P. St. Hill, J. Lipson, & A. Meleis (Eds.), *Caring for women cross-culturally: A portable guide.* Philadelphia: F. A. Davis Co.

Meleis, A. I., & Sorrell, L. (1981). Arab American women and their birth experiences. *American Journal of Maternal Child Nursing, 6*, 171–176.

Nieves, E. (2001, September 28). Recalling internment and saying "never again." *The New York Times.* Retrieved February 22, 2007, from http://www.nytimes.com

Reizian, A. E., & Meleis, A. I. (1987). Arab Americans' perceptions of and responses to pain. *Critical Care Nurse, 6*(6), 30–37.

Rice, V. H., Templin, T., & Kulwicki, A. (2003). Arab-American adolescent tobacco use: Four pilot studies. *Preventive Medicine, 37*(5), 492–498.

Salari, S. (2002). Invisible in aging research: Arab Americans, Middle Eastern immigrants, and Muslims in the United States. *The Gerontologist, 42*(5), 580–588.

Sayed, M. A. (2003). Psychotherapy of Arab patients in the West: Uniqueness, empathy, and "otherness." *American Journal of Psychotherapy, 57*(4), 445–459.

Shaw, I. (2000). *The Oxford history of Egypt.* Oxford: Oxford University Press.

Soliman, A. S., Levin, B., El-Badawy, S., Nasser, S. S., Raouf, A. A., & Khaled, H., et al. (2001). Planning cancer prevention strategies based on epidemiologic characteristics: An Egyptian example. *Public Health Reviews, 29*(1), 1–11.

U.S. Bureau of the Census. (2002). *Ancestry first reported (PCTO24) and ancestry second reported (PCTO25), Census 2000 supplementary suvey summary tables.* Retrieved February 22, 2007, from http://www.factfinder.census.gov/home/en/datanotes/exp_c2ss.html

Zogby, J. (2001). *Testimony of Dr. James. J. Zogby, submission to the United States Commision on Civil Rights, October 12, 2001.* Retrieved February 22, 2007, from http://www.aaiusa.org

Zohry, A., & Harrell-Bond, B. (2003). *Contemporary Egyptian migration: An overview of voluntary and forced migration* (Country Background Papers [WP-C3]). Brighton, United Kingdom: University of Sussex, Development Research Center on Migration, Globalization, and Poverty.

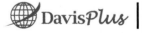 **DavisPlus** For case studies, review questions, and additional information, go to http://davisplus.fadavis.com

Chapter *10*

People of Filipino Heritage

DULA F. PACQUIAO

Overview, Inhabited Localities, and Topography

OVERVIEW

The Philippine archipelago consists of 7107 islands located in southeastern Asia, east of Vietnam. With a landmass of 300,000 square kilometers, it is slightly larger than the state of Arizona. The three major islands of Luzon, Visayas, and Mindanao have mostly mountainous terrain with narrow-to-extensive coastal lowlands. The tropical climate consists of dry and rainy seasons suitable for year-round agriculture and fishing, but it is affected by the seasonal northeastern and southwestern monsoons. In 2005, the total population was estimated at 89.5 million, with an annual growth rate of 2.36 percent. Although the country is rich in natural resources and has a mixed economy of agriculture, light industry, and support services, 40 percent of the population lived below poverty level in 2001 (CIA, 2007).

The Spaniards colonized the country for over 3 centuries, 1565 to 1898, and named the islands *Las Islas Filipinas*, the Philippine Islands. Following the Spanish-American War, the islands were ceded to the United States and given the anglicized name, the *Philippines*. Filipinas (Pilipinas) and Philippines are used interchangeably today. Native speakers refer to the country as *Filipinas* or *Pilipinas* and use *Philippines* when speaking to outsiders or writing in English.

The issue of whether to use *Filipinas* or *Pilipinas* and *Filipino* or *Pilipino* in referring to the country, its people, or its national language is a matter of debate among the country's scholars and historians. There is no letter *F* in the indigenous *Tagalog* language, which is spoken in central Luzon, including Manila, the nation's capital. When

the country gained its independence from the United States in 1946, it adopted the Tagalog-based Pilipino as its national language. In 1959, Pilipino was officially declared the national language. In 1986, however, the national assembly declared the national language as Filipino, based on existing Philippine and other languages. Generally, *Filipino* is used interchangeably with *Filipino American*. The term *Pilipino* is generally used to distinguish indigenous identity and nationalistic empowerment.

Filipino Americans are a diverse group because of regional variations in the Philippines, which influence the dialect spoken, food preferences, religion, and traditions (Fig. 10–1). Generational differences within families are associated with age and time of migration from the Philippines. Other factors influencing diversity include pre- and postmigration level of education, occupation, and intermarriage as well as other primary and secondary characteristics of culture (see Chapter 1). This chapter discusses the major characteristics of mainstream Filipino culture, offering some insights into some differences among groups. The reader should avoid using this information as a universal template for every Filipino.

HERITAGE AND RESIDENCE

The Filipino way of life is a tapestry of multicultural influences superimposed on indigenous tribal origins. The people are predominantly of Malayan ancestry, with overlays of Chinese, Japanese, East Indian, Indonesian, Malaysian, and Islamic cultures. The Philippine culture is distinct from its Asian neighbors largely because of the major influences from the Spanish and American colonizations. The Spaniards introduced Roman Catholicism, which has remained the dominant religion in the country. Spanish colonization spanned 350 years and was followed by 50 years of American domination. The

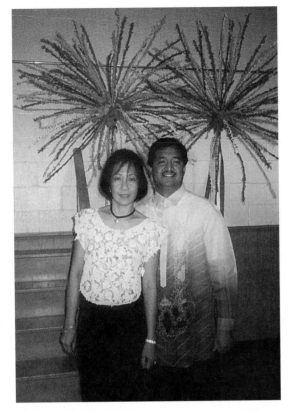

FIGURE 10–1 Traditional Filipino costumes.

Americans introduced public education and English as the medium of instruction to give the Filipinos a common language.

The Filipino way of life has evolved from the everyday situations that the people have to deal with living on scattered islands surrounded by large bodies of water and exposed to natural disasters such as volcanic eruptions, typhoons, floods, and droughts, as well as threats of foreign invasion. The Filipino sense of morality and justice evolved from tribal times. Close-knit, kin-based groups known as *Barangays* emerged to protect communities from outside atrocities. Communal values of collective welfare and solidarity fostered security of its members in an unstable environment. Outsiders to the culture recognize these values in the Filipino traits of collective loyalty, generosity, hospitality, and humility. These basic values are strong components of childhood socialization in the family. Filipinos inculcate a strong sense of family loyalty beyond the nuclear family. Family obligations extend to cousins, in-laws, and others who are intimately linked with the family by ceremonies such as serving as sponsors of marriage or baptisms (Bautista, 2002).

Most Filipinos in North America were born in the Philippines. By 2050, the Asian Pacific Islanders (API) are projected to increase from 4 to 11 percent of the U.S. population. In 2000, Filipinos composed the second largest group (20 percent) of API after Chinese Americans. The majority of Filipino Americans reside in the states of California, Hawaii, Illinois, New Jersey, New York, Washington, and Texas. Filipinos composed the second largest foreign-born population after Mexicans in the United States (Reeves & Bennett, 2004).

REASONS FOR MIGRATION AND ASSOCIATED ECONOMIC FACTORS

The first Filipinos in North America were part of the labor force in Spanish galleons who settled in Louisiana as early as 1753. Filipino immigration to the United States began in 1902, when the Philippines became an American territory. Most of the first groups of migrants were U.S.-sponsored students who completed their college education and then returned to the Philippines. From 1909 until the 1920s, male Filipino laborers were recruited to work on Hawaiian plantations and businesses on the West Coast. These early migrants were ineligible for citizenship and were denied privileges such as employment requiring citizenship, union membership, the right to own land, and the right to marry in states with antimiscegenation laws. The Depression heightened racial animosity toward Filipino workers, and passage of the Tydings-McDuffie Act (Philippines Independence Act) in 1934 virtually ended immigration (Ceniza-Choy, 2003).

In 1946, immigration restrictions for Filipinos were eased and they were granted naturalization rights. Between 1946 and 1965, 33,000 immigrants entered the United States and contributed to a 44 percent increase in the Filipino population in America. The Immigration Act of 1965 initiated a period of renewed mass immigration by promoting family reunification and recruitment of occupational immigrants. Since the passage of the 1965 Act, the Philippines has become the largest source of immigrants from Asia. The post-1965 Filipino immigration consisted of two distinct chains—one deriving from Filipinos who entered the United States before 1965 and the other from the flow of highly trained personnel who began immigration in the 1960s (Espiritu, 2003). A search for better economic and educational opportunities and reunification with family members in the United States continue to be the primary motivating factors for emigration. Working adult children sponsor their older relatives to come to the United States to care for their young children. In turn, older people facilitate the subsequent immigration of other children.

Because the Philippine economy has been unable to provide jobs for college graduates, an estimated 6 million Filipino professionals work overseas and as many as 300,000 Filipinos emigrated in 2006. Export of professional and skilled labor is one of the biggest industries in the Philippines. Remittances sent home by Filipinos overseas contributes as much as 10 percent to the country's gross domestic product, estimated at between 11 and 13 billion pesos in 2006 (IBON Foundation, 2007).

EDUCATIONAL STATUS AND OCCUPATIONS

In the 1900s, Americans introduced public education in the Philippines. Early training of schoolteachers was provided by the Thomasites, forerunners of the U.S. Peace Corps. The development of educational programs in the Philippines was highly influenced and patterned after those in the United States, as in the case of nursing and medicine. Early missionaries and philanthropic organizations such as the Daughters of the American Revolution, the Catholic Scholarship Fund, and the

Rockefeller Foundation were instrumental in the Westernization of health-care education and practice in the Philippines. American nursing educators went to the Philippines, and Filipino nurses were sent to the United States for training. They subsequently returned to the Philippines and assumed leadership positions in nursing schools and hospitals. Since 1970, all nursing curricula have converted to a 4-year degree program leading toward a BSN (Pacquiao, 2004).

The Philippines has one of the highest literacy rates in Asia (96 percent) and is the third largest English-speaking country after the United States and the United Kingdom (Tatak Pilipino, 2003). Schools are either publicly or privately funded. Formal education starts at the age of 7 years, with 6 years of primary education. Nursery school and kindergarten are offered in most private schools. Students get 4 years of secondary education, in either a vocational-technical or an academic school. A high school graduate is 2 years younger than those graduating from U.S. high schools because of the omission of middle school years.

Filipinos view educational achievement as a pathway to economic success, status, and prestige for the individual and the family. A person's profession is always identified when introducing, addressing, or writing about the person (e.g., Doctor Magpantay or Engineer Paredes). A family's status in the community is enhanced by the educational achievement of the children, and a child's education is considered an investment for the whole family. Both male and female children are expected to do well in school, and parents do their best to provide for their children's full-time education. Adolescents who closely identify with their families are found to be concerned with the potential effect of their scholastic achievement on their families' reputation (Salazar, Schuldermann, Schuldermann, & Hunyh, 2000). Family members and other relatives commonly contribute toward the education of their kin. Among lower and middle-class families, siblings take turns going to college in order to maximize resources for one member to finish school, who can then contribute to the education of her or his siblings. One's choice of profession is generally a family decision and is based on potential economic return to the group. Hence, increased demand for nurses abroad attracts higher enrollment in nursing, as families view this occupation as a pathway to economic improvement.

Filipino immigrants since 1965 have had relatively high educational attainment, a high level of labor participation, particularly among women, a high percentage of working professionals, and a low rate of poverty. However, there is a growing concern with the increasing dropout rate among members of the younger generation. Filipino adolescents identified reasons for dropping out of school as intense parental pressure to succeed, fear of not meeting parental expectations, predominance of parental wishes over their own choices, inability to seek support from parents for failures in school, differential parental expectations and attitudes toward their sons and daughters, and experienced tension between assimilation and racism in the outside society (Wolf, 1997).

Filipinos appear to be assimilated and successful and tend to blend into American society, which gives them a reputation as a "model minority." In reality, high educational attainment of American-born and immigrant Filipinos does not guarantee their entry into well-paying or high-status jobs. Significant discrimination confronts native-born and immigrant Filipinos in the American labor market linked with factors such as gender, region of residence, and level of education (Yamane, 2002). As is the experience of many foreign graduates, Filipinos' education and experience are rarely matched with a suitable job because of the restricted labor market, resulting in many individuals competing for low-level jobs for which many are overqualified. Only those who are educated in health-care fields tend to find jobs consistent with their education.

Whereas American nursing education stresses the process of thinking, in the Philippines, mastery of facts and rote learning are emphasized. A defined hierarchy exists in schools, with the teacher as the expert authority. This hierarchy is congruent with the social organization in the broader society, in which age and position are permanent markers of status and power. The younger generations are rewarded for accepting the ideas and counsel of older people and teachers. Challenging authority and asserting one's creative ideas are unnatural predispositions, especially for the young. Nursing faculty have identified the tendency of Filipino students to take things at face value, avoid conflict, communicate nonassertively, and learn by rote memorization. Students' traditional values at home were in conflict with values in school and teacher expectations (Pacquiao, 1996). Facilitating understanding of the dominant cultural values and norms in school, in addition to teaching the subject matter, is essential to facilitate these students' academic success.

Communication

DOMINANT LANGUAGE AND DIALECTS

Over 100 dialects are spoken in the Philippines; the 8 major dialects are Tagalog, Cebuano, Ilocano, Ilonggo, Bicolano, Waray, Pampango, and Pangasinenses. Most Filipinos speak the national language, Filipino, which is based on Tagalog (Tatak Pilipino, 2003). English is used for business and legal transactions, and in school instruction beyond the third grade. Business and social interactions commonly use a hybrid of both Tagalog and English (Tag-Lish) in the same sentence. Tag-Lish is often used in health education.

Many Spanish words are found in the Filipino language such as *sopa* (soup), *calle* (street), *hija/hijo* (daughter/son), and *respeto* (respect). The influence of indigenous Filipino and Spanish languages produces distinct characteristics when Filipinos speak English. There is absence of certain sounds in the Filipino language such as short *i*, long *a*, and long *o*. Hence, *liver* may be enunciated as *lever*, *make* as *mik*, and *flow* as *flaw*. Many Filipinos are unable to differentiate *s* from *sh* (*physiology* as *fishiology*), *u* from short *o* or short *a* sounds (*cut* as *cot* or *cat*; *church* as *charts*). They have a tendency to place emphasis on the second syllable of a multisyllabic word (in ter'fe rence, pen ni'cill in, ro bi'tus sin).

Filipino social hierarchy is evident in the language. Specific nouns rather than pronouns are used to denote a person's age, gender, and position in the social hierarchy. For instance, *Manang* and *Manong* are used to refer to or address an older woman and man, respectively. These nouns are used to address the person or when speaking about her or him. There is absence of the "she/he" in the Filipino language. Rather, generic and gender-neutral pronouns *siya* (singular "she/he") and *sila* (plural "they/them") are used. Hence, many Filipinos may unconsciously use "she" and "he" interchangeably in reference to the same individual.

Although many Filipinos speak English, their ethnic language or dialect, knowledge and use of the English language, and age of migration to the United States often influence enunciation, pronunciation, and accentuation. Older Filipinos who originated from non–Tagalog-speaking regions may understand and speak better English than other Filipinos. In multigenerational Filipino American families, different languages may be used to communicate with family members and friends. Although many Filipinos speak and write fluently in English, they may have difficulty understanding American idiomatic expressions. For example, to a new immigrant, "How are you?" may be interpreted as a question about the person's well-being, requiring an elaboration of one's situation, rather than a mere greeting. Filipinos may have difficulty communicating their lack of understanding to others and may use ritualistic language and euphemistic behavior that appears to be the opposite of how they actually perceive the situation. Saving face, or concealment (Pasco, Morse, & Olson, 2004), is a characteristic pattern of behavior employed to protect the integrity of both parties, which is a consequence of the cultural value on maintaining smooth interpersonal relations. Desirous of group approval, the individual becomes sensitive to the feelings of others and, in turn, develops a high sense of sensitivity to personal insults.

Traditional Filipino communication is highly contextual. The individual is enculturated to attend to the context of the interaction and to adopt appropriate behaviors. Many Filipinos are keenly observant, displaying an intuitive feeling about the other person and the contextual environment during interactions. Contextual variables include the presence of **ibang tao** (outsiders) versus **hindi ibang tao** (insiders) and the age, social position, and gender of the other individual. In the company of insiders, such as one's family, each member develops an intuitive knowledge of the other so that words are unnecessary to convey a message, and meanings are embedded in nonverbal communication. In the presence of outsiders, a child's emotional outburst may be met with adults' stern silence, indifference, or euphemistic grins. These behaviors imply to insiders that emotional outbursts are inappropriate in front of outsiders. One may not disagree, talk loudly, or look directly at a person who is older and who occupies a higher position in the social hierarchy. Honorific terms of address denoting an individual's status within the hierarchy exist in all dialects. In Tagalog, when communicating to an older person or a person of status, he or she is addressed using gender and age-specific honorific nouns such as *Lolo/Lola* (Grandpa/Grandma), and *ate*/kuya (older sister/older brother). Prefixes such as Mr., Mrs., Miss, or Ms.

or the professional title of the person is used in formal interactions.

Filipino interpersonal and social life operates to maintain smooth interpersonal relationships; communication tends to be indirect and ambiguous to prevent the risk of offending others. Filipinos may sacrifice clear communication to avoid stressful interpersonal conflicts and confrontations. As saying no to a superior is considered disrespectful, it predisposes an individual to make an ambiguous positive response. Filipinos are often puzzled, and sometimes offended, by the precision and exactness of American communication. Newly recruited Filipino nurses are stunned by their American coworkers' abrasiveness and open expressions of anger toward each other and their subsequent behavior of sitting down at coffee "as if nothing happened." To many traditional Filipinos, actions speak louder than words. They value respect and might find questions like "Do you understand?" or "Do you follow?" disrespectful. It is preferable for the speaker to say, "Please, let me know if I understood you correctly." When speakers occupy different positions in the social hierarchy, an informal and familiar manner of speaking by the subordinate may be perceived as impolite and disrespectful. Allowing time for a Filipino to respond not only communicates respect but also gives time for translating the dialect into English. Speaking clearly and slowly facilitates appreciation of varying pronunciation and accentuation of the English language across cultures.

CULTURAL COMMUNICATION PATTERNS

Relational orientation has been suggested as the essence of Asian social psychology. Enriquez (1994) posited that the Filipino core values of shame (**hiya**), yielding to the leader or majority (**pakikisama**), gratitude (**utang na loob**), and sensitivity to personal affront (**amor propio**) emphasize a strong sense of human relatedness. These values originate from the central concept of **kapwa**, which arises from the awareness of shared identity with others. *Kapwa* embraces the insider-outsider categories of human relations and prescribes different levels of interrelatedness or involvement with others. **Pakakikipagkapwa** ("being one with others") implies accepting and dealing with the other individual as a fellow human being. *Kapwa* is grounded in the fundamental value of shared inner perception or feeling for another, from which all other attributes for human relations are made possible.

Eight levels of social interactions were identified by Enriquez within the core concept of *kapwa*. These levels demonstrate a hierarchy of human relatedness within the Filipino language and context of meanings. The contextual axis of interactions is conceptualized within a continuum of how the "other" is categorized—whether as an insider or outsider. The degree of sharing and involvement with outsiders may progress from levels 1 to 5, whereas interactions at levels 6 to 8 are observed with insiders. The eight levels are *pakikitungo* (civility, level 1), *pakikisalimuha* (interacting, level 2), *pakikihalok* (participating, level 3), *pakikibagay* (conforming, level 4), *pakikisama* (adjusting, level 5), *pakikipagpalagayang loob* (understanding and accepting, level 6), *pakikisangkot* (getting involved, level 7), and *pakikiisa* (being one with, level 8).

Developing working relationships with Filipinos requires understanding of where one is situated within the insider-outsider continuum. Outsiders can move toward higher levels of interactions by observing cultural norms of communication, using trusted gatekeepers to mediate conflicts, seeking validation of perceptions of behaviors from more acculturated members of the group, and allowing face-saving opportunities to prevent embarrassment and personal denigration. When confronting a Filipino coworker, provide privacy and point out positive attributes as well as the problem. Observing nonverbal behaviors and interpreting them within the Filipino cultural context promotes culturally congruent interactions. Accommodating differential sharing and involvement between insiders and with outsiders shows cultural understanding that enhances development of intercultural relationships. For example, a Filipino speaking Tagalog with another reinforces the value of being one with others. Learning and using some Filipino greetings and honorific terms of address facilitate movement of the relationship to higher levels of involvement. Defining work situations in which Filipino dialects may be spoken demonstrates cultural sensitivity and accommodation. The insider and outsider delineations may be less important to some Filipinos who are highly educated and take pride in their global outlook. Unlike other immigrants who settle in ethnic enclaves, more recent Filipino immigrants acculturate and relate well with people from various cultures.

Smiling and giggling are often observed, especially among young Filipino women. The meanings of these spontaneous and highly unconscious behaviors are embedded in the context of the situation and may range from glee, genuine interest, and agreement to discomfort, politeness, or indifference. It is helpful to point out how the behavior can be misinterpreted by patients and others, if inappropriate to the situation. Behavior change can be expected if correction is done in a timely, respectful, and sincere manner.

Having a heightened sensitivity to personal insults, Filipinos have a remarkable ability to maintain a proper front to protect their self-esteem when threatened. Conflict-avoidance behaviors to conceal discomfort or distress are evident in euphemistic denial of anger, minimization of pain, and silence. However, pent-up emotions and accumulated resentment may result in explosive anger, depression, and somatization. Practitioners should be sensitized to these behaviors and explore the underlying causes by establishing trust and maintaining respectful relationships. Offering pain medications and attending to nonverbal behaviors, rather than waiting for the patient to verbalize his or her needs, are culturally congruent approaches.

First-generation Filipinos in North America have high regard for health-care practitioners (Abe-Kim, Gong, & Takeuchi, 2004) and present themselves in therapy sessions as polite, cooperative, verbal, and engaging. However, agreement with health-care providers does not ensure that clients will follow through with the recommendations. Health-care providers should be comfortable with clients' deferential attitude without resorting to authoritarian approaches, which may be perceived as oppressive and may encourage euphemistic complaint behaviors. Once trust is developed, expression of authentic feelings is possible. Filipinos who are accustomed to indirect communication may perceive focusing on action-oriented strategies and outcomes as intrusive and coercive.

Direct eye contact varies among Filipinos depending on the degree of acculturation, length of time in America, age, and education. Some individuals may avoid prolonged eye contact with authority figures and older people as a form of respect. Older men may refrain from maintaining eye contact with young women because it may be interpreted as flirtation or a sexual advance. Filipinos are comfortable with silence and may allow the other person to initiate verbal interaction as a sign of respect. During a teaching session, a Filipino client's nod may have several meanings that can range from, "Yes, I hear you," "Yes, we are interacting," "Yes, I can see the instructions," or some other message that may be difficult for the client to disclose. Validating a client's response in a sensitive and respectful manner as well as observing her or his behaviors can prevent miscommuniaction.

Touch is used freely, especially with insiders. Greater distance is observed when interacting with outsiders and people in positions of authority. Same-gender closeness and touching, which may be perceived as homosexual adult behavior in America, are considered normal. Young adults of the same gender may hold hands, put one arm over another's shoulder, or walk arm-in-arm. As they become more acculturated, many Filipinos become aware of the differences and adapt to the new culture.

The implicit rules of the social hierarchy are observed when conflicts arise. A subordinate does not confront his or her superiors. Rather, a mediator who is likely to be a trusted individual at the same level of hierarchy as the superior may be employed to mediate and approach the superior on behalf of the subordinate. This behavior may be interpreted as dishonest by Americans who value direct and assertive communication.

VIGNETTE 10.1

Debra Walker, aged 32 years, is a nurse manager in a large Medical-Surgical Unit. She has had a good working relationship with one of the Filipino surgeons, 65-year-old Dr. Amador Mendoza, since they worked together on a project. She considers their relationship as collegial and friendly. She often exchanges stories and jokes with Dr. Mendoza and describes him as "competent, easy to get along with, and has a terrific sense of humor." Debra and Dr. Mendoza attended an administrative meeting to discuss some changes for the unit. Debra remembers this as the last time that Dr. Mendoza was friendly with her. She recalls that at the meeting, she made a joke about what he said. Since then, his behavior toward her has been "cold and formal."

1. How do you explain the change in the doctor's behavior toward the nurse manager?
2. What cultural taboos were violated by the nurse manager?
3. How should the nurse manager deal with the situation?

TEMPORAL RELATIONSHIPS

Filipinos have a relaxed temporal outlook. They have a healthy respect for the past, an ability to enjoy the present, and hope for the future. Past orientation is evident in their respect for older people and dead ancestors (*galang*), and a sense of gratitude and obligation to kin (*utang na loob*). Future orientation is manifested in the family's commitment to provide for the education of the young, parental participation in the care of their children and grandchildren, and a strong work ethic. A strong present orientation is associated with the cultural emphasis on maintaining positive relationships with others. Permanent social bonds with kin and significant others outside of kin are nurtured. Filipinos enjoy their families, fiestas, and life. They spend generously to make family events memorable and enjoyable. Although most Filipinos have adapted to American punctuality in the business sphere, promptness for social events is situationally determined. "Filipino time" means arriving much later than the scheduled appointment, which can be from 1 to several hours. The focus is on the gathering rather than on the schedule. A Filipino host may invite American guests at least 1 hour later than the Filipino guests in the hope that both will arrive at the same time.

Present-time orientation is evident among many Filipino nurses who have difficulty leaving a patient who is upset or when they are in the middle of doing a procedure such as a patient's bed bath. Addressing the present needs of patients, and ensuring smooth relationships with them, may be interpreted by their American coworkers as poor time management and failure to determine work priorities. Newly recruited nurses are distressed by their inability to complete the caretaking tasks that, in their assessment, would clearly please and ensure the comfort of their patients. Differential time orientation between Filipinos and Americans should be made part of job orientations. Defining expressions of these different time orientations can prevent conflicts at work and help provide culturally relevant mentoring.

FORMAT FOR NAMES

The Filipino family is bilineally extended to several generations. Kinship and family affinity can be legally and spiritually claimed equally from both sets of families, giving the child the identity of the extended family. This bilineal kinship is reflected in their names. Children carry the surnames of both parents. For example, Jose Romagos Lopez and Leticia Romagos Lopez are the children of Maria Romagos and Eduardo Lopez. The middle name or initial (R.) is the mother's maiden name, Romagos. After marriage, Jose keeps the same name, whereas his sister's name becomes Leticia L. Lukban (her husband being Ernesto Lukban). Leticia's maiden name, Lopez, is abbreviated as her middle initial.

Many Filipino names are of Spanish origin. Symbolic of Filipinos' Catholic faith, saint names are often used with first names. Filipino females may have a Ma. (for Maria) before their given names: For example, Ma. Luisa stands for Maria Luisa. Although the name Maria is often given to girls, some males may use Maria as a first or second name;

hence, Ma. Jose Romagos Lopez and Jose Ma. Paredes Castro. The saint name is an integral part of the first name; thus, an individual uses both first names, Maria Luisa or Jose Maria. Few Filipino American women keep their own surname after marriage, although this may increase among second- and third-generation Filipinos.

Adults use first names to address young children. Nicknames symbolizing affectionate regard for the person (Nini, Baby, Bongbong) are commonly used instead of the first name. These nicknames may indicate special meanings, positions, and/or outstanding characteristics of the child. First names are avoided when addressing older adults and those occupying higher positions in the hierarchy. In formal business transactions, prefixes such as Mr., Mrs., Miss, or Ms. or the person's professional degree are used before the person's last names (Dr. Abaya or Attorney Abaya).

Family Roles and Organization

HEAD OF HOUSEHOLD AND GENDER ROLES

Since the pre-Spanish era, Filipino women have been held in high regard, having rights equal to those of men (Agoncillo & Guerrero, 1987). In contemporary Filipino families, although the father is the acknowledged head of the household, authority in the family is considered egalitarian. The mother plays an equal, and often major, role in decisions regarding health, children, and finances (Fig. 10–2).

Traditional female roles include caring for the sick and children, maintaining kinship ties, and managing the home. Parents and older siblings are involved in the care and discipline of younger children. In extended family households, older relatives and grandparents share much authority and responsibility for the care and discipline of younger members. Traditional Filipino families may not expect female children to engage in activities that are considered appropriate for men, such as driving, bicycling, and other functions requiring mechanical or technical skills. Blurring of roles between men and women

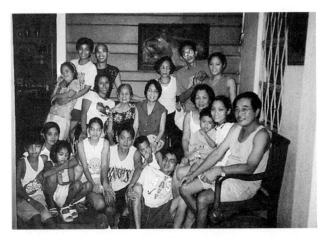

FIGURE 10–2 Members of a Filipino family that is bilaterally extended to three generations. (Photograph by Rowena Legaspi.)

occurs with increased education, urbanization, and emigration to a new culture, as in the United States.

In the United States, Filipino families predominantly consist of married couples with both spouses working. Filipino womanhood has evolved from the Spanish construct of modesty, demureness, and femininity to a contemporary image of a woman who is educated, working, and adept at balancing traditional roles and career demands. Since the 1950s, women represent close to 50 percent of university enrollments and pursue careers in law, medicine, and politics. Traditional Filipino parents expect their male and female children to pursue college education and economically productive careers and also to have a family. Family members and Filipino friends or acquaintances are preferred caregivers of young children when parents are working. Older parents, especially grandmothers, emigrate to the United States in time for the birth of their grandchildren and are expected to take care of them on behalf of their working adult children (Pacquiao, 1993).

PRESCRIPTIVE, RESTRICTIVE, AND TABOO BEHAVIORS FOR CHILDREN AND ADOLESCENTS

The strong in-group consciousness of Filipinos is rooted in the centrality of family and kin, to the exclusion of others, in the socialization of individuals. As the strongest unit of society, the family demands the deepest loyalties and significantly influences an individual's social interactions. Ascriptive and particularistic personal ties with kin are significant in the allocation of rank, authority, and power to individuals. Generational position conditions the status as well as the role performance of individuals. The family and one's familial role define and order authority, rights, obligations, and modes of interaction. Younger generations are taught to be respectful and heed the authority of older siblings and relatives, parents, and grandparents. Respect is manifested in both speech and actions by using honorific terms of address, avoiding confrontation and offensive language, keeping a low tone of voice, greeting older people by kissing their forehead or back of their hand, avoiding direct eye contact when being admonished, offering food, touching, and so forth. Husbands and wives address each other using the honorific terms that they wish to model for their children. In front of the children, a husband will address his wife as *Inay* (mother) and the wife correspondingly refers to her husband as *Itay* (father). Under no circumstance are children permitted to call their parents by their first names. Friends of Filipino children are expected to show respect to adult members of the family when they visit.

Reciprocal obligations among kin are embodied in the value of *utang na loob*, a personal sense of indebtedness and loyalty to kin, which carries an obligation to repay or perform services for one another. Filial respect and obligation for caring for one's parents is the ultimate confluence of generational respect and reciprocal obligation. Childhood socialization to the mechanism of shame (*hiya*) reinforces the value of *utang na loob* and generational respect. Failure to perform or recognize reciprocal obligations, as well as disrespect of older people or people of authority, results in the loss of one's self-esteem and status, as well as incurs shame to one's family.

Children learn early to behave differently toward insiders and outsiders. Private affairs are reserved for close kin and are well guarded from outsiders. Filipino American high school students reported that they were taught to keep problems within the family and that talking to outsiders such as friends, teachers, or counselors would bring shame to the family (Wolf, 1997). Conditions such as mental illness, divorce, terminal illness, criminal offenses, unwanted pregnancy, homosexuality, and HIV/AIDS are not readily shared with outsiders until trust is established. The extent to which a Filipino client may disclose personal information is contextualized. Family presence may act as a barrier to full disclosure of conditions that may be perceived as putting the family at risk for shame.

Dating at an early age is discouraged for young daughters who are advised that a short courtship period may suggest that they are "easy to get." Young men with sincere intent must strive to get on the good side of the family and have patience with a long courtship. Open demonstrations of affection with sexual undertones are to be avoided by the young couple. Ideally, the groom's parents formally ask for the bride's parents' consent for the marriage of their children. Traditional families desire that their daughters remain chaste before marriage. Pregnancy out of wedlock brings shame to the whole family. Modernization and urbanization have changed the social mores in the Philippines; yet, many Filipino American families are still perceived by younger family members as having an overly protective attitude toward children in matters of "hanging out" with friends, dating, and courtship. Girls are subjected to greater limitations than boys, which contributes to higher reports of contemplating suicide by Filipino girls. Studies of second-generation Filipino students in high schools revealed greater parental control over daughters, with more latitude allowed for sons. For many Filipinas, high school achievement was met by parental control over their choice of colleges and pressure to remain close to home and family supervision (Wolf, 1997). Compared with other groups, Filipino American teenagers have the lowest rates of teen pregnancy (U.S. Bureau of the Census, 2002).

FAMILY GOALS AND PRIORITIES

The Filipino family is extended bilineally to several generations with a clear structure and network of relationships. In addition to blood relatives, fictive kinship is established through the *compadrazgo* system in which friends and associates are invited to become godparents or surrogate parents in religious ceremonies, such as baptism and marriage. Fictive kinship is a significant support system for Filipino Americans who left families or relatives in the home country. In times of illness, the extended family provides support and assistance. Sometimes, a family visit to the hospital takes on the semblance of a family reunion.

The family is the basic social and economic unit of Filipino kinship. Family relations strongly influence individual decisions and actions. Relatives and family constitute the reference group for individuals, determining their behavior as well as that of their relatives in any social exchange. Family loyalties and obligations supersede individual interests and residential migration. This is evident in migration patterns of adult children and aged parents, which are planned to maximize the economic welfare and support for group members.

Family emphasis on communal values and generational respect is highly institutionalized. Community activities generally center on the family. Fiestas, weddings, baptisms, illnesses, and funerals are occasions for reinvigorating relations with kin and rekindling local connections, in which the presence and, more importantly, the absence of relatives are viewed as highly significant. Early child-rearing practices are permissive, with emphasis on providing an emotionally secure environment for the child. Priority is placed on promoting the child's well-being and social acceptance. The child is introduced early into various mechanisms designed to impose compliance with family values. A family's prestige is measured by the upbringing of their children, judged by their adherence to traditional cultural values.

The family emphasis on faithfulness to religious obligations is tied with the cultural values of generational respect and reciprocal obligation. Child-rearing practices stress entire family participation in the religious education and adherence to rituals by young members. Older generations share the responsibility for reinforcing these values. Religious sacraments, such as marriage, are embedded in the age-grading activities of the extended family (Fig. 10–3).

As the basic economic unit of society, the family defines the economic obligations of kin to each other. Interdependence within and across generations is fostered. Children are looked upon as economic assets and as sources of support for parents in old age. Thus, educating young members becomes a family priority. The socioeconomic status of the aged is closely linked with the family's wealth; if resources are limited, older people rely on children and relatives. Older parents and grandparents are integrated within the family, thus lessening the impact of advancing age. Traditional Filipinos consider institution-

alization of aged parents tantamount to abandonment of filial obligation and respect for older people. Many older people aspire to return to the Philippines to spend their remaining years with loving kin.

The development of **pakiramdam** (shared perception) and **kapwa** (shared identity) is the defining goal of the family. Group cohesiveness, loyalty, and faithfulness to shared obligation are expectations that transcend distant migration, marriage, and adulthood. Significant evidence exists for the concept of shared perception and identity among Filipinos. Students who feel obligated to maintain their family's reputations believe that effort and interest, rather than ability, can result in school success (Salazar et al., 2000). Filipino American older people have reported experiencing conflict between the maintenance of family obligations, such as babysitting for their grandchildren, and their desire to be more independent from their adult children. Family obligations may result in their inability to meet medical appointments, obtain needed medications, and make meaningful social connections because of lack of independent transportation. Depression has been associated with loneliness, feelings of isolation, and financial difficulty (McBride & Parreno, 1996). Older Filipino Americans identified integration in the family of their adult children, participation in community activities with family and close friends, and maintaining religious functions as highly important (Pacquiao, 1993).

The family provides primary support during illness. It is common to mobilize the extended family support system from the Philippines and in many parts of the United States to care for ailing family members. Many Filipinos believe that mental illness brings a stigma to the individual and the family; hence, support will likely come from family members. This is evident in the underutilization of mental health services and presentation of advanced symptoms by the patient on hospital admission. Among Filipino Americans, religiosity was correlated with seeking help from the religious clergy whereas spirituality was associated with less help-seeking from professional mental health practitioners (Abe-Kim et al., 2004). The first choice is caring by family members, friends, and relatives rather than seeking health professionals (Gong, Gage, & Tacata, 2003).

Diversity exists in the degree to which Filipino Americans adhere to the traditional cultural values. Some middle-aged immigrant Filipino parents do not expect to live with their children in old age. Diversity in family member roles and priorities exists as a result of the financial resources of the family. Reciprocal obligations with kin are expressed differentially based on the capacity of older people and adult children to meet them and include economic, physical, emotional, and social support dimensions.

ALTERNATIVE LIFESTYLES

Traditional Filipino parents seldom provide sex education, and sex is not discussed openly at home. Homosexuality may be recognized and considered an aberrant behavior, but it is not openly practiced in order to save face and prevent shame for the family. In recent

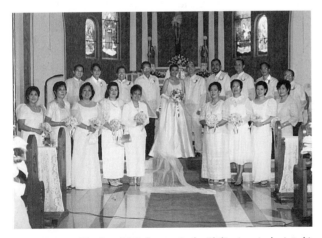

FIGURE 10–3 The Spanish influence in the Philippines is depicted in this Roman Catholic wedding featuring godparents as an important part of fictive kinship development for the couple and their families. (Photograph by Rowena Legaspi.)

years, younger gay, lesbian, bisexual, and transgender Filipinos in the Philippines and in the United States are taking a more active role in being recognized and expressing their rights.

Although the tenets of the Catholic Church have a direct bearing on sexual mores for older generations of Filipinos, they have less influence on younger generations, as is seen in the high incidence of HIV/AIDS among Filipino compared with that of other API. The family may not be the primary source of support for individuals, who may be isolated to prevent stigma to the family. The nuclear family may protect the affected member from outsiders and intentionally remove them from a network of friends and extended family. Providing an atmosphere that fosters the much-needed sense of belonging should be the goal of culturally congruent services.

Divorce can carry a stigma for older and more traditional Filipinos, especially those who are devout Catholics. The stigma may be worse for Filipinos in the Philippines for whom divorces are not allowed and are considered a religious taboo. Divorces among Filipino Americans generally result from failed marital duties, lack of mutual support between partners, and marital infidelity.

Workforce Issues

CULTURE IN THE WORKFORCE

The history of white colonization of the Philippines may influence perceptions of workplace experiences. Experience with racism is a continuing theme voiced by Filipino nurses working with white American nurses (Spangler, 1992). Among Filipino American women nurses and nurses aides, longer residence in the United States was associated with increased stress, evidenced by higher levels of serum norepinephrine, and higher diastolic pressure and lower dips in blood pressure readings during sleep (Brown & James, 2000). The recent business model used in recruiting nurses from the Philippines has removed some of the benevolent provisions for prolonged supportive training that were available to those nurses under the Exchange Visitors Program. The requirement by the American Nurses Association for equal pay for the same job transformed foreign nurse recruitment into a competitive enterprise, in which employers and existing staff expected recruited nurses to be functionally competent on the job as soon as they received their American RN license because they will receive pay comparable with that of other RNs. In reality, providing transitional support for foreign nurses requires a significant commitment of time and financial investment and a prolonged acculturation process (Pacquiao, 2004).

Filipino nurses have been recruited in large numbers to staff mostly evening and night shifts in which acute shortages of American trained nurses exist. This has reinforced the cultural tendency toward collective solidarity by defining the context of interactions within the insider-outsider continuum. Frequent entry of large numbers of new recruits into the same setting has reduced the number of cultural mentors who can help facilitate these nurses' acculturation to the organization and the cultural norms of the society at large. American nurses and administrators of health organizations with large contingents of Filipino nurses are becoming aware of the need for special knowledge and skills in understanding and managing a diverse workforce and in developing culturally specific staff development programs.

Cultural conflicts in the workplace stem from different communication patterns: the dominant norm of assertiveness versus the highly contextual Filipino communication. The cultural concept of shared identity with other Filipinos creates a propensity among Filipino nurses to speak in their own dialect with each other to the exclusion of non-Filipino coworkers and patients. Lack of fluency in speaking and enunciating English words results in anxiety when interacting with outsiders. Nonsupportive reactions from patients and coworkers discourage attempts to speak more English. Assertive communication is difficult for Filipinos, who have been enculturated to avoid conflict. Filipino nurses may consider it impolite and disrespectful to confront or challenge the authority of a superior. When a problem with a manager occurs, a Filipino nurse may communicate through a mediator, usually another Filipino nurse, who is in the same level within the hierarchy as the manager. Communicating disagreement with a physician is difficult for many Filipino nurses. Conversely, Filipino registered nurses expect their subordinates to be deferential toward them.

Conflict can result from different cultural values about caring. Coming from a highly collective orientation, Filipinos define caring in terms of active caring for others. This perspective differs from the American value of self-care. Filipino nurses feel comfortable performing what they perceive as caring tasks for patients that American nurses expect patients to do for themselves. Initially, they may not be inclined to teach and demonstrate procedures to patients because of their traditional belief in doing the caring tasks for patients. Outsiders may misconstrue Filipino nurses' preoccupation with caring tasks as disorganization or lack of assertiveness.

Different views about a valued coworker may be another source of conflict. The Filipino values of shared perception and being one with others create a cooperative, rather than a competitive, outlook. A valued individual produces for the group and puts the group above her or his own personal gain. Humility, hard work, loyalty, and generosity are admired. The business-like and competitive perspectives of Americans, in which behavior is internally motivated by individual gain, may be interpreted as selfish and uncaring. Self-proclamations of accomplishments are viewed as cocky and offensive. Instead, it is up to the group to recognize a member's achievement, which is assessed in terms of how the action benefited the group.

Health-care organizations are cultural entities defined by norms that reflect the dominant values of the host society. Professional schools mirror these dominant societal norms, which are congruent with those of health-care organizations. Among outsiders to the dominant American culture, the experience in nursing schools and health-care organizations is dissonant with previous life experiences, which require an understanding of both cultural and occupational role differences. Bicultural development of Filipino and non-Filipino staff should be the goal of occupational orientation and training. Biculturalism requires awareness of self and others and the ability to adapt behaviors that build positive relationships with others who may be different from oneself (Pacquiao, 2003). Understanding cultural differences and similarities allows for the development of intercultural understanding and skills that promote teamwork. Bicultural mentors who can teach cultural norms of the organization and work with diverse patients and staff will foster the individual's ability to adapt behaviors. Staff development requires training in frame switching—using different frameworks to understand behaviors of others and commitment to the belief that other perspectives are equally sound in explaining our experiences. Impression management is a bicultural skill that is grounded in the ability to interpret behaviors of others within their own cultural context and manifest behaviors that promote relationship and intercultural understanding (Pacquiao, 2001).

ISSUES RELATED TO AUTONOMY

A core Filipino cultural concept is **bahala na**, which consists of the belief and predisposition to trust the Divine Providence and social hierarchy to resolve problems. Filipinos may avoid taking an active role in managing problems because of their fatalistic belief that a "greater power" will prevail. Outsiders may interpret this behavior as a lack of initiative or responsibility. Many Filipino nurses are hesitant to assume leadership roles and assert their points of view, especially with outsiders. After an initial effort, further attempts to resolve the problem are generally left to the leader or hierarchy. Providing support and role modeling help these nurses assert themselves and feel confident in problem solving and conflict resolution. Filipinos are proud people who place importance on maintaining self-esteem and dignity by saving face and avoiding shame. Their sensitivity and attention to other people's feelings are often exhibited as indecisiveness, which many Americans interpret as lack of assertiveness.

Filipinos may achieve power and prestige by acquiring wealth, education, and a distinguished position or by age and through marriage. Although this value has weakened among younger Filipinos, respect for older people and those in positions of power is firmly entrenched among most Filipinos, who are taught not to show open disagreement. Loquacious Americans who uphold egalitarianism and candid expression of feelings and ideas are perplexed by the Filipino deference to authority. Less-acculturated Filipinos may not understand the directness of Americans and, thus, may find it insulting. European American nurses saw the quiet, observant, tactful, patient, and slow-to-respond behaviors of Filipino nurses as unassertive (Spangler, 1992). By contrast, Filipino nurses saw outspoken, impatient, bold, and fast-moving behaviors of European American nurses as crass and insensitive. A Filipino may say "yes" to avoid hurting other people's feelings. Such response should be examined in context to interpret its true meaning.

The Filipino hierarchy and emphasis on collectivity brings a consequent group-oriented sense of responsibility and accountability. The leader is respected, followed, and expected to make decisions on behalf of members. The leader is trusted to act in the best interests of the group. The concept of individual accountability and responsibility in a highly litigious society, such as the United States, may initially be difficult for Filipino nurses to understand. Supportive role modeling in assuming individual accountability is important for Filipino-educated nurses.

Biocultural Ecology

SKIN COLOR AND OTHER BIOLOGICAL VARIATIONS

Variations in anthropomorphic, physical, and biophysiological characteristics of Filipinos exist as a result of ethnocultural and racial intermingling. One of the Filipino aboriginal tribes, the Aeta, is negroid and petite in stature. They are believed to have migrated from Africa through land bridges during the Ice Age. However, like other tribal groups in the Philippines, they are now a minority.

The typical native-born or immigrant Filipino may be of Malay stock (brown complexion) with a multiracial genetic background. Intermarriage of Filipinos with other ethnic and racial groups occurs in many communities across the world. In clinical assessments, a family genogram identifying ethnic or racial blending is useful in tracking predisposition to genetic disorders.

The youthful features of Filipinos make it difficult to assess their age. Common Filipino physical features may include jet black to brunette or light brown hair, dark to light brown pupils with eyes set in almond-shaped eyelids, deep brown to very light tan skin tones, and mildly flared nostrils and slightly low to flat nose bridges. The eye structure may challenge health-care providers in assessment such as observing pupillary reactions for increased intracranial pressure, measuring ocular tension, and evaluating peripheral vision. The flat nose bridge may be overlooked by opticians when fitting and dispensing eyeglasses.

The high-melanin content of the skin and mucosa may pose problems when assessing signs of jaundice, cyanosis, and pallor. This feature also poses difficulty in diagnosing retinal, gum-related, and oral tissue abnormalities. When performing skin assessments, practitioners should consider the complexion and skin tone of the Filipino client. The usual manifestations of anemia (pallor and jaundice) should be assessed in the conjunctiva. Newborns may have mongolian spots (bluish-green discolorations on the buttocks) that are physiological and eventually disappear.

Filipinos range in height from under 5 feet to the height of average Americans. Body weight varies according to nativity and other factors such as nutrition, physical activity, and heredity. Filipinos commonly gain weight when they come to the United States. There are no definitive studies relating nutrition with standard height and weight measures for this population; therefore, it is essential to assess for weight changes on an individual basis.

Filipinos have a small thoracic capacity. Approximately 40 percent have blood type B and a low incidence of the Rh-negative factor (Anderson, 1983). As more interracial families emerge in Filipino communities, changes in their serologic profile will likely occur.

DISEASES AND HEALTH CONDITIONS

Compared with other Asians, Filipino men and women have the highest prevalence of hypertension characterized by sodium sensitivity (Garde, Spangler, & Miranda, 1994). High incidence of hyperuricemia is attributed to a shift from a Filipino to an American diet (McBride, Mariola, & Yeo, 1995). Liver cancer tends to be diagnosed in the late stages of the disease and appears to be associated with the presence of the hepatitis B virus. Silent carriers of the virus are common among Asians, and its presence is detected only when other problems are being evaluated. Health-care providers should routinely screen for hepatitis B virus, especially among recent immigrants. A high incidence of glucose-6-phosphate dehydrogenase (G-6-PD), thalassemias, and lactose intolerance and malabsorption exist among the Filipino population (Anderson, 1983).

Compared with other API and white males, Filipinos are more likely to be diagnosed with advanced-stage colorectal and prostatic cancer. They have the worst survival rates from these cancers (Lim, Clarke, Prehn, Glaser, West, & O'Malley, 2002). Like other API, Filipinos underuse cancer screening tests (Kagawa-Singer & Pourat, 2000). Filipino Americans are at increased risk for type 2 diabetes and have higher visceral adipose tissue (VAT) than whites and African Americans (Araneta & Barrett-Connor, 2005). The three leading causes of mortality among Filipino Americans are cardiovascular disorders followed by stroke and cancer.

Some of the goals of *Healthy People 2010* pertaining to Filipino Americans include (1) reducing overall death rates from cancer (particularly of the breast, cervix, and uterus), coronary disease, and diabetes; (2) reducing the incidence of tuberculosis and diabetes; (3) increasing counseling on tobacco use cessation, physical activity, cancer screening, and adult and adolescent HIV/AIDS prevention; (4) increasing early and adequate prenatal care and reducing rates of low birth weight and gestational diabetes; (5) increasing control of blood pressure among those with hypertension; and (6) decreasing mean cholesterol and low-density-lipoprotein (LDL) levels (Ghosh, 2003).

Lack of insurance, low income, and limited access to care were found to have a significant impact on API's use of health services (Coughlan & Uhler, 2000; Yu, Huang, & Singh, 2004). A Canadian study using the 2001 Community Health Survey revealed that minorities, including Filipinos, were less likely to be admitted in the hospital, tested for prostate-specific antigen (PSA), or given a mammogram or Pap test, despite the fact that they had more contact with a general practitioner than white Canadians (Quan et al., 2006). Among older Filipinas, length of residence in the United States and having had a check-up when no symptoms were present were associated with adherence to cancer screening (Maxwell, Bastani, & Warda, 2000).

Compared with white Americans, Filipinos have higher levels of depression. In contrast, strong ethnic identity characterized by sense of ethnic pride, involvement in ethnic practices, and cultural commitment to one's racial and ethnic identity were significant factors in mitigating depressive symptoms among Filipino Americans (Mossakowski, 2003). Strong bonds with members of the community and access to culturally congruent health services promoted commitment of older Filipinas to planned physical activity (Maxwell, Bastani, Vida, & Warda, 2002).

Although Filipino Americans' experiences with unfair treatment were associated with increased illness, instrumental social support and the city of residence buffered the negative effects of these experiences (Gee et al., 2006). Among Filipina caregivers, significant correlations were found among role stress and overall health, role integration and perceived health, and role satisfaction and psychological well-being (Jones, Jaceldo, Lee, Zhang, & Meleis, 2001).

VARIATIONS IN DRUG METABOLISM

Compared with white Americans, Asians require lower doses of central nervous system depressants such as haloperidol, have a lower tolerance for alcohol, and are more sensitive to adverse effects of alcohol (Levy, 1993). Owing to the sodium-sensitive nature of hypertension affecting Filipinos and the high-sodium content of their diet, use of diuretics should be considered. Culturally congruent stress management in addition to dietary modifications and physical activity should be included in the treatment plan to control high blood pressure.

Because of availability of over-the-counter antibiotics and lack of adequate medical monitoring of these drugs in the Philippines, Filipino immigrants may be insensitive to the effects of some anti-infectives. A positive reaction to tuberculin or the Mantoux test is observed because of the practice of giving bacille Calmette-Guérin (BCG) vaccinations in childhood. Chest x-rays and sputum cultures are recommended for screening and diagnosis of tuberculosis. More research is needed to determine pharmacodynamics among Filipinos, including gender differences. Health-care providers need to assess Filipino clients individually when administering and monitoring medication effects.

High-Risk Behaviors

Gender differences are evident in the Filipino tolerance and acceptance of high-risk health behaviors related to alcohol, drugs, cigarettes, and safe sex, with higher incidences in men than in women. More Filipino men than women are heavy drinkers. Most Filipino Americans report drinking socially, with a small number reporting having three or more drinks per day (Garde et al., 1994). Because denial is closely associated with alcoholism, the frequency and amount of alcohol taken are generally underreported.

Cigarette smoking is more prevalent among Filipino men than women. Smoking rates have been positively correlated with lower educational levels and income and a tendency to think or speak in a Filipino language, and for women, being born in the United States. Most Filipino youths reported living with an adult who smoked, and their first substance of choice was cigarettes, followed by alcohol and inhalants.

Filipinos constitute the largest number of reported HIV/AIDS cases among API in the United States (Reeves & Bennett, 2004). Low knowledge scores on information about HIV transmission and unprotected sex with multiple partners underscore the urgency of HIV and AIDS education and prevention.

HEALTH-CARE PRACTICES

Early Filipino immigrants did not seek health care in the United States until the illness was far advanced. Cultural, social, and economic factors were implicated as reasons for their underutilization of health services. Lacking the rights and privileges of naturalized citizens, early Filipino immigrants remained in poverty and felt shunned and rejected as they grew older. Typical of the ethnically underserved, older people in the United States, many were unaware of available services and were reluctant to access social and health services, particularly when culturally sensitive and bilingual providers were unavailable. Lack of transportation, fear of going to the area where services were located, and inappropriate program design were some of the other reasons for low utilization of services by this group. More recent Filipino immigrants differ significantly from their earlier counterparts in their access and utilization of health services. This group is highly educated and accesses many of the health-care services in the United States.

A study of the experiences of Filipino women with breast screening services identified a pattern of avoidance. Factors contributing to this behavior included cultural beliefs, lack of health insurance, and lack of a familiar source of care (Wu & Bancroft, 2006). Some believe that undergoing the test and attempting to know one's condition could tempt faith, which can bring bad luck. Avoidance of an unpleasant diagnosis and concealment of serious illnesses are consequent behaviors of this belief. Many Filipinos seek a familiar and consistent health practitioner who has established a relationship with them. Gender-congruent practitioners are preferred for conditions specific to women's or men's health. Preference for culturally congruent services and practitioners and the presence of supportive social connections increased participation and commitment among older Filipinas for health promotion (Maxwell et al., 2002).

Older Filipinos generally reside in the household of their adult children. Adult children are responsible for the welfare of their own family and aging parents. Older people's access to health services is influenced by the availability of their adult children who are depended upon to provide transportation, facilitate communication between them and the practitioner, and negotiate with health-care practitioners. Filipino women find the competing demands of caregiving for their children, spouses, and older people as barriers to seeking early screening services.

Family support and caring are central to Filipino health practices. Family members take an active role in health promotion and care during illness. Health beliefs and practices are learned from adults and older family members as well as the community. Whereas Filipinos have high regard for health-care practitioners, advice from family members and trusted friends is also heeded. Adherence to recommended interventions is assured by family commitment and presence of a supportive social network that can draw the individual into action.

Nutrition

MEANING OF FOOD

To the Filipino, food is more than nourishment for the body; it is a fundamental form of socialization. Food and meal patterns are integral to the cultural emphasis on generosity, hospitality, and thoughtfulness that support group cohesiveness. No social gathering of Filipinos occurs without food. Food is offered as a token of gratitude and caring, to welcome others, to celebrate accomplishments and important events, to offer support in times of sickness or crisis, and to reinforce social bonds in everyday interactions. Younger family members are socialized into the closeness of the extended family, the community, and family values. Sharing food with others, or at the very least inviting others to share one's food, is expected of Filipinos and considered a sign of good upbringing. The insider versus outsider context influences the choice of food offered (Enriquez, 1994). Outsiders are served Westernized foods, whereas insiders are served native cuisines.

In the Philippines, traditional Filipino meals are labor intensive, requiring participation of several family members. Meats are costly, so small amounts are cut in pieces and expanded using vegetables and starches to feed an entire family. It is common to offer refreshments and beverages or to invite guests to join in the family's meals. All family members, regardless of age, attend social gatherings at which a variety of dishes are prepared to accommodate individual choices. The hosting family serves large amounts of food to accommodate invited guests and those who happen to be around. Guests customarily linger for several meals as the focus is on the gathering. Late-comers are welcomed and expected to fully participate in the entire meal and the company of other guests. Dishes are served all at once from appetizers to desserts so guests are free to eat their courses without waiting for everyone to arrive. Guests are encouraged to return to the table to join arriving guests. Individual servings are not customary as everyone is expected to partake in what is available. More food means more portions for each one and vice versa.

COMMON FOODS AND FOOD RITUALS

Indigenous Filipino cooking is characterized by simplicity of methods such as boiling, steaming, roasting, broiling, marinating, or sour-stewing to preserve the fresh and natural taste of food. Spanish, Chinese, and American influences are integrated into contemporary Filipino cuisine. Foods may be sautéed, fried, or served with a sauce. Because of the tropical climate of the Philippines, many types of plants and animals flourish. Seafood (fish and shellfish) forms the bulk of the Filipino diet. Fresh, dried, and marinated fish are abundant in the diet.

In the Philippines, animal sources of protein are chicken and pork because cows and water buffalo are primarily used for farming. Because protein-rich foods are costly, meals generally consists of larger portions of carbohydrates, primarily rice. Plants are the second most important food source and include a variety of seaweeds, edible roots, delicate leaves, tendrils, tropical fruits, seeds, and some flowers. Fruits and vegetables are consumed in large quantities in a variety of ways. Rice is a staple food and is eaten at every meal, either steamed, fried, or as a dessert. Less-acculturated Filipinos tend to prepare and serve more traditional Filipino foods at home (De la Cruz, Padilla, & Agustin, 2000). Filipino and Asian food stores are abundant in regions where many API reside.

Except for babies and young children, milk is almost absent in the Filipino diet. This may be partly due to lactose intolerance. However, milk in desserts such as egg custard (flan) and ice cream seems to be tolerated. In the Filipino food pyramid, milk and dairy products are incorporated in the major protein groups rather than as a separate category. Dietary calcium is derived from green leafy vegetables and seafood.

Regional variations in food preparation and use of spices exist in Filipino American households today. Nutrition counseling should take into account these variations when a Filipino needs to alter dietary patterns because of hypertension, diabetes, or other health problems. For instance, coconut milk is a common cooking additive among the Bicolanos of southern Luzon. Salty (soy sauce, fish sauce/*patis*, salted shrimp fry, or fermented fish/*bagoong*) and spicy sauces known as *sawsawan* complement meals. These sauces are distinct from the salt added during cooking.

In the Philippines, breakfast consists of rice, meat or fish and vegetable dishes or dinner leftovers. The breakfast beverage may be coffee, chocolate, or juice. In urban areas, Western-style meals are more common. For many Filipinos, breakfast, lunch, and dinner are not complete without steamed or fried rice served with fish, meat (especially pork), and vegetables. Snacks of bananas, yams, rice cake, and rice-flour cake are served as midday snacks, between meals, and before bedtime. The midday meal is the heaviest meal of the day, although this pattern is becoming more difficult among urban dwellers who cannot go home during lunchtime. Filipinos drink water with meals independently or in addition to another beverage of juice, soda, tea, or coffee.

DIETARY PRACTICES FOR HEALTH PROMOTION

Filipinos believe health is maintained by moderation. Although Filipinos enjoy food and love to eat, they adhere to the wisdom that too much of a good thing can be harmful. In some parts of the Philippines, it is considered polite to leave food on one's plate. For many Filipino Americans, moderation in food intake is a special challenge because of the abundance and great variety of quality products at reasonable costs. Significant increases in weight patterns among new immigrants are associated with changes in dietary.

The principle of hot and cold is observed by many traditional Filipinos to promote health. A warm beverage is served first at breakfast after a long evening fast, and hot soups are served as the first course to enhance digestion. Cold drinks may be avoided when one has a cold or fever to restore balance and promote harmony between the body and its environment. Eating rice is considered to be essential to a healthy life. *Arroz caldo,* chicken and rice soup, is generally offered to promote recovery after an illness. Chicken soup with *malunggay* leaves is believed to cleanse the blood.

Garlic and onions are believed to thin the blood and combat hypertension. Ginger root is boiled and served as a beverage to relieve sore throats and promote digestion. Guava shoots are eaten to treat diarrhea. Drinking coconut juice and water from boiled fresh corn silk promotes diuresis. Bitter melon is eaten as a vegetable to prevent diabetes. Greens such as *malunggay* and *ampalaya* leaves are used in stews to regain stamina for someone believed to be anemic or run down.

NUTRITIONAL DEFICIENCIES AND FOOD LIMITATIONS

In the Philippines, nutrition is greatly affected by socioeconomic factors. Malnutrition persists in the country, especially among the poor and less educated, and is one of the leading causes of infant mortality. In the United States, Filipino immigrants may be at risk for nutritional deficiencies during their adjustment period, especially when they come with limited resources and without a support network of family and friends. Postmenopausal and pregnant women may be vulnerable to calcium deficiency owing to lactose intolerance and decreased intake of seafood and green leafy vegetables that were plentiful in the Philippines but limited in availability and variety in American food stores. Changing food patterns and lifestyle is associated with migration and acculturation. Filipino Americans experience similar problems such as obesity, hyperlipidemia, and diabetes seen in the general population. Knowledge of indigenous food sources and meal patterns, nutritional content of foods, changes in nutritional patterns, and accessibility of traditional ingredients is important for nutritional assessment and counseling.

Pregnancy and Childbearing Practices

FERTILITY PRACTICES AND VIEWS TOWARD PREGNANCY

The Roman Catholic Church and Filipino family values significantly influence childbearing and fertility practices. In marriage, the only acceptable method of contraception is the rhythm method. Abortion is considered a sin and is generally not acceptable. Whereas these beliefs remain strong among many Filipinos, education, global communication, and modernization are causing changes, particularly in metropolitan cities such as Manila. Recent Filipino immigrants who come from large urban areas are more educated and less committed to the Church's position on birth control and premarital sex. Between 1990 and 1997, fertility rates in the Philippines declined from 4.1 to 3.7, partly because of increased contraceptive use among married women. Although female sterilization rates remain stable, use of the contraceptive pill has risen. However, there are high rates of discontinuation of contraceptive methods ranging from 14 percent (intrauterine device) to 60 percent (condoms) (National Statistics Office, Philippines, 2005).

Filipino culture is child-centered, and abortion evokes strong reactions, even among liberal Filipinos. Though some may support the right to abortion, they may have difficulty having one themselves and feel guilty for considering this option. Pregnancy is considered normal and is a time when a woman can demand attention and pampering from her husband and family members. Healthcare providers who do not understand this special period for the pregnant Filipino woman may feel that the client is "lazy and spoiled." Pregnancy and childbirth are times for the family to draw closer together. Everyone assists in anticipation of the new baby, especially the pregnant woman's mother, who has a strong influence during this period. For mother and daughter, this is a special event in which the bond between them becomes closer.

In the Filipino American community, women openly give advice to pregnant women, share their own birthing experiences, and ask personal questions that may be considered rather intrusive by outsiders. Elaborate baby showers are hosted by family members and friends, and it is customary to invite male spouses, relatives, and friends as well as children. Male guests do not join in the activities and congregate separately from the women.

PRESCRIPTIVE, RESTRICTIVE, AND TABOO PRACTICES IN THE CHILDBEARING FAMILY

Filipino practices surrounding pregnancy are influenced by indigenous beliefs, Western practices, and socioeconomic factors. In the Philippines, although most mothers (86 percent) receive prenatal care from a doctor, nurse, or midwife, tetanus toxoid immunization is declining. As two-thirds of births are delivered at home, only 56 percent receive assistance at delivery from a doctor, nurse, or midwife and 41 percent are assisted by traditional birth attendants (*hilots*). Local *hilots* employ massage and are consulted for physical, spiritual, and psychological advice and guidance (National Statistics Office, Philippines, 2005).

After childbirth, the new mother continues to be pampered. Relatives help with the new baby and in running the household. Eighty-eight percent of Filipino babies are breastfed for some time, with a median duration of 13 months. However, supplementation of breastfeeding with other liquids and foods occurs too early, with 19 percent of newborns less than 2 months of age receiving supplemental foods or liquids other than water (National Statistics Office, Philippines, 2005). Lactating mothers are encouraged to take plenty of hot soups (chicken with papaya) to promote milk production (Hawaii Community College, 2005).

Some Filipino American women refuse to take vitamins during pregnancy for fear that these could deform the fetus. Some believe that when pregnant women crave certain foods, especially during the first trimester, the craving should be satisfied to avoid harm to the baby. Some women continue to believe that the baby takes on the appearance of the craved food. Thus, if the mother craves dark-skinned fruit or dark-colored food, the infant's skin will be dark. Pregnant women are protected from sudden fright or stress because of the belief that this may harm the developing fetus. Table 10–1 provides a summary of traditional beliefs and practices observed among some Filipinos in Hawaii. Becoming aware of the pregnant Filipino woman's network of family and community health advisers, whose opinions she respects, is important for building trust and rapport in the client-provider relationship.

Some women prefer to have their mothers rather than their husbands in the delivery room. Mothers of pregnant women serve as coaches and teachers and are often respected over health-care professionals for their experience and knowledge. This may be puzzling to professionals who view pregnancy as an emancipating event. Conflicts are likely to occur if the coach and teacher believe in practices that are contrary to Western childbearing practices.

During postpartum, exposure to cold is avoided. Showers are prohibited because these may cause an imbalance and predispose illness. However, the mother is given a sponge bath with aromatic oils and herbs, or a *hilot* gives an aromatic herbal steam bath followed by full body massage, including the abdominal muscles, stimulating a physiological reaction that has both physical and psychological benefits.

Childbirth experiences of Filipino women immigrants in a hospital in Australia revealed language and communication problems as barriers to seeking antenatal care, perceived discrimination by the hospital staff, and conflicting expectations of delivery practices between the mothers and the practitioners. The women preferred to be examined by female practitioners and assume a squatting position for birthing. Contrary to their birthing practices, practitioners expected the husbands to be with them during delivery. The women felt that they were not consulted about their care and preferred to deliver at home (Asian Pacific Islander Maternity Coalition, 2001).

Death Rituals

DEATH RITUALS AND EXPECTATIONS

In the Filipino culture, death is a spiritual event. Illness and death may be attributed to supernatural and magicoreligious causes such as punishment from God, angry spirits, or sorcery. Religiosity and fatalism contribute to stoicism in the face of pain or distress as a way of accepting one's fate (Lipson & Dibble, 2005). Planning for one's death is taboo and may be considered tempting fate.

| **TABLE 10.1** | *Traditional Filipino Beliefs and Practices Surrounding Pregnancy and Childbirth* |

Prenatal	Postpartum
Eating blackberries will make the baby have black spots.	Use warm water to drink and bathe for a month.
Eating black plums will give the baby dark skin.	Don't name the baby before it is born.
Eating twin bananas will result in twin births.	Don't name the baby after a dead person.
Eating apples will give the baby red lips.	Give money to charity or the needy when a baby comes to your house the first time.
When a woman's stomach is not round, the baby will be a boy.	Eating sour or ice-cold foods may cause abdominal cramps.
If a woman's face is blemished, the baby will be a boy.	Wrap the baby's abdomen with a cloth until the umbilical cord falls off.
Going outside during a lunar eclipse is harmful to the baby.	The mother and baby should not go out for a month except to visit a doctor.
Going out in the morning dew is bad for the baby because evil spirits are present.	Putting garlic, salt, or a rosary near the baby's crib will keep evil spirits away.
Funerals are avoided because the spirit of the dead person may affect the baby.	
Wearing necklaces may cause the umbilical cord to wrap around the baby's neck.	
Sitting by a doorway will make the delivery difficult.	
Sitting by a window when it is dark may let evil spirits come to the pregnant woman.	
Sweeping at night may sweep away the good spirits.	
Knitting might tangle the baby's intestines at birth.	

Source: Adapted from http://www.hawcc.Hawaii.edu/nursing/RN/Filipino, 2005

Hence, many traditional Filipinos are averse to discussing advance directives or living wills (Pacquiao, 2001). When death is imminent, contacting a priest is important if the family is Catholic. Religious medallions, rosary beads, scapulars, and religious figures may be found on the patient or at the bedside. Family members generally wish to provide the most intimate care to the patient.

After death, a wake is planned. In the Philippines, the wake may last 3 days or longer to allow time for relatives to arrive from distant places. In the United States, the wake is much shorter because it is costly. Although a wake is generally held in the home in the rural regions, funeral parlors are used in urban areas and in the United States. Families and friends gather to give support and recall the special traits of the deceased. Food is provided to all guests throughout the wake and after the burial.

The burial rites are consistent with the religious traditions of the family, which may be Judeo-Christian, Muslim, Buddhist, or other religions. Among Catholics, 9 days of novenas are held in the home or in the church. These special prayers ask God's blessing for the deceased. Depending upon the economic resources of the family, food and refreshments are served after each prayer day. Sometimes, the last day of the novena takes on the atmosphere of a *fiesta* or a celebration. Filipino families in the United States follow variations of this ritual according to their social and economic circumstances. Funerals in the Philippines can be simple or elaborate, with a band accompaniment, several priests officiating, and a large throng of mourners. Reciprocal obligation continues in death through the performance of rituals such as the wake, novenas, and establishing a burial site acceptable for the entire family.

On the 1-year anniversary of death, family and friends are reunited in prayer to celebrate this memorable event. Most Filipino women wear black clothing for months or up to a year after the death of a spouse or close family member. The 1-year anniversary ends the ritual mourning. Before this period, family members postpone weddings and other celebrations in deference to the memory of the deceased. Memories and love for the deceased are shown on All Soul's Day, a Catholic feast day celebrated in November, when families visit and decorate the graves of their loved ones. Filipino American families may continue these traditions, particularly when strong kinship is present and the clan lives in close proximity. Many who die in the United States are buried in the Philippines, and the family in that country continues the tradition.

Beliefs related to cremation vary according to individual preference. Ordinarily, bodies are buried, but cremation is acceptable to avoid the spread of disease and limit the high costs of burial plots. In America, some Filipinos who wish to return their deceased family members to the Philippines may choose cremation for practical and economic reasons.

RESPONSES TO DEATH AND GRIEF

Most Filipinos believe in life after death. Caring for the spiritual needs of the dying is one way of ensuring peaceful rest of the soul or one's spirit. Family presence around the dying and immediate period after death to pray for the soul of the departed is considered a priority. If the patient is Catholic, the priest anoints the patient and gives Holy Communion if the patient is able to participate. Caring is shown by providing a peaceful environment, speaking in low tones, and praying with the ill person.

After death, grief reaction varies. Women generally show emotions openly by crying, fainting, or wailing. Men are expected to be more stoic and grieve silently. Young children are admonished for behaving inappropriately because this is considered disrespectful to the deceased. Family members gather together and provide physical and emotional support for each other. Praying for the deceased and following the implicit guidelines of behavior during mourning are ways of demonstrating grief appropriately. Wearing black or subdued colors (gray, white, navy, brown), avoiding parties and playing loud, distracting music, postponing weddings, or devoting time to one's studies to honor the dead are some of the acceptable ways of expressing grief. Honoring the memory of the deceased is a continuing obligation among close kin.

Spirituality

DOMINANT RELIGION AND USE OF PRAYER

The Philippines is the only predominantly Christian country in the Far East. In 2000, Roman Catholics accounted for 80.9 percent of the total population. Other religious groups include Muslims (5 percent), other Christians (4.5 percent), Evangelicals (2.8 percent), Iglesia ni Kristo (2.3 percent), Aglipay (2 percent), and others (2.5 percent) (CIA, 2007). The spread of the fundamentalist movement within Roman Catholicism is becoming more evident. Christianity in the Philippines is a blend of Spanish Catholicism, American Christianity, and surviving indigenous animistic traditions (Fig. 10–4).

Although Filipinos seek medical care, they believe that part of the efficacy of a cure is in God's hands or by some mystical power. Novenas and prayers are often said on behalf of the sick person. Families may bring religious items such as rosaries, medals, scapulars, and talismans for the sick person to wear. Talismans and amulets are believed to protect one from the forces of darkness, one's enemies, and sickness. Performance of religious obligations and sacraments and daily prayers are some of the

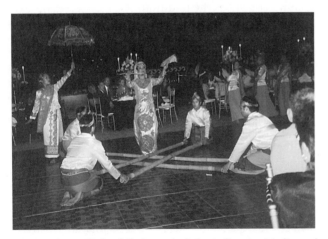

FIGURE 10–4   Filipino folk dance depicting indigenous Muslim and Malayan influences.

ways many Filipinos believe health and peaceful death are achieved. Providing for spiritual needs of Filipino clients requires accommodation to their various ways of practicing beliefs.

MEANING OF LIFE AND INDIVIDUAL SOURCES OF STRENGTH

Filipinos consider a meaningful existence to be a healthy and appropriate relationship with nature, God, and kin. Indigenous Filipino beliefs are embedded in the relationship between humans within the cosmology of the universe. This concept is demonstrated by the integration of supernatural, magicoreligious, and natural phenomena in the belief system and practices toward health and illness. Filipinos do not see themselves as victims, but rather as part of the larger cosmos, subject to both the controllable and the uncontrollable forces of nature. To the traditional Filipino, strength comes from an intimate relationship with God, family, friends, neighbors, and nature. The concept of self is formed from the relationship with a divine being and the social collective.

Many Filipinos find religion a source of strength in their daily lives. Some Filipinos are considered fatalistic in that they tend to accept fate easily, especially when they feel they cannot change a situation. Moreover, the acceptance of fate or destiny comes from their close relationship and healthy respect for nature. The acceptance of events they cannot change is tied to their religious faith. A common expression uttered by Filipinos is *bahala na*, originating from *bathala na* (it is up to God). *Bahala na* is often used when the person has used all resources to deal with a problem, and it is up to a higher power to take care of the rest (Enriquez, 1994). Nevertheless, an element of self-reliance exists among Filipinos, manifested by their confidence that the situation is within their sphere of influence through education and hard work.

SPIRITUAL BELIEFS AND HEALTH-CARE PRACTICES

Holism and integration characterize Filipino health-care beliefs and practices. Religious and spiritual dimensions are important components in health promotion. Belief in harmony between humans and nature and the role of natural and supernatural forces in health and illness are found in their beliefs about causes of illness and healing modalities. Prayers, religious offerings, appeasing natural spirits, and witchcraft may be practiced simultaneously along with biomedical interventions. Despite increasing notoriety and scandal associated with Filipino faith healers, this healing modality is widely sought in the Philippines. Many Filipinos seek biomedical and integrative ways of healing and do not subscribe to the competitive reductionism of the West. They believe in the synergistic relationship of differing modalities and have no problem subscribing to both ways of healing. Many Filipino American health-care professionals participate in religious pilgrimages to Lourdes, France, and the shrine of Fatima in Portugal to pray for good health and healing.

Health-Care Practices

HEALTH-SEEKING BELIEFS AND BEHAVIORS

Filipinos seek out family and close kin first for help when they are ill. When illness is more defined, mobilization of support occurs within the family. Decisions about when, where, and from whom to seek help are largely influenced by the intimate circle of family. Among Filipino older people in the United States, the choice of practitioners is based on accessibility and availability to their working adult children (Pacquiao, 1993). Linguistically and ethnically congruent practitioners are preferred. A dual system of personal health care exists for many Filipinos, including those who are established in American communities. Filipinos may accept and adhere to medical recommendations and may use alternative sources of care suggested by trusted friends and family members. Often, they adhere to Western and indigenous medicine simultaneously, creating more choices to deal with their own or their family's health issues.

Many Filipinos consult an informal network of friends and family members who may be physicians, nurses, pharmacists, or neighbors who have had similar symptoms. Once the person finds the brand name of the "effective" medicine, the person can easily purchase the drug by asking family or friends to purchase medication in the Philippines. Hoarding prescription drugs and sharing medicine may be practiced by Filipinos in the United States. Those who do not believe in wastefulness or who believe that office visits are expensive may practice these behaviors.

When educating Filipino clients about medication, health-care professionals should stress that medications need to be taken as prescribed; medications are ordered specifically for each ailment; unused drugs should be discarded; and the use of medications by individuals other than the intended patient may have serious consequences. Assessing these behaviors and delivering the message in a respectful, courteous, and unhurried manner may enhance the client-provider relationship, especially for traditional Filipino clients.

Health-care practices stress balance and moderation for the Filipino. Health is the result of balance, and illness is the consequence of imbalance. Imbalances that threaten health are brought about by personal irresponsibility or immorality. Care of the body through adequate sleep, rest, nutrition, and exercise is essential for health. A high value is also placed on personal cleanliness. Keeping oneself clean and free of unpleasant body odors is viewed as essential to health and social acceptance. To be slovenly and disorderly is to be shamelessly irresponsible. Aromatic baths are taken both for pleasure and to restore balance.

◉— VIGNETTE 10.2

Alfonso Trinidad, aged 66 years, and his wife Carmen, aged 60 years, moved to the United States to babysit for their young grandchildren. They are devout Catholics. For several years, they lived in the home of their son and daughter-in-law to be near their grandchildren. Once the grandchildren were grown, they moved to the one-bedroom apartment of their youngest daughter, Tessie, who is single.

Recently, Alfonso has been complaining to his wife about persistent low back pain. He also told her that he noted reddish streaks in his stool. He told his wife not to tell Tessie so as not to worry her. He also did not wish to encumber his daughter, who had to take a second job when they moved in with her. He finally requested his daughter to take him to a local Filipino faith healer, who administered several enemas with boiled onions. After a few weeks, the pain increased and Tessie noted that her father was losing weight. She insisted on taking him to the hospital for a checkup. After a diagnosis of colon cancer, Alfonso was operated on immediately. Tessie and her brother have been paying for his surgery, as neither Alfonso nor his wife has medical insurance.

1. What Filipino cultural values predisposed Alfonso's professional help–seeking behavior?
2. Describe the Filipino family kinship system and the roles of older parents and adult children.
3. Identify potential problems of the family and recommend culturally congruent interventions.

RESPONSIBILITY FOR HEALTH CARE

Parents may seek all possible assistance that they can personally generate from family, friends, the church, the community, and the formal health-care system (often in that order) for a child with a serious illness such as cancer, eventually accepting the inevitability of death. From a Western perspective, the outcome may be slightly different than if formal services were accessed as early as possible. Adult children, especially those working in the United States, are responsible for the health care of their aged parents and extended kin. Responsibility may be in different forms such as decision making, accepting financial responsibility, providing supportive presence, performing caretaking tasks, or negotiating with the health-care practitioner and the system.

In general, older adult women provide direct care for younger members. Older men participate in caring tasks such as driving the patient to the clinic. Decisions and financial support are relegated to family members who are deemed qualified and able. The family acts as a unit, and the individualistic paradigm commonly used by American caregivers is replaced by a social ethic of care. Before the decision is made to inform the patient about his or her terminal condition, a discussion among family members occurs, and they may request the doctor not divulge the truth to protect the patient. The ethical principles of beneficence and nonmaleficence take precedence over patient autonomy (Pacquiao, 2003).

Filipino family hierarchy may require consulting with family members before decisions are made. This may pose a problem to Western practitioners who believe in the adult patients' autonomy to make decisions about their own lives. The same perspective of Filipinos may result in their inability to question and assert ideas with physicians, who are regarded to be in a higher position of

TABLE 10.2 *Herbal Medicines Approved by the Department of Health in the Philippines*

Filipino Name/Generic Name	English Name	Uses
Akapulko (*Cassia alata*) "bayas-bayasan"	Ringworm bush	Ringworms and skin fungal infections
Ampalaya (*Momordica charantia*)	Bitter gourd or bitter melon	Non–insulin-dependent diabetes
Bawang (*Allium sativum*)	Garlic	Cholesterol reduction Blood pressure control
Bayabas (*Psidium guajava*)	Guava	Antiseptic to disinfect wounds Mouthwash to treat tooth decay and gum infection
Lagundi (*Vitex negundo*)	Five-leaf chaste tree	Relief of coughs and asthma
Niyog-niyogan (*Quisqualis indica*)	Chinese honeysuckle	Dried matured seeds to eliminate intestinal worms, particularly *Ascaris* and *Trichina*
Sambong (*Blumea balsamifera*)	Blumea camphora	Diuretic, helps in the excretion of urinary stones and treatment of edema
Tsaang gubat (*Ehretia microphylla lam*)		Taken as tea; used in treating intestinal motility and as a mouthwash because leaves have a high fluoride content
Ulasimang bato (*Pepperomia pellucida*) "pansit-pansitan"		Arthritis and gout; may be prepared as tea or eaten as a salad
Yerba buena (*Clinopodium douglasii*)	Peppermint	Analgesic to relieve body aches and pain; may be taken internally or applied locally

Source: Adapted from Department of Health. (2005). Ten herbal medicines approved by the DOH.

authority. Major decisions may be delegated to the physician rather than the patient or family taking an active collaborative role in decision making. Failure to develop a trusting relationship with the practitioner can lead to noncompliance with prescribed regimens because of lack of participation in the decision-making process.

FOLK AND TRADITIONAL PRACTICES

Supernatural and magicoreligious beliefs about health and illness are integrated with scientific medicine. Mental illness may be attributed to an external cause such as witchcraft, soul loss, or spirit intrusion. Illness in infancy and childhood may be attributed to the evil eye. This belief system is consistent with the variety of Filipino folk healers. Healing rituals may involve religious rites (prayers and exorcism), sacrifices to appease the spirits, use of herbs, and massage.

Balance and moderation are embedded in the hot-and-cold theory of healing. The ideal environment is warm, moderate, and balanced. The underlying principle is that change should be introduced gradually. Sudden changes from hot to cold, from activity to inactivity, from fasting to overeating, and so forth, introduce undue bodily stresses, which can cause illness. After strenuous physical activity, a rest should precede a shower; otherwise, the person could develop arthritis. Cold drinks or foods such as orange juice or fresh tomatoes are not served for breakfast to prevent stomach upset. Exposure to sudden cold drafts may induce colds, fever, rheumatism, pneumonia, or other respiratory ailments. Some Filipinos in the United States avoid handwashing with cold water after ironing or heavy labor. Exposure to cold such as showers is avoided during menstruation and the postpartum period.

The Department of Health in the Philippines (2005), through its Traditional Health Program, has endorsed ten herbs that have been thoroughly tested and clinically proven to have medicinal value in the relief and treatment of various ailments (Table 10–2). The Philippine government has encouraged production of these herbal medicines to provide affordable medicines for the populations who have limited or no access to Western health care. Widespread acceptance of these herbal medicines is evident among educated and higher-income groups.

BARRIERS TO HEALTH CARE

Studies of Filipinos in the United States show that, for many reasons, Filipinos generally do not seek care for illness until it is quite advanced. Some take minor ailments stoically and consider them natural imbalances that will run their normal course and disappear. Others claim to watch the progress of their illness so that the appropriate health-care provider can be consulted. Still others may not seek help because of economic reasons, lack of insurance, distrust of the health-care system, religious reasons, lack of knowledge, or an inability to articulate their needs (McBride et al., 1995).

Some Filipinos may not have a primary health-care provider and may rely on emergency services instead. Many Filipinos are reluctant to participate in health-promotion programs such as cancer screening and health education. Aging Filipino veterans may be denied health services because of lack of insurance and consequently referred to various nonprofit community clinics. Older Filipino émigrés did not have adequate health benefits through their place of employment. Thus, they may have been used to postponing seeking care until the illness was quite advanced. In contrast, recent immigrants have health insurance and behave differently, seeking preventive medical services regularly (Garde et al., 1994).

Health-care providers should expect wide variations in health behaviors among Filipino American clients. A nonjudgmental history taking should be well documented. Turning on the "multicultural ear" and listening with care to the context of these actions can provide insight for practitioners, particularly when the practitioner is under time pressure.

CULTURAL RESPONSES TO HEALTH AND ILLNESS

Filipinos view pain as part of living an honorable life. Some view this as an opportunity to reach a fuller spiritual life or to atone for past transgressions. Thus, they may appear stoic and tolerate a high degree of pain. Health-care providers may need to offer and, in fact, encourage pain relief interventions for clients who do not complain of pain despite physiological indicators. Others may have a strong sensitivity to the "busyness" of health-care providers, quietly diminishing their own need for attention so that others can receive care, or they may simply have little knowledge of how pain management can be maximized.

Minimal expression of psychological and emotional discomfort may be observed. The discomfort in discussing negative emotions with outsiders may be manifested by somatic complaints or ritualistic behaviors, such as praying. Exploring the underlying meaning of somatization (loss of appetite, inability to sleep) and observing the client's interactions with others can provide valuable information. Filipino clients may display visible evidence of their religion such as religious medals, prayer cards, and rosary beads to manage anxiety and pain. These artifacts should be incorporated into their treatment regimen. Using cultural mediators or brokers to probe innermost feelings of patients may be helpful if used appropriately. Pain assessment can include the role of prayer by the patient and members of the support network. Questions such as "Do you have someone praying for you?" or "Is there a special prayer to help you deal with pain?" may provide vital information for individualizing care.

Most Filipinos believe that mental illness carries a certain amount of stigma, and some believe that it is hereditary. Family members tend to take care of emotional problems to minimize exposing the problem to outsiders. Among rural residents and less-educated Filipinos in the Philippines, mental illness is generally attributed to external causes such as sorcery, soul loss, or spirit intrusion. Witch doctors, fortunetellers, and faith healers are often sought. Filipinos in the United States seek professional interventions when symptoms are advanced. Psychiatric symptoms are precipitated by a loss in self-esteem, loss of status, and shame related to the stresses of immigration. Separation from family, inability to find suitable employment, uncertainty, lack of money, and other relocation stressors create serious psychological reactions among Filipinos. Talking to a trusted family member or friend, undergoing psychotherapy, staying involved, participating in support and prayer groups, maintaining employment, and taking medication are the preferred treatments.

Using sociocultural behaviors learned early in life, Filipinos have a remarkable ability to maintain a proper front to protect their self-esteem and self-image. However, this front may be fragile, and chronic repression of resentment and anger may build up and erupt violently. Mental health providers should recognize that despite the possibility of a Filipino client's refusing professional mental health services, involving a trusted family member or friends, initiating contact with a Filipino mental health worker, especially a Filipino physician, or using both practices may increase the odds of getting the person into a culturally compatible treatment program. Deference to authority may successfully bring the Filipino client into treatment, with the client's expectation that the authority figure will fix the problem. A family therapy framework can have a more beneficial outcome.

The birth of a child with a developmental disability may be viewed as God's gift, an opportunity to become a better person or family, a curse from some unknown "angry spirit," negligence while pregnant, or a family matter that should be kept private. Health-seeking behaviors are conditioned by the perceived cause. American-born Filipinos may be more inclined to accept rehabilitation services through a homecare program than through institutional placement, such as special schools and long-term care facilities.

The cultural value of reciprocal obligation and the family as the main support exaggerate the burden of caring for a chronically ill family member. Institutionalization may not be readily accepted, causing considerable strains on the family relationships and resources. Self-sacrifice is believed to be virtuous and rewarded spiritually and in future life. Verbalization of caretaking hardships may not be tolerated and may cause guilt feelings on the individual caregiver. Practitioners should be sensitive to the needs of the family caregiver and work with the family unit in finding alternative ways of providing care for the chronically ill members. Reluctance to join support groups composed of outsiders and non-Filipinos can be offset by involving other family members or friends.

BLOOD TRANSFUSIONS AND ORGAN DONATION

The value of blood transfusion is recognized and accepted by Filipinos. However, organ donation may be less acceptable, except perhaps in cases in which a close family member is involved. Many Filipinos who follow Catholic traditions believe that keeping the body intact as much as possible until death is a reasonable preparation for the afterlife. Asian Americans, including Filipinos, hold more negative attitudes toward organ donation. They are less likely to participate in large, urban organ donor program (Alden & Cheung, 2000).

Health-Care Practitioners

TRADITIONAL VERSUS BIOMEDICAL PRACTITIONERS

Western medicine is familiar and acceptable to most Filipinos. Many recent Filipino immigrants are educated in the health-care field. Some Filipinos accept the efficacy of folk medicine and may consult both Western-trained and indigenous healers. Traditional healers are sought more in the rural areas of the Philippines. Folk healers are less common in the United States, with the exceptions of the West Coast and Hawaii. When available, they contribute by facilitating cultural rapport between health-care providers and the client and by increasing utilization of needed health-care services. For example, the *hilot* is often willing to be included in the counseling session and provide support for the patient's compliance with the medical treatment. The *hilot* may provide a special prayer to be incorporated into the medically prescribed treatment plan to increase the client's sense that all available resources are being used. In some areas on the West Coast, the *hilot* has a distinct role and function in the Filipino community. A few Filipino health professionals have learned the *hilot*'s art, skills, and spiritual approach, which they blend into their professional practice.

A practitioner of the same gender and the same culture may encourage more Filipinos to take advantage of disease prevention services. The availability of Filipino primary-care providers and, whenever possible, a bilingual person are critical to improving health care for older Filipinos.

STATUS OF HEALTH-CARE PROVIDERS

Filipinos generally consider the physician as the primary leader of the health-care team, and other providers are expected to defer to the physician. As Filipino families become more acculturated and aware of how health-care services are accessed in the United States, changes in attitude and behavior may be expected.

When ill, Filipinos may first consult a family member or a friend who is a physician or other professional before arranging a medical appointment. Some prefer physicians from their own region, when possible, whereas others indicate preference for physicians who are knowledgeable and competent and have good bedside manners regardless of culture or ethnic background. Factors considered in choosing health-care providers by middle-aged immigrant Filipino women were concern for privacy, feelings of modesty, approval from family members (especially the spouse), and most important, the overall caring environment in the system.

Interactions of Filipinos with Canadian nurses in the hospital reflected their *kapwa*-oriented worldview, which categorized nursing approaches and interactions within the insider-outsider continuum. Sensitivity of nurses to patient's verbal and nonverbal cues allowed them to move toward a more intimate status as insiders, *hindi ibang tao*. Patients based their preferences for which nurses to perform their personal and private tasks or receive information on the nurses' ability to provide spontaneous and unsolicited care and monitoring of their condition. Organizational policies and protocols, in addition to short hospital stays, were identified as barriers toward moving the patient-nurse relationship toward higher intimacy and trust (Pasco et al., 2004).

VIGNETTE 10.3

Jenny Dorn, aged 26 years, has been the primary nurse for 55-year-old Nicanor Abaca, who is hospitalized with a possible myocardial infarction. Jenny welcomes the opportunity to care for Nicanor because he is "not demanding, easy to please, grateful, and enjoys their conversations." After Jenny returned from her day off, she was told by her nurse manager that Nicanor's daughter stated that her father does not want Jenny to be assigned to him anymore. The daughter did not share any explanation with the nurse manager.

1. What precipitated the conflict?
2. How would you describe Nicanor's attempt to deal with the conflict?
3. How should the nurse manager handle the conflict?
4. How should the nurse deal with the conflict?

REFERENCES

Abe-Kim, J., Gong, F., & Takeuchi, D. (2004). Religiosity, spirituality, and help-seeking among Filipino Americans: Religious clergy or mental health professionals? *Journal of Community Psychology, 32,* 675–689.

Agoncillo, T., & Guerrero, M. (1987). *History of the Filipino people* (7th ed.). Manila, Philippines: Garcia Publishing.

Alden, D. L., & Cheung, A. H. S. (2000). Organ donation and culture: A comparison of Asian American and European American beliefs, attitudes, and behaviors. *Journal of Applied Social Psychology, 30*(2), 293–314.

Anderson, J. N. (1983). Health and illness in Pilipino immigrants. *Western Journal of Medicine, 139*(6), 811–819.

Araneta, M. R. G., & Barrett-Connor, E. (2005). Ethnic differences in visceral adipose tissue and type 2 diabetes: Filipino, African-American, and White women. *Obesity Research, 13,* 1458–1465.

Asian Pacific Islander Maternity Coalition. (2001). Retrieved March 3, 2007, from http://www.maternitycoalition.org.au

Bautista, V. (2002). *The Filipino Americans (1763–Present): Their history, culture, and tradition* (2nd ed.). Naperville, IL: Bookhaus.

Brown, D. E., & James, G. D. (2000). Physiological stress responses in Filipino-American immigrant nurses: The effects of residence time, life-style, and job strain. *Psychosomatic Medicine, 62,* 394–400.

Ceniza-Choy, C. (2003). Empire of care: Nursing migration in Filipino American history. Durham, NC: Duke University Press.

CIA. (2007). *World FactBook: Philippines.* Retrieved March 1, 2007, from https://www.cia.gov/cia/publications/factbook/geos/rp.html#People

Coughlan, S. S., & Uhler, R. J. (2000). Breast and cervical cancer screening practices among Asian and Pacific Islander women in the US, 1994–1997. *Cancer Epidemiology Biomarkers and Prevention, 9,* 597–603.

De la Cruz, F. A., Padilla, G. V., & Agustin, E. O. (2000). Adapting a measure of acculturation for cross-cultural research. *Journal of Transcultural Nursing, 11*(3), 191–198.

Department of Health. (2005). Ten herbal medicines approved by the DOH. Retrieved February 27, 2007, from http://herbal-medicine.philsite.net/doh_herbs.htm 2005

Enriquez, V. G. (1994). *From colonial to liberation psychology: The Philippine experience.* Manila, Philippines: De La Salle University Press.

Espiritu, Y. L. (2003). *Homebound: Filipino American lives across cultures, communities and countries.* Ewing, NJ: University of California Press.

Garde, P., Spangler, Z., & Miranda, B. (1994). *Filipino-Americans in New Jersey: A health study.* Final Report of the Philippine Nurses' Association of America to the State of New Jersey Department of Health, Office of Minority Health.

Gee, G. C., Chen, J., Spencer, M. S., See, S., Kuester, O. A., Tran, D., et al. (2006). Social support as a buffer for perceived unfair treatment among Filipino Americans: Differences between San Francisco and Honolulu. *American Journal of Public Health, 96*(4), 677–684.

Ghosh, C. (2003). Healthy People 2010 and Asian Americans/Pacific Islanders: Defining a baseline of information. *American Journal of Public Health, 93*(12), 2093–2098.

Gong, F., Gage, S.-J. L., & Tacata, L.A., Jr., (2003). Helpseeking behavior among Filipino Americans: A cultural analysis of face and language. *Journal of Community Psychology, 31*(5), 469–488.

Hawaii Community College. (2005). Traditional Filipino health beliefs. Retrieved February 27, 2007, from http://www.hawcc.hawaii.edu/nursing/tradfil2.htm

IBON Foundation. (2007). Retrieved September 14, 2007, from http://www.ibon.org

Jones, P. S., Jaceldo, K. B., Lee, J. R., Zhang, X. E., & Meleis, A. I. (2001). Role of integration and perceived health in Asian American women caregivers. *Research in Nursing and Health, 24*(2), 133–144.

Kagawa-Singer, M., & Pourat, N. (2000). Asian American and Pacific Islander breast and cervical carcinoma screening rates and Healthy People 2000 objectives. *Cancer, 89*(3), 696–705.

Levy, R. (1993). Ethnic and racial differences in response to medicines: Preserving individualized therapy in managed pharmaceutical programmes. *Pharmaceutical Medicine, 7*, 139–165.

Lim, S., Clarke, C. A., Prehn, A. W., Glaser, S. L., West, D. W., & O'Malley, C. D. (2002). Survival differences among Asian subpopulations in the United States after prostate, colorectal, breast, and cervical carcinomas. *Cancer, 94*(4), 1175–1182.

Lipson, J. G., & Dibble, S. L. (2005). *Culture and clinical care.* San Francisco: University of California San Francisco Nursing Press.

Maxwell, A. E., Bastani, R., Vida, P., & Warda, U. S. (2002). Physical activity among older Filipino-American women. *Women Health, 36*(1), 67–79.

Maxwell, A. E., Bastani, R., & Warda, U. S. (2000). Demographic predictors of cancer screening among Filipino and Korean immigrants in the United States. *American Journal of Preventive Medicine, 36*(1), 67–68.

McBride, M., Mariola, D., & Yeo, G. (1995). *Aging and health: Asian Pacific Islander American elders.* Stanford, CA: Stanford Geriatric Education Center.

McBride, M., & Parreno, H. (1996). Filipino American families and caregiving. In G. Yeo & D. Gallagher-Thompson (Eds.), *Ethnicity and the dementias.* Washington, DC: Taylor & Francis.

Mossakowski, K. N. (2003). Coping with perceived discrimination: Does ethnic identity protect mental health? *Journal of Health and Social Behavior, 44*(3), 318–331.

National Statistics Office, Philippines (2005). *Index of demographic and health.* Retrieved February 27, 2007, from http://www.census.gov.ph/data/sectordata/datandhs.html

Pacquiao, D. F. (1993). Cultural influences in old age: An ethnographic comparison of Anglo and Filipino elders. Doctoral dissertation, Graduate School of Education, Rutgers University, New Brunswick, NJ. Ann Arbor, MI: University Microfilms, Inc. (number 9320788).

Pacquiao, D. F. (1996). Educating faculty in the concept of educational biculturalism: A comparative study of sociocultural influences in nursing students' experience in school. In V. M. Fitzsimons & M. L. Kelley (Eds.), *The culture of learning: Access, retention, understanding and mobility of minority students in nursing* (pp. 129–162). New York: National League for Nursing Press.

Pacquiao, D. F. (2001). Cultural incongruities of advance directives. *Bioethics Forum, 17*(1), 27–31.

Pacquiao, D. F. (2003). Cultural competence in ethical decision-making. In M. M. Andrews & J. S. Boyle (Eds.), *Transcultural concepts in nursing care* (4th ed., pp. 503–532). Philadelphia: Lippincott.

Pacquiao, D. F. (2004). Recruitment of Philippine nurses to the US: Implications for policy development. *Nursing and Health Policy Review, 3*(2), 167–180.

Pasco, A. C. Y., Morse, J. M., & Olson, J. K. (2004). Cross-cultural relationships between nurses and Filipino Canadian patients. *Journal of Nursing Scholarship, 36*(3), 239–246.

Quan, H., Fong, A., De Coster, C., Wang, J., Musto, R., Noseworthy, T. W., et al. (2006). Variation in health services utilization among ethnic populations. *CMAJ: Canadian Medical Association Journal, 174*(6), 787–791.

Reeves, T. J., & Bennett, C. E. (2004). *We the people: Asians in the US.* Census 2000 Special reports. Washington, DC: U.S. Deptartment of Commerce.

Salazar, L. P., Schuldermann, S. M., Schuldermann, E. H., & Hunyh, C. (2000). The Filipino adolescents' parental socialization for academic achievement in the United States. *Journal of Adolescent Research, 15*(5), 564–587.

Spangler, Z. (1992). Transcultural nursing care values and caregiving practices of Philippine-American nurses. *Journal of Transcultural Nursing, 4*(2), 28–37.

Tatak Pilipino. (2003). *Profile of the Philippines.* Retrieved February 26, 2007, from http://www.filipinoheritage.com

U.S. Bureau of the Census. (2002). The Asian Population: 2000. Retrieved March 2, 2007, from http://www.census.gov/prod/2002pubs/c2kbr01-16.pdf

Wolf, D. L. (1997). Family secrets: Transnational struggles among children of Filipino immigrants. *Sociological Perspectives, 40*(3), 457–483.

Wu, T.-Y., & Bancroft, J. (2006). Filipino American women's perceptions and experiences with breast cancer screening. *Oncology Nursing Forum, 33*(4), 1–11.

Yamane, L. (2002). Native-Born Filipina/o Americans and labor market discrimination. *Feminist Economics, 8*(2), 125–144.

Yu, S. M., Huang, Z. J., & Singh, G. K. (2004). Health status and health services utilization among US Chinese, Asian Indian, Filipino, and other Asian/Pacific Islander children. *Pediatrics, 113*(1), 101–107.

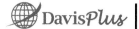 **DavisPlus**

For case studies, review questions, and additional information, go to http://davisplus.fadavis.com

Chapter 11

People of French Canadian Heritage

GINETTE COUTU-WAKULCZYK,
DENISE MOREAU, and DIANE ALAIN

Overview, Inhabited Localities, and Topography

OVERVIEW

Canada, with over 3,800,000 square miles, is larger than the entire United States but has only one-ninth the population. The population is 32,270,507, of which one-quarter have French as their mother tongue and 3 million speak French as a second language (Statistics Canada, 2006). Canada is surrounded by three oceans; the land mass covers six time zones and has fertile agricultural land, vast tundra, dense forests, and mountain ranges. The country is rich in minerals, coal, oil, and gas.

Canada, a member of the Commonwealth of Nations and of the G8, is a federation of 10 provinces, the Northwest and Yukon Territories, and the Nunavut. The Constitution Act of 1981 transferred the Parliament from Britain to Canada; the Canadian constitution is now entirely in the hands of the Canadians. People in each province elect their own premier and provincial legislative government. Even though the Queen of England is also the Queen of Canada, represented by the Governor General, a lieutenant governor is symbolically appointed by the federal government in every province. The 10 provinces in descending order of population are Ontario, Québec, British Columbia, Alberta, Manitoba, Saskatchewan, Nova Scotia, New Brunswick, Newfoundland, and Prince Edward Island; the Yukon Territories and Northwest Territories, which have been subdivided to form the Nunavut.

Based on the 2001 census, Canada's largest cities are Toronto (5,304,100), Montréal (3,635,700), Vancouver (2,208,300), and Ottawa Gatineau (1,148,800), the national capital region (Statistics Canada, 2006). Although more than 9 million people report being able to converse in French (Office of the Commissionor of Official Languages, 2006), the *Francophone* (French-speaking) population remains stable with over 6.6 million, the vast majority of them living in the province of Québec (Statistics Canada, 2002). The presence of the French in North America, beginning in Acadia, has celebrated its 400th-anniversary (1604–2004). Since the early 1980s, Canada has relied on immigration for its demographic growth, with an average of 230,000 newcomers per annum. Since the beginning of the 21st century, the majority come from Asia and Africa (Statistics Canada, 2006).

Before the latter half of the 18th century, most French people immigrating to Canada were Catholics, whereas French Protestants tended to come directly to the United States. After the French Revolution, an increased number of Catholics sought shelter in the United States. The bulk of those coming via Canada settled in the New England states and later dispersed throughout the United States. Peaks of emigration occurred from the Acadian deportation (1755), from the latter part of the 19th century, and just prior to the Great Depression. Most of this latter migration was directly related to economic opportunities and was part of an apparently contagious groundswell of immigration to the United States from Europe via Canada. As of 2000, it was estimated that more than 2.2 million people of French Canadian descent resided in the United States. Nowadays, French-speaking Canadians, unlike those of the 19th century living in the United States, may have been raised within the French culture but descended from a variety of ethnicities. Because French Canadian cultural characteristics vary according to the primary and secondary characteristics of culture (see Chapter 1), assessments must be carefully completed to avoid generalizations based on language and physical or racial traits. In addition, the Multiculturalism Canada Act of 1988 provided guidelines for implementing policies regarding multicultural diversity.

HERITAGE AND RESIDENCE

Before the 1960s, people with French as their mother tongue were identified as *French Canadians*, referring to France as their country of origin. The ancestors of most French Canadians were the French "colons" who established themselves in the St. Lawrence Valley during the 17th and 18th centuries. They brought with them their native language and culture, their customs, songs, stories, and games, which have been enriched over the centuries by contact with indigenous peoples and other immigrant cultures to the region: the Basques, the Scots, and the Irish. The **Métis**, descendants of Native Americans and Europeans, are mainly, though not entirely, French-speaking. Some regard the Métis as a historically and culturally distinct people in their own right. Another major portion of Canada's French-speaking population are the **Acadians**. They are the descendants of the early French colonists, mainly people from west-central France, who settled in the Maritime region of modern-day Nova Scotia and New Brunswick.

Today, the French-speaking population of Canada is far from homogeneous. In many homes, English and French may be used equally. Canadians whose first language is French are called **Francophones**, a designation that broadly encompasses the multiethnic and cultural mosaic of the Canadian population. More recently, Francophones from former colonies under French rule such as Carribeans, Lebanon, Vietnam, Africa, and a smaller number from Eastern Europe (Madibbo & Labrie, 2005) have added to the French population of Canada. Moreover, during the last 20–30 years, many families in Québec have adopted young children mostly from Africa, China, Latin America, and the Middle East. This practice has contributed to the development of an ethnic mosaic within the younger adult population. Although most French-speaking Canadians live in the province of Québec, the French language is used daily for communication within families and communities from coast to coast and as far north as the Yukon. The number increases yearly with the population seeking work in the western provinces.

New France (*Nouvelle France*) was the name given to Canada when it was first settled in the 17th century, a period in which Portugal, Spain, Holland, France, and England all vied for territory. Although religious influences played a part in colonial policies, it was the mercantile system that stimulated exploration of the North American wilderness and the development of trading companies. One of the first permanent colonies in Canada was Québec City. Soon after settling there in 1608, French explorers and traders moved up the St. Lawrence River, established a settlement at Ville-Marie (Montréal) in 1642, explored the Great Lakes (from which the St. Lawrence flows), opened fur-trading centers, and con-

verted the natives to Christianity. In 1718, the French settled at the opposite end of the continent, in New Orleans. In 1750, approximately 80,000 French colonials lived within the vast area between the mouths of the St. Lawrence and Mississippi rivers. The French influence is still visible in large parts of Canada and in cities such as St. Louis and New Orleans in the United States.

Around 1603, other groups of settlers established themselves in **Acadia**, north of what Giovanni da Verrazano, in 1534, referred to as *Arcadia* (note the *r*). This region is known today as Delaware, Maryland, and Virginia. After a devastating experience during the winter of 1604 to 1605, the settlers moved to the Bay of Fundy and founded Port-Royal, which was to become the first coastal settlement and capital of Acadia. By the middle of the 1700s, Acadians were caught in the crossfire of the imperial rivalries of England, France, and inhabitants of the American colonies, finally being absorbed into the British Empire.

With the Treaty of Utrecht in 1713, England secured Newfoundland, Acadia (renamed Nova Scotia), and the extensive region drained by the rivers flowing into the Hudson Bay. As a result of the Treaty of Paris in 1763, France relinquished all its North American possessions east of the Mississippi River to England. Spain ceded Florida to England in exchange for the French territories west of the Mississippi River. Thus, as a geographic area, New France became only a memory. Yet, the French culture, language, and religious institutions remain as an everlasting tribute to the past. The heritage and early French architecture is well preserved through concentrated efforts and pride in restoration. Publication of information about monuments, houses, churches, and ramparts around Québec City keep the public informed about the area's rich French heritage.

As a result of unresolved controversy over several highly contentious oaths of allegiance to the English between 1755 and 1762, a massive deportation occurred, referred to as *le grand dérangement*. French-speaking Catholic Acadians were removed from their homes in Nova Scotia and New Brunswick. Some fled to Québec, others took refuge in the woods, and many died. Still others dispersed to the south: Massachusetts, New York, Pennsylvania, Maryland, Virginia, the Carolinas, Georgia, and Louisiana (Cajun). In 1774, some exiled Acadians returned to the Maritimes and attempted to re-create their lives. Unable to secure their former lands because of British occupation, they directed their energies to settling new areas and gradually explored new activities such as fishing and forestry. Today, 90 percent of the Acadians reside in northern and eastern New Brunswick, southern Nova Scotia, the Acadian region of Cape Breton, and the Evangeline region of Prince Edward Island (Beaudin & Leclerc, 1995).

Throughout Canada, important regional differences exist among the French-speaking population. Outside Québec, the French-speaking population within each province or territory has its own association, which is organized nationally under the Fédération des Communautés Francophones et Acadiennes du Canada (FCFA). An important consideration when health-care providers assess a family's cultural background is the number of mixed marriages leading to the adoption of English as the language spoken in the home and by the majority. French-speaking Canada has become an increasingly diverse society composed of various ethnocultural groups with more than 100 different languages as mother tongue. In 2001, 5,335,000 (1 in 6) allophones (mother tongue other than French or English) immigrated to Canada, up 12.5 percent over 1996, which is three times that of population growth (4.0 percent) (Statistics Canada, 2006). Very much like the situation in the U.S., interethnic marriage patterns have dramatically changed from "... a multiethnic society ... into multiethnic individuals" (Huntington, 2004, p. 299). For example, in Toronto, the Francophones of European descent (*de souche*) are becoming the minority among the Francophones of different ethnic groups (Statistics Canada, 2002).

REASONS FOR MIGRATION AND ASSOCIATED ECONOMIC FACTORS

Economic reasons, including the desire to cultivate the land and exploit fisheries, were the most frequent motivations for French Canadian settlers in the 17th century. Most of these settlers originated from the French regions of Normandy, Perche, and Poitou, and some came from Aunis, Brittany, Ile de France, and Saintonge. During the 17th century in France, many nobles lost their fortune because of changes in France's feudal system and wars; thus, colonization of New France offered possibilities for regaining their prestige and land for their vassals. The richness and the quality of pelts available in the New World promoted fur trading with the Native Americans and attracted merchants and their employees. In addition, missionaries and religious orders were among the earlier settlers. The latter half of the 20th century saw a wide range of reasons for migration including wars, humanitarianism, and appeal for a better life, which is called economic immigration. Today, French-speaking Canadians are represented in all trades and professions.

EDUCATIONAL STATUS AND OCCUPATIONS

Although the overall official literacy rate in Canada approaches 99 percent, the functional literacy rate is lower, and the educational levels of French Canadians represent a broad spectrum, depending on age group and geographic location. Among the older population, illiteracy reaches as high as 50 percent in some regions (Citizenship and Immigration Canada, 2005). In the 2001 national census, despite important progress in accessibility to postsecondary education in the French language, the university education level for Francophones remains below the national average. For example, for Francophones living outside Québec, the rate has increased to 19.6 percent, which is still lower than the national Canadian rate of 22.3 percent (Citizenship and Immigration Canada, 2005).

More recently, educational opportunities at all levels have become available in the French language in Ontario. Nevertheless, the lack of professionals prepared for the delivery of health services in French, as prescribed by the 1989 Ontario Government Law #8, jeopardizes the development of a full network of services in some rural regions.

In order to provide opportunities for the training of health professionals in the French language, the *Consortium National de Formation en Santé* (CNFS, 2001) has put in place mechanisms and organizations in all provinces and Territories outside Québec.

At the beginning of colonization, major occupations such as agriculture, fur trading, and fisheries were important for survival. In the latter part of the 19th century, French-speaking Canadians joined the developing industrial labor force. Factories, mining, forestry, and fisheries took advantage of the numerous hands available among the fertile Canadian families of French ancestry. Despite language barriers, this was a time when the borders of Québec did not stop young families from moving across Canada for work. Throughout Canada, even in the Yukon, the origins of early French-speaking Canadian settlements can be traced to these years. Today, French-speaking Canadians are represented in all trades and professions. However, the older population may have a different life history, depending on their region of origin: Gaspésie, Abitibi, Beauce, Acadia, or the cities of Montréal and Québec.

Communication

DOMINANT LANGUAGE AND DIALECTS

Canada has two official languages, French and English. Regional differences exist in accent, vocabulary, and degree of anglicization. However, French Canadians do not have difficulty understanding one another because the original French spoken in Canada includes some old 17th-century French words and expressions that are no longer used in France. Oral communication, in particular, has undergone assimilation. Indian words have been added and English words are incorporated into a syntax and grammar that is essentially French, resulting in a dialect, **joual** in Québec and **Chiac** in New Brunswick, which is spoken primarily by lower socioeconomic and undereducated groups. Age and location in Canada frequently determine language use and ability.

A population trend analysis in 1983 showed that despite the improved legal status of Francophones in Ontario, urbanization and economic pressures were contributing to a decline in French-speaking Ontarians. This decrease is more noticeable in southern Ontario, with a lesser decline in the northern and eastern counties bordering Québec. As a result of urbanization, the distribution of Francophones in Ontario has become fragmented, although regional cohesion of French-speaking Ontario has remained strongly supported by active networks at the local and provincial levels. Adding to this reality, the 2001 census demonstrated that low birth rate, mixed marriage with bilingualism, and an increase in mean age of Francophones contributed to the fragilized use of French in Canada. For example, in 2001, there were more allophones (732,200 had neither French nor English as mother tongue) in Québec than anglophones (591,400). In Canada, although a little less than a quarter (22.9 percent) reported French as the spoken language in their daily activities, 43.4 percent declared being bilingual (French-English) compared with 9 percent of Anglophones (Statistics Canada, 2002).

Since 1969, the Official Languages Act of New Brunswick guaranteed the availability of government services and education in French and English at all educational levels. Although the Act has increased the political and social utility of French, it has not reversed the Acadians' use of English or the decline in the proportion of Francophones in the province. In an effort to prevent linguistic assimilation, a new policy for language teaching is used in the French schools of heavily Anglicized regions. English as a second language is taught only beginning in grade 5, whereas in Québec since 2000, teaching the second language begins in grade 1. In all provinces except New Brunswick, where the French are the minority, a disproportionate number of young French Canadians are assimilated into the majority English-speaking society. In contrast, on Prince Edward Island, the struggle to obtain education in French remains an ongoing issue.

A recent report prepared by the Official Language Community Development Bureau on behalf of the Consultative Committee for French-Speaking Minority Communities (CCFSMC) states that services in the user's language have benefits that extend far beyond simple respect for the user's culture (Public Works and Government Services Canada, 2001). These services are indispensable for improving the health status of individuals and for community empowerment in matters of health. Studies have shown that the health status of minority Francophones is generally poorer than that of their fellow citizens in any given province. In fact, between 50 and 55 percent of French-speaking minority communities often have little or no access to health services in their mother tongue. Of foremost importance, one of the recommendations is to increase the number of French-speaking health professionals who practice in minority communities and to support the establishment of a pan-Canadian Francophone consortium for the training of French-speaking health professionals and the addition of a school of nursing at Collège Universitaire de St-Boniface in Winnipeg, Manitoba.

The law protecting the French language in Québec may have created another problem for its population. While promoting a false sense of security by maintaining the dominance of the French language, a large portion of Québec's French-speaking population lacks sufficient knowledge of the English language to access the workforce outside their province and may have difficulty in higher-education programs in which readings are mostly in English.

From a health perspective, cultural heritage remains present long after words of the French language have been forgotten. Maintaining the use of French depends mostly on the strength of the local French community. As for other culturally diverse clients, health-care providers must respect the client's preference in choice of language by seeking interpreters when possible; gearing health teaching to the educational level of the client; and supplementing written directions with verbal instructions, demonstrations, and pictures. In the 2001 census, over 100 different languages as mother tongue were identified, although reporting at the same time that French was the primary language; thus, health teaching represents quite a challenge.

CULTURAL COMMUNICATION PATTERNS

Conversation is very important to French people. Among French Canadians, a conversation may be conducted with high voice crescendos, which do not necessarily mean anger or violence. Volume can increase with the importance and the emotional charge invested in the content of the message. Nonverbal communication patterns for French Canadians resemble those of their Latin and Mediterranean ancestors, which encourage sharing thoughts and feelings. Acadians are more reserved, quieter, shy, even self-effacing, and are less likely to share their thoughts and feelings than people from Québec. The use of hand gestures for emphasis when speaking is common. Facial expressions for men and women of all ages are a part of communication, often replacing words. Health-care providers working with French-speaking Canadians need to be attentive to nonverbal and paraverbal communication. These observations provide much of the information on affect, emotion, and mutual understanding between health-care providers and clients.

Spatial distancing for French-speaking Canadians differs among family members, close friends, and the public. When in the intimacy zone, people may touch frequently and converse in close physical space; however, they tend to avoid physical contact in public. When greeting another person, men usually shake hands, which is recommended for health-care providers. Close female friends and family members may greet each other with an embrace. However, in public and more formal situations such as the health-care environment, this is not a recommended practice. Eye contact is an important way for the health practitioner to acknowledge whether the person has understood or is following what is being said. Today, with the many ethnic and cultural groups, this behavior is not always possible. For example, for a student from the Haitian culture, it would be a lack of respect to make eye-to-eye contact with the professor. Hence, training these students to make eye contact with patients may be quite a challenge. Conversely, health professionals should be aware of the wide range of behaviors attached to communication in French among different ethnic cultural groups.

Before radio and television reached the Port au Port Peninsula of Newfoundland, there was a public tradition of storytelling. Narrators were invited to a home where several families had gathered, and an entire evening of storytelling took place. These public performances were time-consuming, followed stylistic conventions and formulas, and made dramatic use of gesturing. Since the 1960s, private storytelling has substantially replaced the public tradition. Stories are told within the confines of a single family or small group and usually last less than an hour, about the length of a television episode. Narrators no longer use stylistic devices, literary formulas, or dramatic gesturing.

TEMPORAL RELATIONSHIPS

For the French Canadian people, relationships take a long time to develop, but once in place, the relationship becomes very important and enduring. Langelier (1996) stated that once one enters the inner sanctum of close friendship, commitment and responsibility ensue.

French-speaking Canadians from Québec have a past, present, and future orientation in their worldview. Balancing the three dimensions depends on traditionalism, generation, religiosity, and urbanization (Pronovost, 1989). More traditional people, and many from rural backgrounds, attach primary importance to living in the present and accepting day-to-day occurrences in a context of fatalism. Many older people, with a strong religious background, maintain a future worldview, regarding life after death, and a past orientation, celebrating death anniversaries of family members and other events. However, many of the younger generation reject past traditions and attempt to maintain a balance by enjoying the present, working, and planning for their future.

FORMAT FOR NAMES

Traditionally, until the late 1970s, women and children took the father's surname. Today, under Québec law, a woman keeps her maiden name throughout her lifetime, although in other parts of Canada, this practice is decided between the spouses. This situation has created tension and self-identity difficulties for some older people. As for children, a Québécois family of two spouses and two children may well include four different surname combinations: One child may have the father's surname or the mother's surname alone or a hyphenated or nonhyphenated surname composed of those of the father and mother. For a second child, the surnames are the same, but in reverse order. The decision for using surnames rests entirely with the parents and must appear on the birth certificate. Today, very few parents adhere to the official use of multiple surnames for children. Women married for several years before the new law often added their maiden name hyphenated with that of their husbands.

Many French-speaking Canadians have dropped the custom of naming the oldest son after the father or the grandfather. Also declining is the custom of adding Joseph to male infants' and Mary to female infants' names. Until the early 1980s, the custom was to use only one name without initials, except on legal documents, which used all three or four names as they appeared on the birth certificate. Another recent change is using names other than those of saints. All of these factors should alert the health-care practitioner to the potential for confusion in the name format for client cultural identification. When in doubt, the health-care provider should ask the patient her or his legal name for record-keeping.

Family Roles and Organization

HEAD OF HOUSEHOLD AND GENDER ROLES

Traditionally, in French-speaking Canadian families, the man was seen as the moral authority and responsible for material well-being, such as economic provider and purveyor of affection and security. The woman served as the family mediator and social director, as well as being responsible for household activities, child care, and health care (Langelier, 1996). The profound social changes encountered after the "Quiet Revolution" of the late 1960s and early 1970s brought important modifications in education and industrialization and increased the role of women in economic activity. Better education for young women, along with the feminist movement, brought forth a desire and opportunities for women to have a career and a family of their own. Furthermore, even without a formal career education, women took the work market path mainly because it was no longer possible to live on one salary. These changes resulted in a new dynamic of family roles and organization that affected every member of the family, be it nuclear or extended. This model shaped family life dynamics and gave birth to a lexicon like "the superwomen or super mom," referring to mothers having two days' work, one outside and one inside the home, and men started to learn about "shared inside home chores." Women not only became producers of domestic goods in the household but also became productive outside the home environment.

Using the husband's income as an index for comparing the family communication and relative independence on marital adjustment among 180 French-speaking couples, Aube and Linden (1991) found that the degree of marital discord was similar across different socioeconomic levels. However, quality of communication accounted for 16 percent of the variance in marital satisfaction among men, and only 13 percent of the variance among women. By the end of the 1980s, marriages changed fundamentally, moving toward equality of husbands and wives, but not necessarily of children and parents. From a socioanthropological perspective, a national survey with 5614 females and 10,965 males demonstrated income differences between genders. Inequality, attributable to career interruptions by women, was estimated along with the importance of factors such as education, occupation, socioeconomic status, and number of hours worked per year. The income difference by gender among native and linguistic minorities in Canada showed that the inequality between sexes was smaller among French-speaking Canadians than among other groups (Goyder, 1981).

According to Langelier (1996), French Canadians have always attributed great value to family relationships and obligations; however, Wu and Baer (1996) found that Francophones were less committed than Anglophones to traditional values concerning marriage and relationships. Those results are consistent with Fong and Guilia's (1990) study showing that French Canadians had more permissive attitudes than English Canadians with respect to marriage, sexual activity, and nonmarried parenthood. Conversely, French Canadians are more traditional than English Canadians when it comes to rating the importance of having children. In addition, Catholicism was positively related to attitudes toward childbearing and differences in these attitudes among French and English Canadians. Recent studies provide clear evidence of a profound transformation in attitudes toward family-related behaviors and gender roles in much of the Western world since the mid-1970s: increased acceptance of divorce, nonmarital cohabitation, unmarried parenthood, permanent nonmarriage, and voluntary childlessness. Norms for gender roles are also changing, with shifts toward gender egalitarianism with respect to the appropriate roles of women and men in the family and workplace.

PRESCRIPTIVE, RESTRICTIVE, AND TABOO BEHAVIORS FOR CHILDREN AND ADOLESCENTS

The greatest source of pride for French Canadian families is to see their children well established with a good education. On this issue, most of the present political elite, educated at religious colleges, share the values and beliefs of their religious professors, not the prescribed behavior for their offspring.

FAMILY GOALS AND PRIORITIES

Traditional French Canadian intergenerational relationships are rapidly disappearing (Fig. 11–1). Urbanization, particularly without adequate social security measures, results in social dislocation of the young and old. Strategies for maintaining cohesion among the generations are required to avoid intergenerational conflict related to competition for scarce resources when survival challenges are real. In Canada, many of the social policies are under provincial jurisdiction. Today, French Canadian families follow the same pattern of declining birth rates as other Canadians. Québec has done the most in formulating a family policy and stimulating a widespread popular debate on the issue. Family policy, when geared toward protecting and fostering a particular type of family, contributes to the detriment of other types of families and becomes a prescribed structure for acceptance. For example, because children who were born out-of-wedlock were being penalized on the basis of their parents' relationship, the legal category of illegitimacy has been abolished in most Canadian provinces. The French Canadian family is more nuclear and autonomous than its counterpart in France.

Starting in 1997, Québec initiated a family policy aimed at promoting family life and increasing the birth rate. Among the most meaningful policies are the monthly allocations granted to each child at birth, for pregnant mothers or for mothers during the breastfeeding period, the right to reprieve from potentially harmful work conditions for the mother and child, parental leave up to 52 weeks for the mother or the father divided between them should they wish to do so, and subsidized

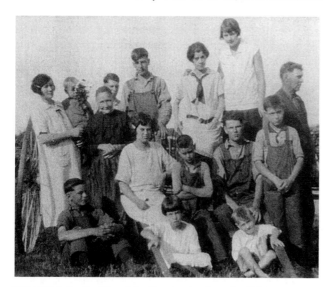

FIGURE 11–1   Traditional family returning from the fields.

day-care centers at a cost of $7.00 a day per child to be paid by parents (Gouvernement du Québec, 2006).

French-speaking Canadian family membership is known for its closeness, and some families are a "closed" family system. Urbanization and smaller families, along with the "Quiet Revolution" in Québec, have encouraged people to open their borders and expand their circle to include others by broadening their family perspective. Nevertheless, within the microcosm of the French Canadian population, the physical and social quality of the microenvironment is more essential to health and survival than wealth and a physical connection (Evans & Stoddart, 1994). House, Landis, and Umberson (1988) reported widespread and strong correlations between mortality and social support networks—friends and family keep French Canadians alive! The sheer number of contacts one has is protective, regardless of the nature of the interaction (Evans, 1994).

Lambert, Brown, Curtis, and Kay (1986), using the 1984 national election study of 3377 Québec inhabitants, explored cognitive differences from a class perspective. English-speaking and French-speaking residents of Québec were surveyed regarding their perceptions of social class, the importance of using characteristics to describe people from diverse social classes, and differentiation of the most important characteristics of social class. Approximately 45 percent stated that the idea of social class had no meaning to them or that they were unsure of its meaning, with English-speaking Canadians being more likely to give this response. Generally, people who said they understood the concept believed that social classes differed materially, whereas those who did not understand the concept preferred to evaluate people on individual characteristics. French-speaking respondents defined social class in the materialistic sense of income and wealth, whereas English-speaking Canadians emphasized individuals in terms of character and ambition and used ascriptive criteria such as country of origin, birth, or ancestry.

ALTERNATIVE LIFESTYLES

Traditionally, the Catholic Church dictated the parameters of sexual behavior, with a high priority placed on marriage and the begetting and raising of children. In the years before 1960 abstinence from premarital sex was encouraged, and a sexual double-standard existed, whereas the 1970s and 1980s witnessed a liberalization of sexual norms and the establishment of more egalitarian relationships between young men and women. At present, there is a growing trend for couples to live together without marrying. Many young couples answer that they cannot financially afford to get married. Yet, many of these same couples insist on having their children baptized and raise them according to Catholic Church principles.

Hobart (1992) studied sexual behaviors and attitudes toward sex, sexually transmitted diseases, and HIV/AIDS among 1775 Anglophone and 493 Francophone Canadian postsecondary students, surveying their expectations about condom use with different sexual partners. Results imply that women's patterns of sexual behaviors were more predictive than men's, but the relationships among variables were neither consistent nor strong. A shift toward greater sexual permissiveness and recognition of female sexuality is apparent. The percentage of sexually active adolescents has increased, from less than 50 percent in the early 1980s to 76 percent in the mid-1990s, with an average age at the time of the first sexual relations of approximately 16 years (Samson, Otis, & Levy, 1996).

An Internet search on gays and lesbians in Canada resulted in numerous Websites devoted to alternative lifestyles. Some Websites were hosted by universities, whereas others were hosted by gay and lesbian organizations (see, e.g., http://www.er.uqam.ca, http://www.clga.ca and http://www.teleport.com). In 1996, the Canadian government extended health, relocation, and other job benefits to same-sex partners of federal employees. During the same year, the Ontario Court of Appeals ruled that same-sex couples must be treated as common-law couples under the Family Leave Act. In 1999, a poll conducted by the Canadian federal government revealed that 53 percent of the Canadian public, across provincial and demographic lines, supported gay people's freedom to marry (International Recognition of Same-Sex Relationships, 2002). Canada is one of the few countries in the world where same-sex marriage is legalized.

Workforce Issues

VIGNETTE 11.1

Michel and Marie Tremblay have moved to the Boston area where they have both found work as aeronautical engineers. Because their life is now more stable with long-term contracts, they decided it was time to have children. Marie is pregnant. Michel is from the Lac St-Jean area of Canada, and Marie was born and raised in Montréal. They located a medical clinic and a physician for health care and the delivery of their baby-to-be. They consider language skills in French as excellent and that they can converse adequately in English for everyday conversations.

1. Do you think their English communication skills will be adequate for meeting their health-care needs? Why? Why not?
2. Name three genetically transmitted diseases for which the Tremblay baby may be at risk.
3. Identify strategies to help the Tremblay family meet their health-care needs in a new culture.
4. Compare the reason the Tremblay family has moved to Boston with the reasons the French immigrated in the 19th century.

CULTURE IN THE WORKPLACE

Among Canadians, workforce issues often correspond to educational background. In this respect, one must not forget the effects of the Durham Report and Law #17, which eliminated public schools' rights to teach in the French language, with the consequence of a high level of illiteracy among French Canadians. This situation was finally reversed with full rights to education in the French language in 1982, based on the Canadian Charter of Rights, article 23 (Denault & Cardinal, 1999). Hence, the overall educational level of French-speaking Canadians is lower than that of their English-speaking counterparts.

Using the Canadian version of the International Literacy Measure, which has a 5-point scale on which "1" is the lowest level and "5" refers to a university level, a survey on 23,000 Canadians provided data on comprehension competency for continued text, schematic text, numeracy, and problem solving. In four provinces (New Brunswick, Québec, Ontario, and Manitoba), the proportion of Francophones aged 16 years and older who obtained a score of 3 or lower was higher than the proportion of Anglophones. A level 3 in comprehension of text equates with understanding, for example, what is written on the label of a medicine bottle (when, how, and numbers of days). The level 3 is considered a basic requirement for active participation in civic life and voting. Of Francophones living outside of the province of Québec, 69 percent chose to be evaluated in the English language (35 percent in New Brunswick; 64 percent in Ontario, and 84 percent in Manitoba). The mean score obtained by those tested in English was higher in text comprehension than their counterparts who chose the French test. However, these differences could be attributable to the educational level, based on the fact that when controlled for educational level, there are no differences between Francophones and Anglophones (National Adult Literary Base, 2005). This information may be useful to health-care professionals when providing written information and prevention education to clients and families.

In addition, the proportion of part-time and casual workers among French-speaking Canadians is higher, especially in Québec hospitals. Labor unions support part-time and casual work as being shared work. However, many male workers are beginning to resent this approach, calling it "shared poverty." This situation resulted in less interest for the younger generation to enter the profession and, combined with 27,000 nurses who emigrated to the United States in the 1990s, resulted in a significant shortage of health-care practitioners (Canadian Nurses Foundation, 2006).

Hofstede (as cited in Punnett, 1991) examined the preferred leadership styles of 113 Anglophone and 77 Francophone managers in Ottawa from the perspective of language and cultural values. The two groups were similar in their preferred style of leadership, but differed significantly in terms of individualism. Differences between this group and an earlier Canadian sample suggest that organizational influences may have more impact on expressed cultural values than do language differences. To a large extent, outside the province of Québec, French-speaking Canadians' patterns of acculturation are intermeshed with educational and work opportunities. From an educational perspective, in the 1970s, a vast movement for French-immersion classes across Canada started changing the views of the younger generation. Also, the long battle for the administrative French school board system has reduced the acculturation process in many areas of Canada without stopping it. The availability of French language higher education outside Québec completes the realm of factors necessary to reverse acculturation and assure health services for French-speaking Canadians wherever they live.

In 1987, Ontario adopted legislation requiring equity in public services and recognized the necessity of looking closely into the principles of equality and equivalence. The designation of a certain number of positions identified as *Francophone* may have opened the door to a new phenomenon, that of ghettos (Denault & Cardinal, 1999). Most of these Francophone positions were created within the areas of essential population services and in the senior positions in the public services. Another aspect of the Francophone positions turns out to be more task elasticity and work overload in the sense that the regular job must be completed in addition to the translation of whatever material is to be produced for the service to be delivered.

ISSUES RELATED TO AUTONOMY

Baccalaureate level education, bilingualism, multiculturalism, and a focus on open-mindedness are the dominant themes in the Canadian workplace. Entry to practice requires a baccalaureate basic training since the early 2000s in the majority of provinces, excluding Québec province. Moreover, in the province of Québec, average yearly salaries may have a difference of nearly $19,000 lower than those paid in Ontario. Another exception relates to the Québec province's position with French as the official language in the workplace. Very few employers outside Québec need to identify English and French as official language; hence, geographic and regional aggregates of people living in specific areas shape the language of services offered.

Nurses' roles and activities remain consistent across Canada; however, changes in the mode of care and the language used in delivering services are apparent. Opportunities for Francophone nurses to function successfully outside Québec are limited if they have not mastered the English language. Frustration occurs among Francophone nurses when the time and effort put into mastering and delivering services in both official languages are not recognized. In addition, the number of Francophone nurses academically prepared to serve in decision-making positions is limited outside the province of Québec. This hinders the type and mode of services offered when decisions become public health policies. Today, with the CNFS contribution and the advancement of distance teaching, the training of health-care professionals in the French language is possible at every level from baccalaureate to doctorate not only in Québec but also all over Canada. Nevertheless, The University of Montréal Faculty of Nursing, founded in 1962, remains the only Francophone international university to offer programs in French from baccalaureate to doctorate. In terms of the number of Francophone students, that Faculty is the most important in Québec and in Canada.

Biocultural Ecology

SKIN COLOR AND OTHER BIOLOGICAL VARIATIONS

Canadians of French descent are white or Caucasian; however, Francophones, as a linguistic group, represent a mosaic of ethnocultural characteristics, including racial differences prompted by acculturation, adoption, and the children of mixed marriages. However, remember that one may change many things in life but one cannot change the biological grandparents (Huntington, 2004). Thus, individuals must be assessed individually for biological risks according to their racial and cultural heritage.

DISEASES AND HEALTH CONDITIONS

Given the limited population density, multiculturalism, and regionalism factors affecting Canadian society, specific risk factors for Canadians of French ancestry are the same as those for other minority groups. The primary causes of death among the Québec population are, in order of prevalence, cancer with an increase of lung cancer in women and cardiovascular diseases. In Québec between 2001 and 2005, death and injuries from road accidents increased by 17 percent. Newborn deaths attributed to the respiratory distress syndrome and neonate septicemia have also increased in Québec (Institut National de Santé Publique [INSPQ], 2006). In Ontario, according to Niday Perinatal Database and Southwest Data Warehouse in 2003, independently of language or culture, 1 in 12 babies are born before term (PPPESO, 2005).

Emard, Drouin, Thouez, & Ghardirian (2001) reported a higher level of prostate cancer among the Francophone population of Québec. Genetic susceptibility to breast cancer in French Canadians has been reported by Krajinovic et al. (2001), who associated the increase with the role of carcinogen-metabolizing enzymes and gene-environment interactions. In addition, Godar (1998) identified major influencing factors of risks for familial and sporadic ovarian cancer among French Canadians, including a family history of breast or ovarian cancer, beginning use of oral contraceptives at a late age, and last childbirth at a late age.

In addition, the suicide rate in Québec is higher than in any other province. On an average, nearly every day four Québecers take their lives, in particularly men between 30 and 49 years of age. Suicide occurs more often in rural areas than in urban areas. From an international perspective, few countries surpass the Québec mortality rate by suicide (INSPQ, 2006). Eighty percent of all suicides reported in 1991 involved men. The male-to-female ratio for suicide risk was 3.8:1 in both males and females; the greatest risk increase between 1960 and 1991 occurred in the 15- to 19-year age group, with a 4.5-fold increase for males and a 3-fold increase for females (Canadian Task Force on Preventive Care, 2003). The high rate of suicide and suicidal ideation, particularly among adolescent and young adult males, is one aspect of mental health that health-care practitioners have yet to address adequately.

Today's French Canadian population suffers from the same endemic conditions and sensitivities to environmental diseases as the Canadian population as a whole. The harsh topography and low winter temperatures are responsible for 19 percent of the population's osteoarthritic disorders, and the prevalence of multiple sclerosis is one of the highest in the world (Société Canadienne de la Sclérose en Plaques, 2005). Allergies related to urban air pollution, smog, and poor air circulation in public buildings affect

13 percent of the population (Pampalon et al., 1990). Distinctive features of idiopathic inflammatory myopathies in French Canadians were also reported by Uthman, Vazquez-Abad, and Sénécal (1996). Pausova et al. (2000) found an association in pedigrees of French Canadian origin. The tumor necrosis factor-α (TNF-α) gene locus contributes to obesity and obesity-related hypertension, and gender modifies the effect of the regional distribution of body fat.

A number of hereditary and genetic diseases more common among Québécois can be traced to early colonists. The regions of Charlevoix et du Saguenay Lac St-Jean are among the most affected in Québec and in Canada, with genetic and hereditary diseases such as spastic ataxia Charlevoix-Saguenay type, cystic fibrosis, tyrosinaemia, cytochrome lipase deficiency (COX), to name but a few. Familial chylomicronemia resulting from the lipoprotein lipase (LPL) deficiency, hyperlipoproteinemia type I, is an autosomal recessive disorder with a prevalence of 1 in 1 million individuals (Brunzell, 1989). Through genealogical research, this hereditary disorder has been traced to migrants from the Perche region of France (DeBraekeleer & Dao, 1994). The distribution of LPL deficiency among French Canadians of Québec reflects the highest frequency worldwide (Ma et al., 1991). Within the French Canadian population of Québec, its prevalence is especially high in the eastern part of the province (Gagné, Brun, Moorjani, & Lupien, 1989). Two separate mutations in the LPL gene introduced by French immigrants in the 17th century have been identified. Although the birthplaces of the obligate carriers were scattered throughout the province, three geographic clusters were identified: the Trois-Rivières-Mauricie region, the Saguenay-Lac-St.-Jean-Charlevoix region, and Beauce region (Dionne, Gagné, Julien, Murthy, et al., 1993). The carrier rate of LPL deficiency is estimated to be 1 in 139 individuals in the province as a whole, but 1 in 85 individuals in eastern Québec, with a peak of 1 in 47 individuals in Saguenay-Lac-St.-Jean (Dionne et al., 1993). With the discovery of a mutation in the human LPL gene, scientists have identified the most common cause of familial chylomicronemia in the French Canadian population (Ma et al., 1991). Furthermore, a single mutation of the fumarylacetoacetate hydrolase gene can lead to hereditary tyrosinemia type I (Grompe, St-Louis, Demers, Al-Dhalimy, Leclerc, & Tanguay, 1994).

Familial hypercholesterolemia (FH), leading to coronary thrombosis, supports the French origin of the French Canadian deletion. One century after settlement in North America, the founders originating from Perche had a large number of descendants. Among the 50 or more fertile couples, 14 came from Perche (Charbonneau, Desjardins, Guillemette, Landry, Légaré, & Nault, 1987). However, it is suggested that the high frequency of this mutation among French Canadian clients with hypercholesterolemia is due to a founder effect rather than to a high frequency within the population (Fumeron et al., 1992). FH is one of the most common autosomal codominant diseases. The frequency of FH among French Canadians in northern Québec is higher than in most other populations (1 in 154 versus 1 in 500) owing to the high prevalence of a few recurrent mutations in the LDL receptor gene (Levy et al., 1997).

A provincewide, long-term longitudinal study on all newborns identified a rare genetic disease among French Canadians. Profiles of phenylketonuria (PKU) in Québec populations show evidence of stratification and novel mutations (Rozen, Mascisch, Lambert, Lamframboise, & Scriver, 1994). To date, five mutations account for almost 90 percent of PKU diagnoses among French Canadians from eastern Québec (National PKU Index, 1992). Time and space clusters of the PKU mutation can be traced to France (Lyonnet et al., 1992). Studies by Vohl et al. (2000) and St.-Pierre et al. (2001) on genetic mutations in the population of French Canadian origin are currently being conducted.

In addition, an increased incidence of cystic fibrosis occurs among French-speaking Canadians (Rozen et al., 1992). Muscular dystrophy, with a worldwide frequency of 1 in 25,000 individuals, occurs in 1 in 154 French Canadians of the Saguenay region (DeBraekeleer, 1991). Health-care providers working with this specialized population of Québecers must screen for these genetic diseases and provide genetic counseling for high-risk clients who express an interest.

VARIATIONS IN DRUG METABOLISM

Research supporting differences in drug metabolism related to race and ethnicity is beginning to identify genetic mutations among descendants of French Canadian settlers from specific areas of France. Although these findings may produce data related to drug metabolism, thus far, little has been published. Risk factors affecting French-speaking Canadians tend to be related to type of work, geographic region, communication, education, and age groups.

High-Risk Behaviors

Special attention must be given to older Francophones living outside Québec. Abuse of alcohol, tobacco, and psychotropic drugs are major health problems among Francophone Québecers. In Québec, the number who use tobacco has been decreasing, down to 24 percent instead of 35 percent in 1995 (INSPQ, 2006). A study with high school students reported that tobacco smoking decreased to 19 percent; yet, marijuana smoking increased to 39 percent (Gouvernement du Québec, 2006).

The French population has a long-standing appreciation of alcohol, with wine being their beverage of choice, dating to the early 17th century. Both French and French Canadians continue to view drinking favorably. Disapproval of women drinking heavily is evident. Francophone youth start drinking at younger ages than do Anglophone youths (DeWit & Beneteau, 1998). Alcohol consumption has increased since the early 1990s, particularly among men, and drinking and driving among young men has reached a summit despite the legal implications (INSPQ, 2006). However, drug use is not associated with personality factors or depression when measured by Rotter's Internal-External Locus of Control Scale Depression Inventory. Tobacco and alcohol use is highest among French-speaking males and is associated with masculine sex roles, higher self-esteem, and an external locus of control. Nonmedical drug use, primarily marijuana and hashish, most frequently involved men and was related to an internal locus of control.

HEALTH-CARE PRACTICES

The aging Francophone population across the country has increased, passing from 11.2 percent in 1996 to 12.5 percent in 2001 (Statistics Canada, 2006). Beliefs about methods for improving one's health are seen as influential factors in health-seeking behaviors. The rate of individuals who do not exercise on a regular basis has increased from 35 percent in 1995 to 26 percent in 2003 despite numerous educational campaign in favor of exercise (INSPQ, 2006). In 2004, half of the population of children aged 4 to 18 years and nearly 60 percent of the adults aged 19 years and older ate at least five portions of fruits or vegetables daily (INSPQ, 2006). According to Wharry (1997), Québécois probably give tobacco its strongest bulwark in the country; in health communication, one has to tailor the message. A communication method that works among the English-speaking populations does not mean it will automatically work among the French. Yet very little has been developed specifically for the French community.

Feather and Green's (1993) study on health behaviors found that good health practices were more prevalent among Canadian men under the age of 25 years and over the age of 65 than among men in their middle adult years. In contrast to men, the prevalence of good health practices among Canadian women increases until the age of 65 and then decreases. In addition, these practices were positively correlated with levels of education in both sexes, adequate income for women, and managerial or professional occupations for men.

Responses of French-speaking Canadians throughout Canada correlated more with the province in which they lived than with the selected cultural group. This correlation could be due to the method of data collection, which is less accurate with a small response rate. The higher proportion of respondents from Québec and New Brunswick may have skewed the statistical outcome. Overall, age was a factor associated with beliefs about one's ability to achieve an improved health status. Results imply that older people focus more on personal well-being than on health practices.

Nutrition

MEANING OF FOOD

For French Canadians, food is associated with hospitality and warmth. Food is part of all meetings and celebrations. The strong influence of nutritional status on health prompted the inclusion of questions on nutritional behaviors and diet changes in the 1990 health promotion survey to identify data among high-risk groups. In this survey, body mass index was used to calculate the ratio of weight relative to height and determine the potential for health risk. Age, gender, and education, rather than culture, were identified as positive influences on the practice of reading labels for nutritional value of food. Regardless

of the reason, this practice demonstrates the importance individuals attribute to food in relation to health.

COMMON FOODS AND FOOD RITUALS

Common vegetables enjoyed by French Canadians include potatoes, turnips, carrots, asparagus, cabbage, lettuce, cucumbers, and tomatoes. Apart from citrus fruits, all other edible fruits, particularly apples and berries grown in gardens or in the wild, are prepared and preserved by French Canadians for the winter. Meat choices are mainly beef, pork, and poultry. Lately, however, lamb has gained popularity. Christmas and seasonal festivities call for the *tourtières and ragoût de boulettes* to go with the turkey. Ham is usually the Easter main dish, along with maple sugar pastery of all kinds. Until the late 1960s, fish was often perceived as a Friday food. However, for the younger generation, this belief is no longer practiced. Increased immigration and fast-food availability have influenced food choices and customs to the point of transforming French Canadians' customs and food practices, with a new phenomenon as *poutine*, fries topped with cheese curds and covered with gravy.

In Acadia, owing to the proximity of the coastal areas, fresh fish and seafood are part of the diet. Common foods include *fricot* (stew made with a special spice called summer savory). Traditional foods such as *poutine réfrapées* (balls of dough made from grated potatoes) and *réfrapure* (grated potato) are not part of the regular diet, but are still enjoyed during special events. The equivalent to the French Canadian pea soup is named *fayots* soup in Acadia.

DIETARY PRACTICES FOR HEALTH PROMOTION

Most men and women report reading nutritional labels on food packages. This behavior is a good predictor of diet changes during the preceding year. As a whole, more Québecers than other Canadians report eating breakfast. Only 10 percent of the French-speaking Canadians report skipping breakfast, which is significantly lower than among respondents from the rest of Canada (Craig, 1993). A similar study conducted with children in grades 1 to 3 yielded similar results in the northern part of Ontario (McIntyre & Doyle, 1992).

NUTRITIONAL DEFICIENCIES AND FOOD LIMITATIONS

In an industrialized country like Canada, six times as many women as men are underweight, yet half as many women as men rated themselves as underweight (Craig, 1993). However, 33 to 50 percent of all Canadians are trying to lose weight. The 1990 health promotion study demonstrates that being overweight is inversely proportional to education and income for both men and women. For men, there was no association between being underweight and education and income, whereas for women, with the exception of the very poor, a positive correlation existed between being underweight and increased income (Craig, 1993). Nevertheless, recent studies tend to show that French Canadians do not escape the overall trend toward being overweight.

Pregnancy and Childbearing Practices

VIGNETTE 11.2

Mrs. Gagné, age 38 years, is of French Canadian heritage. She arrives at the physician's office with complaints of vaginal bleeding and acute unilateral (right side) pain radiating to her shoulder. She has missed her last two menses and believes she is pregnant for the third time. Her two previous pregnancies ended with spontaneous abortions. The physician diagnosed a right ectopic pregnancy, for which she undergoes a salpingectomy. During surgery, she lost a significant amount of blood for which the surgeon wanted to do a blood transfusion. Mrs. Gagné refuses the blood transfusion based on her religious beliefs. The surgeon has ordered treatment with methotrexate, requiring daily follow-up. Because, Mrs. Gagné lives in a rural area, daily follow-up is not an option.

1. Identify culturally congruent counseling strategies to help Mrs. Gagné and her husband work through the grieving process on losing a third baby.
2. Identify possible reasons for the spontaneous abortions.
3. What services would you recommend to assure that Mrs. Gagné can get daily follow-up care?
4. With a high value placed on family and children in French Canadian families, do you think Mr. and Mrs. Gagné would benefit from long-term counseling?
5. How would you foresee their long-term marital relationship if they remain childless?

FERTILITY PRACTICES AND VIEWS TOWARD PREGNANCY

Until the middle of the 20th century, French Canadians maintained high fertility rates, which is uncommon for a population living in an industrialized country. This phenomenon, called the *revenge of the cradles*, has never been explained. Classic interpretations based on the economy, religion, or education do not hold up to scientific examination (Fournier, 1989). The historical co-occurrence of the power of the Church and high birth rates do not prove a causal link. Instead, the "overfertility" of French Canadians appears to be a response to socialization that is distinguished by the prevalence of extended family ties (Fournier, 1989). However, Ansen (2000) found that as education increases, fertility rate within the Francophone group decreases, whereas the contrary is observed within the English group, meaning that as education level increases, so does the fertility rate. For many years, French Canadian fertility practices have been closely tied to the Catholic religion. Before the 1960s, the only acceptable birth control method was abstinence, resulting in a high fecundity rate. From 1851 until the 1960s, Québec families had a mean of 6.84 children per family. The number of children per family started to decline from 3.1 in 1965 to 1.5 in 1990 (Henripin & Martin, 1991), with a current record of 1.2 children per family (Statistics Canada, 2001).

Effective contraception and family planning methods such as the pill, intrauterine devices, and tubal ligation have become available to all women. The pill remains the primary reversible method for birth control (Health and Welfare Canada, 1989). Nowadays contraceptive methods are strongly encouraged. Adolescents by the age of 14 years are legally allowed to obtain a contraception prescription from a physician without a parent's approval. In addition, the "morning-after pill" is available to adolescents in drug stores without a prescription. On the basis of relative frequency, tubal ligation and vasectomy follow the pill as nonreversible methods of fertility control. Diaphragms, foams, and creams are not commonly used for birth control, partially because perceptions imply that women are not supposed to, or do not like to, touch their genitals. The beliefs that condoms reduce the level of sexual feeling during intercourse or that contraception is not a man's responsibility are inversely proportional to the age of men. Many French-speaking Canadians believe that abortion is morally wrong, but it is legally available. The number of annual abortions by language or cultural subdivision is unavailable. Finally, new reproductive technologies are available but are used by a small number of French-speaking Canadians, more because of scarcity than cultural denial or restriction.

Although pregnancy is considered a normal life event, fear of labor and delivery prevails. This learned fear is transmitted to women from childhood and is often reinforced by the health-care system. Midwives have officially been accepted by the government, but the use of midwives and maternity centers (*maisons des naissances*) is far from being the custom. More women are talking about the desire to deliver at home, but the actual use of a midwife throughout labor and delivery at home is quite low. Obstetricians still provide 84 percent of women's health care, family physicians 11 percent; only 4 percent of women's health care is provided by midwives (PPPESO, 2005).

From another perspective, in Canada, age of childbearing has changed with the times. In 1991, women over 30 years of age gave birth to 34 percent of newborns, whereas 10 years later, the rate increased to 41.9 percent, and in Ontario in 2003, the proportion was as high as 55 percent (PPPESO, 2005). Analgesic use and/or local anesthesia such as an epidural for delivery remain high and the rate of cesarean sections has increased to 1 in 4 newborns, for a proportion of 25 percent of total births and 30.3 percent of those in university facilities (PPPESO, 2005). The data do not differ much from those in Québec for cesarian sections over the last 10 years.

PRESCRIPTIVE, RESTRICTIVE, AND TABOO PRACTICES IN THE CHILDBEARING FAMILY

From a clinical perspective, prenatal medical visits are recommended once a month until the end of the seventh month, twice during the eighth month, and weekly during the last month. Since the mid-1970s, prenatal classes are well attended by both the mother and the father-to-be. These classes are generally free of charge and focus on information regarding health and hygiene during pregnancy and on preparation and exercises for labor and delivery.

Alcohol and tobacco use is discouraged for the duration of pregnancy and the breastfeeding period. Intercourse restrictions are not commonly applied during pregnancy unless required for medical reasons. Since the 1970s, fathers have been encouraged to be present in the delivery room. They are invited to assume an active role by assisting the mother and the physician, receiving the baby, and cutting the cord. Most Canadian women still deliver in a dorsal position, even though lying on the back has been shown to be antiphysiological. However, with the advent of birthing rooms, more women are delivering their babies in half-sitting or side-lying positions.

Few French Canadians practice natural childbirth. Although the number of women who are cared for by a widwife is still low, the number is increasing because midwifes have access to hospitals and, in many places, they are part of the health-care team. During hospitalization, rooming-in of the mother and child is a relatively new practice. Many hospitals have made cohabitation a generalized practice, unless the child or mother requires special treatments. Breastfeeding has regained importance after years of bottlefeeding. The mother's general hesitation to breastfeed relates to not having sufficient milk, experiencing sore nipples, losing breast firmness, and muscle wasting after the breastfeeding period. In practice, once the mother has made a decision regarding breastfeeding, the father's support and encouragement are key for a successful outcome.

Differences exist between English-speaking and French-speaking women with respect to breast-feeding. During the Health Survey of 1990, 44 percent of Canadian mothers reported breastfeeding their last child. Of these, 48 percent were Anglophones and 26 percent were Francophones. Craig (1993) found significant regional differences regarding breastfeeding practices. Approximately one-quarter of women from the Maritimes, one-third from Québec, and one-half from Ontario and the western provinces breastfeed their babies. Maternity and paternity leaves are available with pay for a period ranging from 6 to 20 weeks, which may extend up to 12 months without pay. In practice, however, fathers often take only a few days to a few weeks of leave to help the mother care for the new baby and other children.

Some taboo practices related to pregnancy have persisted throughout the years. Although the movement used in washing a floor resembles that of an exercise aimed at strengthening the perineal muscles, this activity in the past was associated with the onset of labor and early or preterm deliveries. Another belief, which is shared by some nurses, is that the full moon plays a role in the onset of labor once the full-term period has been reached. This belief applies to pregnant women who are 2 weeks preterm or postterm. A much less common belief is that pregnant women who experience hyperglycemia give birth to boys and that lack of salt signifies the birth of girls.

Death Rituals

VIGNETTE 11.3

Mr. Bouchard, a widowed Catholic age 70 years, has been on oxygen with chronic obstructive pulmonary disease (COPD) for the last 10 years. A heavy smoker and worker in the mines of Northern Ontario, he has been a socially active individual for many years. He is now confined to his home. His children come to visit as much as they can. His wife cared after him for years, but she now suffers with severe arthritis and has difficulty caring for herself. Their quality of life has greatly diminished.

This morning Mr. Bouchard is giving a press conference to announce his desire to end his life by suicide. He does not want to live another day in this condition. There is no cure for COPD, and living between bed, kitchen, living room, and washroom brings no satisfaction. Even the smallest daily functional activity demands more energy than he has to spare, leaving him continuously overtired. He wishes by this press conference to urge the government to advance the debate on death with dignity, assisted suicide, and euthanasia.

1. How would you assist Mr. Bouchard to identify a source of hope in his life?
2. Discuss the role of spirituality in this family.
3. Discuss Mr. Bouchard's viewpoint on death, end of life, and end-of-life care within the French Canadian culture.
4. Explore culturally appropriate rituals related to death and dying for Mr. and Mrs. Bouchard.
5. To which high-risk health situations are French Canadians most often exposed, and how have they affected this family?

DEATH RITUALS AND EXPECTATIONS

French Canadians do not differ from Canadians of other European origins on issues related to death and death rituals. Expectations are closely related to Christian religious practices, in particular, those of the Roman Catholic Church, of which most French Canadians in or before the first half of the 20th century were members. Whether one is an active church-goer or not, religious funerals are the norm. Values and beliefs related to life after death, the soul, and God vary dramatically across the age span among French Canadians and, even more so, among Francophones. Thus, it is essential to assess each family individually when it comes to death rituals and expectations. For many years, cremation was seen by the Catholic Church as a ritual left for specific circumstances. Currently, the Catholic Church advocates cremation as an acceptable practice.

RESPONSES TO DEATH AND GRIEF

During the second half of the 20th century, long grief and mourning rituals imposed by social norms were adapted to modern lifestyles. Traditional responses to death and mourning periods were influenced by the place women hold in the workforce, the age of the deceased, and other circumstances. Currently, the expression of grief among French Canadians is similar to the stages described by Kübler-Ross (1977). Supports for those who have lost a family member include openly acknowledging the family's right to express grief, being physically present, making referrals to appropriate religious leaders, and encouraging interpersonal relationships.

Spirituality

DOMINANT RELIGION AND USE OF PRAYER

Whereas most French Canadians identify themselves as Roman Catholic and are baptized at birth, they may or may not remain active church members. A growing number of births are registered through civil channels rather than through the traditional Catholic registry and baptism. Despite the sharp decline in actively practicing Catholics, most people from all socioeconomic levels turn to their church for important life events such as marriage and funerals. In some cases, even in a civil ceremony involving previously divorced spouses, the couple may ask a priest to say mass and bless the union. The Catholic Church does not allow a religious remarriage and exchange of solemn vows for divorcees, unless the previous or first marriage has been annulled and judged void by Church's sanction. The abolition of the religious school boards all over Québec will most likely increase nonreligious practices.

Religious holidays honored as civic holidays are New Year's Day, Good Friday, Easter Sunday, and Easter Monday, July 1st (Confederation Day), and Christmas. In the province of Québec, St. John the Baptist Day (June 24) is a civic holiday, and in most Acadian institutions, the national Acadian holiday Feast of the Assumption is celebrated on August 15. All Saints Day (November 1) and the Epiphany (January 6) were dropped as civic holidays in the 1970s.

Older adults are more inclined to use prayers for finding strength and adapting to difficult physical, psychological, and social health problems. In times of illness and tragedy, French-speaking Canadians use prayer to help recovery. Many of the younger generation are not strongly influenced by religious values, beliefs, and faith practices. The younger generations turn toward spitiruality rather than religion. Many French Acadians still request the sacrament of the sick and a visit from the priest.

MEANING OF LIFE AND INDIVIDUAL SOURCES OF STRENGTH

Traditional French Canadians, who view themselves as the core (*gyron*) of the family and who believe that the well-being of their children is more precious than their own life, have faded proportionally with the prevalence of divorce. For hard-working men and women of previous generations, leisure activity was a trivial expression. The little time that could be spared on holidays was dedicated to visiting distant relatives.

SPIRITUAL BELIEFS AND HEALTH-CARE PRACTICES

Although modern health promotion theories suggest that spiritual needs are a critical factor in comprehensive client care, this aspect of family needs has received little attention among French-speaking Canadians. Many health-care providers still equate spirituality with religion, which is often reflected in the patient's history at the time of admission. Renewed interest in spirituality across Canada is being recognized as a source of physical and psychological health (Simard, 2006). Koenig (2000) discussed spirituality, religion, and medicine with applications to clinical social services.

Health-Care Practices

HEALTH-SEEKING BELIEFS AND BEHAVIORS

In the 19th and early 20th centuries, sick people did not readily enter hospitals because mortality rates were high and care was often inhumane. Before the Confederation, resources and preventive health care rested in the hands of religious sisterhoods, United Empire Loyalists, church groups, and local authorities (Allemag, 1995). As pioneers in health services, the Gray Nuns visited the sick and opened hospitals such as Bytown in Ontario in 1845 and St. Boniface in Manitoba in 1847. In 1860, they extended their services to an Indian settlement 400 miles north of Saskatoon, and in 1867, to Fort Providence on Great Slave Lake.

St. Amant and Vuong (1994) surveyed 57 older former psychiatric clients from 14 organizations in New Brunswick on the relationship between cultural affiliation, gender, and satisfaction with health-care services. The findings revealed that women's mental health was more fragile than men's. A positive correlation and higher satisfaction with services was found among those with longer institutionalization. The authors concluded that Francophones in New Brunswick rely more on an informal family support network, whereas Anglophones rely more on professional services.

Results of a 1990 Canadian health survey show that residents of British Colombia and Ontario reported the most favorable assessments of their health, with almost 3 out of 10 reporting excellent health. Lower levels of health were reported in eastern Canada, where 1 in 5 Nova Scotians reported excellent health. Canadians from New Brunswick, followed by those from Québec, were more likely to report fair or poor health, with only 17 percent and 16 percent, respectively, reporting excellent health (Stephens & Fowler Graham, 1993). Good health has been consistently related to education and income, occupation, or both. However, lifestyle showed an inconsistent relationship with income. Among younger adults and older men, social class had little effect on income, whereas among women, the effect of income dominated over social class. Rather than attempting to identify risk factors for specific diseases, it may be more meaningful to identify those factors that affect general susceptibility to risk factors.

RESPONSIBILITY FOR HEALTH CARE

Canada's government-administered health system ensures free, universal health coverage at any point of entry into the system. However, many people in the upper socioeconomic classes call on their family physicians instead of the local community service centers. Among the lower socioeconomic classes of Québec and the Maritimes, many do not seek health care until their health becomes a crisis situation.

Evans and Stoddart's (1994) White Paper, "Producing health, consuming health care," proposed that the determinants of health status are lifestyle, environment, human biology, and health-care organizations. According to this paper, lifestyle and, to a lesser extent, living environments are chosen by the individual. Corin (1994) offered a matrix of stressors for identifying high-risk behaviors within a perspective that avoids victim blaming. Lifestyle behaviors are readily perceived as being under the control of the individual. The broad set of relationships encompassed under the label of "stress" and predictive factors against stress have demonstrated the importance of social relationships for preventing disease and mortality (Sapolsky, 1990).

In 1980, New Brunswick set up a novel program at the Extra-Mural Hospital to provide acute and chronic home-care services to a largely rural province with a small population density and limited financial resources. Because the willingness of clients and family members to participate actively in a plan of care is critical to the success of community-based services, the Extra-Mural Hospital program strongly encouraged self-care with family involvement. Unlike other community initiatives in Canada, such as the Ontario home-care program, the Extra-Mural Hospital does not restrict services within specific boundaries, and offers a comprehensive, provincewide delivery system via a single-agency approach (Cormier-Daigle, Baker, Arseneault, & MacDonald, 1995).

Hagan, O'Neill, and Dallaire (1995) raised the association between health promotion and community health nursing with conceptual and practical issues. In Québec, the infrastructure for public health is different from that in other provinces. The community service centers, or CLSCs, emerged from the Castonguay-Nepveu reform of health and welfare services in the early 1970s. The mission of the Fédération des CLSCs du Québec is to provide health and social services for primary and secondary prevention and rehabilitation. In a survey of health education roles and activities of 631 nurses, Hagan (1991) found that 89 percent of nurses had a humanistic vision of health education. This vision was defined as "teaching and establishing a helping relationship aimed at facilitating individuals' choices of strategies for improving or maintaining their global health" (p. 278).

French-speaking Canadians have joined the current trend toward over-the-counter drug use. However, from the health survey of 1990, their use of analgesics and tranquilizers shows strong provincial differences (Adlaf, 1993). As compared with the national average for the use of narcotic analgesics (11 percent), Québec residents' use is only 5 percent. Residents of Québec (67 percent) are less likely to use aspirin than the average Canadian (76 percent). However, the use of tranquilizers among Québecers is slightly higher than the Canadian average (8 percent versus 5 percent). Drug use followed a pattern similar to that found in the healthy lifestyle practice. Despite the move toward healthy lifestyles, older French Canadian adults have not changed dramatically in comparison with younger age groups. In addition, in the 1990 health survey, the leisure time physical activity (LTPA) index reported a positive relation between adoption of healthy lifestyles and socioeconomic status, although not a smooth, linear one. In particular, the daily LTPA index decreased with increasing education.

FOLK AND TRADITIONAL PRACTICES

Saillant (1992) analyzed the importance, characteristics, and mechanics of women's knowledge of folk medicine in Québec Francophone families at the beginning of the 20th century. This anthropological study focused on domestic activities. The ethnographic data were drawn from 4000 medical receipts dealing with the knowledge of women in folk-healing practices in Québec and abroad to enhance the understanding of the roles played by women in rural society folk-healing tradition. The numerous connections between the culinary and the therapeutic realms of activities bring one to rethink the link between nutrition and health practiced in the early years of the colony.

BARRIERS TO HEALTH CARE

Language differences may have an important impact on the patient, providers, and administrative interactions and may become a barrier to continuity of care. However, language may also be a proxy for issues that can affect access to care. Language is closely related to culture, and language differences may signal variations in values about behaviors or use of health care. Current views toward multiculturalism include removing barriers so that all citizens have equal access and opportunities and cultural diversity needs are to be considered in decision-making and resource allocation. For many older French Canadian adults raised outside the province of Québec, French was the language used in daily living within their cultural environment, except for educational services. In their childhood, they attended English-speaking schools because the public school system was all that was available outside Québec. This situation and other issues present challenges in organizing transcultural health-care delivery. When the spoken language is French, and reading skills (or what is left of them) are often English, adequate communication is limited and complex. Thus, the health-care team may need to supplement written messages and instructions with verbal instructions to ensure understanding. Recruitment teams visiting France in early 2000 did not provide expected results. Once in Québec, the Franchophone nurses did not have similar training or the cultural language background (Old French used by the people) to communicate and deliver care to older people in nursing homes where they were expected to work.

CULTURAL RESPONSES TO HEALTH AND ILLNESS

Choinière and Melzack (1987), using the McGill Pain Questionnaire and a visual-analog intensity scale, assessed acute and chronic pain differences between 68 French-speaking and English-speaking people with hemophilia. The results showed a similarity in the sensory, affective, and evaluative properties between the two types of pain. French-speaking subjects rated their acute pain as more intense than chronic pain and more affectively laden than the English-speaking group. From a different perspective, Rukholm, Bailey, and Coutu-Wakulczyk (1991), studying French and English cultural differences in family needs and anxiety in an intensive care unit (ICU), found that English-speaking subjects rated their distress at seeing a relative in pain more highly than

French-speaking subjects. Though puzzling, this finding deserves attention and additional research to better understand and plan health-care interventions and to assist family members involved with ICU services.

Adam (1989), as part of a broader package of health promotion, developed, implemented, and evaluated a 15-hour community program for French-speaking women living in minority situations, many of whom were socially and economically disadvantaged. The program was designed to increase the participants' ability to take charge of their lives and better manage their physical and mental health. After presenting the program to 29 groups, evaluations showed that women generally reported satisfaction as the program progressed. Most subjects were satisfied with their broader understanding of stress and relaxation techniques for controlling daily stress.

The deinstitutionalized physically and mentally disabled are protected from discrimination and abuse by federal and provincial laws in Canada. Physically disabled people, regardless of their ethnicity, benefit from equal-opportunity regulations. Throughout Canada, official general acceptance and increased awareness have led to the physical adaptation of the environment to facilitate access for the disabled. However, the homeless mentally disabled raise different concerns in regard to the cost of maintaining this segment of the population in the community and the lack of adequate organized services.

Saillant (1990) studied the sick role among a French Canadian sample from a clinical anthropological perspective exploring the relationship between discourse, knowledge, and the experience of cancer within the life story of a patient suffering from cancer. The underlying theoretical model drew on a cultural hermeneutic approach. The client's discourse was analyzed for cognitive and symbolic models used to understand the experience of cancer. The results of this study highlighted the gap between the client's actual medical knowledge and the health professional's perception of the client's experiences and discourse about cancer (Saillant, 1990).

BLOOD TRANSFUSIONS AND ORGAN DONATION

As a cultural group, French Canadians have no official proscriptions against receiving blood or blood products. Those who are members of a religious group that prohibits the acceptance of a blood transfusion are rare in Canada. Organ donation and transplantation are relatively new treatments in Canada. The decision to donate or receive an organ is an individual decision without cultural influence for French Canadians.

Health-Care Practitioners

TRADITIONAL VERSUS BIOMEDICAL PRACTITIONERS

French Canadians have discarded the idea that one goes to the hospital to die. With a publicly administered health-care system in place since the 1960s, the population has benefited from increased accessibility to health care. However, financing this "welfare state" (*état providence*) has imposed a tremendous burden on taxpayers. Although the overall impact on health-care services is minimal, alternative therapies are gaining popularity, which may reflect disillusionment with the biomedical model in Québec.

Men have been members of the nursing profession since the early 1970s. Although male nurses receive the same training as female nurses, they still account for less than 10 percent of professional nurses in Canada. Whereas bedside nursing is gaining in popularity for men, most still hold administrative or teaching positions.

STATUS OF HEALTH-CARE PROVIDERS

In Canada as a whole, health-care practitioners cover a broad realm of specialties and disciplines, each working within an interdisciplinary and intersectorial approach to well-being. However, the system is not ideal, and tension occurs within and among disciplines. Health-care providers hold a favorable status in the eyes of French Canadians, especially among older people. The prevalence study in three home-care community agencies in southern Ontario has demonstrated the implications for cultural sensitivity training (Majumdar, Browne, & Roberts, 1995). To enhance staff knowledge and skills, in spite of their general assimilation, remnants of French cultural heritage must be recognized as both contributing to behavior and influencing the course of clinical intervention.

At the beginning of the 20th century, parents and grandparents were pragmatic and practical people, sharing views about God's power over everyday life. For example, a mother would pray to have at least a priest and a nun among her children, and a physician or a nurse was next in her wish to God. Today, folk and traditional practitioners are almost nonexistent. The current universal health insurance system makes the folk practitioners less appealing. Professionals throughout Canada are vigilant in trying to avoid exploitation by traditional and folk healers, who are viewed as practicing outside the law.

REFERENCES

Adam, D. (1989). Women and stress: A community prevention and health promotion program. *Canada Mental Health, 37*(4), 5–8.

Adlaf, E. (1993). Alcohol and other drug use. *Health and welfare Canada: Canada's health promotion survey 1990.* Technical report. Cat. No. H39-263/2-1990E. Ottawa, Canada: Ministry of Supply and Services.

Allemag, M. M. (1995). Development of community health nursing in Canada. In M. J. Stewart (Ed.), *Community nursing: Promoting Canadians' health* (pp. 2–36). Toronto, Canada: W. B. Saunders Canada.

Ansen, J. (2000). Nationalism and fertility in Francophone Montreal: The majority as a minority. *Canadian Studies in Population, 27*(2), 377–400.

Aube, N., & Linden, W. (1991). Marital disturbance, quality of communication and socioeconomic status. *Canadian Journal of Behavioral Sciences, 23*, 125–132.

Beaudin, M., & Leclerc, A. (1995). The contemporary Acadian economy. In J. Daigle (Ed.), *Acadia of the Maritimes: Thematic studies from the beginning to the present* (pp. 1–44). Moncton, NB: Université de Moncton, Chaire d'Études Acadiennes.

Brunzell, J. T. (1989). Familial lipoprotein lipase deficiency and other causes of the chylomicronemia syndrome. In C. R. Scriver, A. L. Beaudet, W. S. Sly, & D. Valle (Eds.), *The metabolic basis of inherited disease* (pp. 1165–1180). New York: McGraw-Hill.

Canadian Nurses Foundation (2006, Fall). The Facts. *Foundation Focus,* 9.

Canadian Task Force on Preventive Health Care. (2003). Retrieved January 17, 2007, from http://www.canadiancrc.com/Can_Preventive_Care_suicide.htm

Charbonneau, H., Desjardins, B., Guillemette, A., Landry, Y., Légaré, J., & Nault, F. (1987). *Naissance d'une population: Les Français établis au Canada au XVII siècle.* Paris: Institut National d'Études Démographiques.

Choinière, M., & Melzack, R. (1987). Acute and chronic pain in hemophilia. *Pain, 31*(3), 317–331.

Citizenship and Immigration Canada. (2005). *Profil national.récipéré.* Retrieved January 16, 2007, from http://www.cic.gc.ca/français/francophonie/canada/economique1.html

Corin, E. (1994). The social and cultural matrix of health and disease. In R. G. Evans, M. L. Barer, & T. R. Marmor (Eds.), *Why are some people healthy and others not? The determinants of health of populations* (pp. 93–132). New York: Aldine De Gruyter.

Cormier-Daigle, M., Baker, C., Arseneault, A. M., & MacDonald, M. (1995). The Extra-Mural Hospital: A home health-care initiative in New Brunswick. In M. J. Stewart (Ed.), *Community nursing: Promoting Canadians' health* (pp. 163–179). Toronto, Canada: W. B. Saunders.

Craig, C. L. (1993). Nutrition. In T. Stephens & D. Fowler Graham (Eds.), *Canada's health promotion survey 1990.* Technical report. Cat. No. H39-263/2-1990E. Ottawa: Health and Welfare Canada, Ministry of Supply and Services.

DeBraekeleer, M. (1991). Deleterious genes. In G. Bouchard & M. DeBrackeleer (Eds.), *History of a genome: Population and genetics in Eastern Québec* (pp. 343–363). Québec, Canada: Presses de l'Université du Québec.

DeBraekeleer, M., & Dao, T. N. (1994). In search of founders. I: Hereditary disorders in the French-Canadian population of Québec. *Human Biology, 66*(2), 205–224.

Denault, A. A., & Cardinal, L. (1999). L'équité en matière d'emploi en Ontario et les Francophones, de 1986 à 1995. *Recherches Sociologiques, 40*(1), 83–101.

DeWit, D. J., & Beneteau, B. (1998). Predictors of the prevalence of alcohol use related problems among Francophones and Anglophones in the province of Ontario, Canada. *Journal of Studies on Alcohol, 59*(1), 78–88.

Dionne, C., Gagné, C., Julien, P., Murthy, M., Roederer, G., Davignon, J., Lambert, M., Chitayat, D., Ma, R., Henderson, H., Lupien, P. J., Hayden, M. R., & DeBraekeleer, M. (1993). Genealogy and regional distribution of lipoprotein lipase deficiency in French-Canadians of Québec. *Human Biology, 65*(1), 29–40.

Emard, J., Drouin, G., Thouez, J., & Ghardirian, P. (2001). Vasectomy and prostate cancer in Québec, Canada. *Health and Place, 7*(2), 131–139.

Evans, R. G. (1994). Introduction. In R. G. Evans, M. L. Barer, & T. R. Marmor (Eds.), *Why are some people healthy and others not? The determinants of health of populations* (pp. 3–26). New York: Aldine De Gruyter.

Evans, R. G., & Stoddart, G. L. (1994). Producing health, consuming health care. In R. G. Evans, M. L. Barer, & T. R. Marmor (Eds.), *Why are some people healthy and others not? The determinants of health of populations* (pp. 27–66). New York: Aldine de Gruyter.

Feather, J., & Green, K. L. (1993). Health behaviours and intentions. In T. Stephens & D. Fowler Graham (Eds.), *Canada's health promotion survey 1990.* Technical report. Cat. No. H39-263/2-1990E. Ottawa, Canada: Ministry of Supply and Services.

Fong, E., & Guilia, M. (1990). *Neighborhood changes within the Canadian ethnic mosaic.* Ontario, Canada: University of Ontario.

Fournier, D. (1989). Pourquoi la revanche des berceaux? L'hypothèse de sociabilité. *Recherches Sociographiques, 30*(2), 171–198.

Fumeron, F., Grandchamp, B., Fricker, J., Krempt, M., Wolf, L. M., Khayat, M. C., Boiffard, O., & Apfelbaum, M. (1992). Presence of the Canadian deletion in a French patient with familial hypercholesterolemia. *New England Journal of Medicine, 326*(1), 69.

Gagné, C., Brun, L. D., Moorjani, S., & Lupien, P. J. (1989). Primary lipoprotein-lipase-activity deficiency: Clinical investigation of a French-Canadian population. *Canadian Medical Association Journal, 140*(4), 405–411.

Godar, C. (1998). *Health Canada: Ovarian cancer in Canada.* Retrieved January 17, 2007, from http://www.hc-sc.gc.ca

Gouvernement du Québec (2006). *Qu'est-ce qu'une politique familiale?* Ministère de la famille, des aînés et de la condition féminine du Québec, Dernière revision 2006-11-28. Retrieved December 12, 2006, from http://www.mfacf.gouv.qc.ca

Goyder, J. C. (1981). Income differences between the sexes: Findings from a national Canadian survey. *Canadian Review of Sociology and Anthropology, 18,* 321–342.

Grompe, M., St-Louis, M., Demers, S. I., Al-Dhalimy, M., Leclerc, B., & Tanguay, R. M. (1994). A single mutation of the fumarylacetoacetate hydrolase gene in French-Canadians with hereditary tyrosinemia type I. *New England Journal of Medicine, 331*(6), 353–358.

Hagan, L. (1991). Analyse de l'exercice de la fonction éducative des infirmiers et des infirmières des centres locaux de services communautaires du Québec. Unpublished doctoral dissertation, Faculty of Education Sciences, Université de Montréal.

Hagan, L., O'Neill, M., & Dallaire, C. (1995). Linking health promotion and community health nursing: Conceptual and practical issues. In M. J. Stewart (Ed.), *Community nursing: Promoting Canadians' health* (pp. 413–429). Toronto, Canada: W. B. Saunders.

Health and Welfare Canada (1989). *Charting Canada's future: A report of the demographic review.* Ottawa, Canada: Ministry of Supplies and Services.

Henripin, J., & Martin, Y. (1991). *La population du Québec d'hier à demain.* Montréal, Québec: Presses de l'Université de Montréal.

Hobart, C. (1992). How they handle it: Young Canadians, sex and AIDS. *Youth and Society, 23*(4), 411–433.

House, J. S., Landis, K. R., & Umberson, D. (1988). Social relationships and health. *Science, 241,* 540–545.

Huntington, S. P. (2004). *Who are we? The challenges to America's national identity.* NewYork: Simon & Schuster.

Institut national de santé publique (INSPQ) du Québec et Ministère de la santé et des services sociaux du Québec en collaboration avec l'Institut de la statistique du Québec. (2006). *Portrait de santé du Québec et de ses régions 2006: Les analyses- Deuxième rapport national sur l'état de santé de la population du Québec.* Quebec, Canada: Gouvernement du Québec.

International Recognition of Same-Sex Relationships. (2002). Retrieved January 17, 2007, from http://www.hrusa.org

Koenig, H. G. (2000). Religion, spirituality and medicine: Applications to clinical practice. *Journal of the Amerian Medical Association, 284,* 1708.

Krajinovic, M., Ghadirian, P., Richer, C., Sinnett, H., Gandini, S., Perret, C., Lacroix, A., Labuda, D., Sinnett D. (2001). Genetic susceptibility to breast cancer in French-Canadians: Role of carcinogen-metabolizing enzymes and gene-environment interactions. *American Journal of Human Genetics, 59*(3), 633–643.

Kübler-Ross, E. (1977). *Death: The final stage of growth.* Englewood Cliffs, NJ: Prentice-Hall.

Lambert, R. D., Brown, S. D., Curtis, J. E., & Kay, B. J. (1986). Canadians' beliefs about differences between social classes. *Canadian Journal of Sociology/Cahiers Canadiens de Sociologie, 11*(4), 379–399.

Langelier, R. (1996). French-Canadian families. In M. McGoldrick, J. K. Pearce, & J. Giorano (Eds.). *Ethnicity and family therapy* (2nd ed., pp. 477–495). New York: Guilford Press.

Levy, E., Minnich, A., Cacan, S. L., Thibaut, L., Giroux, L.-M., Davignon, J., & Lambert, M. (1997). Association of an exon 3 mutation (Trp66_Gly) of the LDL receptor with variable expression of familial hypercholesterolemia in a French-Canadian family. *Biochemical and Molecular Medicine, 60*(1), 59–69.

Lyonnet, S., De Braekelee, M., Labramboise, R., Rey, F., John, S. W., Berthelon, M., Berthelot, J., Journel, H., & Le Marec, B. (1992). Time and space clusters of the French-Canadian M1V phenylketonuria mutation in France. *American Journal of Human Genetics, 51*(1), 191–196.

Ma, Y., Henderson, H., Ven Marthy, M. R., Roederer, G., Monsalve, M. V., Clarke, L. A., Normand, T., Julien, P., Gagné, C., Lambert, M., Davignon, J., Lupien, P. Jé, Brunzell, J., & Hayden, M. R. (1991). A mutation in the human lipoprotein lipase gene as the most common cause of familial chylomicronemia in French-Canadians. *New England Journal of Medicine, 324*(25), 176–182.

Madibbo, A., & Labrie, N. (2005). La transformation des institutions et des communautés francophones face à l'immigration et à la mondialisation: une étude de cas. *Reflets, 11,* 49–80.

Majumdar, B., Browne, G., & Roberts, J. (1995). The prevalence of multicultural groups receiving in-home service from three community agencies in Southern Ontario: Implications for cultural sensitivity training. *Canadian Journal of Public Health, 86*(3), 206–211.

McIntyre, L., & Doyle, J. B. (1992). Exploratory analysis of children's nutritional program in Canada. *Social Science Medicine, 35*(9), 1123–1129.

National Adult Literary Base. (2005). Retrieved January 17, 2007, from http://library.nald.ca/research/browse/series?name=IALSS+2003+Findings

National de Formation Santé (CNFS). (2001). Retrieved September 14, 2007, from http://www.ami.mr/fr/bulletin 20010902.htm

National PKU Index. (1992). Retrieved September 14 2007, from http://www.pkunewsorg/news/newsix2h.htm

Office of the Commissioner of Official Languages. (2002). *Le français une langue résolument officielle.* Retrieved November 2, 2006, from http://www.clo-ocol.gc.ca/archives /op_ap/facts_faits/fr_canada_f.html

Pampalon, R., Gauthier, D., Raymond, G., & Beaudry, E. (1990). *Health map: A geographical distribution of the Québec Health Survey.* Québec, Canada: Ministere de la Santé et des Services Sociaux.

Pausova, Z., Deslauriers, B., Gaudet, D., Tremblay J., Koetchen, T. A., Larochelle, P., Cowley, A. W., & Hamet, P. (2000). Role of tumor necrosis factor-α gene locus in obesity and obesity-associated hypertension in French-Canadians. *Hypertension, 36*(1), 14–19.

Perinatal Partnership Program of Eastern and Southeastern Ontario (PPPESO). (2006). Retrieved September 14, 2007 from http://www.pppeso.ca/english/niday.html

Pronovost, G. (1989). Transformation in work time and leisure time. In G. Pronovost & D. Mercere (Eds.), *Time and societies* (pp. 37–61). Québec, Canada: Institut Québecois de Recherche sur la Culture.

Public Works and Government Services Canada. (2001). Retrieved January 17, 2007, from http://www.pwgsc.gc.ca

Punnett, B. J. (1991). Language, cultural values and preferred leadership style: A comparison of Anglophones and Francophones in Ottawa. *Canadian Journal of Behavioural Science, 23*(2), 241–244.

Rozen, R., De Braekeleer, M., Daigneault, J., Ferrire-Rajabi, L., Gerdes, M., Lamoureux, L., Aubin, G., Simard, F., Fujiwara, T. M., & Morgan, K. (1992). Cystic fibrosis mutations in French-Canadians: Three CFTR mutations are relatively frequent in a Quebec population with elevated incidence of cystic fibrosis. *American Journal of Medical Genetics, 42*(3), 360–364.

Rozen, R., Mascisch, A., Lambert, M., Laframboise, R., & Scriver, C. R. (1994). Mutation profiles of phenylketonuria in Quebec populations: Evidence of stratification and novel mutations. *American Journal of Human Genetics, 55*(2), 321–326.

Rukholm, E., Bailey, P., & Coutu-Wakulczyk, G. (1991). Needs and anxiety in ICU: Cultural differences in northeastern Ontario. *Canadian Journal of Nursing Research, 23*(3), 67–81.

Saillant, F. (1990). Discourse, knowledge, and experience of cancer: A life story. *Cultural Medicine and Psychiatry, 14*(1), 47–72.

Saillant, F. (1992). Savoir et pratiques des femmes dans l'univers ethnomedical québécois. *Canadian Folklore, 14*(1), 47–72.

St. Amant, N., & Vuong, D. (1994). Quand la language fait une difference: Ce que des "beneficiares" pensent du système de santé mentale. *Sociologie et Sociétés, 261*(1), 179–196.

St.-Pierre, J., Vohl, M. C., Brisson, D., Perron, P., Despres, J. P., Hudson, T. J., & Gaudet, D. (2001). A sequence variation in the mitochondrial glycerol-3-phosphate dehydrogenase gene is associated with increased plasma glycerol and free fatty acid concentrations among French-Canadians. *Molecular Genetics and Metabolism, 72*(3), 209–217.

Samson, J. M., Otis, J., & Levy, J. J. (1996). Risques face au sida, relations de pouvoir et styles de communication sexuelle chez les étudiants des cégeps Francophones du Québec. Rapport de recherche. Montreal, Canada: Département de sexology, Université du Québec à Montréal.

Sapolsky, R. M. (1990). Stress in the wild. Ottawa: Policy, Analysis and Research Directorate Multiculturalism. *Scientific American, 262*(1), 116–123.

Simard, N. (2006). Spiritualité et santé. *Reflets, 12,* 107–127.

Société Canadienne de la sclérose en plaques. (2005). *Communication médicale 17 octobre 2005.* Retrieved October 29, 2006, from www.mssociety.ca

Statistics Canada. (2001). *Une société plus multilingue.* http://www.statcan.com

Statistics Canada. (2002). *Recensement de 2001: serie analyses.* Ottawa, Canada: Ministère de l'Industrie.

Statistics Canada. (2006). *Statistique Canada.* CANSIM, product 91-213-XIB, updated 2006-09-27. Retrieved January 21, 2007, from http://www40.statcan.ca/102/cst01/famil01_f.html

Stephens, T., & Fowler Graham, D. (1993). Overview. In T. Stephens & D. Fowler Graham (Eds.), *Canada's health promotion survey 1990.* Technical report. Cat. No. H39-263/2-1990E. Ottawa, Canada: Ministry of Supply and Services.

Uthman, I., Vasquez-Abad, D., & Sénécal, J. L. (1996). Distinctive features of idiopathic inflammatory myopathies in French-Canadians. *Seminars in Arthritis and Rheumatism, 26*(1), 447–458.

Vohl, M. C., Lepage, P., Gaudet, D., Brewe, C. G., Betard, C., Perron, P., Houde, G., Cellier, C., Faith, J. M., Despres, J. P., Morgan, K., & Hudson, T. J. (2000). Molecular scanning of the human PPAR-_ gene: Association of the L162V mutation with hyperapobetalipoproteinemia. *Journal of Lipid Research, 41*(6), 945–952.

Wharry, S. (1997). Canada: A country of two solitudes when smoking rates among Anglophones, Francophones compared. *Canadian Medical Association Journal, 156*(2), 244–245.

Wu, Z., & Baer, D. E. (1996). Attitudes toward family life and gender roles: A comparison of English and French-Canadian women. *Journal of Comparative Family Studies, 27*(3), 437–452.

Chapter 12

People of German Heritage

JESSICA A. STECKLER

Overview, Inhabited Localities, and Topography

OVERVIEW

Germans are reserved, formal people who appreciate a sense of order in their lives. Their love of music and celebrations has permanently influenced many of the world's cultures. The Christmas tree (*Weihnachtsbaum*) with its brightly decorated ornaments, a universal symbol of the holiday season, is a German creation. Gingerbread houses (*Lebkuchen*), Christmas carols (*Weihnachtslieder*) and cards, the "Easter hare," (*Osterhase*), hot cross buns, valentines (*Freundschaftskarten*), Groundhog Day, chain letters (*Briefe zum Himmel*), the tooth fairy, and *Kaffeeklatsch* or "gossip sessions" have their origins in German culture.

There are 60 million Germans in the United States and 2.7 million in Canada (Wikipedia, 2006a). Ethnic groups of European origin are usually categorized as "white" on applications, in surveys, and in research studies, so there is little culturally specific information available about them. This is unfortunate, because differences in world-view, cultural beliefs, and health-care practices among white ethnic groups hold important implications for health-care providers.

The Federal Republic of Germany (*Bundesrepublik Deutschland*), comprising 16 states, boasts beautiful landscapes, high and low mountain ranges, sandy lowlands, rolling hills, lakelands, and ocean borders. Situated in the heart of Europe, Germany is a link between the East and the West and between Scandinavia and the Mediterranean. Germany has the largest economy in Europe, has the third largest economy in the world, and is the leading per-capita export nation in the world (World

Factbook, 2006). With a population of over 82 million, it is one of the most densely populated countries in Europe. Germany is a member of the United Nations and NATO and is a founding member of the European Union. Most of Germany is located in the temperate zone, with temperatures ranging from 27°F in the mountains to 68°F in the valleys of the south. Temperatures are comparable with the climate in the northwest portion of the United States. The Upper Rhine has a mild climate; Upper Bavaria has warm Alpine winds from the south; and the Harz Mountains have cold winds, cool summers, and heavy winter snows.

HERITAGE AND RESIDENCE

In the 18th century, the New World colonies from New England to the deep South grew and flourished. Even though the colonial settlers shared an Old World heritage, they were a diverse people. German settlers, along with other immigrants from Britain, France, Scotland, and Ireland, shared a love of family and land; a love that would eventually bond them to one another to form a nation of Americans. The earliest German immigrants to the United States settled in the colonies along the eastern seaboard, including William Penn's colony in Pennsylvania. Religious tolerance and equitable land distribution contributed to the success of these Pennsylvania settlements. Mennonites, Dunkers, Amish, and Moravians from Germany made up the new Pennsylvania communities. The area in which they settled, known as *Pennsylvania Dutch Country*, was actually mislabeled by English neighbors who thought the word *deutsch*, meaning "German," stood for "Dutch." One hundred thousand strong, these Pennsylvania Germans were the main carriers of German culture to the mid-Atlantic area (Domer, 1994).

Other religious social idealists from Germany soon flowed into the colonies. Among them were the Harmonists, who broke from the German Lutheran Church under the leadership of George Rapp (Boorstin, 1987). The Harmonists built Harmony, Pennsylvania; Harmony, Indiana; and Economy (Ambridge), Pennsylvania. The Harmonists were followed by other German sects: the Zoars, who settled in Ohio, and the Inspirationists, who originally settled in western New York and later moved west to Iowa by divine command.

The second wave of German immigrants arrived in the United States between 1840 and 1860. They were fleeing political persecution, starvation, and poverty in their homeland and settled on the western frontier (Weaver, 1979). This group of influential Germans was less interested in taking root in the United States than in establishing a German culture. These new immigrants kept the German language in their schools, published newspapers in German, joined their own singing societies and orchestras, and married only other Germans.

The 1930s and 1940s saw a third wave of German immigration. Artists, architects, social scientists, physicists, and mathematicians came to this country to escape the Nazi Holocaust. These new arrivals were highly educated and at the height of their careers. After witnessing the horrors of the Holocaust, they had no desire to transplant Old World institutions or to establish new European-style homelands (Boorstin, 1987). These third-wave immigrants became rapidly acculturated into American life and greatly enriched American culture in the fields of music, psychology, science, and mathematics. Among this prominent group were Albert Einstein and Hannah Arendt, an author and political scientist.

Historians have helped to further our understanding of the diffusion of German immigrants into the American heartland by tracing the existence of the "two-door house." These German-built houses, which architecturally copied their European counterparts, have two front doors. With their movement across the United States, two-door houses appeared in Pennsylvania, Maryland, West Virginia, the Blue Ridge Mountains, Ohio, Indiana, Illinois, Missouri, Iowa, Kansas, Nebraska, Michigan, and Texas (Domer, 1994).

Germans continue to embrace the United States as their own. The desire to become American has been nurtured by the presence of American troops in Germany, and many Germans have entered the United States as spouses of military personnel. For others, business ventures and the promise of career opportunities brought them to this country. Today, about one-fourth of all American citizens can trace their ancestry to German roots. Germans are the dominant ancestral group in St. Louis, Missouri; Milwaukee, Wisconsin; Chicago, Illinois; Cincinnati, Ohio; Buffalo and New York City in New York; and Baltimore, Maryland.

REASONS FOR MIGRATION AND ASSOCIATED ECONOMIC FACTORS

Germans have been very much a part of important events shaping U.S. socioeconomic history. They have been participants, observers, and victims in the Revolutionary War, the Civil War, the influenza epidemic, the Great Depression, both World Wars, the Vietnam War, the Persian Gulf War, and the current global recession. The reasons for their immigration to the United States vary according to historical antecedents and are, therefore, discussed under Heritage and Residence.

EDUCATIONAL STATUS AND OCCUPATIONS

Germans have a deep respect for education. In Germany, credibility, social status, and level of employment are based on educational achievement. In other words, Germans are very class conscious. Germans take pride in their school system, particularly in their craftsmanship and technology. Unlike in the United States, education is free at all levels, except kindergarten, which is optional, but entrance to university education is difficult and accomplished only by passing the *Abitur* examination. Literacy rates of Germany (99 percent) and the United States (98 percent) are comparable (CIA, 2007).

According to S. Maubach (personal communication, December 28, 2006), German children can begin kindergarten at age 3. This is comparable with our preschool. At age 6, they enter grade school, which includes grades 1 to 4. At grade 5, they begin one of three tracks of education: *Hauptschule*, which is special education and the most basic educational path; *Realschule*, which is general education; or *Gynasium*, which is like U.S. college preparatory courses. German students graduate at grade 10 and can then enter into vocational education, which prepares them for a trade or for working in business, or continue college preparation. Those students wishing to go to the universities must pass the *Abitur* test, which is both verbal and written.

Germans who immigrated to the United States in the 19th century influenced American preschool and higher-educational systems. The Johns Hopkins University in Baltimore, Maryland, was founded on the model of Humboldt University in Berlin, Germany (McKinnon, 1993). During this same period, many American historians and political scientists attended German universities, returning with their doctoral degrees, and were instrumental in developing prototypes for American graduate education. Many of the influences of the 19th-century German immigrants on the educational system remain visible today.

By the mid-19th century, *Turnvereins* were taking root in Midwestern German American communities. These political and gymnastic organizations believed in a sound mind and body and provided opportunities to grow both physically and intellectually (Acton, 1994). In this same era, schools—many of which were parochial schools— were established in which only German was spoken. German Catholics also established parochial schools in this era, but unlike the Lutherans, their ethnic identity was not tied to the church (Coburn, 1992).

German immigrants were viewed as an internal threat in the United States during World War II and faced turbulent times. A growing anti-immigrant sentiment leading to calls for immigration restriction intensified the political climate. Some German immigrants' desire to maintain an identity apart from the American culture was expressed through the founding of the National German American Alliance. Many German Americans changed their names, made apologies, and displayed their loyalties in an effort to attenuate suspicions, embarrassments, and persecutions.

Today, German American families continue to value education. Most German Americans have a high school education at minimum. Twenty-four percent have attained post–high school education. However, in the age group 65 and older, 43 percent have less than a high school education (Rowland, 1992); no current information on educational levels of German Americans could be found. Vocational or university education is being sought more frequently by recent high school graduates attempting to prepare themselves for a highly competitive work environment and by adults who are pursuing second and third careers. By German standards, success means being employed, and education is seen as the way to achieve this success (McKinnon, 1993).

The earliest German immigrants were primarily farmers. Tobacco, wheat, rice, cotton, corn, and sugar were among the most widely grown crops. Plantations grew from Virginia to the colonies in the South as a result of these prosperous ventures. Planting and harvesting crops required many workers with strong backs, and because not all Germans could pay for their passage to the New World, many worked as indentured servants. They suffered many hardships and worked long hours at the mercy of their owners. Family members were commonly separated from one another; children were very often sold to pay the debt of their parents.

Between the Revolutionary War and the Civil War, many religious sects, including the Shakers, Harmonists, Zoars, and Inspirationists, founded hundreds of intentional communities (Boorstin, 1987). Known historically as the *Utopians*, they farmed the land; spun flax, cotton, and wool into beautiful textiles; and manufactured fine clocks and furniture. Unlike those who immigrated to the United States before the Revolutionary War, the Utopians formed caring and supportive communities instead of living in isolation from others. They worked happily for the settlement, built simple, strong dwellings, planted bountiful gardens, and established strong trade routes to the American West (Boorstin, 1987).

In the post–Civil War era, Germans who came to the United States often "chain-migrated" to the western frontier. Families and friends would leave one area to join family, friends, and neighbors in another place. These groups became farmers, miners, millers, construction workers, shopkeepers, blacksmiths, and locksmiths. Many were artists and craftworkers who created pottery, leather goods, soap, candles, and musical instruments (e.g., the dulcimer). These Germans established outstanding breweries, beer gardens (*biergarten*) and pubs (*kneipen*) everywhere they settled. They also brought many trades to the United States: butchering, coppering, tailoring, and cabinetmaking. Whereas they dominated the trades, German immigrants were found less frequently in professional and management positions (Schied, 1993).

In the early decades of the 20th century, the Nazi Holocaust drove many German immigrants from their home country. Many who came in the 1930s and 1940s continued their gifted work in the United States. Germans continue to establish their homes in the United States. Newly arriving immigrants are highly educated and vocationally well trained. German workers are among the most skilled in the world. Germany and the United States have similar industries in manufacturing, construction, and service.

Communication

DOMINANT LANGUAGE AND DIALECTS

German, the official language of the Federal Republic of Germany, is spoken in Germany; Austria; and Liechtenstein; large parts of Switzerland and South Tirol; and small parts of Belgium, France, and Luxembourg. German is the native language of over 100 million people, and many literary works have been translated into German (Kappler & Grevel, 1993). Within Germany, there are many dialects. Individuals' home regions can be easily identified through their speech, and citizens from neighboring regions may have difficulty understanding one another because of the differences in regional jargon and accents.

In addition to the German language, German children learn English at grade 5; and at grade 7, learn a third language of their choice. At grade 9, Advanced English or, perhaps, a fourth language can be chosen (S. Maubach, personal communication, December 28, 2006).

English is the dominant language of German Americans. Germans who originally emigrated from Germany learned American English at work, in school, and through socialization. Their children grew up speaking English in public schools and German at home. Parents encouraged their children to learn English only (Wikipedia, 2006a).

Currently, U.S. school children are learning English, and in some schools, Spanish is taught in the grade school. Russian, French, and Advanced Spanish can be chosen in high school, but the opportunity to learn German may not appear until college.

According to the 2000 census, 1.4 million people over age 5 years speak German in the United States. This does not include the number who speak German dialects like Hutterite German, Texas German, Pennsylvania Dutch, and Pautdietsch (Wikipedia, 2006b).

Today, there is a growing awareness of endangered languages. This is true about the dialects of German Americans. A language becomes endangered when there are so few speakers that it may no longer be used often enough and could be lost forever. For example, Texas German, a dialect found in the Texas hill country, is nearly extinct. This resulted from a change in school law mandating the use of English in all schools during World War I (Wikipedia, 2006b). In German American homes where the German language is expected to be spoken and children are faced with speaking English in the schools, intergenerational conflicts result. Parents do not speak English and the children prefer to speak English.

Americans and Germans have some similar patterns of speech behavior. German is a low-contextual language, with a greater emphasis on verbal than nonverbal communication, showing a high degree of social approval to people whose verbal behavior in expressing ideas and feelings is precise, explicit, straightforward, and direct.

Ten percent of more than 47 million German Americans, the largest self-described ethnic population in the United States, can speak German (Wikipedia, 2006b). Individuals in some German American communities mix English and German creatively when expressing humor. In Dubois County, a German American community in Indiana, linguistic competence is measured by a person's ability to switch between German and English to reflect bicultural roots and traditions (Salmons, 1988).

CULTURAL COMMUNICATION PATTERNS

People of German ancestry enjoy discussing topics of interest after dinner. These conversations, sometimes debates, cover a range of issues from politics, religion, food, and work experiences to life in general. Jokes, funny stories, or anecdotes about family members are interspersed within the discussion.

Germans carry on their conversations at three levels. The first, **Gespräch**, is used for casual conversation; the second, **Besprechung**, is conversation carried on in a work setting between employees and supervisors about performance; and the third, **Diskutieren**, is the common form of social discourse used in discussions about various issues (S. Maubach, personal communication, January 11, 2007). Most Americans are often ill prepared to enter the debate on philosophical and political issues that are addressed at this level and are thus placed at a disadvantage. This cultural barrier can prevent Germans from developing deeper relationships with outside groups.

Feelings among Germans and German Americans are considered private and are often difficult to share. Sharing one's feelings with others often creates a sense of vulnerability or is looked on as evidence of weakness. The act of expressing fear, concern, happiness, or sorrow allows others a view of the personal and private self, creating a sense of discomfort and uneasiness. Therefore, philosophical discussions, hopes, and dreams are shared only with family members and close friends. Emotions are intensely experienced but are not always expressed among family or friends. "Being in control" includes harnessing one's emotions and not revealing them to others.

Newer-generation German Americans, influenced by the cultural values of the United States, are more overt in sharing their thoughts, ideas, and feelings with others. They have joined in the American belief that direct confrontation and open dialogue can be productive. In spite of this general pattern of acculturation, pockets of Germans in the United States continue to be reserved when sharing their private affairs, thoughts, and concerns, including their health concerns, with strangers. Their reluctance for socializing may make them appear unfriendly; yet, under their stern exterior, they want to be liked.

Good manners are very important to Germans. A display of politeness and courtesy is viewed as a sign of respect. Social distance, eye contact, touch, and facial expression define boundaries. Failure to adhere to these protocols is considered rude by Germans and may alienate people who are unaware of them. When some people think of the handshake in the context of the German culture, they conjure visions of comics imitating this German greeting—the quick stooping of the shoulders and the clicking of the heels (Friday, 1989). The handshake, still a structured phenomenon in Germany (without the clicking!), has been acculturated into a more casual form by German Americans and is a common method of greeting for both men and women, but the practice is to always shake hands with women first. When families and friends gather, handshaking is practiced along with pats on the arms or back.

Practices associated with personal touch and displays of affection, such as hugging and kissing, vary among German families. In families in which the father plays a dominant role, little touching occurs between the father and the children. This relationship, however, may become more demonstrative as parents and children age. Affection between a mother and her children is more evident. In other German families, there is outward expression of love from both parents, grandparents, and extended family members; hugs and kisses are expected and often demanded as a "reaffirmation of love."

Whereas close friends are often extended warmth through handshakes, brief embraces, and sometimes kisses, strangers are kept at arm's length and greeted formally. As the author recalls from childhood, strangers, particularly those who were not German, were looked on with suspicion, even though some of these "strangers" were in-laws. Generally, Germans are careful not to touch people who are not family or close friends.

The distancing used by Germans to position themselves in relation to others is greater than the distancing used by some other cultural groups in the United States. More acculturated German Americans may control their space in a manner similar to that of other Americans. In health-care situations, providers frequently enter their clients' personal space. German Americans understand the need for this intrusion and voluntarily participate in such encounters while preserving their dignity and privacy.

Germans place a high value on their privacy. Germans may live side by side in a neighborhood and never develop a close friendship. A German neighbor would not be expected to borrow a cup of sugar from another neighbor—doing so would be an admission that she or he failed to adequately stock the pantry. Germans would never consider dropping in on another German neighbor because this behavior is incongruent with their sense of order. Much preparation is completed to ready the house for guests. When invited into the home of a German, the guest may be surprised to find that the distance between pieces of furniture is not conducive to conversation. "German space is sacred" (Hall & Hall, 1990, p. 38). In addition to spacing furniture, Germans use doors to protect their privacy. A closed door requires a knock and an invitation to enter regardless of whether the door is encountered in the home, business, or hospital. A closed door secures a sense of privacy and safety for Germans. Germans guard their privacy, which includes receiving phone calls at home. It is best to wait for an invitation or ask permission before contacting a new German acquaintance at home.

Germans maintain eye contact during conversation, but staring at strangers is considered rude. Even looking into a room from the outside is considered a visual intrusion; the interior of a room should not be entered without permission (Hall & Hall, 1990).

Smiling is reserved for friends and family. Because smiling does not occur during introductions, Germans are often considered unfriendly. Work is considered serious business; thus, Germans smile very little at work. Dealing with illness is also considered serious business, calling for "correct responses" (i.e., reserved, direct, and unsmiling).

Several unacceptable expressions of nonverbal behavior for Germans include chewing gum in public, cleaning one's fingernails in public, talking with one's hands in the pockets, placing one's feet and legs on furniture, pointing the index finger to one's own head (an insult), and public displays of affection. Younger, more nontraditional German American youths may not adhere to these perceptions. Americans cross their fingers for luck, whereas Germans squeeze the thumb between index and middle fingers. However, allowing the thumb to protrude more than its tip length is an offensive gesture (CultureGram, 1994).

TEMPORAL RELATIONSHIPS

Germans use time to buy the future and pay for the past. Their focus on the present is to ensure the future. The past, however, is equally important, and Germans begin their discussion with background information, which always includes history. Americans generally do not understand the German peoples' need to lay a proper foundation for discussion. Conversely, Germans develop a deep understanding of their historical heritage through an intense analysis of past events. Friday (1989) explained this contradiction as the result of a difference in educational emphasis in German and American schools.

Germans pride themselves on their punctuality. Being on time is an obsession. People who expect to be late for appointments should call and explain. If this is not done, the German sense of order is disturbed. Work is completed by setting and meeting deadlines. "Keeping to the schedule" is extremely important. There is a sense of impatience and often intolerance in the German American who encounters a situation in which someone else is not performing on schedule. This impatience can be stirred to anger in the work setting, in the supermarket, on the highway, in the hospital, or in the health-care provider's office. In the mind of a German, who is always on time, there are rarely good excuses for tardiness, delays, or incompetence that disturb the "schedule" of events. Within this cultural continuum model, Western Europeans and North Americans attend to details in a linear, orderly manner measuring days, hours, and seconds. Time has value for both groups, often equated with money.

FORMAT FOR NAMES

Traditionally, Germans keep social relations on a formal basis. Even neighbors of long-standing acquaintance are addressed as *Herr* (Mr.), *Frau* (Mrs.), or *Fräulein* (Miss) and their last name. Those in authority, older people, or subordinates are always formally addressed. Only family members and close friends address each other by their first names. Many German Americans born in the 1930s and 1940s continue to be formal in their social and business interactions. If this consideration is not returned, or if someone presumptuously calls them by their first name, it may be considered a sign of disrespect or poor upbringing. "The taboo against first-naming should not be dismissed as an empty convention" (Hall & Hall, 1990, p. 48). Hall and Hall (1990) describe an old custom, *Brüderschaft-trinken*, in which "two friends formalize their shift to the more intimate form of address. They hook arms and each sips from a glass. Then they shake hands and announce their first names" (p. 49).

Germans combine a person's professional title with *Herr, Frau, Fräulein,* or other titles and their last name. For example, a director of a business is addressed as *Frau* or *Fräulein Direktorin*. The title is often used without the name. A physician may be addressed simply as *Doktor*. Younger generations or more acculturated Germans may be less formal in their interactions. Because of cultural blending, health-care professionals will find that German Americans vary widely in their observance of these rules of etiquette. Therefore, these professionals should ask their clients how they would like to be addressed. This approach lessens the possibility of the provider unintentionally offending the client.

Family Roles and Organization

HEAD OF HOUSEHOLD AND GENDER ROLES

Traditional German families view the father as the head of the household. In the United States, the husband and wife are more likely to make decisions mutually and share household duties. Stay-at-home dads are uncommon in Germany (S. Maubach, personal communication, December 28, 2006). Often, when illness, dependence, and disability interfere and prevent family members from carrying out their roles, others assume decision-making responsibilities either temporarily or permanently.

In Germany, where emphasis is on **Ordnung** (order), and **Gemeinschaft** (community), older people are not expected to be self-reliant. Health and social programs for older people are considered part of the institutional approach of European programs. Because of the comprehensiveness of these benefits, there is less financial reliance on the family. One home may remain in the same family for generations. Often, more than one generation live under the same roof. Older family members who live with their children are included in family celebrations as well as in the daily routine of the families. As they become unable to perform their roles and duties, other family members assume their responsibilities.

Older people within German American families are sought for their advice and counsel, although the advice may not always be followed. They are admired for maintaining their level of independence and their continued contributions to society. Many live alone or with aging spouses. Helping older parents or grandparents to remain in their own home is important to German American families. By providing a helping hand with home maintenance, shopping, and finances, the family is able to safeguard and prolong a state of independence, even when living hundreds of miles away. For those who grow dependent, moving in with children or residing in a retirement nursing home is a viable choice for German American families.

The differences in the family role for older people in Germany and in the United States may be due to the far-reaching mobility of the American population that does not exist in Germany, where families generally live in close proximity. When Americans moved to the western frontier, they were required to adopt attitudes that included a degree of individualism, self-reliance, and initiative not demanded in a more geographically stable and settled society in which families had support because they were geographically close. The emphasis on these traits, as well as the concept of "America, land of unlimited opportunity," has made life in the United States difficult.

The Older Americans Act, Medicare, and Medicaid legislation, which are considered residual approaches for meeting one's social needs, support the context of the German belief in self-reliance and the supportive role of the family. Such residual approaches are offered when the normal channels such as family, marketplace, and church are not sufficient for meeting needs. Strong advocacy groups such as the American Association of Retired Persons and the National Council of Senior Citizens, which have mobilized older Americans as a self-interest group, also support this idea of self-reliance (Gelfand, 1988).

In the United States, 31 percent of older people live alone, whereas in Germany, 16 percent live alone. The significant proportion of older women living alone in both countries can be attributed to the heavy loss of life among German men in World War II. Although families may live close to one another, a significant portion of the older population (24 percent) reports feeling lonely (Rowland, 1992). With both spouses working to maintain economic security, many people have less time available to interact socially with older family members living on their own. An interesting fact is that the Germans love their dogs, and in Germany, it is acceptable to take the family dog everywhere—restaurants, visiting, and the hospital. As is well known, animals, except for seeing-eye dogs, are restricted in most public places in the United States. Other pets found in the households includes cats, rabbits, birds, hedgehogs, and of course, horses (S. Maubach, personal communication, December 28, 2006).

VIGNETTE 12.1

Mrs. Mary Hoffman, a 75-year-old widow and high school graduate, lives in south-central Pennsylvania. Born and raised in York County, Mrs. Hoffman married and had three children. Since her husband died 8 years ago, she has continued to live independently in her own home. Her financial support is from Social Security and from her husband's government pension. Her days are spent crocheting, walking, and watching home-shopping channels and favorite soap operas. She is an excellent cook and prepares many dishes in the Pennsylvania Dutch style.

Her children help her remain in her home by providing assistance with grocery shopping, transportation, and home maintenance. Although she has concerns about her health, she does not always share these with her children. Mrs. Hoffman talks daily with friends in the neighborhood. Occasionally, they share lunch or just visit in each other's homes.

1. Describe Mrs. Hoffman's status and role within her family.
2. What positive socioeconomic factors have helped secure independent living for Mrs. Hoffman?

PRESCRIPTIVE, RESTRICTIVE, AND TABOO BEHAVIORS FOR CHILDREN AND ADOLESCENTS

Prescriptive behaviors for children include using good table manners, being polite, doing what they are told, respecting their elders, sharing, paying attention in school, and doing their chores. Additional behaviors include keeping one's nose clean, eating all food that is placed on their plates, looking at a person who is talking, and sitting up straight. Prescriptive behaviors for adolescents include staying away from bad influences, obeying the rules of the home, sitting "like a lady," and wearing a robe over pajamas. Restrictive and taboo behaviors for children include talking back to adults, talking to strangers, touching another person's possessions, and getting into trouble. Restrictive and taboo behaviors for adolescents include smoking, using drugs, chewing gum in public, having guests when parents are not at home, going without a slip (girls), and having run-ins with the law.

Germany has regulations about noise levels in public areas such as athletic fields where people gather to watch soccer games, tennis, and riding events. These regulations are enforced for both children and adults. On occasion, schools in highly populated areas apply similar restrictions for playground activities (S. Maubach, personal communication, January 11, 2007).

FAMILY GOALS AND PRIORITIES

In Germany, history, family, and lifelong friendships are highly valued. Concern for one's reputation is a strong value. One's family reputation is considered part of a person's identity and serves to preserve one's social position (good and bad). The author recalls her mother admonishing her about the proper behavior for a young woman.

She always pointed out: "You never know whom you will run into." This admonition meant that you might meet someone, at any time and without your being aware, who could draw conclusions from your behavior that might tarnish the family's reputation.

VIGNETTE 12.2

Henry Wolfgang, a 33-year-old father and husband, was transferred by his company in Germany to their subsidiary in Michigan. Henry's wife and two children, 6-year-old Harry and 8-year-old Lilli, recently joined him. With the help of an English tutor, the Wolfgang children attend a public school close to their home.

Six weeks after the family's arrival in the States, Mr. and Mrs. Wolfgang received a call from the school principal asking for a parent teacher conference about their two children. During the conference, Harry's and Lilli's teachers expressed their concerns about the level of socialization and activity they observed in the children. They explained that the children are always seen sitting together, talking softly, and not participating in playground activities.

The teachers offer the help of the school district's psychologist to help the children adapt to their new school environment. Mr. and Mrs. Wolfgang are shocked and indignant.

1. What explanation, from the parents, about German culture would help the teachers better understand the behavior of the Wolfgang children?
2. Do you think the children need a mental health counselor? Why? Why not?

ALTERNATIVE LIFESTYLES

Pregnancy outside marriage results in disapproval, which can be overt or subtle. Because German families are concerned about their reputations in the community, the presence of an unwed mother taints their reputation and may result in the family being ostracized. If marriage follows the pregnancy, less sanctioning occurs, but the fact that pregnancy existed before marriage creates a stigma for the woman, and sometimes the child, that may last for the rest of their lives. The family members rarely forget this embarrassment, although it may never be discussed openly.

Today, acculturation and realignment of the moral rules of society, in which one out of four children is born out of wedlock, have lessened the seriousness of teenage pregnancy. These changes, together with the availability of more options for pregnant teenagers and greater social acceptance for unwed mothers than existed in the 1970s, have not lessened the shock for parents.

When couples delay having children, families may pressure the couple about producing children. Understanding a couple's decision not to have children is often difficult for German American families, and it may never be accepted.

Many middle-aged gay and lesbian German Americans may fear exposure because of the extreme discrimination homosexuals experienced in Nazi Germany. In addition, religious education plays an important role in anchoring family conceptions and leads to denial of homosexual feelings. When health-care providers encounter gays and lesbians who need religious support, a referral to one of the gay and lesbian religious groups may be helpful (see Chapter 2).

Workforce Issues

CULTURE IN THE WORKPLACE

Germans are among the most skilled and educated workers in the world. Much of Germany's success is due to advanced technologies, and it is a leading nation in Nobel Prizes for physiology or medicine. Some of its most important contributions are in rocketry, material science, and chemical products (Solar Navigator, 2006). German workers are educated to meet the needs of a highly industrialized country. The atmosphere of German business is very formal.

Several considerations must be remembered when working with Germans and some German Americans. First, it is important to be on time for work and business appointments and to complete work assignments on time. Second, business communication should remain formal: shaking hands daily, using the person's title with the last name, keeping niceties to a minimum, and avoiding the adjustment of office furniture during meetings. Employees are not addressed by their first names. Third, one should respect privacy by not entering rooms with a closed door before knocking and being invited inside. Fourth, dress, opinions, and activities should be conservative. Finally, learning to speak German is important if an employee is living in Germany and working for a German company (Hall & Hall, 1990).

The current trend toward a global economy has encouraged many American companies to establish sites in Germany and many German corporations to have subsidiaries in the United States as well as other places throughout the world. Many German managers are transferred to the United States by their companies and easily enter and adapt to the American business climate. Others trained in the health professions, the physical sciences and education, and technologies join the ranks of practicing professionals in the United States.

In the workplace, American values and beliefs often oppose German traditions. Friday (1989), in exploring the problems of transcultural adaptation for American and West German managers, noted "that the management style of German and American managers within the same multinational corporation is more likely to be influenced by their nationality than by the corporation culture" (p. 436). Although Friday's work was done outside the health-care industry, some of his findings have implications for relationships across a broad range of work settings, including health-care services. For one, German and American managers hold different perceptions of their relationship with their employer. Germans see themselves as part of the corporate family, whereas many Americans do not identify with their corporation.

Germans anticipate lifelong employment with the same company, whereas Americans may move to other companies should a good opportunity arise. Another difference is that American managers expend much energy to be liked, whereas Germans prefer being credible in their positions to being liked. To satisfy their need to be liked, American managers encourage informality in the workplace, such as by addressing peers, subordinates, or superiors by their first names; by asking personal questions; and by believing in equality and making themselves at home in each others' offices. For the German manager, credentials and education confirm their credibility and lead to power.

ISSUES RELATED TO AUTONOMY

Germans and German Americans expect to receive respect for their work and for their ability to make decisions about their work. They find a hovering supervisor annoying and demeaning. Balancing control and freedom in the workplace is necessary to foster productivity in German and German American workers (Hall & Hall, 1990). American and German managers use different styles of assertiveness. Whereas Americans case their approach within the idea of equality or "fair play," Germans, who have no translation for "fair play," are assertive by putting other people in their place. As in all languages, nuances and jargon can frustrate the individual whose second language comes only from the textbook and who does not understand idioms and colloquial expressions. The Germans' use of two distinctive manners of communication—*Gesprach*, casual talking, and *Besprechung*, the workplace discussion about performance—continues into the workplace.

Biocultural Ecology

SKIN COLOR AND OTHER BIOLOGICAL VARIATIONS

Germans range from tall, blond, and blue-eyed to short, stocky, dark-haired, and brown-eyed. Because many Germans have fair complexions, skin color changes and disease manifestations can be easily observed. For those with fair skin, prolonged exposure to the sun increases the risk for skin cancer.

DISEASES AND HEALTH CONDITIONS

Because Germany is highly industrialized, Germans suffer from many of the same life-threatening diseases that afflict groups from other highly industrialized countries. Leading causes of death for German Americans follow the patterns of the dominant American society and include heart disease, cancer, cerebrovascular disease, and accidents. Because of the poor management of industrial contaminants, people in the Eastern regions often suffer from pollution-related illnesses (CultureGram, 1994). When assessing recent German immigrants, it is helpful for health-care providers to know where in Germany the client resided before entering the United States.

HIV/AIDS are also present in Germany. Germany offers guidance and care to those who are infected as well as a comprehensive prevention program for its citizens (Kappler & Grevel, 1993). Because prostitution is legal in Germany, frequent health checks are required for those in this profession.

In 1998, research localized the genetic cause for a syndrome of symptoms for a new form of myotonic muscular dystrophy. A second study conducted in Minnesota, Texas, and Germany identified the same causative mutation (Mackle, 2001). This new form of the disease, called *DM2*, appears to be most common in Americans of German descent (Mackle, 2001).

Another genetic disease, hereditary hemochromatosis, is also found in German Americans. Hemochromatosis, a toxic level of iron accumulation, can cause diabetes, chronic fatigue, liver disease, impotence, and even heart attacks. The disorder is due to a mutation in the *HFE* gene located on chromosome 6. German Americans can avoid, prevent, and treat these maladies with genetic testing and early diagnosis. Hemochromatosis is treatable through bloodletting. The person can expect a normal life expectancy with aggressive treatment. Diagnosis can be established through a blood test known as an *iron profile*.

Sarcoidosis, a disorder found mostly in women between the ages of 20 and 40, occurs in all races, but people of German descent are at a higher risk (Gottfried, 2001). Sarcoidosis causes persistent cough or no symptoms. The cause is unknown, but doctors speculate that it involves an adverse reaction of the immune system; the diagnosis is often missed.

Dupuytren's disease, a slowly progressive disorder, is a deformity of the hand in which the fingers are contracted toward the palm. This often results in a functional disability. Dupuytren's disease is frequently found in people of German descent. Affecting mostly older males, the disease causes the synthesis of excessive amounts of collagen. The excess collagen is deposited in a ropelike fashion from the palm into the fingers, permanently fixing the fingers in a state of flexion. The current treatment is surgical, but recent medical experimentation with injectable collagenase shows promise (Biospecifics Technologies, 1998).

Although the cause is uncertain, Peyronie's disease is often found in people with Dupuytren's disease (National Kidney and Urology Diseases Information Clearinghouse, 1995). A benign plaque forms within the erectile tissue of the penis, which causes it to bend, resulting in reduced flexibility and causing pain during erection. This can prohibit sexual intercourse. The disease occurs mostly in middle-age men and often in men who are related, suggesting that genetic factors may increase the likelihood of developing this disease. Some researchers have theorized that Peyronie's disease may be an autoimmune disorder. A surgical approach to treatment has had some success. Candidates for surgery are men with curvature so severe that it prevents sexual intercourse.

Lowenfels and Velema (1992) examined the incidence of cholelithiasis in people from Denmark, Germany, India, Italy, Norway, and England. Although the study revealed prevalence rates from each of these centers, Norway ranked first and Germany second for the overall incidence of gallbladder disease. Although the study addresses populations in Germany, the results may be applicable to Germans in other parts of the world.

A cohort study of white men of Norwegian, Swedish, and German ancestry conducted between 1966 and 1986 revealed an increased risk of stomach cancer among foreign-born and first-generation German Americans living in the north-central states (Kneller et al., 1991). This study suggests an interrelationship among ethnic, geographic, and dietary factors as the cause. High concentrations of immigrants from northern Europe, which includes the high-cancer-risk countries of Germany and Scandinavia, settled in the north-central region of the United States. Low educational attainment, employment in laboring and semiskilled occupations, and ingestion of salted fish (at least once a month), bacon, milk, cooked cereal, and apples increased the risk factors for the foreign-born and first-generation individuals. These findings support the theory of ethnic risk. Subjects who smoked 30 or more cigarettes per day exhibited a fivefold risk for the development of stomach cancer. In addition, those who smoked a pipe and chewed smokeless tobacco had an increased risk for stomach cancer (Kneller et al., 1991).

According to Zielenski et al. (1993), an increased incidence of cystic fibrosis (CF) is found among Hutterite German–speaking communal farmers living on the Great Plains of North America. Mutations in the Hutterite population, a genetic isolate with an average inbreeding coefficient of about 0.05, exhibit an increased prevalence of CF carriers. Maternal-child health professionals providing care to this ethnic group can assist clients by encouraging genetic counseling to ensure early diagnosis of CF in their infants.

Hemophilia, a genetic bleeding disease found in Germany and in the United States, can be traced from Queen Victoria of England, who through a gene mutation, passed hemophilia to her son and through her daughters (Kilcoyne, 2004). The disease was then spread into Europe through the royal families including the House of Hohenzollern. The House of Hohenzollern comprised kings and emperors of Prussia, Germany, and Romania. World War I lead to the German Revolution and the House of Hohenzollern abdicated, ending the monarchy. Historians believe that the source of hemophilia in the United States is a woman in Plymouth, New Hampshire, most likely English. There are currently over 20,000 people in the United States with hemophilia, accounting for over 75 percent of all cases of hemophilia (Kilcoyne, 2004). As in the United States around 1993, those with hemophilia in Germany were contaminated with the AIDS virus through the administration of blood products and anticlotting factors. Health-care providers may want to be mindful of the German history of hemophilia and the AIDS issues while diagnosing bleeding issues in newly arrived German immigrants.

S. Maubach (personal communication, December 28, 2006) described the back pain experienced by school children who must carry their books everywhere during school sessions. No lockers are provided in the school building, so all supplies including books are carried all day long. Only public transportation is available to transport children to school, and children must carry their books and personal belongings with them. Again, during medical examinations of newly arrived immigrant children complaining of back pain, the health-care provider should question whether this situation existed in their former school.

VARIATIONS IN DRUG METABOLISM

Few research studies have been completed on variations in drug metabolism and interactions specific to people of German ancestry. Aggregate data on white populations report that there are no slow metabolizers of alcohol in this population (Levy, 1993). One study reported that 5 percent of Germans are poor metabolizers of debrisoquine (Levy, 1993), and therefore, this group may need lower dosages of propranolol to control blood pressure.

High-Risk Health Behaviors

Germans are known for their breweries and their *Gasthäuser*, or "restaurant that serves spirits." Beer is also served at the pubs (*kneipen*). In Germany, drinking beer is a way of life. German youth can legally drink beer at 16 and drive at 18 years of age. Beer is served with meals, whereas water is rarely consumed. Sparkling mineral water (*mineralwasser*) is commonly served if water is requested by a patron. Even lactating mothers are encouraged to drink malt beverages to increase breast milk production. This long-standing tradition of beer consumption is not without its abuses.

HEALTH-CARE PRACTICES

Germans, whether born in Germany or in the United States, share a love of nature. They enjoy the great outdoors. Fresh air and exercise are highly valued. Hiking, walking, swimming, skiing, cycling, soccer, horseback riding, and playing tennis are just a few of the activities enjoyed by people of German ancestry. Walking is a way of life. Sports are played for exercise and the pleasure of participating in group activities. Water sports are very popular and are encouraged among older people, disabled people, mothers, and small children. Because many German Americans are joiners, health club memberships appeal to German Americans.

Ruhezeit, or quiet time, is nearly sacred in Germany. This time-honored tradition occurs between 1 p.m. and 3 p.m. Monday through Saturday and all day Sunday. During this time, older Germans take naps and older retired German Americans may follow this ritual as well. Stores in Germany close over this time period. Neighbors and friends are expected not to create noise, telephone, or interrupt in any other manner. This quiet time is often followed by *Kaffe and Kuchen*, coffee and cake time, around 4 p.m. (German Connection, 2006).

Nutrition

MEANING OF FOOD

Food is a symbol of celebration for Germans and is often equated with love. Food and food rituals are powerful identification symbols for ethnic groups. The diet of immigrants is modified by the availability of foods and their financial status. The desire to maintain ethnic food habits has prompted children and grandchildren of immigrants to retain their ethnic heritage.

COMMON FOODS AND FOOD RITUALS

Traditional methods of food preparation with high-fat ingredients add to nutritional risks for many German Americans. Real cream and butter are used in German cooking. Gravies and sauces that are high in fat content, as well as fried foods, rich pastries, sausages, and boiled eggs, are only a few of the culinary favorites. Germans have traditional ways to prepare their favorite foods. Meats, turkey, chicken, pork, and fish are stewed, roasted, or marinated and are often served with gravies. Vegetables (fresh is preferred) are often served in a butter sauce. Foods are also fried in butter, bacon fat, lard, or margarine. *Bratwurst* (*currywurst*) served with curry ketchup and *pommes frites* (French-fried potatoes) with mayonnaise are found at the top of the list in Germany.

One-pot meals such as string beans and potatoes, *snipply* cabbage and potatoes, chicken pot pie, pork and sauerkraut, stews, and soups are served as family meals. Casseroles are also popular. Foods prepared with vinegar and sugar as flavorings are also favorites. Potato salad, cucumber salad, coleslaw, chow, pickled eggs, pickled cucumbers, cauliflower, tongue, and herring are common examples of favored foods prepared with these flavorings. Sour cream, mayonnaise, and mustards are used frequently in food preparation.

The nutritional habits of some Germans may be a significant health risk factor. Food is an integral part of a German's life. Food is served at celebrations and during visits and is taken on trips. The German infatuation with food can lead to overeating, which results in obesity. Children are rewarded for good behavior with food. Those who are ill receive Jell-O, egg custards, ginger ale, or tomato soup (not creamed) to settle their stomachs. Sending food with loved ones who will be away from the family for a time is quite common: Homemade cakes, cookies, and jams are a few of the offerings.

Nothing pleases German cooks more than witnessing people with hearty appetites at the table. Generous amounts of food are prepared, and second helpings are encouraged. Burping, with an apology, to honor the good food is acceptable at the German table (S. Maubach, personal communication, 2006). In choosing foods for German Americans, the health-care provider should consider cutting portion size, overcoming harmful food rituals, and reducing fat intake.

Some German American food practices reflect acculturation. For example, rice pudding enjoyed by many German Americans is originally a European American dish. However, unlike European Americans who serve rice pudding as a common dessert dish, German Americans reserve it for special occasions such as weddings. Celebration versions of rice pudding often contain dried fruit, such as raisins or currants, rum for flavoring, or a meringue topping.

Corn, frequently served as a vegetable in North America, is not eaten in Germany, where it is considered food for farm animals. Visitors from Germany are often startled when corn is served to them, but once they taste it, they are easily converted. Many early German immigrants turned to farming to conquer starvation, raising grains (including corn), fruits, and vegetables that were popular in North America. Foods associated with special events such as weddings, holidays, and religious occasions are the last to yield to acculturation. German cooks produce their best culinary efforts for holidays. Weeks of baking and preparation often precede the actual holidays. Selection of foods for the meal, proper preservation, and artistic presentation of tasty dishes are attended with care.

Table 12–1 lists common foods in the German American diet, based on the author's experience, personal interviews, the literature, and a marketing analysis conducted at a meeting of a local DANK (*Deutsch Amerikanischer National Kongress* [German American National Congress]) for a new food chain planning an international market concept.

DIETARY PRACTICES FOR HEALTH PROMOTION

Because of apartment living in Germany, many Germans love to garden. They bring this love to the United States. Gardening provides the fresh vegetables that Germans enjoy. What is not eaten is canned, pickled, dried, or frozen for future use. Having a full larder is very important to Germans and German Americans.

A few foods are used to prevent or treat illnesses. Prune juice is given to relieve constipation. A special soup from fresh tomato juice is used to treat a migraine headache. Ginger ale or lemon-lime soda relieves indigestion and settles an upset stomach. After gastrointestinal illnesses, a recuperative diet is administered to the sick family member, beginning with sips of ginger ale over ice. If this is retained, hot tea and toast are offered. The last step is coddled eggs, a variation of scrambled eggs prepared with margarine and a little milk. If these foods are tolerated, the sick person returns to the normal diet. Garlic and onions are eaten daily to prevent heart disease.

NUTRITIONAL DEFICIENCIES AND FOOD LIMITATIONS

The literature does not report any enzyme deficiencies or food intolerances specifically related to Germans. However, those of lower socioeconomic status may lack the financial ability to purchase foods essential for a nutritious diet.

VIGNETTE 12.3

Hyde Pfiefer, a retired 70-year-old German American, has lived in the United States for the last 50 years. A widower of 5 years, Mr. Pfiefer prepares his own meals following his wife's recipes from the old country. Nine months ago, Mr. Pfiefer was told that his cholesterol is elevated and he was instructed about a low-fat diet. His most recent test results show his values to be unchanged.

1. Discuss the meaning of food in the German culture.
2. Using the predominant health beliefs of people of German ancestry, how might you help Mr. Pfiefer reduce his cholesterol level?

TABLE 12.1 *Common Foods in the German American Diet*

Beverages	*Fish*	*Saage* (veal)
Coffee (with sugar and cream)	Anchovy paste	Tongue
Herbal teas	Carp (*karpfen*)	Veal
Kümmel (caraway seed)	Dover sole	Venison
Light and dark beers	Pickled herring	*Vonname* (smoked pork chop)
Schnapps	Roe	*Weissbratwurster*
Steinhager (juniper beverage)	Rollmops	Wild boar
White wine	Smoked cisco	
		Preserves
Breads, Noodles, and Dumplings	*Fruits*	Apple butter
Rolls	*Apfel* (apple)	Crabapple jelly
Dumplings	Dried apples	
Knöpfle	Dried pears	*Vegetables*
Potato dumplings	*Madelkerr* (fruits)	Beets
Pretzels	*Nüsse* (nuts)	Cabbage
Pumpernickel	Prunes	Carrots
Ribbles		Celery roots
Spätzle	*Meats and Fowl*	Mushrooms
	Bacon	Onions
Cheese	Beef	Potatoes
Camembert	Bratwurst	Sauerkraut
Limburger	Chicken	White asparagus
	Duck	White radishes
Desserts	Frankfurter	
Baumkuchen (tree trunk cake)	Game bird	*Miscellaneous*
Kranz (almond and hazelnut cake)	*Gänseleberwurst* (goose liver)	Caraway seeds
Lebkuchen (honey cakes)	Goose	Castor sugar (pearl sugar)
Lübecker marzipan	Knockwurst	Cilantro
Pfannkuchen	Liver dumplings	Honey
Pfefferkuchen (gingerbread)	Mettwurst	Juniper berries
Rice pudding	Mutton	Molasses
Springerle (cookies)	Pork	Paprika
Stollen	Salami	Vanilla beans
Strudel		

Pregnancy and Childbearing Practices

FERTILITY PRACTICES AND VIEWS TOWARD PREGNANCY

In her book, *Life at Four Corners*, Coburn (1992) captured a bit of the history of maternal-child health in Block Corners, Kansas, a German Lutheran settlement of the mid-19th century. She provided a glimpse into the daily life of a woman in the Midwest: "A woman's role within the family centered on supporting the farm economy, childbearing, child rearing, and providing continuous services to feed, clothe, and nurture all family members" (p. 88).

Coburn's research showed that large families were common in Block Corners. Farms needed a labor force and a large family often addressed that need. First-generation Block Corners women had at least seven or eight children. Babies were born every 2 years; miscarriages and stillbirths were common. Accidents and disease claimed the lives of many children. An average of 6.5 children was born to second-generation women, but only 2.5 children were born to third-generation women. This drop in birth rate of the third generation is attributed to assimilation.

Bearing large numbers of children, coupled with the hard life of supporting a farm economy and continuously providing food, clothes, and nurturing, caused physical strain on women, which often limited their longevity. In spite of these hardships, birth control was not sanctioned by the church until the 1930s and was not openly discussed. Educational information was passed verbally from one woman to another. Although it was known that breastfeeding decreased the likelihood of pregnancy, little else about pregnancy prevention was known.

Large families are rare in Germany. Most couples have only two children. This may be a result of limited living space; most Germans rent apartments rather than own homes. The German government recognizes the importance of family and provides child-rearing allowances and work leaves. The state pays a monthly allotment for each child up to 18 months of age and allows a child-rearing leave of 3 years for each child. Employers cannot sever parents from their employment, and leave time counts toward their pension. These benefits also apply to the care of sick family members (Helmert, Beck, Marstedt, Muller, Muller, & Hebel, 1997; Kappler & Grevel, 1993). Family leave legislation in the United States is more restrictive. Although maternity or paternity leave may be available after childbirth, it is often provided without pay and for a shorter duration.

A variety of birth control practices and interventions for improving fertility among Germans are readily available. On the one hand, the German respect for authority and love for scientific facts and data encourage the use of methods to control, as well as to enhance, fertility practices. On the other hand, the use of medication or devices might be viewed as interrupting the natural progression of things. "These approaches may be contradictory to the German love and appreciation of the world of nature" (Cathy Seibold, personal communication, March 25, 1995).

For German Catholics, the influence of religious beliefs on birth control matters should not be overlooked. Heterologous artificial insemination, use of contraceptive pills, and unnatural contraception are forbidden. In addition, therapeutic or direct abortion is forbidden as the unjust taking of innocent life. Teachings of Protestant sects on fertility control vary from no official position to forbidding the behavior (see the discussion under Spirituality).

PRESCRIPTIVE, RESTRICTIVE, AND TABOO PRACTICES IN THE CHILDBEARING FAMILY

Germans share some of the prescriptive, restrictive, and taboo practices of other cultures concerning pregnancy. Some examples of prescriptive practices include getting plenty of exercise and increasing the quantity of food to provide for the fetus. Some restrictive practices include not stretching and not raising the arms above the head to minimize the risk of the cord wrapping around the baby's neck.

Predicting the sex of the child was, and may still be, an important practice. For example, if the child is carried low, it is a girl; if the child is carried high, it is a boy. If the mother is "all out in the front," it is a girl; and if the mother is broad in the back, it is a boy.

A review of the literature and personal interviews did not reveal any prescriptive, restrictive, or taboo practices related to the birthing process. Birthing rooms that allow fathers and other family members to be present are popular among German Americans. In Germany, midwives commonly deliver babies (H. Morton, personal communication, February 1995).

The author's grandmother, who assisted with many home deliveries in the 1930s and 1940s, related one belief concerning the delivery of an infant. A child born with the membrane (the amniotic sac, also known as a *veil*) over its head is believed to be a special child, a belief shared by many cultures.

Prescriptive practices for the postpartum period include getting plenty of exercise and getting fresh air for the baby; if the mother is breastfeeding, she should eat foods that enhance the production of breast milk. Many believe that a new baby will soon arrive in the household that is visited first by a newborn. The author's mother often said, "Come visit us, but go somewhere else first."

Death Rituals

DEATH RITUALS AND EXPECTATIONS

Germans and German Americans traditionally observe a 3-day period of mourning activities after the death of a family member. The body of the deceased is prepared and "laid out" in the home, where support from family and friends is readily available. Neighbors come to do the chores and to sit with the family of the deceased until the burial. A short service is held in the home before the body is taken to the church, where family and friends can attend a funeral service. After the church services, the body is taken to the cemetery for burial. After a short graveside service, the minister invites everyone at the graveside service to the home of the deceased for food.

As embalming practices emerged at the turn of the 20th century and funeral homes became more popular, particularly in the urban areas, this tradition changed. Today, German Americans usually have a family funeral director. The family may go to the funeral home together to select a coffin. Following the directions of loved ones about what should be done after their death is very important. Careful selection of the clothes to be worn by the deceased and the flowers that represent the immediate family is equally important. These selections are based on their knowledge of the deceased's way of life and on preserving the family's reputation and good name. Even in death rituals, Germans are quick to judge the quality of attention given to these details. The author can recall her family's suspicion about the possibility that a certain family in the community took shortcuts to decrease the cost spent on the funeral process. The insinuation was that the family pocketed the money instead of honoring the family member.

RESPONSES TO DEATH AND GRIEF

The viewing provides an opportunity for family, friends, and acquaintances to view the body, offer their condolences, and extend their offers of assistance should the family need help in the future. Crying in public is permissible in the author's family, but in some German American families, the display of grief is done privately. A tradition of wearing black or dark clothing when attending a viewing or a funeral may be expected of both family and friends. Another expectation is that the bereaved family limits socialization activities for the following several months.

The traditions that surround the provision of food for the mourners have changed over the years. From the 1940s through the early 1960s, women in the neighborhood prepared the food and served it as people arrived at the home following the burial. More recently, families have become the primary providers of food and may hire caterers to prepare food or use a restaurant as is done in Germany, where homes are too small to accommodate large groups of people.

For Germans and German Americans, death is seen as part of the life cycle, a natural conclusion to life. Individuals who embrace a set of religious beliefs may look forward to a life after death, often a better life. Death is a transition to life with God. Because illness is sometimes perceived as a punishment, the length and intensity of the dying process may be seen as a result of the quality of the life led by the person.

Spirituality

DOMINANT RELIGION AND USE OF PRAYER

Martin Luther launched the Reformation in the early 16th century. Ninety percent of the population has some religious affiliation. Protestants and Catholics share equal portions of the population (33 percent). Other religions of German Americans include Judaism (the third largest population of Jews in Western Europe), Islam, and Buddhism (Solar Navigator, 2006). Similar to the United States, Germany has no state church; church and state remain separate. Religion is seen as a personal matter for German Americans, but those with an active interest in religion often discuss their beliefs with others (CultureGram, 1994).

A provision made by the Basic Law of Germany guarantees that "freedom of faith and conscience as well as freedom of creed, religious or other beliefs, shall be inviolable. The undisturbed practice of religion shall be guaranteed" (Kappler & Grevel, 1993). Although there is no state church in Germany, churches, as independent public corporations, have a partnership relationship with the state. They can claim state grants, which in turn, support schools and kindergartens. Churches can levy taxes on their membership, but the taxes are collected by the state. German churches also serve a charitable and social purpose by running nursing homes, retirement centers, hospitals, schools, training centers, and consultation and caring services.

Table 12–2 reflects the formal positions or the relationships between spiritual beliefs and health practices of several Protestant religions and the Roman Catholic Church. The Jewish, Mennonite, Muslim, and Greek Orthodox faiths are addressed in other chapters. Health-care providers must recognize that individuals' decisions may vary from the formal position of their religious groups. Therefore, the table serves only as a guide, not as an exclusive basis for decision-making in health care.

Most German religious philosophies do not divorce physical health from the actions of God. Many hold the view that God works through health-care providers as well as through the resources of medicine. Prayer is used to ask for healing, for effectiveness of treatments, for strength to deal with the symptoms of the illness, and for acceptance of the outcome of the course of the illness. Prayers are often recited at the sick bed, with all who are present joining hands, bowing their heads, and receiving the blessing from the clergy.

Reading the Bible is also an important spiritual activity. Most German and German Americans have a family Bible, which is passed down through the generations. It serves as spiritual comfort and as a reservoir of family historical data such as the dates of births, marriages, and deaths.

MEANING OF LIFE AND INDIVIDUAL SOURCES OF STRENGTH

Individual sources of strength for most Germans and German Americans are their beliefs in God and in nature. Although they may not attend church on a regular basis, a Germans' faith is deep. Family and other loved ones are also sources of support in difficult times. Home, family, friends, work, church, and education provide meaning in life for individuals of German heritage. Family loyalty, duty, and honor to the family are strong values.

SPIRITUAL BELIEFS AND HEALTH-CARE PRACTICES

Teachings of the churches joined by German people provide direction and counsel on many health-care issues. Many of these churches have taken a formal position on abortion, artificial insemination, and prolongation of life. The church prescribes when individual choice is important in deciding on accepting or refusing treatments and provides advice when seeking spiritual counseling.

Health-Care Practices

HEALTH-SEEKING BELIEFS AND BEHAVIORS

Germans receive regular medical and dental checkups, immunizations, and routine screening because most of the population is covered by statutory health insurance. Germany has one of the slowest-growing economies in Europe. Supporting the East German modernization, high unemployment, and a growing aging population since the mid-1990s has stressed the economy. In addition, Germany has faced health-care reform, embracing an approach that mirrors the U.S.'s HMOs with protest from the German physicians, similar to the reactions of physicians in the United States. The health-care systems are sharing more similarities than in the past. Germans are facing challenges of access experienced in the United States.

RESPONSIBILITY FOR HEALTH CARE

Although health care in Germany is considered "the individual's own responsibility, it is also a concern of the society as a whole" (Kappler & Grevel, 1993, p. 353). The average life expectancy in Germany is 75.81 years for men and 81.96 years for women versus 74.8 years for men and 80.1 years for women in the United States. Germany's infant mortality rate of 7 per 1000 infants is comparable with the U.S.'s infant mortality rate of 8 per 1000 (Arias, 2003).

Women in the family often administer remedies and treatments. In traditional families, the mother usually

TABLE 12.2 *Positions of Roman Catholic and Selected Protestant Religions Regarding Various Health-Care Practices*

Health-Care Practice	Baptist	Roman Catholic	Brethren	American Lutheran	Missouri Methodist	Presbyterian	Synod Lutheran	Wisconsin Lutheran	Church of Christ	Salvation Army
Administration of drugs, blood, and vaccine	Acceptable	Justifiable as long as for the good of the whole	Acceptable	Acceptable	Acceptable	Acceptable	Acceptable	Acceptable	No position	Acceptable
Biopsies	Acceptable	Acceptable	Acceptable	Encouraged	Acceptable	Acceptable	Acceptable	Acceptable	No position	Acceptable
Loss of limb	Acceptable	Acceptable (principle of totality)	Acceptable	Acceptable	Acceptable	Acceptable	Has no position	Acceptable if done to save a life	No position	Acceptable
Transplants	Acceptable	Permissible	Acceptable	Encouraged	Acceptable	No position	Acceptable	Acceptable	No position	Acceptable
Prolongation of life	Discouraged in clearly terminal cases	Advocates taking into consideration benefit and burden to patient	Allowed to preserve individual's freedom and dignity	Extraordinary and heroic efforts sometimes deemed justifiable	When death inevitable, allows freedom to direct or encourage a physician to remove artificial support systems	Quality of life viewed as more important than length of life	Permitted only in extraordinary cases after careful deliberation	Disapproves of prolongation of the agony of death	No position	Acceptable if prolongation of life is desired by individual; comfort and appropriate measures should be provided
Euthanasia	Left to individual choice for no extraordinary measures	Not permissible	Decision left to doctor and family	Advocates death with dignity	Discouraged	Favors right to die	Opposed	Advocates use of drugs to relieve pain	Favors death by natural means and processes	Unacceptable
Donation of body parts	Encouraged	Deemed justifiable	Acceptable	Encouraged	Encouraged	No official position	No position	Acceptable	No position	Acceptable
Autopsy	Encouraged	Permissible	Acceptable	Strongly approved	Encouraged	No position	Left to individual choice	Relatives encouraged to give permission	No position	No restriction
Disposal of body	Burial or cremation permitted	Burial favored; cremation permitted if unusual circumstances exist (e.g., infection)	Left to individual or family	Burial favored, but cremation acceptable	Burial and cremation permitted, and customary procedures for disposal of body after use for research	Burial favored, but cremation acceptable	Allowed if done with honor	Burial favored, but cremation permitted under epidemic conditions	No position	Left to individual and family

	1	2	3	4	5	6	7	8	9	10
Eugenics, genetics	No position	Opposed	Advised for assessment of serious illness	Acceptable; marriage and procreation discouraged if offspring likely to inherit hereditary defects	Research and parental counseling encouraged	No position	No position	Viewed as great blessing	No position	No position
Birth control	Left to individual choice	Only natural means permitted	Acceptable	Disapproved	Family planning favored	Acceptable	No position	Unacceptable, except if hereditary defects likely to occur	No position	Acceptable within marriage bond
Artificial insemination	No restrictions for mates	Viewed as illicit	Left to individual choice	Acceptable	Theological barriers	No position	No position	Left to husband and wife; adoption acceptable	No position	No position
Sterility tests	Acceptable	Permissible	Left to individual choice	Approved if necessary to ensure health of mother	Acceptable, but counsel with physician and pastor encouraged	No position	Left to individual choice	Acceptable	No position	Acceptable
Therapeutic abortion	Left to individual choice	Permitted only indirectly (e.g., removal of uterine cancer)	Left to individual choice	Approved if necessary to ensure health of mother	Acceptable, but counsel with physician and pastor encouraged	Justifiable by circumstances (e.g., rape or incest)	Permitted to save life of mother	Justifiable to save mother's life or in case of rape or incest	Decision of physician accepted	Opposed
Abortion on demand	Left to individual choice	Prohibited	Opposed	Opposed	Same as above	Deemed justifiable by circumstances (e.g., rape or incest)	No position	Opposed	No position	Opposed

sees that children receive checkups, immunizations, and vitamins. German Americans use a variety of over-the-counter drugs. C. M. Weicksel (personal communication, February 1995) summed up the practice as "people tend to self-medicate with over-the-counter drugs until these medications are ineffective, then they go to the doctor." The use of over-the-counter drugs may stem from the belief that individuals are responsible for their own health and from the beliefs and traditions about the treatment of sickness learned within the family system. In Germany, however, over-the-counter drugs can be purchased only from a pharmacy, which increases the cost to the consumer. Therefore, over-the-counter drugs are not as accessible to Germans as they are to German Americans. Today, prescription drugs are more complex, and numerous over-the-counter medications have become more accessible to German Americans. The two, used in combination, may lead to dangerous drug interactions for those who practice self-medication. Thus, health-care providers need to ascertain if over-the-counter and folk remedies are being used to determine whether there are contraindications with prescription medications.

FOLK AND TRADITIONAL PRACTICES

Among the early German immigrants, women practiced folk medicine, which often included singing and the laying on of hands. Families passed this knowledge on from mother to daughter. Common natural folk medicines included roots, herbs, soups, poultices, and medicinal agents such as camphor, peppermint, and spirits of ammonia. The author's mother and grandmother had an arsenal of remedies that were a combination of folk and over-the-counter preparations to treat a variety of ills. A list of these remedies and their uses can be found in Table 12–3.

Magicoreligious folk medicine includes "powwowing," use of special words, and the wearing of charms. Some stories told by the author's mother referred to the pow-wow sessions she attended as a child to cure her frequent ear infections and her inability to gain weight. She attempted to cure a plantar's wart by rubbing it with a sliced onion and burying the onion where water flowed. The expectation was that as the onion deteriorated, so would the wart. When this failed, an appointment with the podiatrist soon followed. Another belief is that carrying a buckeye guarantees health. Some individuals have a strong belief that being hexed brings bad luck, which can manifest itself as illness. The extent to which today's German American population continues to follow these practices is unknown.

BARRIERS TO HEALTH CARE

Germans have varying degress of access to health care (S. Maubach, personal communication, 2006). Because this is also true in the United States, newer immigrants may experience economic difficulties in securing care or in purchasing health-care insurance. Access to care is also limited for those who live in rural areas. Although efforts are being made to reduce these barriers, economic and geographic barriers to health care continue to exist for a large number of German Americans.

TABLE 12.3 *German Folk Remedies for Various Afflictions*

Affliction	Remedy
Abrasions, burns	Vaseline
Boils	Black salve
Bumps and burns	Butter
Cleaning cuts and abrasions	Hydrogen peroxide
Colds	Vicks as chest rub or placed in a vaporizer
Colds	Camphorated oil (chest rub; soft cloth covered with oil is placed over chest and neck area)
Colic in infants	Catnip and fennel (diluted in water and flavored with a little sugar)
Constipation	Castor oil
Cuts	Mercurochrome
Diaper rash	Cornstarch
Diarrhea	Paregoric in water
Earache	Warm oil
Headaches	Warm oil
Menstrual cramps	Hot tea
Muscle aches	Alcohol with wintergreen
Muscle stiffness	Hot or cold compresses
Nervousness	Spirits of ammonia in water
Sunburn	Noxzema
Teething in infants	Whiskey in water (rubbed on infant's gums)
To enhance health	Cod liver oil
Toothache	Oil of cloves
Upset stomach	Hot tea with peppermint oil

CULTURAL RESPONSES TO HEALTH AND ILLNESS

When asked to describe a German's response to pain, the word most often used is "stoic." Even when Germans are experiencing pain, they may continue to carry out their family and work roles. Research reveals that older German Americans are less likely to complain, more accurate in their description of pain, and more likely to follow the physician's advice (Wright, Saleebey, Watts, & Lecca, 1983). Although results of studies that examine ethnicity and pain remain problematic, one significant finding does exist: Regardless of the degree of acculturation, individual expressions of pain may follow those of the more traditional members of the culture. Thus, health-care professionals may not be able to identify verbal or nonverbal clues among Germans. Careful interviewing and astute observation must be used to accurately assess the level of pain experienced by Germans.

Although both Germany and the United States provide care for the mentally ill, mental illness may continue to be viewed as a flaw and is perhaps not as acceptable to German Americans as it is for some other cultures. If this is accurate, members of this group may be slow to seek help because of the lack of acceptance as well as the stigma attached to needing help. German people's discomfort with expressing personal feelings to strangers may impede the counseling process and influence the counseling methods used. The German need to discuss the past without expressing their feelings should be recognized within the counseling process.

Even though the mentally ill have been assimilated into American culture, many may remain stigmatized in the German American culture. Since the passage of the Americans with Disabilities Act, more people are aware of the needs of the physically disabled, including acculturated German Americans. Physical disabilities caused by injury are more acceptable to German Americans than those caused by genetic problems. The latter brings feelings of guilt and a sense of responsibility.

Returning people to the highest level of health possible appeals to the German nature. The European American culture believes in helping people, including older people, to recover their health. Rehabilitation has become an integral part of patient care in both Germany and the United States, and rehabilitation facilities abound in both countries. In Germany, rehabilitation is also a vital component of care in psychiatric facilities (Wuerth, 1993). For Germans, the rapid return to their roles in society is paramount, and rehabilitation represents the transition to these roles.

Once others become aware of illness, sick individuals are excused from their responsibilities. Even through German Americans are allowed to assume the sick role, some individuals may have difficulty doing so. The stoicism of some may delay their seeking medical care and allow the problem to become more severe or chronic. This may result in the need for more complex treatments for relief of symptoms. As individuals recover, they are expected to relinquish the sick role and resume their normal responsibilities. It is important to note that it is the physician in Germany who determines whether a person can attend work. The physician determines the length of absence from work, and the employer must provide employees with their salaries. There is no accruing of sick time as we do in the United States (S. Maubach, personal communication, December 28, 2006).

BLOOD TRANSFUSIONS AND ORGAN DONATION

German Americans identify blood transfusions, organ donation, and organ transplants as acceptable medical interventions. Many religions followed by German Americans provide guidance on each of these issues. See Table 12–2 for a more complete description of these beliefs and practices.

Health-Care Practitioners

TRADITIONAL VERSUS BIOMEDICAL PRACTITIONERS

In Germany, folk medicine and midwifery are highly revered. Midwifery is a "family-based tradition" (Coburn, 1992, p. 93), with skills passed from mother or close female relatives to daughters. Through interviews with

the residents of Block Corners, Kansas, Coburn was able to describe the work of a local midwife, Grandma Block. In addition to her midwifery, she passed along folk remedies for a variety of illnesses. The local physicians respected Grandma Block. She knew when their skills and knowledge were needed, and if she called them, they knew to come immediately (Coburn, 1992). Adolescent girls were pressed into service when illness and childbirth occurred. Older or widowed women also provided help in preparing food, cleaning house, and nursing the sick in families of both relatives and nonrelatives. Currently, in Germany, medical-care regulations deem that a physician must have a midwife (*Hebamme*) present during a birth. However, a physician does not have to be present if the midwife is doing the delivery (Wikipedia, 2006c). This is opposite of the practice in the United States, where a physician must be present if the birth is complicated. In Germany, alternative medicine such as acupuncture and homeopathy is used also during childbirth to control pain.

The use of certified nurse-midwives is currently growing in the United States. Choosing a nurse-midwife over an obstetrician is a personal, not a cultural, decision for German Americans. German Americans accept the care of health-care practitioners of the opposite gender. However, this is probably due to cultural indoctrination rather than an ethnic mandate.

STATUS OF HEALTH-CARE PROVIDERS

Health-care providers hold a relatively high status among Germans. This admiration stems from the German love of education and respect for authority. German Americans appreciate the status symbols of money, power, and institutional affiliations held by these professionals. German families are proud to have a health-care professional in their midst, and it is common for family members to seek counsel from them. Because Germans may find asking for help difficult, they may feel more comfortable confiding in a family member.

Health-care providers' strange language, unusual practices, and "secret" body of knowledge often create barriers to forming relationships with clients. Because of their indoctrination into the culture of the health professions, health-care providers can become short-sighted and fail to meet the personal needs of German clients. To deliver culturally conscious health care, providers must understand their own ethnic and professional culture as well as the ethnic cultures of their clients.

Today, the entry of more women into nontraditional work roles in health care has forced changes in the health-care environment in the United States. The same may not be true in Germany, where hospital libraries are reserved for doctors and patients only and are closed to nurses (Wuerth, 1993).

REFERENCES

Acton, R. (1994). A remarkable immigrant: The story of Hans Reimen Claussen. *The Palimpsest, 75*(2), 87–100.

Arias, E., (2003). United States Life Tables, 2003. *National Vital Statistic Reports, 54*(14), 3–6.

Biospecifics Technologies. (1998). *Annual report*. Retrieved November 2001, from http://www.biospecifics.com/annualreport98.html

Boorstin, D. J. (1987). *Hidden history*. New York: Harper & Row.

CIA. (2007). *World Factbook: Germany*. Retrieved March 29, 2007, from https://www.cia.gov/cia/publications/factbook/geos/gm.html

Coburn, C. K. (1992). *Life at four corners*. Overland Park, KS: University of Kansas Press.

CultureGram. (1994). *Germany '95*. Provo, UT: David M. Kennedy Center for International Studies.

Domer, D. (1994). Genesis theories of the German-American two-door house. *Material Culture, 26*(1), 1–35.

Friday, R. (1989). Contrasts in discussion behaviors of German and American managers. *International Journal of Intercultural Relations, 13*(42), 429–446.

Gelfand, D. (1988). Directions and trends in aging services: A German-American comparison. *International Journal of Aging and Human Development, 27*(1), 57–68.

German Connection. (2006). *Autrata family's home page—Behavioral norms in German: Siestas and Sundays*. Retrieved January 10, 2007, from http://www.actrata.com/expart/siestas.html

Gottfried, M. (2001). *Duff's a true model patient*. Life and Breath Foundation. Retrieved November 2, 2002, from http://www.lifeand-breath.org/newbook.html

Hall, E. T., & Hall, M. R. (1990). *Understanding cultural differences*. Yarmouth, ME: Intercultural Press.

Helmert, U., Beck, B., Marstedt, R., Muller, G., Muller, H., & Hebel, D. (1997). Effects of decreasing sick leave benefits: –Results of a survey of social health care insurace members. Retrieved January 25, 2007, from http://www.ncbi.nlm.nih.gov/entrez/query.fcgi?cmd=Retrieve&db=PubMed&list_uids=9440911&dopt=Abstract

Kappler, A., & Grevel, A. (1993). *Facts about Germany*. Frankfurt, Germany: Westermann, Braunschweig.

Kilcoyne, R., (2004). Hemophilia, musculoskeletal complications from E. Medicine, Web MD. Retrieved September 14, 2007, from http://www.emedicine.com/ radeo/topic 909. htm

Kneller, R. W., McLaughlin, J. K., Bjelke, E., Schuman, L. M., Blot, W. J., Wachoulsder, S., Gridley, G., Cochien, H. T., & Fraumeni, J. F. (1991). A cohort study of stomach cancer in a high-risk American population. *Cancer, 68*, 672–678.

Levy, R. (1993). Ethnic and racial differences in response to medicines: Preserving individualized therapy in managed pharmaceutical programmes. *Pharmaceutical Medicine, 7*, 139–165.

Lowenfels, A. B., & Velema, J. P. (1992). Estimating gallstone incidence from prevalence data. *Scandinavian Journal of Gastroenterology, 27*(11), 984–986.

Mackle, B. (2001). *New gene found for myotonia muscular dystrophy: Unusual mutation involved*. MDA News. Retrieved November 3, 2001, from http://www.mdaa.org/news/010803dm_mutation.html

McKinnon, M. (1993). In the American grain: The popularity of living history farm. *Journal of American Culture, 3*, 168–170.

National Kidney and Urology Diseases Information Clearinghouse. (1995). *Peyronie's disease*. Retrieved November 2, 2001, from http://www.niddk.nih.gov/health/urolog/pubs/peyronial/peronie.htm

Rowland, D. (1992). A fine nation. *Health Affairs, 11*(3), 205–215.

Salmons, J. (1988). In the social function of some southern Indiana German-American dialect stories. *Humor, 1 & 2*, 159–175.

Schied, F. M. (1993). *Learning in a social context*. DeKalb, IL: LEPS Press.

Solar Navigator. (2006). Retrieved January 25, 2007, from www.solarnavigator.net

Weaver, W. (1979). Food acculturation and the first Pennsylvania-German cookbook. *Journal of American Culture, 2*(3), 420–429.

Wikipedia. (2006a). *Distributor of ethnic German*. Retrieved December 19, 2006, from http://en.wikipedia.org/wiki/Ethnic-German

Wikipedia. (2006b). *Immigrant languages*. Retrieved December 19, 2006, from http://en.wikipedia.org/wiki/languages_in_the_United_States

Wikipedia. (2006c). *Midwivery*. Retrieved December 16, 2006, from http://en.wikipedia.org/wiki/Hebamme

Wikipedia. (2006d). *Texas German*. Retrieved January 4, 2007, from http://en.wikipedia.org/wiki/Texas_German

World Factbook. (2006). *World Factbook: Germany Economy*. Retrieved December 19, 2006, from http://worldfactboook.com

Wright, R., Saleebey, D., Watts, R., & Lecca, P. (1983). Attitudes toward disabilities in a multicultural society. *Social Science and Medicine, 36*, 616–620.

Wuerth, U. (1993). An open psychiatric unit in the U.S. and Germany. *Journal of Psychosocial Nursing, 31*(3), 29–33.

Zielenski, J., Fujwara, T. M., Markiewicz, D., Paradis, A. J., Anacleto, A. I., Richards, B., Schwartz, R. H., Klinger, K., Tsui, L., & Morgan, K. (1993). Identification of the M1101K mutation in the cystic fibrosis transmembrane conductance regulator (CFTR) gene and complete detection of cystic fibroses mutations in the Hutterite population. *American Journal of Human Genetics, 52*, 609–615.

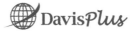

| | For case studies, review questions, and additional information, go to http://davisplus.fadavis.com |

Chapter 13

People of Haitian Heritage

JESSIE M. COLIN and GHISLAINE PAPERWALLA

Overview, Inhabited Localities, and Topography

OVERVIEW

Haiti, located on the island of Hispaniola between Cuba and Puerto Rico in the Caribbean, shares the island with the Dominican Republic. With a population of 8.5 million inhabitants, Haiti covers an area of 27,750 square kilometers (10,714 square miles), about the size of the state of Maryland. The capital and largest city, Port-au-Prince, has a population of over 800,000. The per capita annual income is $450, with a daily wage rate of $3 (World Bank Annual Report, 2006). Widespread unemployment and underemployment exist; more than two-thirds of the labor force do not have formal jobs owing to the marked decrease in assembly sector jobs, plummeting from a high of 80,000 in 1986 to 17,000 in 2006. About 80 percent of the population lives under the poverty line, with 57.4 percent living in abject poverty. The yearly inflation rate has fallen from 42.7 percent in 2003 to 15 percent in April of 2006. Nearly 70 percent of all Haitians depend on the agricultural sector, mainly small-scale subsistence farming, and remain vulnerable to damage from frequent natural disasters, exacerbated by the country's widespread deforestation. The infant mortality rate is high with 95.23 deaths per 1000 live births, the average life expectancy is 53 years, and only 13 percent of the people have access to potable water (CIA, 2006).

Columbus landed on the island in 1492 and named it *Hispaniola*, which means Little Spain. Haiti, or *Ayti*, meaning "land of mountain," was given its name by the first inhabitants, the Arawak and the Caribe Indians. Before 1492, there were five well-organized kingdoms: the

Magua, the Marien, the Xaragua, the Managua, and the Higuey (Dorestant, 1998). Two-thirds of Haiti contains mountains, great valleys, and extensive plateaus; small plains mark the rest of the country.

The Haitian population in the United States is not well documented; this may be because of the U.S. Bureau of the Census's failure to track the large numbers of undocumented immigrants. According to the 2000 census, 548,199 Haitians live in the United States. An additional 122,000 live in Canada, of which 90 percent live in Quebec (Statistics Canada, 2006). In 2001, 7,200 immigrants from Haiti were living in Canada for 5 years or less. However, Haitian leaders and activists believe that close to 1.5 million Haitians live in the United States: 500,000 in New York; 150,000 each in Boston and Chicago; 100,000 in California; and the rest scattered throughout the United States (H. Frank, personal communication, December 2006). An estimated 267,689 documented Haitians live in Florida. However, if the undocumented population is included, this number may be as high as 400,000 (Elliot, 2001).

Haitians, like other ethnic groups, are very diverse. They come from urban and rural Haiti and represent all socioeconomic classes. Factors affecting Haitians' acculturation and assimilation include the primary and secondary characteristics of culture (see Chapter 1).

HERITAGE AND RESIDENCE

Before the time of Columbus, the various indigenous tribal groups intermarried. With the arrival of Europeans, and then Africans, the people of Haiti became more diverse. Today, Haitians range from light- to dark-skinned, and social identity is shaped by sharp class stratification and color consciousness.

In 1697, Haiti came under French rule. By the end of the 18th century, the slave population numbered 500,000. In 1791, a slave insurrection broke the chain of slavery, and on January 1, 1804, Haiti gained its independence from France. The French plantation owners were removed and replaced by the generals of the indigenous Haitian Army, which ruled mercilessly (Louis-Juste, 1995). Agricultural workers and peasants were trapped in a semifeudal system: They were exploited by landowners, terrorized by the section chiefs of police, and forced to obey laws explicitly. The coffee fields of the peasants served as the primary source of revenue for the government coffers, thereby guaranteeing all government debt payments between 1826 and 1932 (Louis-Juste, 1995). These harsh conditions did not prevent the peasants from rising up against injustice and exploitation, as evidenced by the Goman uprising in 1820, the Acaau in 1880, and the peasant movement of Jean Rabel (Louis-Juste, 1995).

Haitian immigrants have a sense of national pride, including a high level of self-esteem regarding their blackness, although in both public and private discourse, they may focus on color and class division—two painful wedges within Haitian society.

Haiti's independence from France in 1804 did not resolve the division among the descendants of French colonists, the African slaves, and the core of the population, who were largely of African descent and culture. Many members of the upper class used the markers of **mulatto** (color), the French culture, and the French language to differentiate themselves from the lower class, who were mostly black and **Creole** and spoke a predominantly African language.

Ti Manno, a Haitian singer who migrated to New York, used satire and irony to expose and deride the type of thinking that divides Haitians in Haiti and abroad. The following song depicts the turmoil and struggle that promote the division within the Haitian society (Jean-Baptiste, 1985):

The Black Man

> *Neg Kwens dil pa Kanmarad neg Brooklyn.*
> *Neg Potopwens dil pa anafe ak neg pwovens.*
> *Mon Che se-m nan fe yon ti pitit.*
> *M'rayi ti pitit la*
> *A fos li led.*
> *Li nwa tankou bombon siwo.*
> *Nen-l pa pwenti.*
> *Ti neg mwe ala nou pa gen chans o.*
> *La vi nou toujou red o.*
> *Nou deyo, pi red.*
> *Se neg nwe cont milat o.*
> *Nou deyo nap soufri.*
> *Nou lakay se pi red.*

Haitians in Queens feel superior to those who live in Brooklyn.
Haitians in Port-au-Prince despise those who live in the provinces.
My dear, my sister had a little baby.
I hate this little kid.
This baby is ugly.
He is as dark as sugarcane syrup cake.
His nose is not pointy.

We Haitians, we are so unlucky.
Life is always hard for us.
Away from home we suffer more.
It's black against mulatto.
Abroad we suffer.
At home it is even worse.

Despite independence, colonial prejudices about skin color have persisted. Internal social rivalries and the scale of Haitian mobility are tied to a European color, race, and class model. This model relates to skin pigmentation, hair texture, the shape of the nose, and the thickness of the lips. Whereas the structure of Haitian society continues to be built on a neocolonial model, relationships based on color are extremely complex. For example, dark skin color tends to be associated with underprivileged status. Although more black-skinned people have entered the circle of the privileged, most blacks are poor, underprivileged, and unemployed.

Haiti defines itself as a black nation. Therefore, all Haitians are members of the black race. In Haiti, the concept of color differs from the concept of race. The Haitian system has been described as one in which there are no tight racial categories, but in which skin color and other phenotypic demarcations are significant variables.

In the 1940s, a black middle class emerged in Haiti and claimed to represent the majority. The development of this class and its rhetoric served as a springboard for Francois Duvalier, a rural physician who was elected president for a 4-year term in 1957. In 1964, he became president-for-life, using the issue of black empowerment and a promise to eliminate the color and class privileges of the mulattos. By the late 1970s, a group of dark-skinned, primarily American-educated and English-speaking technocrats had attained positions of prominence and influence in the government. However, the mulatto retained social prominence, and color continued to play a major role in the perception of class in Haiti.

REASONS FOR MIGRATION AND ASSOCIATED ECONOMIC FACTORS

Haitian immigration and travel to the United States have continued for many years. Most, but not all, of those who emigrated were members of the upper class. Before 1920, Haitians traveled to North America and Europe only for educational purposes. In 1920, the United States occupied Haiti; the first wave of Haitian migration to North America soon followed. Over the next decade, more than 40,000 Haitian peasants were forced to go to Cuba and the Dominican Republic to cut sugarcane in the *bateys* (plantations). Haitian land was taken and used for apple and banana plantations, and many acres of land throughout Haiti were controlled by the United States. The atrocities that accompanied the American occupation resulted in a small group of Haitians leaving Haiti and settling in the Harlem section of New York City, where they assimilated into American society.

The late 1950s showed signs of weakness in Haitian agriculture. The peasants started leaving the provinces in search of work and a better life. Migrating to the capital,

Port-au-Prince, they established Lasalin, the first slum of Port-au-Prince (Aristide, 1995). Today, approximately 1.5 million people live in and around the capital (Regan, 1995), many in large slums such as Cite Soley, Lasalin, Karidad, Dedye, Delwi, and Fo Mekredi.

A significant turning point in Haitian migration occurred in 1964 when Duvalier was elected president-for-life. As a result of his government, many Haitians began fleeing the island. These emigrants were primarily relatives of politicians who opposed the political philosophy of Duvalier. When Duvalier died in 1971, his son, Jean Claude, age 19, was appointed president-for-life. In addition, during this era, Haiti was suffering from economic deprivation, which motivated a major exodus of urbanites and peasants. Because many Haitians were unable to pay for their transportation, passports, and visas, some covertly emigrated to the United States in small sailboats.

From 1980 to the present, Haitian immigrants have been divided into two groups: those who have arrived in the United States legally and those who have entered through the underground. An explosion of immigration took place in 1980, in part because of a short-lived (April to October) change in U.S. immigration policy during the period of the Mariel boat lift from Cuba. The influx of Cuban refugees required that a special status be created by the State Department called "Cuban-Haitian entrant: status pending." According to Health and Rehabilitation Services, Haitian refugees were included in this status to prevent the policy from being discriminatory. This group of immigrants were labeled **boat people**, a term associated with extreme poverty. Today, this term does not evoke as much negativism, although it continues as a reminder of a painful emigration period in Haitian history.

From 1990s to the present, political unrest, coups, and protests occurred. The tides of history were changing, Jean-Bertrand Aristide was elected in the first democratically held election in many years. The democratic process did not last; in that same year, a coup d'état on Aristide and a hemisphere-wide embargo was imposed on Haiti. In 2001, Aristide was re-elected in a flawed election. In February 2004, an armed rebellion led to the departure of President Jean-Betrand Aristide; an interim government took office to organize new elections under the auspices of the United Nations Stabilization Mission in Haiti (MINUSTAH). Continued violence and technical delays prompted repeated postponements, but Haiti finally did inaugurate a democratically elected president, Rene Preval, and parliament in May of 2006. The Prime Minister, Jacques-Edouard Alexis, is appointed by the president and ratified by the National Assembly to serve a 5-year term, with new elections in 2010.

In Haiti, most major industries are owned and operated by the government. Unemployment is 66 percent. Those who are employed often work under such poor conditions that they have become unmotivated and take little pride in their work, which results in low productivity. In general, Haitians are entrepreneurial, operating their own shops, marketplaces, or schools. Among these entrepreneurs, the motivation, spirit, and pride in their work are readily apparent.

EDUCATIONAL STATUS AND OCCUPATIONS

Following Haiti's independence in 1804, the new rulers of Haiti began advocating French cultural patterns and replicating the French value system. A French model of education was informally adopted and codified in 1860, in accord with the Roman Catholic Church. This resulted in two major changes: The Catholic Church became the official church of Haiti, and Catholic missionaries became responsible for education. The accepted language for communication was now French. During this era, **Creole**, the language of the uneducated, was perceived as inferior. Social mobility was possible only for French-speaking Haitians. While the educated elite became acculturated into the European value system, the illiterate masses tended to perpetuate the traditional values and customs of their African heritage.

Even though Haitians value education, only 15 percent are privileged enough to attain a formal education. In the past, the government appropriated only 1.8 percent of the total budget for education. The Haitian school system is based on the French model and offers free primary and secondary education. Public schools include those operated and controlled by religious orders as well as those under the direct jurisdiction of the Minister of Education. Children from families with financial means attend private schools. The educational model emphasizes liberal arts and humanities rather than technical and vocational studies.

The Haitian educational system continues to emphasize 19th-century values, which promote good manners, the classics, literature, philosophy, Latin, and Greek. It de-emphasizes the physical and social sciences. The Haitian educational system is based on a two-level curriculum. In the first level, the student receives a certificate of primary education. To receive this certificate, the student must sit for a rigorous test, which includes spelling, reading comprehension, composition, Haitian history and geography, general knowledge, arithmetic, and biology. At this level, the student can speak, read, and write French at the basic level.

The next level consists of two parts: The first is reached after 6 years of secondary education. To receive this diploma, the student must pass examinations in French, English, and Spanish; Haitian literature and history; mathematics; and sciences such as physics, chemistry, biology, and botany. Students in the classical track also take Latin and Greek examinations. A student who has received the first-level certificate should be able to enter the first year of college in American schools. The second-level baccalaureate is likened to the first year of college in North America; the emphasis is on the liberal arts. Again, the student must pass an examination in all the areas covered in the first level plus philosophy. The results of these national examinations are announced on the radio over a 2-day period.

Although Haiti has several universities, they are mainly located in Port-au-Prince. Most of them are state universities. With proper credentials, anyone can enter the university system. However, since the early 1980s, only those in positions of influence have been able to benefit from the state universities. Haitian professionals mirror those of American society; they are lawyers, physicians, nurses, engineers, educators, electricians, plumbers, and construction workers.

The literacy rate, which means that those age 15 and over can read and write, is 52.8 percent. The level of illiteracy continues to be a major concern in Haiti. Since 1940, the government has conducted several literacy programs. In 1948, Haiti had its first experience with community education. This public educational system was based on the growth model of development, a UNESCO education project, which duplicated experiences in Latin America (Jean-Bernard, 1983).

Among Haitian immigrants, women work in hotels, hospitals, and other service industries in domestic and nursing assistant roles. Men work as laborers and factory helpers. Many more Haitians are in the workforce today than there were in the early 1980s, although data for the years 1974 and 1994 from the U.S. Immigration and Naturalization Service (2006) revealed that a disproportionate number of legal Haitians were not employed. In addition, when comparing data by specific groups, a dramatic increase in the number of Haitians in all work environments is found. Data about the work structure of undocumented people are not available because these people technically are "underground" and do not exist.

Communication

DOMINANT LANGUAGE AND DIALECTS

The two official languages in Haiti are French and Creole. Creole, a rich, expressive language, is spoken by 100 percent of the population, whereas French is spoken by 15 percent of the population. Since 1957, Creole has been the unofficially accepted language in the internal affairs of the Haitian government, and in 1987, it was designated in the Haitian Constitution as one of the official languages. Because Creole is the official language, it is used for internal communication within the island.

In contemporary society, the Haitian dilemma can best be understood through this dual-language system. Language is one of the vehicles used to depersonalize those of the lower classes. French is the dominant language of the educated and the elite, whereas Creole is the language of those who are suppressed, the lower classes. The emphasis on French served as a barrier to the early social dynamism that permitted Creole to develop and serve as a unifying force among the African slaves, who came from many different tribes and spoke different languages. In spite of its suppression in formal education, Creole has inspired a very rich and interesting oral literature comprising songs, proverbs, and tales. This oral literature is the most significant aspect of Haitian folklore.

Understanding the language dilemma and the literacy issues assists health-care practitioners in developing creative tools for educating Haitians. Some of these tools may include video programs, audiocassettes, and radio programs in Creole. Because of the masses of people who are unable to read, printed literature in Creole is not a helpful educational tool.

CULTURAL COMMUNICATION PATTERNS

Haiti has an oral culture with a long tradition of proverbs, jokes, and stories reflecting philosophical systems. These are used to pass on knowledge, convey messages, and communicate emotions. For example, *Pale franse pa di lespri pou sa* means "To speak French does not mean you are smart." *Crayon Bon Die pa gin gum* ("God's pencil has no eraser") conveys the concept of fatalism. Another proverb frequently used is *sonje lapli ki leve mayi ou* ("remember the rain that made your corn grow"), which means that one must show gratitude to those who have helped them or done good for them.

Haitians are very expressive with their emotions. By observing them, one can tell whether they are happy, sad, or angry. Haitians' communication patterns include loud, animated speech and touching in the form of handshakes and taps on the shoulder to define or reconfirm social and emotional relationships. Pain and sorrow are very obvious in facial expressions. Most Haitians are very affectionate, polite, and shy. Uneducated Haitians generally hide their lack of knowledge to non-Haitians by keeping to themselves, avoiding conflict, and sometimes, projecting a timid air or attitude. They smile frequently and often respond in this manner when interacting with Americans or when they do not understand what is being said. Many may pretend to understand by nodding; this sign of approval is given to hide their limitations. Therefore, health-care providers must use simple and clear instructions. One strategy to ensure proper understanding is to ask family members to assist with translation and interpretation if an interpreter is not available. Because Haitians are very private, especially in health matters, it is inappropriate to share information through friends. Many may prefer to use professional interpreters who will give an accurate interpretation of their concerns. Most importantly, the translator should be someone with whom they have no relationship and will likely never see again.

Voice intonations convey emotions. Haitians speak loudly even in casual conversation among friends and family; the pitch is moderated in formal encounters. When the conversation is really animated, the conversants speak in close proximity and ignore territorial space, especially when emphasizing a point or an issue. Sometimes, the conversation is at such a high pitch and speed that, to an outsider, the conversation may appear disorganized or angry. Haitians love political discussions. In these instances, the conversation may appear stressful and hostile; however, to the participants, the conversation is enjoyable, motivating, and meaningful.

Traditional Haitians generally do not maintain eye contact when speaking with those in a position of authority. In the past, maintaining direct eye contact was considered rude and insolent, especially when speaking with superiors (e.g., children speaking with parents, students with teachers, or employees with supervisors). However, the influence of American education seems to be changing this trend. Most adults maintain eye contact, which means "We are on equal terms, no matter who you are. I respect you and you respect me as an equal human being." For children, however, the custom of not maintaining eye contact with superiors remains deferential. Thus, health-care providers may need to assist children in dealing with conflicting messages.

Haitians touch frequently when speaking with friends. They may touch you to make you aware that they are speaking to you. Whereas Haitian women occasionally walk hand-in-hand as an expression of their friendship, this trend is disappearing both in Haiti and in Haitian communities in North America. This behavior may be changing because of the concept of homosexuality, which is taboo within the Haitian culture.

Haitians greet each other by kissing and embracing in informal situations. In formal encounters, they shake hands and appear composed and stern. Men usually do not kiss women unless they are old friends or relatives. Children greet everyone by kissing them on the cheek. Children refer to adult friends as uncle or auntie out of respect, not necessarily because they are related by blood.

TEMPORAL RELATIONSHIPS

The temporal orientation of Haitians is a balance among the past, the present, and the future. The past is important because it lays the historical foundation from which one must learn. The present is cherished and savored. The future is predetermined, and God is the only Supreme Being who can redirect it. One hears *Bondye Bon* ("God is good"), meaning if you conduct yourself conservatively and the right way, God will be there for you. The future is left up to God, who is trusted to do the right thing. In a study by Prudent, Johnson, Carroll, & Culpepper (2005), several of the informants voiced their belief in God's will when talking about whether or not they would survive being HIV positive and/or having AIDS.

Haitians have a fatalistic but serene view of life. Some believe that destiny or spiritual forces are in control of life events such as health and death, so they say, *Si Bondye Vle* ("If God wants"). Given the belief in a predetermined path of life, one can understand this view. Haitians believe that they are passive recipients of God's decisions. Health-care practitioners must be clear, honest, and open when assessing Haitian individuals' perceptions and how they perceive the forces that have an influence over life, health, and illness. Acceptance of these beliefs is an important factor in building trust and ensuring compliance.

Most Haitians do not respect clock time; flexibility with time is the norm, and punctuality is not valued. They hold to a relativistic view of time, and although they try, some find it difficult to respond to predetermined appointments. Arriving late for appointments, even medical appointments, is not considered impolite. In North America, Haitians may be more readily compliant with business appointments; but socially, the margin around expected time is very wide—anything or anyone can wait. It is not unusual to see an invitation to a social function listed with an invitation time an hour earlier than the actual time of the function. For example, a wedding invitation may reflect a 6:00 p.m. wedding when, in fact, the ceremony is actually scheduled for 7:00 p.m. to ensure that all invitees are there for the start of the ceremony.

Health-care practitioners should be mindful of this time orientation by making reminder calls for appointments and encouraging the client in a respectful and caring manner about the importance of timeliness. A thorough assessment of time and temporal view helps practitioners to plan appointments so that clinic or office backlogs and disruptions are minimized.

FORMAT FOR NAMES

Haitians generally have a first, middle, and last name: for example, Marie Maude Guinard. Sometimes the first two names are hyphenated as in Marie-Maude. The family name, or *nom de famille,* is very important in middle- and upper-class society; it helps to promote and communicate tradition and prestige. However, friends call individuals by their first names. Families usually have an affectionate name or nickname for individuals. The father, mother, grandparent, or any close family member gives this affectionate name at birth.

When a woman marries, she takes on her husband's full name. For example, if Marie-Carmel Guillaume marries Charles Guy Lespinasse she is always called Mrs. Lespinasse. In an informal setting, she might even be called Mrs. Charles. She loses her name except on paper. Her name and identity are subsumed by her husband's name. This is a reflection of Haitian society in which women are considered subservient to men. Haitian names are primarily of French origin, although many Arabic names are now heard since the migration of Arabs to Haiti in the 1920s. Haitians are formal and respectful and, as such, should be addressed by their title: Mr., Mrs., Miss, Ms., or Doctor.

Family Roles and Organization

HEAD OF HOUSEHOLD AND GENDER ROLES

Traditionally, the head of the household was the man, but in reality, most families today are matriarchal. Haitian men prefer and choose to believe that they make the decisions, but most major decisions are made by the wife and/or mother, with the man remaining a distant figure with a great deal of authority. Today, joint decisions are common. The man is generally considered the primary income provider for the family, and governance, rules, and daily decision-making are considered his province. Sociopolitical and economic life centers around men. Men are expected to be sexual initiators, and the concept of *machismo* prevails in Haitian life. Women are expected to be faithful, honest, and respectable. Men are usually permitted freedom of social interaction, a freedom not afforded to women. The opportunities offered in North America for women to become income providers, together with their observations of different male-female interactional styles, have encouraged many Haitian women to reject their native, subservient role. This change in the marital interaction has created much stress on marital relationships and an increase in domestic violence, although domestic violence remains one of those closeted issues that are not publicly discussed.

PRESCRIPTIVE, RESTRICTIVE, AND TABOO PRACTICES FOR CHILDREN AND ADOLESCENTS

Children are valued among Haitians because they are key to the family's progeny, cultural beliefs, and values. Children are expected to be high achievers because *Sa ki lan men ou se li ki pa ou* ("What's in your hand is what you have"). In other words, education can never be taken away. Children are expected to be obedient and respectful to parents and elders, which is their key to a successful future. They are not allowed to express anger to elders. **Madichon** is a term used when children are disrespectful; it means that their future will be marred by misfortune. Another proverb used to scare and compel children to behave is *ti moun fwonte grandi devan baron* ("an impudent or insolent child will grow under the Baron's eye [Baron Samedi is the guardian of the cemetery in the voodoo religion] and therefore won't have a long life").

Physical punishment that is often used as a way of disciplining children is sometimes considered child abuse by America's standards. Fear of having their children taken away from them because of their methods of discipline can cause parents to withdraw or not follow through on health-care appointments if such abuse is evident (e.g., bruises or belt marks). Haitians need to be educated about American methods of discipline and laws so that they can learn new ways of disciplining their children without compromising their beliefs or violating American laws.

Many parents feel confused about how to raise their children in the United States. Their authoritarian behavior is challenged in American society, which they perceive as being too permissive. They feel powerless in understanding how to raise their children in America, while retaining Haitian traditions. The liberal American approach to child rearing poses a great dilemma for Haitian children. They find themselves living in two worlds: the American world, which allows and supports self-actualization and oneness, and the Haitian world, which promotes silence, respect, and obedience.

In the summer, Haitian parents engage their children in certain health-promotion activities such as giving them *lok* (a laxative), a mixture of bitter tea leaves, juice, sugarcane syrup, and oil. In addition, children are also given *lavman* (enemas) to ensure cleanliness. This is supposed to rid the bowel of impurities and refresh it, prevent acne, and rejuvenate the body.

Because Haitian life is centered on male figures, the education of boys is different from that of girls. The family is more indulgent of the behavioral deviations of boys. Boys are given more freedom and are even expected to receive outside initiation in social and sexual life. However, girls are educated toward marriage and respectability. Their relationships are closely watched. Even when they are 16 or 17 years of age, they cannot go out alone because any mishap can be a threat to the future of the girl and bring shame to her family. These beliefs increase Haitians' frustrations and challenges of rearing their children, especially girls, in America.

Health-care practitioners need to be aware of these various challenges and be prepared to assist children and family members to work through these cultural differences, while conveying respect for family and cultural beliefs. Health-care practitioners can play a significant role by helping children and their parents to better understand American practices.

FAMILY GOALS AND PRIORITIES

The family is a strong component of the Haitian culture. The expression "blood is thicker than water" reflects family connectedness. An important unit for decision-making is the *conseil de famille*, the family council. This council is generally composed of influential members of the family, including grandparents. The family structure is authoritarian and includes linear roles and responsibilities. Any action taken by one family member has repercussions for the entire family; consequently, all members share prestige and shame.

The family system among Haitians is the center of life and includes the nuclear, consanguine, and affinal relatives, some or all of whom may live under the same roof. Families deal with all aspects of their members' lives, including counseling, education, crises, and marriage. Each family has its own traditions, which form the basis for a family's reputation and are generalized to all members of the family. The prestige of a family is very important and is based on attributes such as honesty, pride, trust, social class, and history. Even families who experience economic difficulties are well respected if they are from a *grande famille*. Wealthy families who have no historical background or tradition are referred to as *nouveaux riche* and find it difficult to marry into the more well-established *grandes familles*, even though they have money.

The **family** is an all-encompassing concept in the Haitian culture. By including family members in the care of loved ones, health-care practitioners can achieve more trusting relationships, which foster greater compliance with treatment regimens. Haitians believe that when family members are ill, there is an obligation to be there for them. If a family member is in the hospital, all family members try to visit. Many visitors may cause concern to health-care practitioners who are not accustomed to accommodating large numbers of visitors. Practitioners need to be patient with them and facilitate their visits.

When grandparents are no longer able to function independently, they move in with their children. The house is always open to relatives. Elders are highly respected and are often addressed by an affectionate title such as aunt, uncle, grandma, or grandpa, even if they are not related. Their children are expected to care for and provide for them when self-care becomes a concern. The elderly are family advisers, babysitters, historians, and consultants. Migration to America poses a tremendous challenge in caring for elderly Haitians. The nursing home concept does not exist in the Haitian culture; therefore, Haitians are generally very reluctant to place their elderly family members in nursing homes.

ALTERNATIVE LIFESTYLES

Homosexuality is taboo in the Haitian culture, so gay and lesbian individuals usually remain closeted. If a family member discloses that he or she is gay, everyone keeps it quiet; there is total denial. Gay and lesbian relationships are not talked about; they remain buried. There are no gay bars in Haiti, and overt homosexual conduct is not publicly displayed.

Although divorce is common among Haitians, before it becomes final, family members, friends, the church, and elders try to counsel the couple. Health-care providers must approach this issue carefully and establish a trusting relationship before discussing divorce.

Single parenting, widespread in Haiti, is well accepted and closely tied to the issue of concubinage. In Haitian society, a well-accepted practice is for men to have both a wife and a mistress, with the latter relationship referred to as *placage*. Both women bear children. The mistress raises her children alone and with minimal support from the father. These children are often known by the man's family, but are not known to the wife. Haitian women in general know that their husbands are involved in extramarital relationships but pretend not to know. Health education, birth control, and safe sex are issues that should be approached with sensitivity and acceptance within cultural boundaries.

Workforce Issues

VIGNETTE 13.1

Mrs. Solange Perard, a 42-year-old Haitian, migrated to the United States 15 years ago. She lives with her two daughters, ages 16 and 17, in a two-bedroom apartment in North Miami, Florida, in a predominantly Haitian community. They feel supported by and secure with their Haitian neighbors. Mrs. Perard takes comfort in knowing that her neighbors share her culture and beliefs.

Mrs. Perard is a Haitian graduate diploma nurse who initially worked in the pharmacy department as a courier for a local hospital. As her English improved, she transferred to a Patient Care Technician position in the oncology unit. Mrs. Perard speaks Creole and English but prefers to speak Creole with her coworkers. She also works for a home health agency on her days off and weekends in order to send money to her mother in Haiti. Mrs. Perard has attempted unsuccessfully to pass the NCLEX-RN twice. Owing to her multiple jobs, she is unable to dedicate the necessary time to her studies. Her coworkers praise her hard work and for being a supportive coworker.

1. Is Mrs. Perard's acculturation hindered because she lives in a Haitian-predominant neighborhood? Why? Why not?
2. Describe the differences between the Haitian nursing educational system and the nursing educational system in the United States.
3. Is it common for Haitian workers to socialize with other Haitian coworkers in Creole? Do you feel that this is done to upset members of other cultures?

CULTURE IN THE WORKPLACE

Haitians living in America have demonstrated a very strong motivation for work and a continued commitment to the entrepreneurial spirit. They can be found in every sector of the American workforce. They are hard workers, and many work two jobs to provide for their American family while sending money to Haiti for those left behind. In the first year of migration, they are generally forced to take lower-status and low-paying jobs. These jobs are used as stepping stones to better jobs until they are able to communicate in English and legalize their immigrant status. A literature search did not reveal official statistics, or even rough estimates, on the income distribution of Haitian immigrants. Work is a necessity, and they conform to the rules and regulations of the workplace. Haitian immigrants have taken menial, low-paying jobs that many Americans would not accept even when unemployed. Haitians appreciate comfort, and they work to be able to afford the necessities of life. The economic survival of Haiti is closely tied to the financial support provided to family members in Haiti by Haitians who have migrated to the United States and Canada.

ISSUES RELATED TO AUTONOMY

In America, educated Haitians seek job opportunities in their fields. Those who have a trade try to find employment in that area. Uneducated, undocumented, and illiterate individuals experience much more difficulty in entering the job market, where employment opportunities are restricted to working in places in which there is overcrowding, poor ventilation, and high pollution, all of which place them at high risk for occupational diseases.

Immigrants from various Haitian villages and cities tend to settle in clusters with their relatives or neighbors from their areas of origin. This pattern of settlement by area of origin helps immigrants adapt to the demands of their new environment and assure that they have someone living nearby whom they can call on in time of illness or other crisis. However, when people live and work primarily in an ethnic enclave, the native culture becomes a barrier to assimilation and acculturation into the dominant society.

The educational level of health-care professionals in Haiti is different from that in America. For example, medical education is not research-based, and nursing programs for the most part are at the diploma level with an apprenticeship. The only nursing baccalaureate program is the *Faculté des Sciences Infirmiere de L' Universite Episcopal D'Haiti* (Faculty of Nursing Science of the Episcopal University of Haiti), in Leogane on the southern coast of the island. Establishing this school and adopting this name was a major accomplishment. Nursing is finally accepted on par with the medical community as well as with the other professional schools. All other professional schools start with those three words "*Faculté des Sciences . . .*" and continues with whatever the science is (e.g., medicine, law, engineering).

Haitian health-care professionals who migrate to the United States have experienced a great deal of difficulty in obtaining licensure to practice. Those who learned their profession in Haiti were taught in French and the test-taking approach is different; multiple-choice examinations are a new and difficult concept for Haitians.

Haitian nurses are very skilled clinically; however, sometimes, they may experience difficulty in applying theoretical knowledge to practice. This may be due in part to language barriers and their diploma education, which focuses on tasks and skills development. Haitian professionals struggle with professional cohesiveness and collegiality. Many groups have established professional societies whose goals are to support each other, to promote professional development, and to promote collegial relationships. Some examples of these professional groups are the Haitian Nurses Association, the Haitian-American Medical Association, the Haitian Educator Association, the Haitian-American Engineers, and the Haitian-American Lawyers.

Sometimes, Haitians in the workplace greet each other in their native tongue because it is easier to articulate ideas and feelings and to express support in their native language. This may be irritating to non-Haitians who consider it rude.

Biocultural Ecology

SKIN COLOR AND OTHER BIOLOGICAL VARIATIONS

Different assessment techniques are required when assessing dark-skinned people for anemia and jaundice. One must examine the sclera, oral mucosa, conjunctiva, lips, nailbeds, palms of the hands, and soles of the feet when assessing for cyanosis and low blood hemoglobin levels. To assess for jaundice, one must examine the conjunctiva and oral mucosa for patches of bilirubin pigment because dark skin has natural underlying tones of red and yellow.

DISEASES AND HEALTH CONDITIONS

VIGNETTE 13.2

Jean-Claude Auguste, a 25-year-old with a history of attention deficit hyperactivity disorder (ADHD), has been overactive since early infancy. His parents initially attributed his behavior to the natural tendencies of being male. Mr. Auguste's parents tried to control his behavior by corralling him in his crib, verbally disciplining him, and occasionally, spanking him. His parents realized that he had a problem when he was about 3 years of age. He was hyperactive, impulsive, and unable to follow simple directions. Throughout his preschool years, he was repeatedly suspended from school. Jean-Claude's mother initially accepted the use of medication, but stopped it and refused to consider any other medication when side effects placed him into a "zombie-like" state that included sluggishness, difficulty sleeping, and loss of appetite. In his community, he developed a reputation for being *mal élevé*—a French term for "badly reared"—which in turn, reflected negatively on his parents within their extended family and community.

When his parents halted his medication, school staff registered their concern with the Department of Social Services by filing a child neglect report. His parents were placed on the defensive and began to feel threatened, stating, "the focus was no longer on [their] child's condition, but rather on [their] parental abilities." Unable to navigate the different agencies that had become involved with their family, and believing a more disciplinary and controlled environment might help, his parents sent Jean-Claude to Haiti to live with grandparents who eventually sent him to a Haitian boarding school. Neither environment had an effect on his behavior. Two years later, he returned to live with his parents in the United States. With much difficulty, he graduated from high school but continues to be hyperactive and unfocused. His parents are finally convinced that medication would be beneficial, but Jean-Claude refuses to take medications and denies his disorder.

1. Is ADHD a recognized and understood illness in the Haitian community?
2. Why were his parents not able to manage Jean-Claude?
3. Within the Haitian belief system, is ADHD considered a natural or an unnatural illness? Why?
4. What approach might social services have taken to assist his family?

Because Haiti is a tropical island, prevalent diseases include cholera, parasitosis, and malaria. Haiti has no mosquito control, so newer immigrants should be assessed for signs of malaria such as chills, fever, fatigue, and an enlarged spleen. Other diseases of increased incidence among Haitian immigrants are hepatitis, tuberculosis, HIV/AIDS, venereal diseases, and parasitosis from inadequate potable water sources in their homeland. Actual tuberculosis rates for Haitians are misleading because, until a few years ago, Haitians living in Haiti were routinely vaccinated with *Bacille bilié de Calmette-Guérin*, thus making all subsequent skin tests positive, even though they may not actually have had the disease. Unfortunately, upon immigration, many Haitians continue to live in overcrowded areas, are malnourished, and live in very poor sanitary conditions, factors that increase their risk for infectious diseases.

Haitians are prone to diabetes and hypertension—a reflection of genetics and their diet, which is high in fat, cholesterol, and salt. Data on the prevalence of diabetes and hypertension among Haitian Americans are difficult to assess because they are categorized as black. In addition to type 1 and type 2 diabetes, there is a type 3 malnutrition-related diabetes, also known as *tropical diabetes*. The prevalence ranges from 2 to 8 percent, accounting for different parts of the island (Pan American Health Organization, 2001). In addition, Haitians experience a high incidence of heart disease. Cerebrovascular diseases are the third leading cause of death; other cardiopathies are in fifth place, and arterial hypertension is in eleventh place. More deaths are registered among females than males. In addition to cardiovascular diseases, there is a high incidence of cancer. The National Cancer Institute statistics showed that the most frequent type of cancer treated was cervical cancer, representing 40 percent of cases. Breast cancer ranked second with 30 percent. Nasopharygeal cancer ranked in third position with 10 to 15 percent of the cases (Pan American

Health Organization, 2001). Both cancer and heart disease are related to a high-fat diet. Today, Haitians in Haiti and in the United States are very conscious of the need to limit the fat content in their diets; as a result, the Haitian diet is not as fatty as it once was.

Attention-deficit/hyperactivity disorder (ADHD) is a commonly diagnosed chronic mental condition in Haitian children (Prudent, Johnson, Carroll, & Culpepper, 2005). This disease has a large genetic component (McCann, Scheele, Ward, & Roy-Byrne, 2006). In the Haitian culture, there is no conceptual term for ADHD, nor is there a Creole term to describe it. Unfortunately, in the Haitian culture, the behavior displayed with this diagnosis may be interpreted as an ill-behaved or a "poorly raised" child or a psychically victimized child suffering from an "unnatural" condition. Parents may believe that this behavior can be controlled by parental discipline, or they may seek an alternative health consult such as a *Hougan* or voodoo priest. Although medications are the preferred treatment for ADHD, which may be combined with psychological intervention, Haitians are fearful of psychoactive drugs because they see them as the cause of substance abuse and even possibly mental illness (Prudent et al., 2005). Therefore, assessing the parents' perceptions of the cause of the ADHD behavior and assisting them in holistic treatment are important.

VARIATIONS IN DRUG METABOLISM

The literature reveals no studies on drug metabolism specific to Haitians or Haitian Americans. When Haitians are included in drug studies, it is assumed that they are included under the category of African American. Therefore, health-care providers may need to start with the literature for this broad category of ethnicity to posit and test theories of ethnic drug metabolism among Haitian Americans.

High-Risk Behaviors

VIGNETTE 13.3

The St. Fleur family is well respected in the Haitian community because they are religious with great moral values. They moved to the United States because of political issues in Haiti. Ronald, the youngest son of this family, is 27 years old and lives at home with his mother and father. Recently, he began having fevers and subsequently developed pneumonia. He was admitted to the hospital, where laboratory tests were HIV positive. Ronald was in shock when the doctor informed him that he was HIV positive. He confessed to the doctor that he was gay but he could not tell his family. He said that he did not want to bring shame to the family. Because he couldn't be in a formal relationship owing to his family and the Haitian community's view of homosexuality, he has been very promiscuous over the years.

1. What are Haitians' views of homosexuality?
2. If Ronald's parents were to learn of his positive HIV status, how might they react if they are religious and traditional?
3. Identify three major culturally congruent strategies to address in designing HIV-prevention practices in the Haitian community?

Haitian refugees are one of the most at-risk populations living in the United States. Therefore, it is important for health-care practitioners to consider a number of factors in providing health-care services. An in-depth assessment of the person's environmental, occupational, socioeconomic, demographic, educational, and linguistic status enables the development of strategies that are culturally appropriate, adequate, and effective. As a new group of immigrants, Haitians bring to the health-care system a different set of beliefs and values about health and illness. These differences challenge health-care practitioners who must try to explain treatments while acknowledging, but not changing, their clients' cultural convictions. Attempts to change firmly held beliefs are counterproductive to establishing trusting provider-client relationships.

Behaviors that may be considered high risk in American society are generally viewed as recreational or unimportant among Haitians. Alcohol, for example, plays an important part in Haitian society. Drinking alcohol is culturally approved for men and is used socially when friends gather, especially on weekends. Women drink socially and in moderation. Cigarette smoking is another high-risk behavior practiced by Haitian men, whereas Haitian women have a very low rate of tobacco use. The trend toward decreasing cigarette use in America has not influenced Haitian society. Drug abuse among Haitians used to be low; however, there seems to be an increase in drug abuse, concentrated in the adolescent population.

In 1982, Haiti became the first developing country to be blamed for the origin of AIDS. As a result, Haitians have had to endure the stigma associated with the belief that Haitians are "AIDS carriers." Unfortunately, HIV/AIDS has continued to spread in the Haitian community in Haiti and in the United States. Heterosexual transmission is the primary source mode of HIV transmission in the Haitian community and is rapidly becoming a disease of women and children (Santana & Dancy, 2000). Health professionals need to recognize the impact the stigma has had on male-female relationships as well as familial relationships in the Haitian community. Health professioanls must be mindful of the impact the stigma has had on Haitians. Health professionals must broaden their scope and approaches to HIV prevention by incorporating societal, contextual, and economic factors designed to modify traditional gender roles germane to influencing beginning negotiations of safer sex practices.

High-risk behavior in the Haitian culture includes the nonuse of seat belts and helmets when driving or riding a motorcycle or bicycle. Most cars in Haiti do not have seat belts, and there are no laws regarding the use of seat belts and helmets. Haitian cities are extremely overpopulated and traffic laws are very loose, resulting in hazardous driving conditions. Everyone tries to gain the upper hand. Haitian Americans must be educated about traffic laws, seat belt use, car seats for youngsters, and the need for helmets. Health-care practitioners may have to use graphic videos or skits when instructing clients about these safety practices. Practitioners may also use Haitian radio stations for educational programs when they are available. Other strategies that may be used to help promote behavioral changes are through church and community group activities. Through these avenues, health-care providers can have a significant impact on health promotion and health risk prevention among Haitian Americans.

HEALTH-CARE PRACTICES

To Haitians, good health is seen as the ability to achieve internal equilibrium between *cho* (hot) and *fret* (cold) (see also Nutrition and Health-Care Practices). To become balanced, one must eat well, give attention to personal hygiene, pray, and have good spiritual habits. To promote good health, one must be strong, have good color, be plump, and be free of pain. To maintain this state, one must eat right, sleep right, keep warm, exercise, and keep clean.

Haitians who believe in voodoo and other forms of folk medicine may use several types of folk healers. These healers include a voodoo practitioner, a *docte fey* (leaf doctor), a *fam saj* (lay midwife), a *docte zo* (bonesetter), and a *pikirist* (injectionist). Depending on whether the individual believes that the illness is natural or unnatural, she or he may seek help other than Western medicine from one of these healers.

Nutrition

MEANING OF FOOD

For many Haitians in lower socioeconomic groups, food means survival. However, food is relished as a cultural treasure and Haitians generally retain their food habits and practices after emigrating. Food practices vary little from generation to generation. Most Haitians are not culinary explorers. They prefer eating at home, take pride in promoting their food for their children, and discourage fast food. When hospitalized, many would rather fast than eat non-Haitian food. Haitians do not eat yogurt, cottage cheese, or "runny" egg yolk. Haitians drink a lot of water, homemade fruit juices, and cold fruity sodas.

COMMON FOODS AND FOOD RITUALS

The typical Haitian breakfast consists of bread, butter, bananas, and coffee. Children are allowed to drink coffee, which is not as strong as that consumed by adults. Generally, the largest meal for Haitians is eaten at lunch. At lunchtime, a basic Haitian meal might include rice and beans, boiled plantains, a salad made of watercress and tomatoes, and stewed vegetables and beef or cornmeal cooked as polenta. Table 13–1 lists popular foods in the Haitian community.

DIETARY PRACTICES FOR HEALTH PROMOTION

Hot and cold, acid and nonacid, and heavy and light are the major categories of contrast when discussing food. Illness is caused when the body is exposed to an imbalance of cold (*fret*) and hot (*cho*) factors. For example, *soursop*, a large green prickly fruit with a white pulp that is used in juice and ice cream, is considered a cold food and is avoided when a woman is menstruating. Eating white beans after childbirth is believed to induce hemorrhage. Foods that are considered heavy, such as plantain, cornmeal mush, rice, and meat, are to be eaten during the day because they provide energy. Light foods, such as hot chocolate milk, bread, and soup, are eaten for dinner because they are more easily digested. Table 13–2 presents a classification of hot and cold foods.

To treat a person by the hot-and-cold system, a potent drink or herbal medicine of the class opposite to the disease is administered. Cough medicines, for example, are considered to be in the hot category, whereas laxatives are in the cold category. Certain food prohibitions are related to particular diseases and stages of the life cycle. Teenagers, for example, are advised to avoid drinking citrus fruit juices such as lemonade to prevent the development of acne. After performing strenuous activities or any activity that causes the body to become hot, one should not eat cold food because that will create an imbalance, causing a condition called *chofret*. A woman who has just

TABLE 13.1 *Popular Foods in the Haitian Community*

Bouillon	Soup made with beef broth mixed with various green vegetables (e.g., spinach, cabbage, watercress, string beans, carrots), meat or poultry, plantain, sweet potato, and Malaga, a sweet aromatic wine
Chiquetaille	Codfish or smoked herring, unsalted, shredded finely, mixed with onions, shallots, finely chopped hot pepper, vinegar, and lime
Fritters	*Marinade:* flour, water, eggs, parsley, onions, garlic, salt and pepper, chicken, hot pepper, and a pinch of baking soda powder, mixed together to pancake consistency and deep-fried
	Acra: chopped parsley, eggs, garlic, and onion mixed with Malaga; finely shredded codfish or smoked herring and hot pepper may be added
	Beignet: sweet ripe banana, sugar, and eggs, mixed with cinnamon, milk, margarine, flour, nutmeg, and vanilla extract
Green plantain	Boiled or fried, usually eaten with *griot*
Griot	Marinated pork cut up in small pieces and fried
Lambi	Conch meat softened and prepared in a sauce
Legume	Vegetables such as chayote and eggplant cooked with meat
Patee	Pastry dough filled with choice meat, chicken, or smoked herring
Pumpkin squash soup	Meat or poultry mixed with vegetables and pureed cooked squash and spices
Tomtom	Similar to dumplings, cooked and made into round balls and eaten with beef stew and okra

TABLE 13.2 *Haitian Hot and Cold Food Classification*

Very Cold (−3)	Quite Cold (−2)	Cool (−1)	Neutral (0)	Warm (+)	Very Hot (+2)
Avocado	Banana	Tomato	Cabbage	Eggs	Rum
Cashew nuts	Grapefruit	Cane syrup	Conch	Pigeon	Nutmeg
Mango	Lime	Orange	Carrot	Soup	Garlic
Coconut	Okra	Cantaloupe	Watercress	Bouillon	Tea
Cassava	Watermelon	Chayote	Brown rice	Pork	Cornmeal mush

Source: Adapted from M. S. Laguerre (1981, pp. 194–196).

straightened her hair by using a hot comb and then opens a refrigerator may become a victim of *chofret*. This means she may catch a cold and/or possibly develop pneumonia.

When they are sick, Haitians like to eat pumpkin soup, bouillon, a special soup made with green vegetables, meat, plantain, dumplings, and yams. The Haitian diet is high in carbohydrates and fat. Eating *right* entails eating sufficient food to feel full and maintain a constant body weight, which is often higher than weight standards medically recommended in the United States. Men like to see "plump" women. Furthermore, weight loss is seen as one of the most important signs of illness. Additional components of what Haitians consider a healthy diet are tonics to stimulate the appetite and the use of high-calorie supplements such as *Akasan*, which is either prepared plain or made as a special drink with cream of cornmeal, evaporated milk, cinnamon, vanilla extract, sugar, and a pinch of salt.

A thorough nutritional assessment is very important to effectively promote nutritional health. Understanding food rituals assists health-care providers in designing individualized dietary plans, which can be incorporated into the diet to facilitate compliance with dietary regimens that promote a healthier lifestyle.

NUTRITIONAL DEFICIENCIES AND FOOD LIMITATIONS

Many Haitian women and children who come from rural areas have significant protein deficiencies owing to Haiti's economic deprivation. A cultural factor contributing to this problem is the uneven distribution of protein among family members. However, the problem is not one of net protein deficiency in the community but, rather, the unwise distribution of the available protein among family members. Whenever meat is served, the major portion goes to the men, under the assumption that they must be well fed to provide for the household. This same pattern exists today among Haitian immigrants. Being aware of this cultural factor enables health-care practitioners to prepare nutritional plans that meet clients' dietary needs.

Another major concern in this area is that of food insecurity and short intervals between births, chronic malnutrition, and anemia, which are widespread among Haitian women of childbearing age. These health inequalities result in a high prevalence of low birth weight, estimated

at 15 percent; anemia, ranging from 35 to 50 percent; a body mass index under 18.5 kg/m^2, estimated at 18 percent; and a high maternal mortality rate, estimated at 456 per 100,000 live births (Pan American Health Organization, 2001).

Pregnancy and Childbearing Practices

FERTILITY PRACTICES AND VIEWS TOWARD PREGNANCY

Pregnancy and fertility practices are not readily discussed among Haitians. Most Haitians are Catholic and are unwilling to overtly engage in conversation about birth control or abortion. This does not mean that these two practices do not occur, but rather, that they are just not openly discussed. Abortion is viewed as a woman's issue and is left to her and her significant other to decide. Accurate assessments and teaching related to these sensitive areas require tact and understanding. Initially, health-care practitioners should be cautious in assessing and gathering information related to fertility control. Pregnancy is not considered a health problem, but rather, a time of joy for the entire family. Pregnancy does not relieve a woman from her work. Because pregnancy is not a disease, many Haitian women do not seek prenatal care. Pregnant women are restricted from eating spices that may irritate the fetus. However, they are permitted to eat vegetables and red fruits because these are believed to improve the fetus's blood. They are encouraged to eat large quantities of food because they are eating for two. Pregnant women who experience increased salivation may rid themselves of the excess at places that may seem inappropriate. They may even carry a "spit" cup in order to rid themselves of the excess saliva. They are not embarrassed by this behavior because they feel it is perfectly normal.

Fifty percent of women living in Port-au-Prince give birth in a hospital, compared with 31 percent of births in other urban areas, and only 9 percent of births in rural areas. The leading causes of maternal deaths are obstructed labor (8.3 percent), toxemia (16.7 percent), and hemorrhage (8.3 percent). The high maternal mortality rate is mainly the result of inadequate prenatal care (Pan American Health Organization, 2001).

The most popular methods of contraception are the birth control pill, female sterilization, injections, and condoms (3 percent each). Among sexually active women, 13 percent use a modern method of contraception and 4 percent relied on traditional methods. Among sexually active men, 17 percent used a modern method (6 percent used condoms) and 16 percent relied on traditional methods (Pan American Health Organization, 2001).

PRESCRIPTIVE, RESTRICTIVE, AND TABOO PRACTICES IN THE CHILDBEARING FAMILY

During labor, the woman may walk, squat, pace, sit, or rub her belly. Generally, Haitian women practice natural childbirth and do not ask for analgesia. Some may scream or cry and become hysterical, whereas others are stoic, only moaning and grunting. What they need is support and reassurance; for example, applying a cold compress on the woman's forehead demonstrates caring and sensitivity on the part of the practitioner. Since migrating, some Haitian women have adopted American childbearing practices and request analgesics. Cesarean birth is feared because it is abdominal surgery. Women in higher social strata are more amenable to having cesarean deliveries. Fathers do not generally participate in the labor and delivery, believing that this is a private event best handled by women. The woman is not coached; female members of the family give assistance as needed.

The crucial period for the childbearing woman is postpartum, a time for prescription and proscription. The woman takes an active role in her own care. She dresses warmly after birth as a way to become healthy and clean. Haitians believe that the bones are "open" after birth and that a woman should stay in bed during the first 2 to 3 days postpartum to allow the bones to close. Wearing an abdominal binder is another way to facilitate closing the bones.

The postpartum woman also engages in a practice called *the three baths*. For the first 3 days, the mother bathes in hot water boiled with special leaves that are either bought or picked from the field. She also drinks tea boiled from these leaves. For the next 3 days, the mother bathes in water prepared with leaves that are warmed by the sun. At this point, the mother takes only water or tea warmed by the sun. Another important practice is for the mother to take a vapor bath with boiled orange leaves, a practice believed to enhance cleanliness and tighten the internal muscles. At the end of the 3rd to 4th week, the new mother takes the third bath, which is cold. A cathartic may be administered to cleanse her intestinal tract. When the process is completed, she may drink cold water again and resume her normal activities.

In the postpartum period, Haitian women avoid white foods such as lima beans, as well as other foods, including okra, mushrooms, and tomatoes. These foods are restricted because they are believed to increase vaginal discharge. Other foods are eaten to give the new mother strength and vitality. Foods associated with this prescriptive practice are porridge, rice and red beans, plantains boiled or grated with the skins and prepared as porridge (the skin is high in iron, which is good for building the blood), carrot juice, and carrot juice mixed with red beet juice.

Breastfeeding is encouraged for up to 9 months postpartum. Breast milk can become detrimental to both mother and child if it becomes too thick or too thin. If it is too thin, it is believed that the milk has "turned," and it may cause diarrhea and headaches in the child and, possibly, postpartum depression in the mother. If milk is too "thick," it is believed to cause impetigo (*bouton*). Breastfeeding and bottle feeding are accepted practices. If the child develops diarrhea, breastfeeding is immediately discontinued. Practices that do not put the mother or the child at risk should be supported and encouraged. Respecting the clients' cultural beliefs and practices helps to establish trust between the client and the caregiver and demonstrates caring. By being familiar with these health practices and beliefs, health-care practitioners can assist women in making culturally safe decisions related to pregnancy and plans for delivery.

Another prescriptive postpartum practice among Haitian women is to feed their infant a *lok* similar to the one administered to the older children in the summer. The laxative is administered as the initial feeding and is intended to hasten the expulsion of meconium. Because Haitians are fearful of diarrhea in children, health-care providers should stress the risks associated with *lok* and any other type of bowel-cleansing cocktails in infants and children. It is important to stress the impact of laxative use on the body system and educate the woman about the need to prevent dehydration.

VIGNETTE 13.4

Natasha Saint-Fleur, a 32-year-old Haitian-American, is 9 months' pregnant. She lives with her husband and parents. During her pregnancy, Mrs. Saint-Fleur has been very happy and excited about the upcoming birth of her first baby. Although Mrs. Saint-Fleur has had no prenatal complications, she has stopped working until the arrival of her new infant. Natasha eats four small meals a day and her mother feels that it is inadequate and feels this is why her daughter has not gained enough weight during her pregnancy. She fears that the baby's blood will not be "strong."

Natasha delivers a healthy baby. Upon her discharge to home, her mother takes full responsibility for the care of the baby and the afterbirth rituals. One day postpartum, Natasha is wearing shorts and a small tank top, the air conditioner is set at 70°F, and she is drinking a soft drink with a lot of ice. When Natasha's mother sees this, she is very upset.

1. Is it common practice for Haitian women not to work when pregnant?
2. Why does Natasha's mother feel that the baby's blood will not be strong? What diet might be adequate, in her opinion?
3. During the postpartum period, what is a common Haitian ritual provided to the mother?
4. Why did the grandmother take over care of the infant?
5. What types of foods do you expect Mrs. Saint-Fleur to eat after childbirth?

Death Rituals

DEATH RITUALS AND EXPECTATIONS

Generally, Haitians prefer to die at home rather than in the hospital. Since migrating to America, many have accepted death in a health-care facility to alleviate the heavy burden on the family during the last stage of the loved one's life. When death is imminent, the family may pray and cry uncontrollably, sometimes even hysterically. They try to meet the person's spiritual needs by bringing religious medallions, pictures of saints, or fetishes. When the person dies, all family members try, if possible, to be at the bedside and have a prayer service. If possible, and if it is not too disturbing to other clients, health-care practitioners should encourage this practice and involve a family member in the postmortem care.

RESPONSES TO DEATH AND GRIEF

Death in the Haitian community mobilizes the entire family, including the matrilineal and patrilineal extensions and affines. Death arrangements in America are similar to those in Haiti. Generally, a male kinsman of the deceased makes the arrangements. This person may also be more fluent in English and more accustomed to dealing with the bureaucracy. The kinsman is responsible for notifying all family members wherever they might be in the world, an important activity because family members' travel plans influence funeral arrangements. In addition, he is responsible for ordering the coffin, making arrangements for prayer services before the funeral, and coordinating plans for the funeral service.

The preburial activity is called *veye*, a gathering of family and friends who come to the house of the deceased to cry, tell stories about the deceased's life, and laugh. Food, tea, coffee, and rum are in abundant supply. The intent is to show support and to join the family in sharing this painful loss. Another religious ritual is called the *dernie priye*, a special prayer service consisting of 7 consecutive days of prayer. Its purpose is to facilitate the passage of the soul from this world to the next. It usually takes place in the home. On the 7th day, a mass called *prise de deuil* officially begins the mourning process. After each of these prayers, a reception/celebration in memory of the deceased is held.

Haitians have a very strong belief in resurrection and paradise; thus, cremation is not an acceptable option (Father Darbouze Gerard, personal communication, September 2001). Haitians are very cautious about autopsies. If foul play is suspected, they may request an autopsy to ensure that the patient is really dead. This alleviates their fear that their loved one is being *zombified*. According to this belief, this can occur when the person appears to have died of natural causes but is still alive. About 18 hours after the burial, the person is stolen from his or her coffin; the lack of oxygen causes some of the brain cells to die, so the mental facilities cease to exist while the body remains alive. The zombie then responds to commands, having no free will, and is domesticated as a slave.

Spirituality

DOMINANT RELIGION AND USE OF PRAYER

Clients' cultural beliefs and religion can have a great impact on their acceptance of health care and compliance and, therefore, on the outcomes of treatment. Catholicism is the primary religion of Haiti. Since the early 1970s, however, Protestantism has gained in popularity throughout the island and has seriously challenged the Catholic Church, especially among the lower socioeconomic classes. Even though Haitians are deeply religious, their religious beliefs are combined with **voudou** (voodooism), a complex religion with its roots in Africa (Fig. 13–1). Voudou, in the most simplistic sense, involves communication by trance between the believer and ancestors, saints, or animistic deities. Voudou is not considered paganism among those who practice it, even though many of the rituals resemble paganism. Participants gather to worship the *loa or mystere*, deities or spirits who are believed to have received their powers from God and are capable of expressing themselves through possession of a chosen believer. With their great powers, the *loa* or *mystere* can provide favors such as protection, wealth, and health to those who worship and believe in them.

MEANING OF LIFE AND INDIVIDUAL SOURCES OF STRENGTH

The family system among Haitians is the center of life and includes the nuclear, consanguine, and affinal relatives. They may all live under the same roof. The family deals with all aspects of a person's life, including counseling, education, crises, marriage, and death.

The best way to understand and assess the spiritual beliefs and needs of Haitian American clients is to understand their culture. This is especially important because

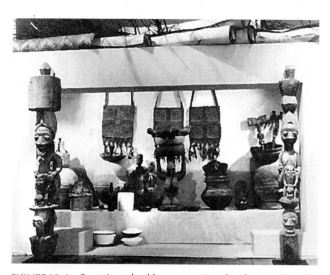

FIGURE 13–1   Santeria evolved from two main cultural antecedents: the worship of *orisha* among the Yoruba tribe of Nigeria and the cult of saints from the Roman Catholicism of Spain. (Retrieved September 15, 2007, from http://archive.nandotimes.com/prof/caribe/ShangoAltar.html)

Haitian clients may express their concerns in ways that are unique to their cultural and religious beliefs. To ensure accurate assessments of these clients, it is essential to ask questions carefully and to completely understand the answers in order to gain an understanding of clients' perceptions of health and illness as dictated by their culture and religious beliefs. By recognizing and accepting clients' beliefs, health-care providers may alleviate barriers and clients may feel more at ease to discuss their beliefs and needs.

SPIRITUAL BELIEFS AND HEALTH-CARE PRACTICES

Voudou believers may often attribute their ailments or medical problems to the doings of evil spirits. In such cases, they prefer to confirm their suspicions through the *loa* before accepting natural causes as the problem, which would lead to seeking Western medical care. For Haitian clients, the belief in the power of the supernatural can have a great influence on the psychological and medical concerns of the client.

Health-Care Practices

HEALTH-SEEKING BELIEFS AND BEHAVIORS

For Haitians, illness is perceived as punishment, considered an assault on the body, and may have two different etiologies: natural illnesses, known as *maladi Bondye* ("disease of the Lord"), and supernatural illnesses. Natural illnesses may occur frequently, are of short duration, and are caused by environmental factors such as food, air, cold, heat, and gas. Other causes of natural illness are movement of blood within the body, disequilibrium between hot and cold, and bone displacement. Supernatural illnesses are believed to be caused by angry spirits. To placate these spirits, clients must offer feasts called *manger morts*. If individuals do not partake in these rituals, misfortunes are likely to befall them. Illnesses of supernatural origin are fundamentally a breach in rapport between the individual and her or his protector. The breach in rapport is a response from the spirit and a way of showing disapproval of the protégé's behavior. In this instance, health can be recovered if the client takes the first step in determining the nature of the illness. This can be accomplished by eliciting the help of a *voudou* priest and following the advice given by the spirit itself. To accurately prescribe treatment options, health-care providers must be able to differentiate between these belief systems.

Physical illnesses are thought to be on a continuum beginning with *Kom pa bon* ("I do not feel well"). In this phase, the affected person is not confined to bed; illness is transitory, and the person should be able to return to his or her normal activities. The next phase is *moin malad* ("I am sick"), in which the individuals stay at home and avoid activity. The third phase is *moin malad anpil* ("I am very sick"). This means that the person is very ill and may be confined to bed. The final phase is *Moin pap refe* ("I am dying").

Haitians believe that gas (*gaz*) may provoke pain and anemia. Gas can occur in the head, where it enters through the ears; in the stomach, where it enters through the mouth; and in the shoulders, back, legs, or appendix, where it travels from the stomach. When gas is in the stomach, the client is said to suffer *kolik*, meaning stomach pain. Gas in the head is called *van nan tet* or *van nan zorey*, which literally means "gas in one's ears," and is believed to be a cause of headaches. Gas moving from one part of the body to another produces pain. Thus, the movement of gas from the stomach to the legs produces rheumatism, to the back causes back pain, and to the shoulder causes shoulder pain. Foods that help dispel gas include tea made from garlic, cloves, and mint; plantain; and corn. To deter the entry of gas into the body, one must be careful about eating "leftovers," especially beans. Since migrating to the United States, Haitians have begun eating leftovers, which is believed to cause many of their ailments. After childbirth, women are particularly susceptible to gas, and to prevent entry of gas into the body, they tighten their waist with a belt or a piece of linen.

RESPONSIBILITY FOR HEALTH CARE

Haitians engage in self-treatment and see these activities as a way of preventing disease or promoting health. Haitians try home remedies as a first resort for treating illness. They are self-diagnosticians and may use home remedies for a particular ailment, or if they know someone who had a particular illness, they may take the prescribed medicine from that person. They keep numerous topical and oral medicines on hand, which they use to treat various symptoms. For example, an individual who suspects a venereal disease may buy penicillin injections and have someone administer them without consulting a physician. In Haiti, many medications can be purchased without a prescription, a potentially dangerous practice. However, health-care providers must be very discrete in assessing, teaching, and guiding the client toward safer health practices. Admonishing clients may cause them to withdraw and not listen to instructions. Haitians may also lead practitioners to believe that they are interested, when in fact, they have already discredited the practitioner. When taking the client's history, the practitioner should inquire if the patient has been taking medication that was prescribed for someone else. Moreover, when prescribing a potentially dangerous drug, the practitioner should be sure to caution the client not to give the medication to ailing friends or relatives. Even though the practitioner may not be completely successful at stopping the practice of exchanging medications, with continued reminders, she or he may be successful later.

FOLK AND TRADITIONAL PRACTICES

Haitians may use others' experiences with a particular illness as a barometer against which to measure their symptoms and institute treatment. If necessary, a person living in the United States may ask friends or relatives to send medications from Haiti. Such medications may consist of roots, leaves, and European-manufactured products that are more familiar to them. Therefore, it is very important to ascertain what the client is taking at home to avoid serious complications.

Constipation, referred to as *konstipasyon*, is treated with laxatives or herbal tea. Sometimes, Haitians use enemas (*lavman*). Diarrhea is not a major concern in adults; however, it is considered very dangerous in children and sometimes interpreted as a hex on the child. Parents may try herbal medicine, may seek help from a *voudou* priest, or *hougan*, or if all else fails, may consult a physician. It is very important to assess the child carefully because he or she may have been ill for quite some time.

A primary respiratory ailment is *oppression*, a term used to describe asthma. However, the term really describes a state of anxiety and hyperventilation rather than the condition. *Oppression* is considered a cold state, as are many respiratory conditions. Clients say *M' ap toufe* or *mwen pa ka respire*. A home remedy for *oppression* is to take a dry coconut and cut it open, fill it with half sugarcane syrup and half honey, grate one full nutmeg and add it to the syrup mix, reseal the coconut, and then bury it in the ground for a month. The coconut is reopened, the content is stirred and mixed, and 1 tablespoon is administered twice a day until it is finished. By the end of this treatment, the child is supposed to be cured of the respiratory problem.

BARRIERS TO HEALTH CARE

Because orthodox medicine is often bypassed or perceived as a second choice among Haitians, the potential delay of medical care can pose an increased risk to clients. The view that physicians of conventional medicine do not understand *voudou*, and therefore, cannot cure magical illness, or that an illness worsens if the bewitched person seeks a physician, is enough to persuade these individuals to seek unconventional modes of therapy with which they are more comfortable. The health-care team should understand some of the basic principles and practices of folk medicine, particularly root medicine, because this can play a significant role in determining the progress of the client's health status.

Many Haitians are in low-paying jobs that do not provide health insurance, and they cannot afford to purchase it themselves. Thus, economics acts as a barrier to health promotion. In addition, for those who do not speak English well, it is difficult for them to access the health-care system, fully explain their needs, or understand prescriptions and treatments.

CULTURAL RESPONSES TO HEALTH AND ILLNESS

The *root-work system* is a folk medicine that provides a framework for identifying and curing folk illnesses. When illness occurs, or when a person is not feeling well or is "disturbed," root medicine distinguishes whether the symptoms and illness are of natural or unnatural origin. An imbalance in harmony between the physical and the spiritual worlds, such as dietary or lifestyle excesses, can cause a natural illness. For example, diabetes is considered a natural illness; however, most Haitians do not seek

immediate medical assistance when they detect the symptoms of polyuria, excessive thirst, and weight loss. Instead, they attempt symptom management by making dietary changes on their own by drinking potions or herbal remedies. When the person finally seeks medical attention, she or he may be very sick. At this point, the practitioner should be cautious in explaining the condition and use a culturally specific approach when explaining the medical regimen, diet, and medications.

Pain is commonly referred to as *doule*. Many Haitians have a very low pain threshold. Their demeanor changes, they are verbal about the cause of their pain, and they sometimes moan. They are vague about the location of the pain because they believe that it is not important; they believe that the whole body is affected because disease travels. This belief makes it very difficult to accurately assess pain. Injections are the preferred method for medication administration, followed by elixirs, tablets, and finally, capsules.

Chest pain is referred to as *doule nan ke mwen*, abdominal pain is *doule nan vent*, and stomach pain is *doule nan ke mwen* or *doule nan lestomak mwen*. Oxygen should be offered only when absolutely necessary because the use of oxygen is perceived as an indicator of the seriousness of the illness.

Nausea is expressed as *lestomak/mwen ap roule, M santi m anwi vomi, lestomak/mwen chaje*, or *ke mwen tounin*. Those who are more educated may express their discomfort as nausea. Because of modesty, they may discard vomitus immediately so as not to upset others. Specific instructions should be given regarding keeping the specimen until the practitioner has had a chance to see it.

Fatigue, physical weakness known as *febles*, is interpreted as a sign of anemia or insufficient blood. Symptoms are generally attributed to poor diet. Clients may suggest to the health-care provider that they need special care—that is, to eat well, take vitamin injections, and rest. To counteract the *febles*, the diet includes liver, pigeon meat, watercress, bouillon made of green leafy vegetables, cow's feet, and red meat.

Another condition is fright or *sezisman*. Various external and internal environmental factors are believed to cause *sezisman*, thereby disrupting the normal blood flow. *Sezisman* may occur when someone receives bad news, is involved in a frightful situation, or suffers from indignation after being treated unjustly. When this condition occurs, blood is said to move to the head, causing partial loss of vision, headache, increased blood pressure, or a stroke. To counteract this problem, the client may sit quietly, put a cold compress on the forehead, drink bitter herbal tea, take sips of water, or drink rum mixed with black, unsweetened coffee.

Haitian Americans may strongly resist acculturation, taking pride in preserving traditional spiritual, religious, and family values. This strong hold on cultural views sometimes creates stress leading to depression. The stigma attached to mental illness is strong, and most Haitians do not readily admit to being depressed. A major factor to remember is the strong prevalence of *voudou*, which attributes depression to possession by malevolent spirits or punishment for not honoring good protective spirits. In addition, depression can be viewed as a hex placed by a jealous or envious individual. Factors that may trigger depression are memories of family in the homeland, thoughts about spirits in Haiti, dreams about dead family members, or guilt and regrets about abandoning one's family in Haiti for the abundance in America. Health-care providers need to be sensitive to the underlying causes of problems and ascertain the need for comfort within specific religious beliefs.

In the case of an unnatural illness, the person's poor health is attributed to magical causes such as a hex, a curse, or a spell, which has been cast by someone as a result of family or interpersonal disagreement. The curse takes place when the intended victim eats food containing ingredients such as snake, frog, or spider egg powder, which cause symptoms of burning skin, rashes, pruritus, nausea, vomiting, and headaches (Fishman, Bobo, Kosub, & Womeodu, 1993). These symptoms often coincide with psychological problems manifested by violent attacks, hallucinations, delusions, or "magical possession." Because, under Western medical standards, an evil spirit would be classified as a true psychiatric problem with "culturally diverse manifestations" and not as an actual case of possession, the health-care practitioner is challenged in assessing and making the appropriate intervention (Fishman et al., 1993). If the practitioner is aware of witchcraft, *voudou* practices, and the symptoms associated with them, it may prevent (1) incorrectly diagnosing an individual as mentally ill, (2) giving advice that frightens or confuses the patient into thinking an illness is unnatural in origin, or (3) initiating symptomatic treatment that does not reach the underlying stress. The role of the health-care provider is to be sensitive and understanding toward the patient who holds a belief in these traditional practices. Health-care providers should realize that hesitating to offer a specific diagnosis might be more detrimental to the client than a negative diagnosis.

BLOOD TRANSFUSIONS AND ORGAN DONATION

Most Haitians are extremely afraid of diseases associated with blood irregularities. They believe that blood is the central dynamic of body functions and pathological processes; therefore, any condition that places the body in a "blood-need" state is believed to be extremely dangerous. Clients and their families become emotional about blood transfusions. Thus, these are received with much apprehension. In addition, as in all societies, blood transfusions are feared because of the potential for HIV transmission. Health-care providers should explain the need for a blood transfusion factually and carefully clarify the procedure along with the involved risks. Practitioners should involve clients and their families in the care as much as possible. Precautionary measures that have been taken to prevent blood contamination should also be explained.

Because Haitians hold strong religious beliefs about life after death, the body must remain intact for burial. Thus, organ donation and transplantation are not generally discussed. Since migrating to the United States, some Haitians have, with considerable distress, participated in organ transplantation. A prime concern is transference, believing that through the organ donor, the donor's per-

sonality will "shift" to the recipient and change his or her being. Health-care providers should assess Haitian clients' beliefs about organ donation and involve a religious leader to provide support and help facilitate a decision regarding organ donation or transplantation. Because some Haitians' knowledge and understanding in this area is limited, the health-care provider should be proactive by promoting health education.

Health-Care Practitioners

TRADITIONAL VERSUS BIOMEDICAL PRACTITIONERS

In general, most Haitians resort to symptom management with self-care first and then spiritual care. They commonly use traditional and Western practitioners simultaneously (see Spirituality and Folk Practices).

STATUS OF HEALTH-CARE PROVIDERS

Haitians are very respectful of physicians and nurses. Physicians are men and nurses are women. Nurses are referred to as Miss. By incorporating culturally specific strategies in their program, practitioners inspire confidence and trust. Haitian clients who have had limited contact with American health-care systems may have limited understanding of biomedical concepts. Health-care providers need to take the time to explain and re-explain relevant points to compensate for clients' knowledge deficit or language limitations. Health-care providers who show compassion and sensitivity toward Haitian clients achieve greater success in educating clients, families, and the community.

REFERENCES

Aristide, M. V. (1995). Economics of liberation. *Roots, 1*(2), 20–24.
CIA. (2006). *World Factbook: Haiti.* Retrieved December 12, 2006, from http://www.odci.gov/cia
Dorestant, N. (1998). *A look at Haitian history from a Haitian perspective.* Retrieved February 3, 2007, from http://www.geocite.com
Elliot, A. (2001, August 6). South Florida Caribbean population has almost doubled. *The Miami Herald.* Retrieved February 3, 2007, from http://www.miamiherald.com
Fishman, B. M., Bobo, L., Kosub, K., & Womeodu, R. J. (1993). Cultural issues in serving minority populations: Emphasis on Mexican Americans and African Americans. *American Journal of Medical Science, 306,* 160–166.
Jean-Baptiste, A. R. (1985). *The black man: Ti Manno in public.* New York: St. Aude Records.
Jean-Bernard, L. (1983). *Impossible alphabetization.* Port-au-Prince, Haiti: Des Antilles SA.
Laguere, M. S. (1981). Haitian Americans. In L. Sana (Ed.), *Handbook of immigrant health* (pp. 194–196). New York: Springer Publishing Co.
Louis-Juste, A. (1995). Popular education and democracy. *Roots, 2*(1), 14–19.
McCann, B. S., Scheele, L., Ward, N., & Roy-Byrne, P. (2006). Childhood inattention and hyperactivity symptoms self-reported by adults with Asperger syndrome. *International Journal of Descriptive and Experimental Psychopathology, Phenomenology and Psychiatric Diagnosis, 39,* 45–54.
Pan American Health Organization. (2001). *Regional core health data systems.* Retrieved November 22, 2006, from http://www.paho.org/English/SHA/glossary.htm

Prudent, N., Johnson, P., Carroll, J., & Culpepper, L. (2005). Attention deficit disorder: Presentation and management in the Haitian American child. *Primary Care Companion Journal Clinical Psychiatry, 7*(4), 190–197.

Regan, J. (1995). Behind the invasion more misery. *Roots, 1*(2), 7–13.

Santana, M. A., & Dancy, B. L. (2000). The stigma of being named "AIDS carriers" on Haitian-American women. *Health Care for Women International, 21*, 161–171.

Statistics Canada. (2006, February 8). Ethnic origin. *The Daily.* Retrieved December 18, 2006 from http://www.statcan.ca

U.S. Immigration and Naturalization Service. (2006). *Statistical yearbook of the Immigration and Naturalization Service 2005.* Washington, DC: U.S. Government Printing Office.

World Bank Annual Report. (2006). *Countries eligible for borrowing from World Bank.* Retrieved January 30, 2007, from http://www.worldbank.org

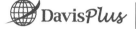

Chapter *14*

People of Iranian Heritage

HOMEYRA HAFIZI, MARYAM SAYYEDI, and
JULIENE G. LIPSON

Overview, Inhabited Localities, and Topography

OVERVIEW

Iran is a geographically and ethnically diverse, non–Arabic-speaking, Muslim country. Iran's 1979 Revolution generated a steady wave of immigration to North America, Europe, and Australia. Prior to the 1979 Revolution, the main reason for immigration was educational advancement. The few who immigrated had little impact on the host country's social make-up and the health-care system. But in the past 10 to 15 years and with the marked increase in immigration, some Iranian communities, such as that in Los Angeles, have begun to influence the regional economy.

Since the 1979 Revolution, Iran's socioeconomic and political instability has spurred emigration. Among immigrants, a deep generation gap, both within the family unit and with the larger population, frequently occurs. First-generation Iranian-born immigrants often live between the two worlds. Their age and reason for immigration are mitigating factors. The generation gap has widened as each subgroup adopts the new culture, tries to fit into the environment, and garners new ways of self-expression. A study of Iranian immigrants in New South Wales, Australia, noted that women's roles were changing slowly from the more traditional roles of home manager and nurturer to those of education and employment (Omeri, 1997). In another study conducted in Los Angeles, Iranian women who left Iran at a young age had more liberal attitudes toward sex and intimate relationships and more conflicts between their Iranian and American iden-

tities (Hanassab, 1998). Evidence suggests that, in general, women acculturate at a faster rate than men and begin to undermine the patriarchal and sexist cultural values (Darvishpour, 2002).

Many Iranian immigrants face considerable ethnic bias in the United States, with an intensity directly linked to the ongoing events in the Middle East. Anger and prejudice toward Iranians began in November 1979 with the 14-month occupation of the U.S. Embassy in Tehran. The hostility was manifested in many ways and experienced by Iranians of all ages. Some trilingual immigrants identified themselves by their ethnicity rather than their place of origin. For example, one would identify himself or herself as Turkish rather than as an Iranian Turk. The tragic events of 9/11, the ongoing instabilities in the Middle East, the current Iran's nuclear ambitions, and the Iraq war have marginalized the Iranian immigrant. By virtue of its location, predominant religion, and the central government's reaching out to neighboring countries, Iran is a figure in international policy making. The U.S. media overemphasize the influence of Islamic fundamentalism, and the public tends to view Middle Eastern immigrants as a homogenous population. In actuality, most Iranians are more secular and nationalistic than people from Sunni Arab nations, who may hold a more common Islamic identity (Sayyedi, 2004).

The U.S. Bureau of the Census estimates the number of Iranians in the United States at 400,000. Unofficially, the estimate is closer to 1 million. The political climate discourages Iranian immigrants from disclosing their native origin; hence, they self-identify as "other" or "Caucasian." The 2002 Census described the California Iranian American population as largely concentrated in the Los Angeles area, which consequently has the largest concentration of Iranians outside of Iran. Totaling 159,016 persons, this population is larger than the combined number of Iranians in 20 other states. The Los Angeles population is ethnically and religiously diverse. Although Muslims are still the majority, the Armenian, Jewish, and Baha'i communities have a strong presence (Bozorgmehr, Sabagh, & Der-Martirosian, 1993). Divided by political, religious, and social class differences, most live in small social networks.

In this chapter, the terms *Persian* and *Iranian* are used interchangeably. For mainly political reasons, some immigrants call themselves *Persian*. In 1935, the country's name was changed from Persia to *Iran* (from the word *aryana*) to present an image of progress and to unify the many ethnicities, tribes, and social classes. The original Persians were an Indo-European group, the Aryans of India. The Persian Empire, founded by Cyrus the Great in 559 BC, covered an area from the Hindu Kush (now in Afghanistan) to Egypt. Iranians are proud of their heritage, which includes ancient empires, the Zoroastrian religion, and some of the world's greatest poets and leaders in philosophy, astronomy, and medicine.

Even though the focus of this chapter is on cultural commonalities, health-care providers must recognize that Iranians are a highly diverse population. We encourage readers to carefully assess each client's and each family's beliefs and circumstances. Overemphasis on culture, religion, and ethnicity as the defining factors in the expression of health and illness, treatment-seeking behaviors, and health-maintenance practices can lead to stereotyping (Hollifield, 2002).

Iran covers an area of about 636,000 square miles and is bordered by the Caspian Sea on the north and the Persian Gulf on the south. Neighboring countries are Turkmenistan, Azerbaijan, Armenia, Turkey, Iraq, Afghanistan, and Pakistan. Iran is home to many agricultural communities, nomadic tribes with livestock, and several highly industrial regions. Fertile agricultural lands are found in the southwest and on the Caspian Sea shore. The dry lakes of the interior regions are less conducive to farming. Both northern and southern shores are extremely humid. A large area of the country is mountainous. The climate varies with altitude, including hot, dry summers and extremely cold, snowy winters.

Iran has a population of over 70 million, three-quarters of whom are under the age of 30 and live in urban areas. The annual population growth rate is 1.4 percent. Almost one-fifth of the inhabitants live in an impoverished state with no basic public-health infrastructure, including drinking water, electricity, and sewage. The overwhelming majority of the people practice Shiite Islam. Christianity, Judaism, and Zoroastrian, an ancient Persian faith, are recognized in Iran, and adherents enjoy a degree of pseudo-freedom. However, the Baha'i community has experienced discrimination since the religion was established in the 19th century.

HERITAGE AND RESIDENCE

In Iran, ethnic groups with differing dialects and strong heritage coexist in a somewhat conflict-free environment, and the many groups embrace and identify with the core of the Iranian culture and the Persian civilization. For example, regardless of ethnicity or religion, the country unifies around **Eid Norouz** as a symbol of national identity and as a significant cultural event. The practice of visiting during *Eid Norouz* is an important expression of care, both within the family structure and as a community activity (Omeri, 1997). As commonly practiced in Iran, immigrant families continue to gather for important occasions such as weddings, births, and funerals.

Iran is divided into regions, each inhabited by people of differing ethnicities and traditions. For example, **Iranian Turks** live in the northwest, **Kurds** live along the western borders, and **Arabic-speaking Iranians** live in the south and southwest. Ethnic interdependence is being cautiously tested by the central government in Iran. The many years of occupation by the Greeks, Arabs, Mongols, and Turks have made Iranians cautiously resilient; the Iranians developed an uncanny ability to assimiliate without a complete loss of the collective self or their national identity.

Most Persians remained **Zoroastrian** until the **Sunni Arabs** conquered the land in the 7th century. Consequently, Iranians, except for the **Shiite sect**, converted to **Islam**. Iran is the only **Muslim** country in the Middle East that uses the solar calendar and celebrates *Eid Norouz* at the spring equinox in celebration of the New Year without any religious undertones. Centuries of occupation and the void of a central government committed to the country's welfare placed Iran at economic and industrial disadvantage. The reality became painfully noticeable to the people of Iran in the early 1900s when trading expanded to Europe and the West. The awareness marked the very slow beginning of emigration.

In the mid-1900s, several political parties—Nationalist, Communist, and Religious in ideology—literally pushed Iran toward becoming a more independent nation. To this day, even though it was short-lived, the nationalistic movement of Dr. Mosadeq resonates fondly in people's minds. The Pahlavi Dynasty (father and son) followed this movement, but it was mired in corruption and unethical alliances with foreign governments. Moreover, Mohammed Reza Shah reinstituted the secret police and did not tolerate political opposition. The 1979 Revolution and the establishment of the Islamic Republic of Iran were direct consequences of Pahlavi's management of the country. However, some powerful social and economic reforms were instituted during Pahlavi's reign, such as national public health, literacy programs, and a creation of a more secular society with decreased power for the religious clergy. Women's rights advanced until they were fully enfranchised in 1963. The 1979 Revolution drove the social and secular gains underground. Today, Iranian society is facing one of its greatest challenges; this time the occupying force has originated from within and its people are trapped by friendly fire.

To this day, a central tenet of Iranian social life and personal development is the boundary between inside/private (*baten*) and outside/public (*zaher*). Stimulated by the long history of occupation, the most private and true self is always kept for intimate spaces and trusted relations. "Inside" and "outside" define both individuals and families, in which honor and social shame play powerful roles.

REASONS FOR MIGRATION AND ASSOCIATED ECONOMIC FACTORS

Three waves of immigration contribute to the diversity of Iranians in the United States and elsewhere. In addition, each wave of immigrants appears to respond differently to the stress of migration. The first two waves of immigrants, 1950s to 1970 and 1970 to 1979, are demographically more cohesive. The second wave was more varied in social class and included a higher proportion of minority Iranians, such as Baha'is and Jews. The second wave included mostly young urban technocrats, scientists, professionals seeking advanced education, and adolescents of upper-middle class or privileged families who came to study at U.S. universities. Fluent in English, familiar with Western culture, and financially supported by government grants, scholarships, or family wealth, these individuals were better able to adjust to life in the United States. For this population of immigrants, a primary source of stress was distance from family and friends (Jalali, 1996).

The third wave immigrated from the early 1980s to the mid-1990s to escape the Iran-Iraq war and/or the Islamic government's political persecution. They were forced rather than voluntary migrants; some sought refugee status and continue to consider themselves in exile. This wave includes older individuals, fewer professionals, a higher percentage of high-ranking members of the pre-Revolution Iranian armed forces, owners of mid-size businesses, industry managers, and clerks.

Challenges particular to this older population of Iranian immigrants have been learning the language, adapting to the new culture and lifestyle, and redefining the relationship between parents and children (Emami, Benner, & Ekman, 2001). Older immigrants often express their ambivalence about being in the United States and may strongly believe they immigrated for the sake of their children and to provide emotional and financial support, similar to that of older immigrants in Sweden (Emami, Torres, Lipson, & Ekman, 2000). Older people often feel isolated, and their desire to return home keeps them from making permanent commitments. They are concerned about how their children will fare as they adopt less appealing aspects of the new culture. Older people view lack of respect for older people, loose family ties, and insufficient social support as examples of an unfavorable Western culture (Omeri, 1997). At times, to avoid isolation and to emulate the past, some immigrants "befriend" other Iranians despite having little in common but their national heritage and language; hence, creating a community weak in infrastructure and ties.

In summary, lack of fluency in the English language, education, and familiarity with Western culture are characteristics that differentiate the last wave of immigrants from those who immigrated prior to the 1980s (Bozorgmehr, 1997). The third wave has experienced multiple losses and witnessed role reversals between parents and children. These families left Iran under duress and lost their financial assets and status. Many experienced a profound degree of hardship, such as fleeing Iran by relying on smugglers and other high-risk means only to seek refugee status (Koser, 1997).

EDUCATIONAL STATUS AND OCCUPATIONS

Iranians greatly value education and expect their children to do well. Individuals who immigrated before the 1979 Revolution have most often obtained college degrees and are professionally successful and active. Iranian immigrants strive to maintain a social façade of affluence and upper-class status because family judgment and social shame weigh heavy on their decision-making. These issues have rarely been mentioned in studies addressing the health and mental health needs of immigrants in the United States (Sayyedi, 2004).

Many middle-aged immigrants who held white-collar positions in Iran were unable to find comparable work in the United States. As a result, they are self-employed in businesses such as pizza parlors or gas stations, using their business acumen to maintain a middle-class or better lifestyle. In Los Angeles, 61 percent of Iranian heads of household claimed to be self-employed in 1987 and 1988 (Dallalfar, 1994); 82 percent of Iranian Jews were self-employed. Only 10 percent reported employment in blue-collar jobs (Bozorgmehr et al., 1993). Health-care providers should not assume education and social class from occupation alone.

Communication

DOMINANT LANGUAGE AND DIALECTS

Farsi (Persian) is the national language of Iran, and all school children are taught in Farsi. An indication of modern Iran's Indo-European heritage is found in words similar to English words. As mentioned previously, nearly half the country's population speaks different languages and dialects, such as Turkish, Kurdish, Armenian, or Baluchi. Well-educated and well-traveled immigrants and those who might have stayed in an intermediate country prior to entering another country may speak three or more languages.

CULTURAL COMMUNICATION PATTERNS

The health-care provider should attempt to distinguish cultural patterns from individual personality characteristics. Communication among Iranians must be understood within the context of their history, the personality styles valued in the culture, and the structure of social relationships. Iranians are very cautious in their interactions with outsiders.

Not verbalizing one's thoughts is viewed as a customary and useful defensive behavior. This form of communication, also known as **ta'arof**, can effectively hinder open exchange of feelings with the health provider. Time to complete assessment, history-taking, and therapeutic approaches must be planned accordingly. Clearly implemented in the practice of *ta'arof* is the road map to communication whereby being other-centered, not self-centered, is expressed with distinct and respectful forms of speech and behavior. Whereas the constant offers of hospitality and compliments may sound insincere to non-Iranians, the dynamic is hard at work to set the boundaries of the relationship (Sayyedi, 2004).

Bagheri (1992) described such highly valued personality characteristics in Iranians as indirectness, subdued assertiveness, modesty, and politeness. Iranians are very concerned with respectability, a good appearance of the home, and a good reputation. Social behavior is also influenced by a constant awareness of others' judgment. Spontaneity is limited by rules that clearly define how and when to approach people of different ages and members of the opposite gender.

Communication also occurs on a continuum anchored by **baten** (inner self) and **zaher** (public persona). *Baten* is personal feelings, and *zaher* is a collection of proper and controlled behaviors. What lies in between is a buffer zone. The Persian language and its nonverbal accompaniments have evolved to help the expression of this complexity. *Ta'arof* is an example of a tool in verbal communication.

Health-care providers should be aware of the manner in which Iranians handle potentially disturbing information. Discussing serious diagnoses must be handled with respect to the family dynamics. Care is expressed in supportive gestures and by maintaining family relationships in times of health and need. Frequent visiting and keeping in contact by any available means are care practices (Omeri, 1997).

More traditional married couples do not display outward affections to each other in public. Greeting is often accompanied by a kiss on each cheek and/or a handshake. Strangers and health-care providers may be greeted with both arms held at the sides. A slight bow or nod while shaking hands shows respect. Iranians generally stand when someone enters or leaves the room for the first time. It is appropriate to offer something with both hands. Crossing one's legs when sitting is acceptable, but slouching in a chair or stretching one's legs toward another is considered offensive; showing the sole of one's foot is rude. Nonverbal beckoning is done by waving the fingers with the palm down. Tilting the head up quickly means no. Tilting the head to the side means what?, and tilting it down means yes. Extending the thumb (like thumbs-up) is considered a vulgar sign.

As in other Mediterranean cultures, personal distance is generally closer than that of Americans or Northern Europeans. The strength of the relationship affects how freely participants touch each other.

Iranians maintain intense eye contact between intimates and equals of the same gender. This behavior may be observed less in traditional Iranians. Conversations are expressive, as body language is used and the tone is loud.

TEMPORAL RELATIONSHIPS

Time orientation is a combination of emphasis on the present and on the future. In other words, time is continuous; what is anticipated in the future shapes the current lived experience. The ideal is to maintain a balance between enjoying life to the fullest and ensuring a comfortable future. Iranians' understanding of time as a contextual and directional phenomenon enhances the effectiveness of health promotion and education. At the same time, a fatalistic theme among many Iranians' may hinder their understanding of health risk assessment and risk reduction. Continuity and balance in life is the definition of health and well-being. Obtaining the diagnosis of a chronic or terminal illness is tolerated as an expected outcome of aging. Any disappointments in and derailments from the culturally accepted process of caring are reasons for ill health (Emami et al., 2001).

Iranians are feeling oriented. Interestingly, in business, they portray a strong work ethic; they are time-conscious and intensely competitive. Although social time is extremely flexible, Iranians respond to time requirements at work.

FORMAT FOR NAMES

Iranians refrain from calling older people and those in higher status by their first names. A man may wait before extending his hand to a woman as a measure of respect for her comfort with the practice. One is expected to greet every member of the family. To begin an interaction, the younger person initiates the greeting process.

Family Roles and Organization

Consistent with traditional collectivistic cultures, Iranian families value harmony within an established patriarchal hierarchy. Also valued are avoidance of open conflict, unconditional respect for parents, and indirect and figurative communication to maintain social hierarchy and group harmony. As a norm, they tend to be fatalistic and have an external locus of control and destiny (Daneshpour, 1998).

HEAD OF HOUSEHOLD AND GENDER ROLES

In this patriarchal and hierarchical culture, the father has authority and expects obedience and respect. In the father's absence, the oldest son has authority. Traditionally, families were large in Iran, with male children being highly desirable. Today's families have fewer children, and the authority figure may be a working female adult. As a father ages, he may give control of the business and all property to the oldest son. In more traditional families, older male siblings have the authority to make decisions about their younger siblings, even in the father's presence. However, more acculturated families are more flexible. Most sibling relationships are deep, trusting, and lively. Health-care providers should understand the decision-making dynamics of the family. The process is highly collaborative in enlisting trusted friends and relatives who are subject-matter experts.

Young people are free to select their life (marriage) partners, but families prefer to have the voice to approve. Husbands are often a few years older than their wives. Male immigrants experience emotional stress when they lack social status, which is tied to finances and occupation.

PRESCRIPTIVE, RESTRICTIVE, AND TABOO BEHAVIORS FOR CHILDREN AND ADOLESCENTS

Most immigrant Iranian families are child-oriented, sometimes to a fault, as they become overprotective.

Manners are considered important even outside the home. Children and teens are usually included in adult gatherings. Young children are rarely left with babysitters as families rely on friends and family suppport.

Taboo behaviors for teens in Iran and in the United States differ only in degree and intensity. In Iran, parents are concerned about smoking, drugs, alcohol, and sex. Young women are expected to remain virgins until they marry, but sexual activity by men outside marriage is tolerated. Dating is not allowed in the most traditional Iranian families but is tolerated in more acculturated families.

Whereas many Iranian adolescents in the United States resemble their American counterparts in dress and outward behavior, they often behave more respectfully toward family members, particularly older people and other highly respected individuals. The fear of shaming the family and losing face in public acts as a strong social constraint.

FAMILY GOALS AND PRIORITIES

The family is the most important institution in the Iranian culture. Members often live in close proximity to minimize isolation and to maintain strong intergenerational ties. The intensity of such strong relationships can be a double-edged sword; it brings comfort as it generates conflict. The key is to find a healthy balance.

A strong family unit ensures the continuation of the family name and lineage. If parents are able, they support their children financially by providing assistance with educational expenses, home buying, or starting a business. The children's academic or career achievement is considered the family's.

Parenting values and behaviors vary dramatically across immigrant Iranian families. Parents are conscientious in meeting their children's needs for comfort, safety, and success, but similar to parents from other collectivistic and traditional cultures, they expect their children's absolute devotion to the ancestral lineage. Since the mid-1990s, immigrant parents have become interested in improving their parenting skills by challenging some of the more traditional views. They attend parenting classes taught by Iranian American psychologists, social workers, and marriage and family therapists and are learning to rely on such behavioral modification techniques as rewards or time-outs for discipline (Sayyedi, 2004).

Some Iranians have clothing that is worn only inside the home. Often, they remove their shoes at the door and wear slippers inside. Outside the home, they tend to dress conservatively. Religious women living outside Iran may avoid bright colors, cover their arms and legs, and conceal their heads with head covers or scarves (hejab). In Iran, wearing the hejab is mandatory.

Age is a sign of experience, worldliness, and knowledge. Regardless of kinship or relationship, an older person is treated with respect. Older people are cared for at home. Skilled nursing facilities are viewed negatively. Despite their esteemed role within the Iranian family, older immigrants with minimal language skills feel isolated when their adult children work and the grandchildren are in school. Loneliness and isolation among older people are particularly common in neighborhoods where transportation is unavailable or walking is unsafe. In some enclaves of Southern California and Sweden, Iranians have established adult day-care centers in response to this issue (Emami et al., 2000).

Iran does not have a formal caste system; however, social status is both inherited and gained. Some are born into the upper class, but one can also ascend the class hierarchy through higher education and attainment of professional status. Parents often try to arrange marriages with families of higher status.

ALTERNATIVE LIFESTYLES

The religion of Islam has a conservative point of view about the male-female relationship, as is true of the Iranian society. Most Iranians strongly disapprove of the practice of living together before marriage. Although divorce is viewed negatively, the rate has been increasing among Iranians abroad, partly as a result of the many stressors of immigration and an increase in intercultural marriages. Rezaian (1989) found that intraculturally married Iranians reported more marital satisfaction than Iranians married to Americans or other intraculturally married Americans. One reason may be that cultural mores advocate for ignoring minor marital discord to maintain family stability. Collectivist cultures place greater emphasis on one's role in a kinship structure.

In Iran, out-of-wedlock teen pregnancy is neither talked about nor prevalent, and it can have a devastating outcome. Although homosexuality undoubtedly occurs in Iranians as frequently as in any other group, it is highly stigmatized. Iranian gays and lesbians do not easily disclose their sexual orientation because they are going against both a religious and a cultural norm. Since 1979, when the judicial system became one with the religious doctrine, homosexuality, which is considered unnatural and sacrilegious, is a crime punishable by death (Clark, 1995). Members of an Iranian gay support group in the San Francisco Bay area use anonymity and pseudonyms to protect themselves from potential physical harm by fundamentalist groups. In contrast to the older generation, younger Iranians are increasingly tolerant of alternative lifestyles.

Workforce Issues

CULTURE IN THE WORKPLACE

Iranian immigrants face several difficulties, among them are acquiring legal residency and suitable employment opportunities. For example, a physician who works as a plebotomist experiences continual bitterness that manifests itself either outwardly as anger and discord or internally with serious outcomes to personal health and familial relations.

Iranians may perceive and actually experience a degree of bias at work. Prejudice is less evident in highly multicultural and metropolitan areas. There is a general lack of understanding that the countries of the Middle East and their people are very different in ethnic identity and culture. For the most part, Iranians are secular and nationalistic and do not adhere to an Islamic identity common to the Arab nations (Biparva, 1994). More acculturated immigrant professionals respond flexibly in the workplace. For example, when one of the authors (Hafizi) perceives that a client is uncomfortable with her background or overtly expresses dislike, she uses *ta'arof*. Using formal speech, she addresses clinical tasks with minimal personal touch and interaction. Efficiency and efficacy supersede personal communication and human connection.

ISSUES RELATED TO AUTONOMY

Most newcomers may not be familiar with American vernacular or slang. An ongoing stressor is the condescending attitudes directed at individuals with a strong accent. For example, a nurse with a master's degree described her first year in the United States as follows:

> I was seen as an ignorant nurse's aide who couldn't even speak English. One nurse used to follow me around, checking everything I did. I resented being treated that way, and my own self-esteem suffered (Lipson, 1992, p. 16).

Biocultural Ecology

SKIN COLOR AND OTHER BIOLOGICAL VARIATIONS

Iranians are white Indo-Europeans. Their skin tones and facial features resemble those of other Mediterranean and Southern European groups. Their coloring ranges from blue or green eyes, light brown hair, and fair skin to nearly black eyes, black hair, and brown skin.

DISEASES AND HEALTH CONDITIONS

In Iran, the estimated 2006 birth rate was 17 per 1000 people, and the infant mortality rate was 40.3 deaths per 1000 (CIA, 2007).

Heat and humidity in some provinces provide fertile ground for the spread of cholera, including new and mutant strains. Malaria is widespread in Baluchistan (in the southeast), with serologic test results sometimes showing more than one strain in a single client. In rural areas that lack standardized sanitary systems, viral and bacterial meningitis, hookworm, and gastrointestinal dysenteries caused by parasites are prevalent. Hypertension is widespread, and in Tehran, 22 percent of adults are affected (Azizi, Ghanbarian, Madjid, & Rahmani, 2002).

Ischemic heart disease is on the rise secondary to the stress of living under economic and social constraints. Health-care providers should screen newer immigrants for diseases and illnesses common in their home country.

The most common health problems in Iran are linked to underdevelopment, the recent economic downturn, mental stress, and lack of coordination of scarce resources.

Examples of common health conditions are malnutrition (caused by protein and vitamin deficiencies), hepatitis A and B (caused by poor sanitary conditions, such as poor aseptic technique, or public-health measures), rising rates of tuberculosis and syphilis, genetic problems (owing to interfamily marriages), and genetic blood dyscrasias. Interfamily marriage used to be common; however, increasing urbanization and scientific data have resulted in a decline.

The head of Iran's Institute of Mental Health estimates that 1.2 million people in Iran suffer from acute psychological illnesses. Forty to 60 percent of all Iranians suffer from an episode of mental illness that requires specialized medical intervention. The prevalence of diabetes is 1.5 percent, but about 50 percent of those diagnosed were unaware of having this disease despite clear symptoms. Thalassemias, prevalent in the northern and eastern provinces, are now being addressed through premarital screening for carriers and through genetic counseling. Individuals are also tested for vitamin B_{12} or folic acid deficiencies linked to an enzyme deficiency. Mediterranean glucose-6-phosphate dehydrogenase (G-6-PD) deficiency is also common among people of Iranian heritage and can precipitate a hemolytic crisis when fava beans are eaten; it can also affect drug metabolism, such as increasing sensitivity to primaquine.

In the United States, many Iranians experience stress-related health problems from culture conflict and loss, homesickness, and the previous conditions of war. Although Northern California Iranians in Lipson's study (1992) were generally healthy, many expressed their ongoing stress somatically, through intermittent physical discomfort. Several articulated a direct connection between their worries and their illness; for example, three of the first seven people interviewed had suffered from ulcers and attributed their "stomach problems" to their "worries" and "troubles." Others complained of headaches, backaches, a racing heart, or other manifestations of anxiety or depression. Iranians often focus their acute generalized stress on the alimentary system, attributing illness or its severity to something eaten (Emami et al., 2001).

High-Risk Behaviors

Iranians' high-risk health behaviors are similar to those in the general population. Among both men and women, smoking is more prevalent in Iran than in the immigrant population residing in the United States. In general, health education, through the media and the influence of their children, encourages many to quit smoking. A degree of alcohol and recreational drug use occurs in the Iranian immigrant population, but the rate is no higher than that of the population at large. Alcohol is prohibited by the **Qur'an**, Holy Book of the Islamic faith. However, Iranians who are not devoutly religious drink socially, a few to excess. In Iran, the most popular street drug among the older generation is opium, traditionally used for medicinal purposes. However, years of opium use has created both a psychological and a physical addiction. The prevalent drugs in Iran are heroin and opium, mostly used by younger, unemployed adults. Family responses to drug use range from complete support of the family member to disownment. However, more families support their child to reduce the social burden and to save face.

Moderate alcohol use is openly accepted among immigrant Iranians. Substance abuse in this population is related to low levels of acculturation, a perception or experience of prejudice, and a sense of helplessness and loneliness. Sometimes Iranian men demonstrate their "masculinity" by claiming to "hold" their liquor well. The need to assert masculinity combined with a poor self-esteem increases the risk of alcohol addiction and spousal abuse.

HEALTH-CARE PRACTICES

Because of city planning and self-contained neighborhoods, walking is a great form of mobility in Iran. Soccer remains a passion, regardless of age and gender. Men continue to play soccer and encourage their children's participation to promote family activity. Iranian women participate in a wide range of physical activities such as walking, swimming, or aerobics depending on finances and time availability.

Mandatory seat belt use on intercity highways in Iran was instituted in the 1990s; compliance is periodically monitored and enforced. Radio and TV stations are state owned and, therefore, at the state's disposal for any form of campaign. In the United States, most Iranians comply with safety laws such as wearing seat belts and using child seats and restraints.

Nutrition

MEANING OF FOOD

Food is a symbol of hospitality and kinship. Iranians prepare their best dishes and insist on the consumption of several servings. More food than necessary is prepared and presented to preserve public face and to show respect. Tea is the hot beverage of choice and is offered with cubed sugar, dates, pastries, fruits, and nuts.

COMMON FOODS AND FOOD RITUALS

Iranian food is flavorful, with a lengthy preparation time. Working immigrants have created shortcuts and healthier versions of traditional recipes. Presentation is important. At any given table, a pleasing mixture of foods of different colors and ingredients, composed of a balance of **garm** (hot) and **sard** (cold) (see Dietary Practices for Health Promotion), are usually served. Tea, fruit, and pastries are served both before and after each meal. Iranians prefer fresh ingredients, although cost and availablity are determining factors. Canned, frozen, and fast foods are perceived to be less nutritious and contain preservatives harmful to health and well-being. Eating fast food is less common, especially among older immigrants, mainly owing to poor nutritional value, associated cost, and taste preference.

The most common carbohydrates are rice and sheet breads (wheat and white). The art of preparing rice is the measuring stick of a good cook. Long-grained white rice is preferred. The bread of choice is flat like *lavash* or pita. Corn and potatoes are used but are less favored. Beans and legumes (e.g., pinto, mung, kidney, lima, and green beans; and split and black-eyed peas) make up a high proportion of the dietary intake and are commonly used in rice mixtures.

Dairy products are dietary staples, particularly eggs, milk, yogurt, and feta cheese. Dairy by-products, such as *doog*, yogurt soda, and *kashk*, milk by-product, are other favorites. Meat and protein choices are beef, lamb, poultry, and fish. Shellfish is also consumed, but it is a regional favorite of Iran's southern region. Fresh fruit is always found in Iranian homes. Green, leafy vegetables are used in cooking, and herbs such as parsley, cilantro (coriander), dill, fenugreek, tarragon, mint, savory, and green onions are served fresh at a meal or included in stews served over rice.

Similar to Judaism, Islam has a strict set of dietary prescriptions, **halal**, and proscriptions, **haram**. Slaughter of poultry, beef, and lamb must be done in a ritual manner to make the meat *halal*. Strict Muslims avoid pork and alcoholic beverages; a few avoid shellfish. Historically, pork was prohibited for hygienic reasons. Compliance with proscriptive food and beverage items is seen less frequently among the younger generations.

Health-care providers can make simple adjustments to accommodate traditional food practices of Iranians by making provisions for home-cooked meals or identifying more appealing foods on the hospital menu. One of the authors (Hafizi) noted by experience that hospitalized Iranian older people would identify and select one or two food items for the duration of their stay and greatly appreciated any form of spice to add flavor to their hospital meal. A simple slice of lemon or a cup of hot tea are pleasing items.

DIETARY PRACTICES FOR HEALTH PROMOTION

Based on humoral theory, Iranians classify foods into one of two categories, *garm* (hot) and *sard* (cold). The categories sometimes correspond to high-caloric and low-caloric foods. The key to humoral theory is balance and moderation. The belief is that too much of any one category can cause symptoms of being "overheated" or "chilled." Therefore, symptoms are treated by eating foods from the opposite group. Becoming overheated is manifested by sweating, itching, and rashes as a result of eating too many walnuts, onions, garlic, spices, honey, or candy. Conversely, the stomach may become chilled, causing dizziness, weakness, and vomiting after eating too many grapes, rhubarb, plums, cucumbers, or too much yogurt. Susceptibility is believed to be gender-dependent. Women are more susceptible to *sardie*, caused by eating too much cold food, than to *garmie*, a digestive problem from eating too much hot food. Health-care providers may need to incorporate Iranian foods and dietary practices into health teachings in order to improve compliance with special dietary restrictions.

The diabetic nurse educator is teaching Mrs. Bahrami, a newly diagnosed insulin-dependent Iranian immigrant aged 65 years who immigrated from Iran in 1986. She has three adult children who live independently of their parents; two are attending college in another state and the oldest is working as a pharmacist. Mr. Bahrami, aged 72 years, is a retired educator who is experiencing a new onset of mild dementia. The family lives in a neighborhood with minimal access to Iranian markets. The family owns an automobile and Mrs. Bahrami is able to drive; however, her husband has lost his driver's license owing to his health condition.

1. What specific cultural communication strategies should the nurse use in teaching Mrs. Bahrami about her diabetes?
2. How would you go about assisting Mrs. Bahrami with balancing her diabetic diet with *garm* and *sard* food properties?
3. What problems do you foresee with transportation for food purchasing and appointments with her physician?
4. If Mrs. Bahrami cannot afford or find fresh foods that she prefers, what might the nurse suggest?

NUTRITIONAL DEFICIENCIES AND FOOD LIMITATIONS

Economic problems and unemployment in Iran have made certain foods unavailable, resulting in an increased incidence of protein and vitamin deficiencies. Although influenced by food marketing campaigns and younger people who have traveled abroad, the older generation's basic food beliefs remain mostly unchanged. Almost all ingredients used in Iranian cooking are available in Middle Eastern markets or via the Internet. The same is true for medicinal herbs. Health food stores stock some of the items but at a higher price.

Pregnancy and Childbearing Practices

FERTILITY PRACTICES AND VIEWS TOWARD PREGNANCY

Iran adopted a national family planning program in 1967 at a time when traditional values and low literacy prevented people from clearly understanding the impact of rapid population growth. High fertility was valued for religious and economic reasons and as insurance against potential loss of children and poverty in old age. In 1989, the plan was revitalized by the Islamic Republic; however, this time the populace was markedly educated and urbanized, and the plan was fully supported by the religious and political leaders. As a result of this plan's evolution over the years and a combination of modern and traditional contraceptive use, the fertility rate is on the decline (Mehryar, Roudi, Aghajanian, & Tajdini, 1997). Vasectomies are slowly beginning to gain acceptance.

Traditional Iranian beliefs and practices are influenced by Galenic or humoral medicine, particularly with regard to hot and cold temperament and the conditions of pregnancy and birth. Menstrual blood is believed to be unclean; therefore, menstruating women refrain from participating in religious activities and intercourse. Menstruation is also considered a time of great fragility for woman.

Historically, infertility was blamed on the woman. Baluch, Al-Shawaf, and Craft (1992) found that reasons for seeking infertility treatment differed for men and women: Men wanted children to ensure future support, and women wanted to fulfill social expectations of having babies, especially early in the marriage.

PRESCRIPTIVE, RESTRICTIVE, AND TABOO PRACTICES IN THE CHILDBEARING FAMILY

Food cravings during pregnancy are believed to result from the needs of the fetus; thus, cravings must be satisfied. Women generally avoid fried foods and foods that cause gas; fruits and vegetables are recommended, with special attention given to the balance of hot and cold. Heavy work is believed to cause miscarriage. Sexual intercourse is allowed until the last months. The pregnant woman receives considerable support from female kin both during the pregnancy and postpartum.

During the birthing process in the more traditional families, the father is usually not present. The choice for delivery is mainly based on the medical status of the mother and child. The postpartum period can be as long as 30 to 40 days. Some families believe in keeping an infant home for the first 10 to 15 days, after which time, the infant is strong enough to handle environmental pathogens. The more-acculturated families utilize mother and child education classes to prepare for delivery, but their choices greatly depend on the assistance of close family and friends.

Death Rituals

DEATH RITUALS AND EXPECTATIONS

Family members and friends gather to support the dying person and one another. Among devote Muslims, the deathbed, or at least, the patient's face, is turned to face Mecca. In the 1980s and early 1990s, Muslim burial services were few and scattered. In some instances, family members assisted in preparing the body for burial. This is less common because more facilities have been established to handle the many rituals of preparing a body for burial. For example, when using soap and water, washing proceeds from the head to the toes and from front to back. The body is then wrapped in a special white cotton shroud while prayers are read.

Death and dying is an anticipated and expected process in the cycle of life among Iranianas (Emami et al., 2001). In a fatalistic culture and Islam, the locus of control is outside one's power and ability, commonly referred to as the *will of God*. Withdrawal of life support may be considered as "playing God." However, there may be no objection to beginning life support, viewing it as a gift of medical technology (Klessig, 1992). As cultural meanings and practices evolve over time, so will one's perception of health and illness; therefore, assessing the patient and the family's beliefs within the context of life changes and experiences is essential (Emami et al., 2001).

No specific religious rules against autopsy exist. However, the reason to proceed must be clear and legitimate; some families may still refuse. In Iran, embalming is not practiced, and coffins are not used. The body is buried quickly and directly in the earth to facilitate the transition from "dust to dust." Cremation is not practiced in Iran. It is unlikely for Iranians outside of their mother country to practice cremation.

RESPONSES TO DEATH AND GRIEF

Loss of a loved one is met with strong and expressive grieving among family and friends. Death is perceived as a beginning in which the mortal life gives way to the spiritual existence and unification with God.

After burial, relatives, friends, and acquaintances gather on the 3rd, 7th, and 40th days. Special foods are served, and grieving may be expressed outwardly and loudly. Attendance at funerals is a sign of caring as well as a socially expected way to pay respect to the dead and to support survivors. Black is the customary color for clothing. On the anniversary of the death, the family gathers again. Some families donate money to charity in lieu of a ceremony. In either case, relatives observe the date by visiting the gravesite, especially on the first anniversary. Spouses or parents regularly visit the grave site.

Spirituality

DOMINANT RELIGION AND USE OF PRAYER

Islam exerted its influence on Iran and its culture in terms of temporality, fate, and dietary practices (Pliskin, 1987). However, certain culturally embedded norms, such as family loyalty and respect for older people, transcend religious and ethnic boundaries. During the month of **Ramadan**, individuals fast from sunrise to sundown, although pregnant women, the young, older people, and those who are ill are exempt from fasting. The beliefs and practices of Jewish, Christian, and Baha'i Iranians may be significantly different and must be specifically addressed.

MEANING OF LIFE AND INDIVIDUAL SOURCES OF STRENGTH

Family, friendship, and social support are sources of strength and comfort, particularly in times of illness or crisis (Omeri, 1997). Iranians are highly affiliative and thrive on social relationships. Given the importance of such contact, health-care providers may need to adjust visiting policies.

SPIRITUAL BELIEFS AND HEALTH-CARE PRACTICES

Taqdir means God has power over one's fate in life and death. The belief is more characteristic of older immigrants than the younger ones. Hafizi's research (1990)

illustrated this concept and the integration of religion and health. In the words of a highly educated and devout Muslim man:

> To ask me what health means is to ask me how I see myself in relation to God, my family, the society as a whole, and my relation to my material body. Man is the embodiment of the unworldly being. To excel through this journey, the body and spirit work as a unit. The mortal life represents only one stage of this voyage, while death another. Death is not the end, death signifies one's "graduation" to a higher level. I believe in God and His plan for the future. Simply said, being sick is not having a cold; rather it is not having the vision and the ability to deal with the cold (Hafizi, 1990).

Health-Care Practices

HEALTH-SEEKING BELIEFS AND BEHAVIORS

Traditional Iranian health beliefs and therapeutic practices are a combination of three schools of medicine: **Galenic** (**humoral**), **Islamic** (**sacred**), and **modern biomedicine**. In classic humoral theory, illness arises from an imbalance, excess or deficiency, in the basic qualities, hot and cold or wet and dry. The purpose of treatment is to restore balance. The Galenic-Islamic tradition of humoral medicine is widely practiced throughout Iran and continues to influence the beliefs of the immigrant population. In Galenic thought, every individual has a distinctive balance of four humors, or *mezaj*, resulting in a unique temperament, or *tabi'at*. An emotional upset can cause physical illness and vice versa. Climate and weather are believed to significantly affect health. For example, wetness and wind are avoided. Ears might be covered on a windy day because wind is believed to cause earache or infection. Sacred medicine is from the Qur'an and *hadith*, in which holy men are considered healers. The sacred tradition includes beliefs in the evil eye and *jinns* as evil spirits. Healing is reached through manipulating impurities or by prayers.

Among Iranians, *narahati* is a general term used to express a wide range of undifferentiated, unpleasant emotional or physical feelings such as feeling depressed, uneasy, nervous, disappointed, or generally speaking, not well. Iranians often use somatization to communicate emotional distress. In doing so, they construct an illness that is culturally sanctioned and socially understood. The stressor can be personal, social, spiritual, or psychological. *Narahati* allows individuals to distance themselves from the actual problem while putting the responsibility and focus on the metaphoric body. Because Iranians generally shy away from overt expressions of "personal self," the "somatic self" becomes a focal point in the health-care encounter. The concepts of *zaher* (and *baten*) once again manifest themselves in the health arena, creating a safe communication tool. The ritual of *ta'arof* creates the same safety zone in social, nonmedical interactions.

Somatization is also expressed in a cultural syndrome called *ghalbe gerefteh* (*narahatiye ghalb*, or distress of the heart). Good's classic study (1977) in rural Iran found that two-thirds of women of all ages reported experiencing heart distress, the same proportion found in Lipson's study (1992) of immigrants in California. Heart distress was attributed to having great sadness, being homesick, or having problems that are overwhelming or seem impossible to resolve. One woman stated, "I get it when I read Persian newspapers about the situation in Iran."

A widespread belief among Iranians is that fright or being startled by bad news negatively affects health outcomes. Symptoms caused by fright range from mild to extreme fatigue accompanied by chills and fever. When appropriate, identify the family spokesperson for communicating matters of grave concern, because losing hope is the greatest illness.

In some instances, a sudden ailment may be attributed to the evil eye, **cheshm-i-bad**, the belief that negative thoughts and jealousy can cause illness. *Cheshm-i-bad* can be the result of an intentional or unintentional thought projection. Acculturated immigrants use the terminology in everyday speech and encounters; however, most do not fully believe in the concept.

Cheshm-i-bad and other folk syndromes are better understood by viewing the body in the context of its social and supernatural environment. Similar to somatizing, which distances an individual from the actual problem, *cheshm-i-bad* attributes illness to an outside person or force. In reality, the evil eye gives meaning to an occurrence of puzzling origin and puts the blame on something other than the affected person.

Hafizi's research (1990) found that Iranians' concepts of health represented two of Smith's (1983) four domains: the clinical view, health as absence of disease, and the adaptive view, health as the ability to cope successfully. Healthy people are able to cope successfully with their changing world and have a harmonious exchange between available resources and their ability to use them. Health is a lifestyle marked by demands and adaptations (Hafizi, 1990). Similar health concepts were found among older Iranian people in Sweden (Emami et al., 2000).

Iranians accept both biomedical diagnoses and cultural illness categories. The concept of the body is viewed in relation to its total environment: society, God, and the supernatural. When someone has a discomforting symptom, the first question is often whether she or he ate something that did not agree with her or his *mezaj*, humoral temperament. If the answer is no, then other causes are explored.

RESPONSIBILITY FOR HEALTH CARE

Iranians often seek treatment relatively soon after the onset of symptoms. If within their ability, they will "shop around" until they find a provider of choice. They will seek advice from acquaintances or family in the medical field and will use home remedies for symptom management.

Self-medication, prescription, over-the-counter, and homemade herbal remedies are commonly used simultaneously. Antibiotics, codeine-based analgesics, mood-altering drugs in the benzodiazepine family, and intramuscular vitamins are available over the counter in Iran. Immigrants commonly bring these medications for personal use. Medication self-adjustment is also a common practice,

especially when finances are an issue or symptoms are not resolved. Health-care providers should carefully consider dosage and medication type. In some instances, because of previous inappropriate use, a first-generation antibiotic may not affect the microorganism because of inappropriate and repeated use.

When ill, Iranians are more inclined to be passive and to seek care and attention from family members. The patient may behave passively, while the family appears demanding. This unceasing and, at times, overbearing attention is an expected behavior for caring. If a patient is hospitalized, visiting is frequent, sometimes excessive according to some. Dealing with the patient's right to privacy and the good intentions of the visiting relatives is a balancing act.

Two cultural traits among the more-traditional and less-acculturated immigrants can complicate help-seeking behaviors. *Ta'arof* may keep patients from sharing their personal feelings. *Zaher*, a social façade of decorum and composure to hide one's unwanted negative feelings or attitudes, may further preclude the communication necessary for a meaningful assessment. More-acculturated immigrants tend to be more open and direct.

FOLK AND TRADITIONAL PRACTICES

Herbal remedies are used in a complementary manner to prevent illness, to maintain health, and to manage symptoms. Iranians believe strongly in combination therapy. Herbal remedies became increasingly popular in post-Revolutionary Iran because of the economic embargo and scarcity of biomedical supplies.

Common herbal remedies include dried flowers, seeds, leaves, and berries steeped in hot or cold water and drunk for digestive problems, coughs, aches, and pains, fevers, nerves, or fear. Some common herbal medications include *gol-i-gov zabon*, dried foxglove flowers, for digestive problems or nervous upsets, which is sometimes taken with *nabat*, a concentrated sugar (Lipson, 1992). *Khakshir* (flat, brown rocket seed) is used for stomach problems; *razianeh* is used for halitosis; quince seeds are sucked or used to create a thick syrup with hot water for sore throats; and *sedr* is used to prevent or treat dandruff.

BARRIERS TO HEALTH CARE

Lack of adequate language skills, inadequate financial resources, lack of insurance, immigration status, and lack of transportation are the top five barriers for accessing health care for most Iranians. Physicians and nurses should work with social workers and community agencies to help decrease these barriers.

CULTURAL RESPONSES TO HEALTH AND ILLNESS

Iranians are expressive about their pain. Some justify suffering in the light of rewards in the afterlife. For example, the grandmother of a young women with a slow-growing brain tumor consoled herself and her granddaughter with the statement that "suffering in this world assures her a place in heaven."

Mental illness is highly stigmatized and is believed to be genetically predisposed. Mental illness is likely to be called a "neurological disorder" or *narahati-e-asa'b* in order to emphasize the physical ailment. Bagheri (1992) found that Iranians consider psychopharmacological treatment to be most effective for somatic illness.

Iranian immigrants experience numerous stressors related to resettlement in a foreign culture. As measured by the Health Opinion Survey, 44 percent of Lipson's (1992) newer immigrant interviewees experienced medium or high stress compared with 14 percent of the long-term-resident group. With reference to mood, about 35 percent of the informants answered yes when asked if they considered themselves to be "nervous," and about the same percentage stated that they did not have "peace of mind." The reasons were adjusting to their new life in the United States, missing family members, and having concerns about relatives left behind. Despite these problems, most Iranian immigrants had no plans to seek counseling or treatment, preferring to rely on family support (Lipson & Meleis, 1983). However, in recent years, psychotherapy and counseling have become acceptable treatment modalities, particularly in dealing with children (Sayyedi, 2004).

Since the return of the injured soldiers from the Iran-Iraq war, physical disability has begun to receive attention. Before then, the handicapped and the mentally challenged were kept at home with few care and treatment options. The outcome of the war and the World Health Organization's Year of the Disabled stimulated Iran to promulgate the civil rights of people with disabilities and to guarantee access to health care. Today, physical therapy and art and music therapy are used as adjunct treatments.

VIGNETTE 14.2

Mrs. Rastinpour is a 46-year-old Iranian immigrant. On admission, she self-identified as being Jewish. She and her family (immediate and extended) immigrated to the United States in 1981. She is 2 days' postoperative for mitral valve replacement and is scheduled for discharge in 2 days. Her wound is healing well. She has a clear understanding of her plan of care at home. Today, the nurse noticed a degree of anxiety, especially when discussing discharge plans. When the nurse approached her, she became tearful. Mrs. Rastinpour assured the nurse that both her children are a great help and that they have a complete understanding of her limitations. When the nurse asked about her husband, Mrs. Rastinpour avoided eye contact and squirmed in her chair, stating her husband is super busy with business; her close friend and the many relatives will gladly fill in the gap. Later that day, the nurse discussed her concerns with the discharge coordinator. The day of discharge, while meeting with the coordinator and Mr. and Mrs. Rastinpour, the nurse asked Mr. Rastinpour if he had any particular concerns or questions that had not been addressed. Mr. Rastinpour angrily replied, "Since my wife has been cut, she is now imperfect. I refuse to share my bed with any woman who has a scar on her chest."

1. What cultural versus personal issues might exist between Mr. and Mrs. Rastinpour?

2. What recourse does the nurse have with Mr. Rastinpour's comment made on discharge?
3. What religious issues might be present?
4. Should the nurse get the Rastinpour children involved at this stage?
5. How might the nurse determine the role of extended family and friends in the care of Mrs. Rastinpour?

BLOOD TRANSFUSIONS AND ORGAN DONATION

Blood transfusions, organ donations, and organ transplants are widely accepted among Iranians. In Iran, donation of organs has become a business transaction—if a kidney is needed, it can be purchased (Zargooshi, 2001).

Health-Care Practitioners

TRADITIONAL VERSUS BIOMEDICAL PRACTITIONERS

Iranians appreciate state-of-the-art facilities, high-technological equipment, and skilled professionals. At the same time, the expense of health care is a widespread concern. Immigrants are confused by differences in the mannerisms and attitudes of the health-care providers in Iran versus those abroad. According to one woman, "Doctors here don't listen to you, they are always careful of malpractice; they don't want to be specific" (Lipson, 1992). Many Iranian clients expect to receive a prescription for medication and quick results. Iranian women are modest in front of men; if possible, male health-care providers should not ask women to undress fully for an examination or procedure.

STATUS OF HEALTH-CARE PROVIDERS

Religious and folk practitioners are generally not sought by most Iranian immigrants. The most respected health-care provider is an educated and experienced male physician. In Iran, medical imaging equipment, such as computed tomography scanners, is scarce. The government of Iran has supported medical school admissions based on influential kin rather than merit; therefore, graduates are of mixed quality.

Nursing as a profession in Iran remains in its infancy. Nurses are accorded less respect compared with physicians and, as a whole, receive mixed reviews. Whereas nursing education has evolved from an apprenticeship to a baccalaureate degree, nurses are still striving for acceptance and recognition as professionals (Nasrabadi, Lipson, & Emami, 2004). Immigrants have repeatedly stated that nursing care in the United States is far more interactive, communicative, and people-oriented than it is in Iran.

VIGNETTE 14.3

Hamid, his pregnant wife, Jaleh, and their two children moved to the United States within 5 years of the 1984 revolution. The third pregnancy was problematic, and without the support of her sisters and mother, Jaleh's recovery has been slow and troublesome. Jaleh is 2 months' postpartum, but her mental and physical states have continuously declined. She feels their situation is worse than what they would, and could, have had if they had remained in Iran. Hamid works long hours and is rarely home before 8 p.m. The family lives in a neighborhood isolated from friends and family.

Unfortunately, as Hamid continues to work harder and longer, Jaleh becomes even more depressed and nonattentive to the three children. Hamid has decided to seek help from a friend, but the friend is so concerned that he has convinced Hamid to have Jaleh admitted to the hospital and assessed for depression. The nurse assigned to Jaleh notices that Hamid and the three children, ages 10 and 8 years and 2 months, are nearby. Hamid is overtly upset, the two children are holding hands, and the baby is starting to fuss.

1. Should the nurse talk with Jaleh alone or with the family present? Why? Why not?
2. How might the nurse develop a trusting relationship in order to ask Jaleh personal questions?
3. How might Jaleh perceive her changing behaviors and mood?
4. What is the name of the Iranian concept of depression and how is it explained from a cultural perspective?
5. What should the nurse do with Hamid and the children while the nurse is admitting Jaleh?

REFERENCES

Azizi, F., Ghanbarian, A., Madjid, M., & Rahmani, M. (2002). Distribution of blood pressure and prevalence of hypertension in Tehran adult population: Tehran Lipid and Glucose Study (TLGS), 1999–2000. *Journal of Human Hypertension, 16*(5), 305–312.

Bagheri, A. (1992). Psychiatric problems among Iranian immigrants in Canada. *Canadian Journal of Psychiatry, 37*, 7–11.

Baluch, B., Al-Shawaf, T., & Craft, I. (1992). Prime factors for seeking infertility treatments amongst Iranian patients. *Psychological Reports, 71*, 265–266.

Biparva, E. (1994). Ethnic organizations: Integration and assimilation vs. segregation and cultural preservation with specific reference to Iranians in the Washington, D.C. metropolitan area. *Journal of Third World Studies, 11*, 369–404.

Bozorgmehr, M. (1997). Internal ethnicity: Iranians in LA. *Sociological Perspective, 40*(3), 387–409.

Bozorgmehr, M., Sabagh, G., & Der-Martirosian, C. (1993). Beyond nationality: Religio-ethnic diversity. In R. Kelly (Ed.), *Irangeles: Iranians in Los Angeles* (pp. 59–79). Berkeley: University of California Press.

CIA. (2007). *World FactBook: Iran.* Retrieved February 14, 2007, from https://www.cia.gov/cia/publications/factbook/geos/ir.html

Clark, D. (1995, January 27). Small Iranian group maintains anonymity. *The Washington Blade*, p. 14.

Dallalfar, A. (1994). Iranian women as immigrant entrepreneurs. *Gender and Society, 8*(4), 541–561.

Daneshpour, M. (1998). Muslim families and family therapy. *Journal of Martial and Family Therapy, 24*(3), 355–390.

Darvishpour, M. (2002). Immigrant women challenge the role of men: How the changing power relationship within Iranian families in Sweden intensifies family conflicts after immigration. *Journal of Comparative Family Studies, 33*(2), 270–296.

Emami, A., Benner, P., & Ekman, S.-L. (2001). A sociocultural health model for late-in-life immigrants. *Journal of Transcultural Nursing, 12*(1), 15–24.

Emami, A., Torres, S., Lipson, J., & Ekman, S.-L. (2000). An ethnographic study of a day care center for Iranian immigrant seniors. *Western Journal of Nursing Research, 22*, 169–1.

Good, B. J. (1977). The heart of what's the matter. *Culture, Medicine and Psychiatry, 1*, 25–58.

Hafizi, H. (1990). *Health and wellness: An Iranian outlook.* Unpublished master's thesis, University of California, San Francisco.

Hanassab, S. (1998). Sexuality, dating and double standards: Young Iranian immigrants in Los Angeles. *Iranian Studies, 31*, 65–76.

Hollifield, M. (2002). Accurate measurements in cultural psychiatry: Will we pay the costs? *Transcultural Psychiatry, 39*(4), 419–420.

Jalali, B. (1996). Iranian families. In M. McGoldrick, J. Giordano, & J. K. Pearce (Eds.), *Ethnicity & Family Therapy*, 2 ed., (pp 347–363). New York: Guilford Press.

Klessig, J. (1992). The effect of values and culture on life-support decisions. *Western Journal of Medicine, 157*(3), 316–322.

Koser, K. (1997). Social networks and the asylum cycle: The case of Iranians in the Netherlands. *International Migration Review, 31*(4), 591–612.

Lipson, J. (1992). Iranian immigrants: Health and adjustment. *Western Journal of Nursing Research, 14*, 10–29.

Lipson, J., & Meleis, A. (1983). Issues in health care of Middle Eastern patients. *Western Journal of Medicine, 139*, 854–861.

Mehryar, A., Roudi, F., Aghajanian, A., & Tajdini, F. (1997). Repression and revival of the family planning program and its impact on fertility levels and demographic transition in the Islamic Republic of Iran. Retrieved February 14, 2007, from http://www.erf.org.eg/html/blabor8.pdf

Nasrabadi, A., Lipson, J., & Emami, A. (2004). Professional nursing in Iran: An overview of its historical and sociocultural framework. *Journal of Professional Nursing, 20*, 396–402.

Omeri, A. (1997). Culture care of Iranian immigrants in New South Wales, Australia: Sharing transcultural nursing knowledge. *Journal of Transcultural Nursing, 8*(2), 5–17.

Pliskin, K. (1987). *Silent boundaries: Cultural constraints on sickness and diagnosis of Iranians in Israel.* New Haven, CT: Yale University Press.

Rezaian, F. (1989). A study of intra- and inter-cultural marriages between Iranians and Americans. Unpublished doctoral dissertation, California Institute of Integral Studies, San Francisco.

Sayyedi, M. (2004). Psychotherapy with Iranian-Americans: The quintessential implementation of multiculturalism. *The California Psychologist*, p. 10. Retrieved February 14, 2007, from http://www.ocpapsych.org/downloads/Jan2004.pdf

Smith, J. A. (1983). *The idea of health: Implications for the nursing profession.* New York: Teachers College.

Zargooshi, J. (2001). Iranian kidney donors: Motivations and relations with recipients. *Journal of Urology, 165*, 386–392.

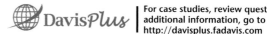

DavisPlus | For case studies, review questions, and additional information, go to http://davisplus.fadavis.com

Chapter 15

People of Japanese Heritage

SUSAN TURALE and MISAE ITO

Overview, Inhabited Localities, and Topography

OVERVIEW

Nihon, or **Nippon**, as Japan is called in the Japanese language, is a 1200-mile chain of islands in the northwestern Pacific Ocean. Japan's neighbors are Russia, Korea, and China, and its modern history has been shaped by conflict with these countries.

Japan's territory extends generally from northeast to southwest, covering an area slightly smaller than California in the United States. The northern and westernmost areas have a climate similar to that of northern United States, with some heavy falls of snow in wintertime; the Ryukyu Islands in the south are subtropical. The climate of the Tokyo region, where most of the population is clustered, is similar to that of Washington, DC. Winters are moderate, with snows that seldom accumulate except in the north, whereas summers are hot and steamy.

The population of around 127.4 million resides mainly on the four largest islands (U.S. Department of State, 2006): Honshu, Kyushu, Hokkaido, and Shukoku. Tokyo, on Honshu island, is the capital and largest city with 35.3 million people residing in its greater metropolitan area and 8.4 million in the city proper. The Japanese, who refer to themselves as **Nihonjin**, share a strong sense of nationalism and pride in ethnic purity. Japanese citizenship is not readily obtained, and currently, there are 2 million foreign residents in Japan, required to register as aliens. The inclusion of even third-generation Korean residents in the category of foreigners has received considerable adverse international press in recent decades. However, some changes are on the way as Japan has begun acknowledging that a long-revered sense of

ethnic homogeneity may not be sustainable. Globalization, low birth rate, an aging population, and increasing labor shortages are causing the country to rethink its immigration policies. However, this has to be balanced against tensions arising from growing international terrorism; and therefore, stricter controls on immigration have been instigated (Kashiwazaki & Akaha, 2005).

HERITAGE AND RESIDENCE

The original inhabitants of Japan most likely migrated from the Korean peninsula. The marked Chinese cultural influence began in the late 400s and included the Chinese system of writing, the calendar, Confucianism, Buddhism, and East Asian beliefs about health and illness. Following World War II, from 1945 to 1952, Japan was an occupied territory of the United States. As a bitter legacy of that war, the northernmost Kuril Islands are still claimed by Russia, and today, Japan still has U.S. military bases on its soil, in part to counteract perceived threats from neighboring countries.

Japanese citizens residing in North America have tended to locate in large commercial and educational centers. With the establishment or purchase of factories in the Midwestern and Southern states by Japanese companies, communities of Japanese expatriates can now be found in smaller cities as well.

REASONS FOR MIGRATION AND ASSOCIATED ECONOMIC FACTORS

In the late 1800s, Japanese people began to migrate to the United States and Canada, and from 1891 to 1924, more than 250,000 Japanese immigrated, settling primarily in the Territory of Hawaii and along the Pacific coast (Yanagisako, 1985). By 2004, however, an estimated 369,639 Japanese nationals lived in the United States, of whom 240,000 were considered long term and 129,600 permanent (UN Secretariat, 2005). Japanese love overseas travel, and in 2005, more than 3.9 million of them visited the United States and spent 16.5 billion U.S. dollars on goods and services (U.S. Commercial Service, 2006).

EDUCATIONAL STATUS AND OCCUPATIONS

Education is highly valued in Japan, where the illiteracy rate is only about 1 percent (U.S. Department of State, 2006). Completion of the 12th grade by more than 95 percent of young people ensures a highly competent workforce. For instance, calculus is part of the mandatory junior high school curriculum, and high school graduates complete 6 years of English instruction. Many youngsters preparing for high school or college entrance examinations attend proprietary *juku*, or cram, schools, in the evenings or on weekends, which creates enormous pressure on youth to succeed in schooling.

About 40 percent of all young people go on to higher education at over 1200 universities, junior colleges, and technical schools. Entrance examinations for high school and college are very competitive. Because the alumni network helps to provide job placements, the school one attends determines to a great extent where one is employed after graduation. To gain higher education degrees, Japanese commonly study at the university where they earned their undergraduate degree rather than to go to different universities like their American counterparts do.

Whereas the concept of adults returning to college is still new, self-improvement is a huge industry. Hobbies are taken very seriously and often entail formal study to seek "perfection" in a particular hobby: For example, the traditional Japanese arts, such as *chadō* or *sadō* (tea ceremony), *ikebana* (flower arranging), *bonsai*, *kimono* wearing, *shodo* (calligraphy), painting, wood carving, and even doll making, are studied diligently by large numbers of women and by some retired men.

Sales of books, periodicals, and daily newspapers in Japan are among the highest among industrialized nations, and there is an increasing love of *manga*, comics or print cartoons. In fact, almost half of all periodicals or books are *manga* (Japan Media Review, 2006). Popular *manga* are adopted into *anime* (or animation), and at any time of day, one can witness the very young to middle-aged crowding train stations, bookstores, or convenience stores voraciously reading their favorite comics, some with explicit sexual or violent content. This has a significant impact on the way in which messages are passed on culturally. Health professionals need to consider the use of *manga* and *anime* when promoting health education to Japanese clients. The national broadcasting system, NHK, offers high-quality radio and television news and entertainment, and cable TV is increasingly popular.

Although culture reflects Japan's recent agrarian past, at present, only 2 percent of Japanese are engaged in agricultural occupations because a significant amount of foodstuffs is imported. In the United States, **issei** (first-

generation immigrants) originally tended to work in agriculture or as small-business owners. More recent immigrants work in business, the professions, service industries, and manufacturing. Second- (**nisei**) and third-generation (**sansei**) Japanese Americans tend to be highly educated professionals. Most Japanese nationals living in the United States are well-educated executives, visiting scholars, individuals with technical expertise, or students.

Communication

DOMINANT LANGUAGE AND DIALECTS

Japanese is the language of Japan, with the exception of the indigenous *Ainu* people. The Japanese spoken in Tokyo is the national standard heard in media broadcasts; however, regional variations to the language do exist. Because high school graduates in Japan complete 6 years of English instruction, even newer Japanese immigrants and sojourners can understand, read, and write the English language to some degree. The biggest problem, however, is conversational English; whereas many Japanese may have studied the language for many years, they often lack strong conversational skills and are frequently embarrassed to try their language ability with foreigners.

In the United States, *issei* vary widely in their English language ability. *Nisei* and *sansei* have been educated under the American educational system to the extent that they were permitted; for example, educational access was limited or segregated during the World War II internment of American citizens of Japanese ancestry. Although the language barrier may be an obstacle to understanding verbal instructions or explanations in English-speaking health-care settings, Japanese clients are likely to use written materials effectively. More recent immigrants to the United States are likely to understand English but may need prompting in conversation skills.

CULTURAL COMMUNICATION PATTERNS

Japanese society is both highly structured and traditional. Politeness, personal responsibility, loyalty, and people working collectively for the greater good of the group are very important. One complexity of the Japanese language is the customizing of speech according to relative social status and gender. The Japanese sensitivity to relative status and the need to constantly gauge one's behavior accordingly is one reason the circle of intimates with whom one can truly relax is quite limited. In addition, men tend to speak more coarsely and women with more gentility or refinement.

Light social banter and gentle joking are mainstays of group relations, serving to foster group cohesiveness. Polite discussion unrelated to business, often over *o-cha* (green tea), precedes business negotiations, and *sake* parties are common during the negotiation period. *Sake*, a fermented beverage with a history of over 2000 years in Japan, is integral to culture and society. Relationship building and respect for personal privacy are important aspects of working relationships in all sectors.

In a densely populated society that values group harmony above all else, open communication is discouraged, making it difficult to learn what people think (Doi, 1971). In particular, among people of Japanese descent, saying no is considered extremely impolite; rather, one should let the matter drop.

A high value is placed on "face" and "saving face." Asking someone to do something that he or she cannot do induces loss of face or shame. For people to be shown to be wrong may be deeply humiliating. People may feel shame for themselves and their group, but they are expected to bear that shame in stoic silence. In fact, Japan is considered to have a shame-based culture rather than a guilt-based culture (Leonardsen, 2004), unlike many Western cultures. Suicide over shame is a common theme in Japanese literature, lore, and media. Regular reporting of suicides occurs in the daily media, often mentioning the name of the suicidee who has committed the act after embarrassment, shameful deeds, allegations of corruption, or bullying in the workplace or at school. Because of ethnic homogeneity, an ingrained sensitivity to the feelings of others, and close contact with one's family, classmates, and work group, Japanese believe that vague, intuitive communication, called *hara wo yomu* (belly talk), is well understood by fellow group members.

In Japan, presenting a person with choices is regarded as a burden, and it is a kindness to spare people the burden of decision-making. For example, a hostess may serve already-poured drinks to spare her guests the burden of deciding what they would like. Professors do not offer a choice of learning activities to their students; a teacher may arrange employment for a former student; a physician will tell the client what to do about a health problem. These actions are motivated by concern for the well-being of the person in one's care. Japanese society is sometimes described as a web of *giri* (mutual obligations) that serves to ensure societal integrity and harmony.

Etiquette and harmony are very important, and many Japanese people exhibit considerable control over body language. Anger or dismay may be quite difficult for Westerners to detect. Smiling and laughter are common shields for embarrassment or distress. However, one need only see tearful family partings at train stations to know that, contrary to Western assumptions, Japanese people do show their feelings, but often do not hug or kiss one another at such partings, as is so common in many other cultures.

Prolonged eye contact is not polite even within families. Social touching occurs among group members but not among people who are less closely acquainted. In general, body space is respected. Intimate behavior in the presence of others is taboo. When people greet one another, whether for the first time or for the first time on a given day, the traditional bow is performed. The depth of the bow, its duration, and the number of repetitions reflect the relative status of the parties involved and the formality of the occasion. An offer to shake hands by a Westerner is reciprocated graciously. With an introduction, *meishi* (business cards) are exchanged first, enabling the parties to assess their relative status.

TEMPORAL RELATIONSHIPS

An awareness of Japanese history and legend, a high regard for older people, the value of family honor, and veneration of dead ancestors suggest a strong connection with the past. However, the overall orientation of the Japanese people, who are known for their postwar economic miracle, is toward the future. The population made huge sacrifices in the decades after the war for the good of the nation, enabling it to become a world power. Parents encourage their children to study hard so that their futures will be bright. Housewives are diligent savers for future family expenses. Companies plot their growth, and the government anticipates needs decades in advance. Whereas Zen calls its practitioners to attend to the here and now, this tenet actually has few adherents in Japan. Health-care providers may find that Japanese clients are astonishingly motivated in health-related decision-making by considering their children's needs and the economic future for their family.

Punctuality is highly valued among the Japanese: Commuter trains run to split-second timing; people are expected to be in attendance at the exact start of meetings. In an interesting contrast, the clinic system of health care pervades even the private sector in Japan. Clinic services are not expected to be efficient, and hospital stays are still longer than in many Western countries, although the average number of hospitalization bed-days per illness is falling owing to economic problems and some shortages of qualified nurses.

FORMAT FOR NAMES

In Japan, family names are stated first, followed by given names. Seki Noriko would be the name of a woman, Noriko, of the Seki family, and often women's names end with -*ko*. The family names of both men and women, married or single, are designated by the suffix, -*san*, but one does not use that designation when referring to oneself. Women generally assume their husband's family name upon marriage. School children may use given names when speaking to one another, also designated with -*san*. Work groups and business associates tend to use family names. Infants and young children are called by their first names followed by -*chan*. Schoolboys are usually referred to by their first or last names followed by -*kun*, whereas schoolgirls' first names are usually followed by -*chan* or -*san*. Elders are referred to respectfully. The designation *sensei* (master) is a term of respect used with the names of physicians, teachers, bosses, or others in positions of authority.

— VIGNETTE 15.1

With encouragement from their daughter and son-in-law, Mr. and Mrs. Kawamura have agreed to come to day care at your local community center to attend the craft and art classes. They have been feeling isolated, especially because all members of their family have to go to work each day. They are first-generation Japanese who are both now in their early 80s and very traditional in outlook. The community nurse has been asked by the occupational therapist to help her plan for their introduction to the center.

1. How would you address this older couple in a culturally sensitive fashion?

2. How would you introduce them to others?
3. What elements of communication might be important to make this couple feel welcome?
4. What kinds of activities might be appropriate for them?
5. What kind of foods and drinks might be appropriate for them?

Family Roles and Organization

HEAD OF HOUSEHOLD AND GENDER ROLES

The predominant family structure among the Japanese is nuclear, accounting for 60 percent of families in 2005, with 28 percent of households composed of one person (Ministry of Internal Affairs and Communications, 2006). This contributes to problems in social isolation, particularly among older people, because the number of households in which three generations are present is falling. In feudal Japan, a bride had very limited contact with her own family after marriage, and the mother-in-law dominated the household. Now, wives often determine the household budget, their husbands' pocket money, investments, family insurance, real-estate decisions, and all matters related to child rearing.

Even today, with higher education widely available to women, the role of wife and mother remains dominant. Young women in the workplace may have jobs with little substantive responsibility, even if they are college graduates (Orenstein, 2002), but matters are slowly changing. The Ministry of Internal Affairs and Communications (2006) reported that the ages for first marriages are rising (30 years for men and 28 for women), and now around 45 percent of women under 30 are single. Further, in 2005, the natural increase rate per 1000 population showed −0.2, the first minus recorded since statistics-gathering began in its present form in 1899. With this knowledge, the government is attempting to reduce the strong social pressure confronting women who try to continue working after motherhood, primarily because of Japan's need for skilled workers.

Longevity Japan (2006) described a new law in 2005 that gave workers the opportunity to take leave to care for sick children and other family members, developed corporate strategies to support workers or other family members who take care of children, permitted shorter working hours for workers who are raising a young child, and allowed more generous family-care provisions. The effects of this law are yet to be seen as it is still difficult to return to work after childbearing. An equal rights amendment has been part of Japan's constitution since the U.S. occupation of Japan. Whereas Japan has protected women's interests in matters such as property ownership and voting, women are treated far from equally in the workplace. Conversely, increasing numbers of child-care centers assist families in which both parents are working, and a few of the larger corporations have begun to offer child care. Daily newspapers are filled with discussions about how Japan can increase its birth rate, and any reforms to date have failed to stop the trend of increasing numbers of working women, women who choose not to marry, or couples who choose to have few or no children at all. The difficulty of paid employment or a career after motherhood and the desire for two incomes to maintain a middle-class lifestyle often cause couples to delay having a family.

Wives in Japan care for their husbands to a degree that many Western women would not tolerate. Japanese men are presumed not to be capable of managing day-to-day matters, and some salarymen (white-collar workers) or office workers may leave for work at 7 a.m. and return after 10 p.m., Monday through Saturday. On Sundays, men may be so exhausted that they sleep a good part of the day, or they may be obligated to socialize with colleagues. Wives and children often stay behind when husbands are transferred by their companies within Japan or overseas, leaving women to raise children singlehandedly. Not surprisingly, one focus of the Ministry of Health, Labour and Welfare in addressing the low birth rate is to convince men to assume more responsibility for child care and housework and for companies to change policies to keep families from being separated.

The paramount family concern is for the children's education, and it is the mother's responsibility to oversee the completion and quality of homework. When the children grow up and leave home, women tend to become involved in volunteer activities, community groups, travel, arts, and the previously mentioned self-improvement classes.

VIGNETTE 15.2

Mrs. Seike, a 38-year-old mother and housewife, has been living in the United States for 2 years. Her husband, a busy executive, spends a great deal of his time away from the family home in Chicago. Mrs. Seike, therefore, has the major role caring for the home and their sons, ages 8 and 12. She has become very stressed about her life in general and is homesick. Her Japanese friend brings her to the community health center where you are the nurse. She reveals that her 12-year-old son is having difficulty adjusting to school and is quiet and withdrawn. Mrs. Seike seems very hesitant to talk about her problems and does not readily make any decisions on her own.

1. What cultural factors need to be considered in this situation?
2. How can the nurse help Mrs. Seike and her son adjust to life in America?
3. What agencies or persons could you call for assistance?

Western observers would be wrong to presume that married Japanese couples do not love each other. But in Japan, love has not been valued highly as a prerequisite for a successful marriage, and men and women have tended to be more motivated by duty to fulfill societal expectations than by the desire for spousal companionship. Conversely, domestic violence has begun to be openly acknowledged. The Gender Equality Bureau (2006) explained that in 2001, the Law for the Prevention of Spousal Violence and the Protection of Victims was implemented and then amended in 2004. Under this law,

120 shelters for victims were established and counselling programs offered. Moreover, restraining orders and orders to vacate are now issued at a rate of about 100 a month. With this law, a number of public education programs are in place and a few women's shelters are opening. In a society marked by strict norms differentiating the public and the private realms, couples have lacked resources to learn how to deal with tension and conflict.

Health-care providers need to be aware of differences in spousal relationships when assessing the quality of family dynamics and communication, sexual health, and sensitivity to risk for sexually transmitted infections. Health-care providers who work with college-age and young adults may find that Japanese youth are less autonomous than their American counterparts. Conflicts between traditional and American values may arise among these young people and within their families.

PRESCRIPTIVE, RESTRICTIVE, AND TABOO PRACTICES FOR CHILDREN AND ADOLESCENTS

The primary relationship within a Japanese family is the mother-child relationship, particularly that of mothers and sons. It is customary for the mother, and sometimes both parents, to sleep with the youngest child on *futons*, or mattresses, on the floor or in adult beds (Fukumizu, Kaga, Kohyama, & Hayes, 2005) until a child is age 10 years or older. When a new baby is born, the older sibling may sleep with the father or a grandparent. A special child bed is used for neonates to prevent the parents rolling on the child during sleep. Fukumizu et al. (2005) found that 80 percent of Japanese parents sleep with their young infants and young children. The primacy of the mother-son relationship and the absence of fathers contribute to the known problem of mother-son incest. Father-daughter incest occurs, but a stronger taboo prohibits public discussion of it (Kanazumi, 1997), and so it is very difficult to find data on it. Despite the occasional occurrence of family dysfunction in this area, health-care providers working with childbearing couples and children need to be aware of Japanese family sleeping practices and refrain from judgment.

The maternal role is so important for women in Japan that it is not unusual for a young mother to spend hours watching her infant sleep. If she observes the reflexes of urination, she changes the diaper immediately. Babies are not allowed to cry; they are picked up instantly. Women constantly hold their babies in carriers on their chests and sleep with them (Sharts Engel, 1989). "Skinship" or direct contact, is a value to be desired.

Young Japanese children tend to be indulged, especially if they are single children. At the same time, they are socialized to study hard, make their best effort, and be good group members. They are taught to take care of each other, and girls are taught to take care of boys. Self-expression is not highly valued.

Corporal punishment has been more accepted in Japan than in some Western cultures, and the word *punishment*, for example, is often used in the daily English newspapers to describe actions to counteract the transgressions of government workers. Cases of punishment by school officials or *ijime* (bullying) by their peers at school have resulted in the suicide of young children recently—matters debated hotly in the local press. The fears are that bullying is reaching epidemic proportions. Children who are bullied by schoolmates typically have different looks, interests, or family structures, and health professionals need to be aware of this among Japanese-American children.

The Ministry of Education in 2006, under directives of the new Prime Minister, Abe, has begun a review of school education across the country, intending to incorporate content on national values. The government has also begun to address ways for families and schools to more effectively foster the development of Japanese children. One important aspect is that it is now mandatory for teachers and health professionals to report child abuse cases, a matter that has radically increased the reports of child abuse, most of which have involved violence and neglect. As of yet, strategies to identify and intervene or educate the public about child abuse have not been implemented.

Despite strong social pressure to conform, many adolescents in Japan have their rebellious streaks and use popular music, pornography, way-out clothing, and illicit drugs and alcohol to escape social restrictions. Increasing numbers of young people are expressing themselves through their clothing, hair, and makeup, but vandalism is a minimal concern in the country. Teenagers and college students in Japan generally do not date to the degree that Western youth do. They typically join clubs, membership in which is taken seriously; most social activities, such as ski trips, are club activities. However, sex education in school and/or university settings is minimal, despite teenagers having sexual encounters. The use of contraceptives as a preventive measure is not common among teenagers, and about 2 percent of Japanese girls have had abortions by the time they reach their late teens. The rash of abortions in women in their early 20s continues to increase annually (Sato & Iwasawa, 2006). Japan, however, has one of the lowest incidences of births to teenagers in the world. American health-care providers cannot assume that dating holds the degree of concern for Japanese young people as it does for American teenagers; nor can they assume that Japanese youth are well-informed about sexuality and sexual health risks.

Other health concerns among young people include the pressures to conform within a peer group and to perform well in school, pressures that may lead to depression and suicide risk (Takakura & Sakihara, 2000). Interest in studying eating disorders is increasing, although research indicates lower rates among Japanese youth than among U.S. youth and in college students rather than high school students in Japan (Makino, Hashizume, Yasushi, Tsuboi, & Dennerstein, 2006). One reason for this may be young students' increasing identification with skinny models from the West, increasingly portrayed in the media.

After graduation from high school or college, young adults are traditionally expected to be employed through their network of school contacts or family friends. Young women now typically live with their parents for many years after school, wheras young men are likely to live in company housing until marriage, and even after.

FAMILY GOALS AND PRIORITIES

Promoting success in school is the mother's main focus in child rearing. Children compete for their junior and senior high school admission, and high schools vary in the caliber of universities to which their graduates are admitted. The schools from which individuals graduate determine such major issues as career prospects for men and the status of husbands whom young women are likely to marry.

Children are highly valued and motherhood traditionally has been revered in Japan. The recent extreme drop in the birth rate has taken the society by surprise, although in prior decades, the expense of rearing and educating children triggered its beginning. Nothing is permitted to interfere with child-rearing responsibilities. Japanese women may be less likely than North American women to engage in activities, including health-care appointments, that require them to leave their children with babysitters.

The ideal of romantic love plays less of a role in marriage in Japan than in the United States, and the marriage rate was 5.7 per 1000 population in Japan, lower than in the United States with 7.5 per 1000 population (Ministry of Internal Affairs and Communications, 2006). About 30 percent of marriages are arranged, often by employers or family friends. The o-miai is the ritual of the first arranged meeting between prospective partners.

As mentioned previously, Japanese couples are marrying later in life. The groom's goals for marrying focus on advancement of his career and a desire to be cared for. For the bride, economic security and child rearing are traditional goals. A "honeymoon baby" is becoming less common, and couples are delaying having a family early in the marriage. Few Japanese women bear children outside of marriage, and abortion is one of a number of contraceptive practices, with the use of condoms more prevalent than the use of the contraceptive pill.

Japanese couples place less emphasis on companionship and sexual fulfillment than do North American couples and are far less likely to live together without being married. The divorce rate has declined: in 2005, there were 2.08 divorces in Japan per 1000 population compared with 3.6 in the United States (Ministry of Internal Affairs and Communications, 2006).

The Japanese family (especially the eldest son, who has a sense of obligation to his parents) has traditionally cared for and respected older people and children. However, with the drift to living in urban areas in small apartments and with more couples working, it is increasingly difficult to care for older parents. Retirement and nursing homes are growing in number across the country, although many of the latter have a poor public image and are poorly regulated. With the longevity of its people, Japan is aging more rapidly than any other nation. The government has begun to address how to care for older people, who now account for 20 percent of the total population. North American health-care providers must be sensitive to Japanese clients' sense of obligation and commitment. Helping families network within the Japanese American community both for social support and for resources or good long-term-care facilities is a useful strategy.

Elements of social status include age, gender, educational background, and work group affiliation of oneself or one's husband. Though there is a peerage system and some old families are known to be descendants of *samurai*, Japan is largely a meritocracy. Exceptions include Korean descendants or descendants of the **burakumin**, the untouchable caste who cared for the dead and tanned leather in feudal times. In this largely middle-class society, school children can reasonably expect to study hard and go on for higher education if that is the family goal.

Biases that may be evident among Japanese people who reside in North America are directed at minority groups such as African Americans, Jews, and individuals with limited education, as well as women in high-status positions. This prejudice is seldom overt, but it may threaten the comfort of Japanese people, who are likely to encounter such diversity among health-care providers in North America.

ALTERNATIVE LIFESTYLES

In Japan, a small segment of women have long lived outside the usual constraints for their gender. Women of "the floating world," or the entertainment industry, enjoy a fair degree of autonomy. The most traditional of these, the *geisha*, live in all-female communal arrangements, but they are reducing in number annually. *Geisha* are not prostitutes, but are considered highly skilled artists, and they are now recognized as a cultural treasure. However, other women in the entertainment industry fulfill men's need to relax in a society highly constrained by social norms; therefore, the sex trade is flourishing and occasional mention is made of the sex slave trade in Japan. Hostesses at bars look after their male customers, pour their drinks, and listen to them. In earlier eras, concubines were accepted within families. Today, infidelity by married men is more tolerated than in North America, but much less so for married women.

An increasing number of the Japanese population remains single throughout life, and only a few men and women enter monastic life. The small proportion of heterosexual couples who live together outside of marriage find greater tolerance in urban settings in Japan. Marriage of a Japanese person to a foreigner is less tolerated than it is in the United States. The existence of a gay and lesbian social network and of cross-dressing clubs is evident in English-language publications in Tokyo.

Workforce Issues

CULTURE IN THE WORKPLACE

Japanese employees in North American institutions need to be carefully oriented to the legal and professional requirements of client autonomy and of accountability in reporting, solving, and documenting problems that occur. An overview of dominant American society values may prepare them for the directness of communication they will encounter.

Claims for medical malpractice are growing slowly in Japan but are far less common than in the United States;

for example, in 2003 in Japan, only 1019 newly accepted lawsuits in the Supreme Court were associated with medical malpractice across the country (Ehara, 2005). American practices designed to avoid liability, such as informed consent, are not routinely implemented in Japanese health-care settings. Client autonomy is recommended in health-care settings; however, the real priority in Japan is meeting dependency and recuperation needs.

Like most Japanese workers, nurses in Japan work long hours, often between 8 and 10 hours per day 5 days per week. Nurses often work extra time after their shift without pay. Their pay is low in relation to their cost of living compared with that of other health professionals. With the advance of a university education, nursing is slowly becoming a respected profession. Staffing is complicated by federal restrictions on shift work among women, although change is underway because Japan, like North America, is experiencing a nursing shortage.

The mix of people providing nursing care in Japan represents many levels of educational preparation, and nurses may be prepared for registered nursing practice in a number of different ways. Baccalaureate degrees, representing 4 years of education at university, are growing across the country, with over 130 such programs now in existence. However, registered nurses are still being prepared in colleges of nursing and schools attached to hospitals offering diploma and associate degree programs. In the face of the nursing shortage and the growing health-care needs of a rapidly aging population, aides are likely to be used more extensively, and Japan is now actively seeking to recruit nurses from selected Asian countries, especially The Philippines.

After registered nurse preparation, an additional year's course prepares individuals for certification as midwives or as public-health nurses. A recent nursing role is that of clinical specialist in a variety of settings. In addition, the number of masters and doctoral degree programs across the country has experienced a strong growth over the last decade. Like nursing students, medical students enter medical school immediately after high school, and after graduation they complete a clinical residency.

ISSUES RELATED TO AUTONOMY

Japanese workers are quite sensitive to the desires and expectations of colleagues and superiors. Because saying no or delivering bad news is extremely difficult, they may avoid issues or indicate that everything is fine rather than state the negative. Of course, sensitive Japanese workers, who are attuned to nonverbal cues, may understand the true situation. In addition, many Japanese workers tend not to leave work before their boss does nor do they take their full complement of paid vacation time each year, which may contribute to worker stress and tiredness. North American employers should explicitly discuss expectations about starting and quitting times and vacation leave with Japanese employees. Japanese workers do not assert individual rights. Japanese professionals working in North America accept the need to assert themselves if it is presented within the context of legal and professional requirements to protect their clients.

Japanese nurses are less likely than North American nurses to confront or question physicians or to suggest strategies. Workers tend to do what the head of the group tells them to do and make every effort to do it very well. Japanese health-care workers seeking to practice in the United States have studied English from grade 7 throughout professional school, and will have passed an examination certifying minimal competency, but their verbal skills may still be weak. Specific approaches to documentation, such as problem-oriented record-keeping, are now being more widely taught and used in Japan. However, these may still be unfamiliar to some nurses and need to be addressed specifically in employees' orientation.

Biocultural Ecology

SKIN COLOR AND OTHER BIOLOGICAL VARIATIONS

Racial features of Japanese people include the epicanthal skin folds that create the distinctive appearance of Asian eyes, a broad and flat nose, and "yellow" skin that varies markedly in tone. Hair is straight and naturally black with differences in shade. Health-care providers who are not accustomed to assessing racially diverse client groups may need to rely on color changes in the mucous membranes and sclerae to assess oxygenation and liver function in Japanese clients. The average stature of Japanese adults is smaller than that of Americans, although the gap has steadily decreased as national wealth has increased and a greater percentage of the population are able to improve their dietary practices.

The Ainu people of northern Japan, who number only about 15,000, are a fair-skinned people whose racial and linguistic origins are unknown. The Okinawan people of the Ryukyu Islands are darker-skinned than "mainlanders" and have a stockier build.

DISEASES AND HEALTH CONDITIONS

The three leading causes of death in Japan are malignant neoplasms, heart diseases, and cerebrovascular diseases. These account for over 50 percent of deaths in both sexes. In descending order, other causes are pneumonia, accidents, traffic accidents, suicide, renal disease, liver disease, diabetes mellitus, hypertensive diseases, and tuberculosis (Ministry of Health, Labour and Welfare, 2006). Moreover, men have a life expectancy of 78.5 years, whereas women have a life expectancy of 85.5 years, making the Japanese the longest living people in the world. An increasing focus is on reducing suicide, particularly among depressed men, because Japan ranks ninth in the world for suicides (Nakao & Takeuchi, 2006). Asthma and other allergic reactions related to dust mites in the *tatami* (straw mats that cover floors in Japanese homes) are considered some of the few endemic diseases along with illnesses related to air pollution in urban areas. In rural areas, allergic reactions to the pollen from numerous *sugi* (cedar) trees are a seasonal problem.

VARIATIONS IN DRUG METABOLISM

In general, drug dosages may need to be adjusted for the physical stature of Japanese adults, and racially linked genetic differences in drug metabolism can be important. More Asians than whites are poor metabolizers of mephenytoin and related medications, potentially leading to increased intensity and duration of the drugs' effects (Levy, 1993). Asians tend to be more sensitive to the effects of some beta blockers, many psychotropic drugs, and alcohol. A greater proportion of Japanese people rapidly metabolize acetylate substances, which has an impact on the metabolism of tranquilizers, tuberculosis drugs, caffeine, and some cardiovascular agents. Asians often require lower doses of some benzodiazepines, such as diazepam, and neuroleptics. Opiates may be less-effective analgesics, but gastrointestinal side effects may be greater than those among whites. Health-care providers need to take all clients' body mass into consideration in dosing; even with that precaution, clients' responses to drugs need to be monitored carefully.

The pornography industry thrives, and prostitution is big business. Rape and other sexual abuses are acknowledged in Japanese society and are now being more openly discussed. In fact, there have been a number of incidences since 2005 regarding harrassment; rape and murder cases are on the increase. In Tokyo, commuter trains for women now run at night to combat sexual harassment. Health education about avoiding rape and inappropriate touching, when approached in a matter-of-fact way, is very appropriate for Japanese in North America.

High-Risk Behaviors

The smoking rate for Japanese men has declined since the mid-1990s to around 57 percent of all men in 2004 aged over 20 years, but it is on the increase in women (13 percent). Around 20 percent of women in the 20- to 39-year-old age group now smoke (Ministry of Health, Labour and Welfare, 2006). Many restaurants, aware of the dangers of passive smoking, now offer nonsmoking areas, and plans are to make them smoke-free in the not-too-distant future. Public facilities, hospitals, transport, and many office situations are now smoke-free, and a series of fines can be levied in certain parts of Tokyo for people caught smoking. Cigarettes are easily available in vending machines and shops but are banned for sale to those under 20 years of age.

Alcohol has ritual significance. For example, in the marriage ceremony, the bride and groom drink *sake* or *saki* (rice wine), which is also an appropriate offering at **Shinto** shrines and at the *butsudan*, or household ancestral shrine. In addition, alcohol is part of many social rituals, such as picnics to celebrate cherry blossoms, autumn leaves, or moon viewing. Adults commonly drink beer and *sake* in the home, and college students drink beer when they socialize, although the legal age for drinking is 20 years.

The most serious concerns about alcohol use reflect the informal work requirement for men in Japan to socialize after hours and on Sundays. Considerable alcohol may be consumed, and it is common to see intoxicated salarymen snoozing on the trains or stumbling home late in the evening. In part, this extensive use of alcohol reflects the stress of Japanese corporate life and the rigid protocols that dictate social interactions. Once alcohol is consumed, workers can relax and speak freely. This is called *bureiko*, which means a gathering at which one can speak freely about what is on one's mind; people are forgiven for what they say because of the alcohol. Although diminished in the recent economic downturn, entertaining is expected in the Japanese business culture, and drinking is tolerated as an obligation to one's company.

Public acknowledgment of alcoholism is limited, and alcoholism rates are very difficult to determine. According to the Ministry of Health, Labour and Welfare (2006), in the period 1965 to 1999, the average rate of alcohol consumption per head of population rose from 5.86 to 8.30 L. The rate of youth abuse of alcohol is increasing (Tsuchiya & Takei, 2004). Over several decades, the Maryknoll Missionaries established alcohol treatment centers throughout the country and were among the first to publicize the problem of alcoholism among housewives, opening the first treatment center for women in the mid-1980s. Health-care providers need to be aware of the prevalence of smoking and heavy alcohol consumption among Japanese people, particularly men. An effective strategy for curtailing these abuses is to give individuals specific medical reasons why they must abstain, thus providing a socially acceptable excuse to do so.

VIGNETTE 15.3

Mr. Akutagawa, a 58-year-old business executive, has led a very busy life building up the family business with offices in both the United States and Japan. This has involved a lot of travel, long hours of work, and entertainment of clients. He has recently been diagnosed with gastric ulcers, and it is clear that he needs to modify his diet, change his lifestyle, and reduce his alcohol consumption.

1. What are the culturally sensitive elements to consider when advising Mr. Akutagawa about his alcohol consumption and diet?
2. Who needs to be involved in the decision-making about a plan for his lifestyle changes?

Over the last few years, Japan has witnessed a soaring abuse of illicit drugs by young people, particularly in high-density urban districts. The drugs used are mostly narcotics and stimulants, which have caused an increase in mental health problems, school drop-out rates, and drug-related crimes. The most serious is methamphetamine use, which has been connected to mental illness, and its use has been increasing since the 1990s. Distribution of methamphetamine is believed to be controlled by the *yakuza*, the Japanese mafia (Tsuchiya & Takei, 2004). Also increasing are serious crimes involving guns, which have often been smuggled into the country. In 2003, the Government instituted the *New Five Year Drug Abuse Strategy* and increased efforts to combat the smuggling of drugs and guns into the country by sea (Customs and Tariff Bureau, 2006). Punishment is harsh and swift, and there is no popular sentiment for liberalization. Despite such problems, the crime rate is quite low, and in most cities, the streets are safe at all hours.

Students and workers in Japan also make heavy use of over-the-counter stimulants. Students and young salary-men are commonly seen consuming high-dosage caffeine elixirs at train stations in the morning.

Groups of Japanese businessmen may be treated to a sex tour in Bangkok or other Southeast Asian cities. The implications for transmission of HIV to wives and children back home are clear, but societal acknowledgment of this risk has been slow to develop. In Japan, as in a number of Western countries, the rate of new cases of HIV and AIDS is on the increase, with sex between men identified as being responsible for 60 percent of the transmissions (UNAIDS, 2006), indicating the need for more effort in early discovery and treatment and in education on prevention. Every health-care contact with Japanese businessmen or their wives is an opportunity to state the facts about infectious disease risk. The United States is perceived as a place high in HIV risk, and concerns among Japanese who come to the United States tend to focus on casual contact as a possible modality.

Other growing concerns are the rise in inactivity and obesity levels of Japanese children. Success in the educational system demands long hours of study each day, thus reducing participation in physical activities, and this is compounded by the growth in the fast food industry and the predeliction for computer and electronic games usage among the young. Another problem is the prevalence of dental caries, which is high owing to unfluoridated water supplies across the country.

HEALTH-CARE PRACTICES

Japanese people are likely to attribute their generally high level of well-being to the centuries-old tradition of the daily bath. The *o-furo* (Japanese bathtub) is deep enough for an adult to enjoy a leisurely soak in neck-deep water, and the temperature is typically set around 105°F. The purpose of the bath is relaxation. Scrubbing for cleanliness and thorough rinsing are done before climbing into the tub. Families share the same water; in fact, they may soak together in the bath. Bath water may be reheated for several days before the tub is drained; depending on the type of bath, the water may be recycled for washing clothes or watering plants. Herbs or bath salts with therapeutic properties are sometimes added.

Young people in Japan do not drive until age 18, and an expensive and lengthy course of instruction is mandatory. Driving under the influence of alcohol or reckless operation of a vehicle carries stiff penalties. Rigorous inspection standards mean that people drive recent models of vehicles that are fully equipped with standard safety features. One major problem, however, is the rise in injury by rear seat passengers not using seat beats, a common feature in busy traffic, even though Japanese generally exhibit a high degree of public-safety consciousness.

Traditional housing materials and the close proximity of buildings have made fire a common and large-scale

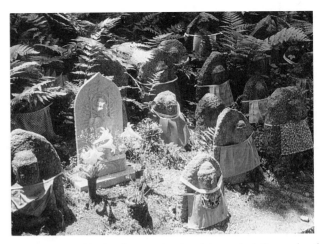

FIGURE 15–1 Misuko jizu are implored to protect the souls of aborted fetuses in the Japanese Buddhist tradition.

hazard. Each neighborhood has modern fire stations. Japanese readily use public services. Explicit instructions for accessing the local police, fire station, paramedics, and an emergency medical facility in a given North American community may be necessary, as well as the circumstances under which access is appropriate.

Nutrition

MEANING OF FOOD

Many Japanese social and business interactions begin or end (or both) with the serving of *o-cha* (coffee and snacks), or an *o-bento* (boxed lunch) (Fig. 15–1). Business entertaining can be lavish. Part of the atmosphere of congeniality depends on the artistic presentation of the food.

COMMON FOODS AND FOOD RITUALS

In Japan, all food groups are well represented, even in small shops, and the national diet is steadily becoming more Western, particularly among young people. In a wealthy, cosmopolitan society in the big cities, one can find just about any food or drink in common use in North America and Europe.

Large-scale agricultural production within Japan provides rice, beef, poultry, pork, seafood, root vegetables, cabbage, persimmons, apples, and *mikan* (tangerines). Rice, or *gohan*, the mainstay of the traditional diet, is included in all three meals as well as snacks. The electric rice cooker is a household necessity.

A traditional breakfast includes fish, pickles, *nori* (various seaweeds used to flavor or garnish meals), a raw egg stirred into the hot rice, *miso* (soybean-based) soup, and tea. Some people prefer a Western breakfast of toast or cold cereal and coffee.

School children lunch on their *o-bento*, packed with rice, pickles, vegetables, and meat or fish. Elementary schools generally provide a school lunch for pupils. A popular lunch among working people is *o-bento*, which can be ordered to be delivered quite cheaply to workplaces, or cold noodles on a hot summer day. Instant broth, or instant noodles, though high in sodium, is another popular quick lunch.

An example of a traditional dinner would be a pot of boiled potatoes, carrots, and pork seasoned with *mirin* (sweet *sake*), garlic, and soy sauce; or a stir-fried meat and vegetable dish. In major cities, Japanese housewives and working people have easy access to an enormous range of take-out food or home-delivery service, including Japanese, Chinese, and Western selections. American or Japanese fast food hamburger chains can be found in all cities. The daily intake of sweets can be high and often includes European-style desserts, sweet breads and cookies, sweet bean cakes, soft drinks, and heavily sweetened coffee, which may contribute to the high incidence of tooth decay.

For people in Japan, rice has a symbolic meaning related to the Shinto religion, analogous to the concept of the "bread of life" among Christians. One of the Emperor's duties is to ceremonially plant the first rice in the spring and harvest the first rice in the late summer. A staple of school children's *o-bento* is a bed of white rice garnished with a red plum pickle, reminiscent of the Japanese flag. Meals combine elements of land and sea. Office workers commonly have an *o-bento* box delivered to their workplace by one of the many *bento* companies in existence.

Holidays and family celebrations are times for ritual use of food. *O-bon*, in the summer, is a holiday for remembering family members who have died and a time when many travel to their family home, causing transport congestion across the country. Vegetables, especially *daikon* (large white radishes), are carved into animals, which are said to carry dead ancestors back to the afterlife after the holiday. Likewise, the new year's festival, *O-shogatsu*, is a 3-day celebration with food that has been prepared in advance. Japanese may ring in the new year by literally standing in line at a Shinto shrine to ring a gong, and then drinking a cup of warm *sake*. Another traditional new year's food is *mochi*, a ball of sticky rice dough that celebrants take turns pounding out with a heavy mallet. Red rice, or rice with red beans, is a celebratory food, as are various sweet bean desserts. A meal customarily begins with the simple grace, *Itadakimasu*, with the palms of hands facing together, and ends with the compliment, *Gochisosama deshita*. Western food rituals, including birthday cakes, wedding cakes, Christmas cakes, Valentine's chocolates, and Halloween trick or treats, have been incorporated into Japanese life, no doubt spurred on by a consumer-driven market economy.

DIETARY PRACTICES FOR HEALTH PROMOTION

Increasingly Westernized food tastes, resulting in higher fat and carbohydrate intake, have contributed to the rise in obesity, particularly in young children, in modern Japan as it has in many Western countries (Wang & Lobstein, 2006). These dietary changes and other lifestyle factors are causing great concern about an increase in conditions such as diabetes and heart disease. A huge Japanese diet industry has arisen that includes weight-loss clinics and programs and an amazing array of diet foods

and medications in supermarkets and pharmacies. Public education programs continue to warn the public about the high sodium content of soups and the overuse of food additives, soy sauce, and table salt. General principles of nutrition are the same in America as in Japan, although the food preferences may differ significantly.

Green tea, although high in caffeine, is a good source of vitamin C. Garlic and various herbs are widely used for their medicinal properties. In larger cities, health-food stores offering organically grown produce are available, and 10 percent of the population now use dietary supplements (Ishihara, Sobue, Yamamoto, Sasaki, Akabane, & Tsugane, 2001).

NUTRITIONAL DEFICIENCIES AND FOOD LIMITATIONS

Although some Asian people, including the Japanese, may have difficulty digesting milk products owing to lactose intolerance, increasing amounts of dairy products, including milk, cream, cheese, butter, ice cream, and yogurt, are on sale throughout the country, although these are not used to the same extent as in Western diets. Reduced-lactose milk is now available, as are low-fat milks and cheeses. Calcium is supplied in other foods such as *tofu* (soybean curd) and small, unboned fish. Water supplies are not fluoridated, and dental caries continue to be widespread. Fluoridated dental products can be recommended to Japanese clients, with the rationale for their use provided. Iron deficiency anemia is a concern among young women and can be alleviated with dietary counseling or dietary supplements. *Nori* (seaweed) is a traditional food source for iron.

Pregnancy and Childbearing Practices

FERTILITY PRACTICES AND VIEWS TOWARD PREGNANCY

After a national debate that lasted nearly 40 years, oral contraceptives became legal in Japan in 1999, shortly afterwards sildenafil citrate (Viagra) was quickly approved. The use of oral contraceptives, however, still remains fairly limited, and they are still not often used to treat menstrual cycle problems. In fact, Japan has managed to achieve a low birth rate without the major use of contraceptive pills. Condoms remain the most common contraceptive method used in Japan. Many women, both married and unmarried, have several abortions during their fertile lives. Although the number of reported abortions has steadily declined each year in Japan (just over 250,000 in 2003), the incidence is rising in the 15- to 24-year-old age group (Sato & Iwasawa, 2006). Some temples have *jizo* shrines where women give offerings of gifts and money to attendants who watch over aborted or miscarried fetuses (Orenstein, 2002), and often, a woman or a couple will place a *gizo* at a temple or shrine in memory of their aborted or miscarried fetus (Fig. 15–2).

The decline in the Japanese birth rate is regarded as a national crisis, and the economic implications are

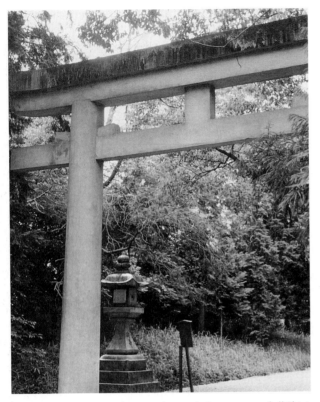

FIGURE 15–2   Torii are the gates that mark the entrance of all Shinto shrines.

devastating as the country ages. An educated female population, in a society in which women are oppressed, has asserted itself in a way that has certainly caught the nation's attention. As a result, many social structures and policies regarding female labor laws and child-care and social support systems are under scrutiny. Japan's status as a "low-birth-rate country" has created great interest in assistive reproductive technology within the last few years, and the Ministry of Health, Labour and Welfare has targeted infertility treatment as a priority. In the past, male infertility was too shameful to address.

Within traditional Japanese culture, pregnancy is highly valued as a woman's fulfillment of her destiny. Women may enjoy attention and pampering that they get at no other time, and our observations are that they take their role as mother-to-be very seriously, including health and diet. When a pregnancy is first detected in Japan, it is registered with the local government office, which distributes a special mother/child handbook that becomes a comprehensive longitudinal health record for the child right up until kindergarten. Some Japanese nationals living in the United States might want to receive and complete this handbook.

Maternity clothes are now often very fashionable. Some believe that keeping one's feet warm will promote uterine health. Pregnant women may undergo a ceremony involving the wrapping of an *hara obi* (a bleached cotton abdomen sash) obtained and purified at a Shinto shrine. The sash is wrapped around the abdomen for protection as part of a small ceremony performed on the Day of the Dog in the 5th month of pregnancy (Ito &

Sharts-Hopko, 2002). Because dogs give birth easily, the Chinese word for "dog" may be drawn on the *obi* by the obstetrician or midwife before they wrap it on the woman. Some women wear this sash throughout the rest of the pregnancy, but others may use a maternity girdle, a stomach band, or a special amulet to ensure a safe delivery.

Continuity of care throughout pregnancy is generally different in the United States and Japan. In Japan, a woman usually receives medical care and birthing support, including ultrasonography and physical examinations, from the same medical staff. In the United States, these may occur in different locations. Japanese women often return to their mother's home for the last 2 months of their pregnancy (called *satogaeri bunben*) and through the first 2 months' postpartum. Alternatively, mothers may come to stay with their daughter during this period, even traveling abroad to be with her. Although this trend may be lessening, it is still important for health providers to consider. American healthcare providers should explore a Japanese woman's expectations during pregnancy and the possibility that she might return to Japan. Finding another Japanese woman who has experienced childbearing in the United States and who can share her experiences can provide support for the pregnant client.

VIGNETTE 15.4

Keiko Okuni is a 29-year-old Japanese woman living in a high-rise apartment in your city and is 4 months' pregnant, having moved to the United States 6 months ago. She is not working and has no social or family supports here apart from her husband. You meet her at the antenatal clinic and are responsible for helping her to plan for the delivery of her baby.

1. What specific factors would you need to take into consideration when trying to ensure that her prenatal care is culturally and socially appropriate?
2. How could you help her find appropriate ways to learn about the American health system, particularly in relation to prenatal and postnatal care?
3. What are some of her health beliefs that need to be taken into consideration during her pregnancy, labor, and the postpartum period?
4. What kinds of information do you think needs to be supplied to her husband in relation to pregnancy and childbirth?

PRESCRIPTIVE, RESTRICTIVE, AND TABOO PRACTICES IN THE CHILDBEARING FAMILY

Health teaching for pregnant women in Japan emphasizes rest and restraint from stressful activities. Women who are found working until late in their pregnancy are given special considerations in the workplace. Loud noises, such as trains or very loud music, are believed to be bad for the baby. Shinto shrines sell amulets for conception and easy delivery, and women may pray for their safe delivery at these shrines. Some women now attend exercise classes for pregnant women but are rarely accompanied by their husbands.

In the past, it was not so common for husbands to attend the births of their children; however, this is changing and varies considerably across Japan. Some hospitals still do not allow husbands to be present. Most Japanese women choose private obstetric care and give birth in 1 of the 2500 maternity hospitals in which most births occur with a physician delivering the baby. Certified nurse-midwives often give perineal massages during childbirth. They may deliver the baby, sometimes observed by a physician who assists if complications occur. However, the strong tradition of local community-based midwifery, with independent midwives offering services at their own birth houses, is regaining popularity. Currently, about 350 of these across the country cater to about 2 percent of the births. Birthing houses are quite separate from hospitals and are supported by the community. Birthing at home is quite rare in Japan.

Episiotomies may still be performed for first deliveries, but shaving and the use of enemas predelivery are not common in Japan. In addition, Japanese midwives often use perineal massage. Oxytocics are common in the second stage of delivery if contractions are weak, and antibiotics are often prescribed after delivery even though there may be no sign of infection. Pregnant women are educated about balanced natural foods, and easily digested foods are preferred during the first stage of labor.

The differences in birthing procedures need to be explained to women giving birth in the United States, especially when they may have knowledge only of procedures in their home country. It is important for midwives and obstetricians in the United States to remember that Japanese families want to keep the dried umbilical cord that falls from the newborn's abdomen. This is very special, and it is stored by the family for many years in boxes made of *kiri* (paulownia) wood; sometimes, it may be given to the bridegroom on marriage.

Physicians are skilled at mid- and high-forceps deliveries because cesarean delivery is viewed as hard on the mother; such surgery is reserved for emergency cases. Vaginal deliveries are usually performed with minimal medication, and the mother tries to be very stoic, using the breathing exercises taught during pregnancy. Ito and Sharts-Hopko (2002) explained that Japanese women prefer nonpharmacological interventions such as the Lamaze method whenever possible. To give in to pain dishonors the husband's family, and mothers are said to appreciate their babies more if they suffer in childbirth.

Japan enjoys one of the lowest rates of infant and maternal mortality in the world. Maternal mortality, at 7.3 per 100,000 births in 2003, is most commonly caused by hemorrhage, and is associated with delivery in small, single-physician birthing hospitals (Ministry of Health, Labour and Welfare, 2006).

Japanese women in the United States are not likely to have a birth plan when they are admitted to a health-care facility. They prefer natural methods of child delivery as they would in Japan and to avoid cesarean delivery and pain relief whenever possible. Their husbands may choose not to attend the actual delivery, in which case, women will need additional supportive nursing care.

In the postpartum period, time to recover from childbirth is taken seriously. In Japan, a woman may stay in the hospital 5 days to 1 week while learning to breastfeed and attending daily mother-care classes. Japanese hospitals vary about allowing rooming-in of babies. Culturally, postpartal women often do not wash their hair for a few days postpartum. Because the new mother often stays with her mother, the new father may not see his baby for a few months until he comes to take the mother and baby home from the grandmother's house. Because of the perceived risk of infections, it is unusual to see infants in public before the age of 3 months.

Mothers will often be asked about the feeding method they used for their baby, for example, on kindergarten admission forms. Maternal rest and relaxation are deemed essential for success. Lactation nurses are widely available, and breast massage is one of their strategies for promoting milk production and flow. A number of promotional campaigns have been held recently to encourage women to breastfeed, and concerns do exist about its decline when women choose to re-enter the workforce.

Japanese women who give birth in the United States may resent the American expectation that they will resume self-care and child-care activities quickly, which they believe is harmful to them and their relationship with the baby. Although American health-care providers cannot provide the length of hospital stay the women would have experienced in Japan, they can explain the expectations for postpartal care, exercise sensitivity, and help plan for assistance upon discharge.

Death Rituals

DEATH RITUALS AND EXPECTATIONS

In Japan, open discussions about death, serious illness, and mental illness are usually not common subjects for discussion, but recently, the daily media include more awareness and discussion about depression, HIV/AIDS, and dementia. Most Japanese people still hesitate to reveal serious mental illness in their family. However, physicians are more commonly revealing diagnoses of cancer or other life-threatening illnesses to patients, whereas in the past, patients were rarely told of the possibility of their impending death. This paternalistic approach was meant to relieve the patient of emotional suffering. In recent years, the biomedical literature has begun to reflect open discourse on pain management in terminal illness, the need for greater national investment in intensive-care services, the need to increase organ transplantation, and the need for end-of-life decision-making.

Under the Organ Transplant Law of 1997, organ transplantation is not permitted in children under the age of 15 nor are children permitted to donate organs. Brain death is not considered a legal means by which ventilators can be turned off by medical staff. Recently, controversial decisions have been made to charge medical staff who have done so.

RESPONSES TO DEATH, GRIEF, AND SUFFERING

When considering the death and grief reactions of Japanese, one must not neglect the close intertwining of Buddist and Shinto beliefs at large in the population. In Shinto, death is believed to be impure and one should not spend time dwelling on it. According to the first Noble Truth of Buddhism, all human beings suffer. When a Japanese person is dying, the family should be notified of the impending death so they can be at the dying person's bedside. Traditionally, the eldest son has particular responsibility during this time.

Many homes have a Buddhist altar, *butsudan*, where deceased family members are honored and remembered. Photographs of the deceased are displayed, floral arrangements are placed within and outside of the home, and a special altar may be constructed when a person dies. A bag of money is hung around the neck of the deceased to pay the toll to cross the river to the hereafter (Shinto Online Network Association, 2006). An alternate version of this custom dictates that if the dead is satisfied with the amount of money, then the inheritance is freed for the survivors. Visitors bring gifts of money and food for the bereaved family. White flowers are the symbol of death in Japan and are used at funerals; therefore, these should not be sent to someone who is ill.

Modern corporate life in Japan does not allow for taking more than a few days off from work for official mourning. However, in terms of religious practice, the mourning period is 49 days, the end of which is marked by a family prayer service and the serving of special rice dishes. At this time, the departed has joined those already in the hereafter. Perpetual prayers may be donated through a gift to the temple. In addition, special prayer services can be conducted for the 1st, 3rd, 7th, and 13th anniversaries of the death. The common belief is that the dead need to be remembered and failure to do so can lead the dead to rob the living of rest. Proper funeral rites and reassurance that they are remembered during temple and family prayers alleviate the agitation of the dead.

VIGNETTE 15.5

Mrs. Kobayashi, aged 78 years, was admitted to the local hospital with a myocardial infaction. She lapsed into a comatose state and died. The community nurse has been visiting Mrs. Kobayashi's frail husband in their apartment over the last 3 months. She was his main caregiver, and they were both very traditional in their beliefs and outlook on life, even though they had lived in the United States for 25 years. The nurse and the social worker from the local health center are very concerned for Mr. Kobayashi. He wants to remain in his apartment until his son arrives from Tokyo.

1. In order to help Mr. Kobayashi to deal with his wife's death, what culturally appropriate rituals could the nurse and the social worker suggest to assist him?
2. Who could be called to help Mr. Kobayashi?
3. What are some challenges the nurse might encounter while working with Mr. Kobayashi?

Spirituality

DOMINANT RELIGION AND USE OF PRAYER

Japan does not have a clearly articulated theology or religious belief system. Tradition holds that the Japanese people are descendants of the Sun goddess and that the emperor is a God (Keene, 1983), although the Occupation forces required Hirohito to publicly renounce this status after World War II ended. Some say that the demotion of the emperor from God to mortal has left the Japanese with a spiritual vacuum. Reischauer and Jansen (1995) believed this secularization of Japanese society began when Confucianism, imported during the 9th century, grew in influence during the 17th century. Confucian values, including faith in education, hard work, and the emphasis on interpersonal relationships and loyalty, continue to be important today.

Shinto, the indigenous religion, is the focus of joyful events such as marriage and birth. Many *matsuri* (festivals) are marked by offerings, parades through the streets, and a carnival on the grounds of the shrine. **Buddhism**, brought to Japan in the 6th century, has permeated Japanese artistic and intellectual life. Very few Japanese people regularly attend services, but most are registered temple members, if only to ensure a family burial plot. One percent of Japanese people are Catholic or Protestant in nearly equal numbers, and Christianity has been known, although at times not well tolerated, in Japan since the 16th century. Most Japanese do not identify themselves solely with one religion; even a baptized Christian might have a Shinto wedding and a Buddhist funeral. These days, some young people get married in a commerical-style chapel that looks like a Christian chapel but has nothing to do with religion.

MEANING OF LIFE AND INDIVIDUAL SOURCES OF STRENGTH

This crossover of Shinto and Buddhist beliefs and customs may be a surprise to visitors from overseas. Many Japanese believe in reincarnation, a Buddhist belief, and also accept the Shinto recognition of the eternal life of the soul, which needs purification in the earthly life. Ancestor worship is widespread, and many Japanese believe that their ancestors can be called back to earth. Such beliefs play a large part in mourning the dead. Other valid interpretations include honoring one's family and country, working hard, being a good group member, and joining one's deceased ancestors (Woss, 1992).

SPIRITUAL BELIEFS AND HEALTH-CARE PRACTICES

Japanese religions play a significant role in health-care practices. People or objects such as cars are taken to special shrines for purification from evil by priests. People often buy protective *omamori* (amulets) at shrines or temples for a wide variety of reasons. Some shrines and temples specialize in specific illnesses. *Kampo* (pharmacists or traditional healers) often set up shop in the vicinity. At the temple or shrine, a person might be seen scooping incense smoke onto an ailing body part or praying for good health. Prayer boards might bear requests for special healing. Gifts of toys or devices used in child care may be left with Buddha statues. Newborns are taken to a shrine for a blessing. Children are taken for blessings on November 15, when they are 3, 5, or 7 years old (the *shichi-go-san*). Visits to shrines and temples in Japan are social, recreational, and spiritual outings. Souvenirs and refreshments are usually available, and the hike into the prayer area provides exercise, with access to many temples or shrines involving a climb up steps.

Various types of diviners, soothsayers, and prophets may be present at shrines, temples, and even along the most fashionable streets in Tokyo. Statues depicting folktale heroes, often animals, are believed to bring luck. Americans may have difficulty understanding and accepting the reliance of sophisticated and well-educated people on what may be viewed as superstitions. But these measures appear to be more sources of comfort than deciding factors in health-care decision-making. They should be accepted as a very important part of what it means to be Japanese.

Health-Care Practices

HEALTH-SEEKING BELIEFS AND BEHAVIORS

The general health of the populations of Japan and the United States are similar, with a shift in leading causes of morbidity and mortality from infections to chronic illnesses and diseases. However, behaviors and underlying belief systems differ markedly between Japan and the United States. The Japanese are more tolerant of self-indulgence, even during minor illnesses. Because Japanese are less likely to express feelings verbally, this indulgence may be a way for people to affirm caring for one another nonverbally. Hypochondriasis among the Japanese has been described in the medical literature and is more tolerated. Bodily flaws, for example, birthmarks, are a source of concern; and body piercing is now becoming more fashionable in the young.

In Japan, people seem less inclined to seek correction of minor orthopedic and dental variations than those in middle-class American society, although immigrant families make full use of services offered in the United States. Health-care providers engaged in health promotion and screening need to be aware of this difference. Function, rather than appearance, may be a more appropriate emphasis.

Humankind is a part of nature, subject to its forces, and a person is an integrated whole. Whereas Chinese tradition calls for a restoration of balance when one is ill, Shinto calls for purging and purification. Both influences operate in modern Japan. In the past, Shinto was the source of principles of prevention, whereas Buddhist priests healed the sick. Centuries before the germ theory was known, Shinto effectively distinguished between spaces and body parts that were dirty versus those that were clean and pure. For example, taking off one's shoes at the doorway keeps one's home clean, and people wear slippers inside. However, only stockinged feet or bare feet are used on grass matting or *tatami*. Family members will also change their slippers when entering bathroom or toilet areas. Mothers carefully teach young children to fear dirt. People with colds in Japan customarily wear disposable surgical masks in public to shield others from their infection.

Preoccupation with germs and dirt is not likely to interfere with daily life. It may account for prejudices among some Japanese against certain categories of workers, including nurses. Americans who visit Japanese homes should usually assume that outside shoes are taken off before entering the home, and the hostess will usually offer guests slippers to wear. The same thing may occur in special types of businesses, in some restaurants, or in areas in aged-care homes or special clinics.

RESPONSIBILITY FOR HEALTH CARE

Newsstands and vending machines, particularly in commuter rail stations in Japan, provide large quantities of flavored caffeine elixirs, high-potency vitamin elixirs, and electrolyte replacement drinks. These products are promoted to give workers and students an edge in their daily work. Health-care providers need to ask specifically what remedies are being used and why. Japanese clients in North America find general principles of nutrition to be the same as those taught in Japan, although their food preferences may differ.

The health of pregnant and nursing mothers and of children has the highest priority in the Japanese health-care system, and all school children and workers have comprehensive annual check-ups at the expense of their school system or employer. National insurance is available to all Japanese, including foreigners, for a sliding-scale fee, and covers both medical and dental care. Treatment by osteopaths, chiropractors, and traditional practitioners is covered if clients have been referred by a physician; in fact, acupuncture, moxibustion (heat applied to acupuncture sites), and other traditional modalities of care are still part of the national university curriculum for physical therapists. Older people and people with certain chronic conditions receive free treatment, whereas low-income people may be eligible for subsidized services. The municipal government handles enrollments.

Japanese residents in the United States frequently carry Japanese health insurance. Japanese nationals working for American institutions or companies may be eligible for the same coverage as other employees, but they often need assistance in understanding how their benefits work. Students and others can continue their Japanese national health insurance while in America, but they may need assistance in seeking care and understanding the American billing and payment process.

Many American over-the-counter medications, or their Japanese equivalents, are widely available in Japanese pharmacies. In addition, many pharmacies stock traditional herbal *kampo* preparations, as well as a large amount of stomach preparations for gastric upset.

Japanese people make liberal use of both modern medical and traditional providers of health care. Influenced by German and American medical science, the Japanese health-care system incorporates local primary care, neighborhood hospitals, specialty clinics, academic medical centers, and national research institutes. Most hospital beds are found in tiny, unregulated, physician-owned neighborhood clinics, and it is not common for patients to have their own room, even if they have private insurance. A sophisticated public health system offers prenatal and well-child care, school health initiatives, visiting nursing services, home health services, senior centers, and health education at little or no cost to the public.

Japanese residents in the United States have Internet and mail order access to traditional medications, if they are not available locally. As with any client population, a complete health assessment includes inquiry about home therapies. From the second generation of immigrants onward, the tendancy is to rely fully on the American health-care system.

FOLK AND TRADITIONAL PRACTICES

Morita therapy, one of the most popular indigenous models of psychotherapy in Japan, is used to address **shinkei shitsu**, excess sensitivity to the social and natural environment. Morita therapy focuses on constructive physical activities that help clients adjust to and accept the reality in their lives and the interconnectedness to others (Tamura & Lau, 1992). This form of psychotherapy is very different from Western psychotherapy in that it tries to avoid introspection and deep analysis of self in an individualistic sense. *Naikan* **therapy** is another indigenous psychotherapy of reflection on how much goodness and love is received from others and is very much focused on well-being in Japanese culture. A third indigenous therapy, **Shinryo Naika**, focuses on bodily illnesses that are emotionally induced.

Within the last several decades, Western-style psychiatry has been fully incorporated into Japanese health-care services. Indeed, psychiatric care in Japan in the early 1990s was predominantly given in overcrowded institutions. Today, it is moving toward a community-based emphasis. However, according to Tsuchiya and Takei (2004), substantial changes are needed in forensic psychiatry, child and adolescent psychiatry, substance misuse, and the naming of psychiatric disorders. One major problem is inadequate provision of mental health care for children and adolescents. Japan today has 348,966 psychiatric beds for a population of nearly 27 million people, approximately three times higher than the 10 psychiatric beds per 10,000 population in the United Kingdom in 1998 (Ministry of Health, Labour and Welfare, 2002). Despite the greater availability of psychiatric inpatient care, increased stress and violent attacks in the community continue to fill the daily newspapers without any sign of improvement. This is of great concern to Japanese people at large, especially when Tsuchiya and Takei (2004) pointed out that there is no special provision for violent mentally ill offenders other than in regular psychiatric hospitals.

Health-care providers need to be sensitive to workplace or family issues that may underlie illnesses among Japanese clients, as among all clients. If a provider believes that psychotherapy is indicated, the therapist must be someone familiar with the Japanese culture. Guidance in locating resources may be obtained through large academic medical centers or universities in coastal (particularly the Pacific Coast) cities, as well as through professional associations, Japanese churches, or other religious organizations.

Health care is easily obtained in Japan. However, the system of referrals is unique. When a physician leaves medical school, she or he becomes part of that school's "family." She or he is unlikely to refer patients to specialists or hospitals outside the "family" of her or his fellow alumni or former professors. Personal acquaintance is essential for doing business in Japan, and it is also reflected in health-care practice.

Japanese people may be unlikely to assert themselves in American settings, and their efforts to do so may seem inappropriate to American health-care providers. Their high regard for the status of physicians decreases the likelihood of asking questions or making suggestions about their care. The idea that clients should be given care options may be alien. Health-care providers need to provide ample opportunity for dialogue and explain the choices that are offered. Japanese and Japanese American health-care providers may be an important resource in bridging gaps in understanding.

VIGNETTE 15.6

Mayuko is a 19-year-old Japanese student studying at the local university in your city. She has been referred to the mental health clinic by one of her tutors because she has been missing classes, appears not to be taking care of herself, and is withdrawn and uncommunicative. She would not visit the health center at the university or visit her local doctor. When the nurse meets her, it is clear that she seems depressed and unhappy and says she is missing her family in Japan.

1. What specific cultural factors could be contributing to Mayuko's present state?
2. Why has she been reluctant to seek help?
3. How could the nurse provide education about depression to her in a culturally sensitive fashion?

CULTURAL RESPONSES TO HEALTH AND ILLNESS

Pain, *itami*, may not be expressed, and bearing pain is considered a virtue and a matter of family honor. Medications that specifically relieve pain are used less frequently in Japan than in the United States; narcotic use in particular is restricted. Addiction is a strong taboo in Japanese society. Biomedical researchers are beginning to study the comfort needs of dying patients (Morita, Tsunoda, Inoue, & Chihara, 2000), but the use of hospices, as they are known in the Western sense, is not common in Japan. Those that do exist often combine the comfort of the dying with intrusive medical care. Davis, Konishi, and Mitoh (2002) pointed out that terminal care of the dying in Japan is much different. Some hospices may be attached to acute-care hospitals, and most patients are not told of their diagnosis or prognosis because the ethical notion of health professionals is that protecting the patient from distressing news is the moral thing to do.

American health-care providers may use a schedule of analgesic administration rather than an as-requested or a patient-controlled approach to ensure adequate pain management. Japanese clients may respond positively to the information that physiological status and healing are actually enhanced by pain control.

Physically and intellectually handicapped children and adults are not commonly seen in public in Japan. In fact, most handicapped children, if they attend school, go to special schools rather than being integrated in the public school system. In addition, many public areas in Japan are not designed to cope with people with disabilities, making it very difficult for people who use wheelchairs or other assistive mobility devices. However, recently, the number of public toilets with facilities for handicapped people has increased. Many Japanese families hide knowledge of deformity or disability in family members because of shame, and there are still instances of people with physical handicaps—for example, cerebral palsy—being admitted to psychiatric hospitals owing to a lack of suitable facilities elsewhere. Japanese families residing in the United States need encouragement to avail themselves of community resources and to understand that shame associated with disability is not as prevalent in American society.

Assumption of the sick role is highly tolerated by families and colleagues, and a long recuperation period is encouraged by Japanese health-care providers. For example, in Japan, a client with a myocardial infarction may be hospitalized for a month, with outcomes comparable with those found in the United States (Kinjo et al., 2004). However, changes to the national insurance system to extend care for rehabilitation, to shorten hospital stays, and to provide for more rehabilitation are now starting to have an effect, particularly in rehabilitation after stroke (Miyoshi, Teraoka, Date, Kim, Nguyen, & Miyoshi, 2005). Rehabilitation to achieve the full level of activities of daily living after serious illness or injury is less aggressive than in the United States. However, the number of higher education programs to train occupational and rehabilitation specialists is slowly growing across the country, and the importance of rehabilitation is becoming more recognized and implemented.

BLOOD TRANSFUSIONS AND ORGAN DONATIONS

Giving blood is encouraged in the Japanese culture. The Japanese Red Cross is a very active and highly respected organization that runs 92 Red Cross hospitals in the country and collects blood in 77 centers, using over 340 blood mobiles, which travel around the country (Japan Red Cross, 2006). Donees are not paid for their contributions. Blood usage is accounted for by 100 percent of domestic usage; however, blood products for hemophilia have to be imported. People with negative blood types account for less than 1 percent of the population; therefore, RhoGam, used to protect an Rh-positive fetus from antibodies from an Rh-negative mother, is not commonly stocked in Japanese hospitals.

Critical-care technology has not received the emphasis in Japan that it has in the United States. Moreover, Ohaki, Yano, Shirouzu, Kobayashi, Nakagomi, and Tamura (2006) explained that in Japan, organ donation following diagnosed brain death was legalized in 1997, except for children under 15 years of age. Japan now has the strictest laws on organ donation in the world. Very few organ transplants have been from brain-dead donors; the number of transplants needed is vastly more than the organs available. Japanese people, including health professionals, may be distrustful of the diagnosis of brain death, which may be thought of as a persistent vegetative state. Critical care and organ transplantation and donation issues need to be approached sensitively with Japanese residents in the United States. Health-care providers must be cautious in initiating extraordinary measures with Japanese family members. Japanese people rely more heavily on the physician's opinion, and the family may have difficulty negotiating for cessation of treatment. The concept of advance directives has not been implemented in Japan, and upon admission to an American hospital, families need to understand what this means.

VIGNETTE 15.7

Kyoko Moromoto, aged 10 years, was admitted to intensive care following a serious car accident in which she sustained ruptured kidneys as well as other injuries. She is currently on renal dialysis, and her attending and other physicians believe she requires a kidney transplant. Kyoko was on holiday with her Japanese parents when the accident happened in New York.

1. Given that Kyoko and her parents are Japanese, what are some cultural issues that may be involved in this case?
2. What specific information should be given to the parents about organ donation in the United States, particularly in relation to organs donated from people who were diagnosed with brain death?
3. What may cause Kyoko's parents to hesitate about approving a kidney transplant for their daughter?

Health-Care Practitioners

TRADITIONAL VERSUS BIOMEDICAL PRACTITIONERS

In modern Japan, physicians are clearly in charge of the health-care team. Some physicians may have a high degree of understanding of *kampo*, or Japanese herbal medicine, and may offer patients a choice between Western medicine and *kampo*. However, Teramoto (2000) noted that only about 10 percent of the population uses herbal medicines today and that Japanese medical students may now receive poor training in its use. *Kampo* may be used in psychiatric care and care of older people;

traditional practitioners may refer clients to the medical establishment and vice versa. Japanese health practitioners who come to the United States face a different type of health-care system, with greater diversity and autonomy for many professionals. The authority of insurers to dictate care is novel for them, as is the extent of concern for malpractice liability.

STATUS OF HEALTH-CARE PROVIDERS

Physicians, referred to as *sensei*, are highly esteemed. Self-care as a philosophy is not evident in Japan. Being told what to do by the physician or *kampo* practitioner is expected, and his or her authority is not questioned. Physicians control most health-care delivery in Japan, running public and private hospitals and owning most private hospitals. Hospital administration is not an established field, and administrators in public hospitals are generally physicians elected to their post.

In Japan, females account for only about 15 percent of physicians, and male nurses account for about 6 percent. However, the professions and their interrelationships generally tend to reflect traditional gender roles. In the past, nurses were titled according to gender, *kango-shi* if a male, and *kango-fu* if female. The former means approximately "Mr. Nurse," whereas the latter means "Ms. Nurse." However, the title of nurse is pronounced the same as the former one, but it is literally different in meaning in Kanji. The unified *Kango-shi* literally means "person to be a nurse by profession" and has the same written Kanji character as doctor and pharmacist.

Nurses in Japan today believe that nursing is still not highly regarded in Japanese society, but the raising of educational levels to a baccalaureate will undoubtedly change this, as has been the case in the United States. However, as noted previously, Japanese women do not hold high status in society, so this reflects strongly on the status of a largely feminine occupation. The proliferation of various types of health-care providers and technicians is less in Japan than in the United States (Anders, 1994; Tierney & Tierney, 1994). Japanese residents in the United States need considerable assistance in understanding how the health-care delivery systems work and the functions of the different health-care providers they encounter. In particular, they need to understand the autonomy of a diverse group of health professionals. Home care, and the orchestration of many community-based providers, may be overwhelming for Japanese residents who expect longer recuperations in the hospital.

Japanese health professionals working in the United States need careful orientation to laws and institutional regulations about appropriate male-female interactions and professional requirements for accountability in communicating problems. Japanese residents seeking health care in America may be surprised by the assertiveness and autonomy of nonphysician professionals. An overview of the details of their care and who will be doing various aspects of that care can be helpful. Japanese residents in the United States may need assistance in seeking care. Their verbal English skills may be an impediment to making their needs known and to understanding the care

they are offered, although their ability to understand written information is very good. Japanese people tend to believe that they are physiologically different from non-Japanese people, and they may be skeptical of recommendations. They may also be very unwilling to discuss family members with mental health problems for fear of stigma. Calling on the local Japanese community for support and encouragement may be a useful strategy with these clients.

REFERENCES

Anders, R. L. (1994). An American's view of nursing education in Japan. *Image: Journal of Nursing Scholarship, 26,* 227–230.

Customs and Tariff Bureau. (2006). *Trends in illicit drugs and firearm smuggling in Japan: 2005 report.* Toyko: Ministry of Finance.

Davis, A., Konishi, E., & Mitoh, T. (2002). The telling and knowing of dying: Philosophical bases for hospice care in Japan. *International Nursing Review, 49*(4), 226–233.

Doi, T. (1971). *The anatomy of dependence* (J. Bester, Trans.) Tokyo: Kodansha International Ltd.

Ehara, A. (2005). Lawsuits associated with medical malpractice in Japan [Letter to the editor]. *Pediatrics, 115*(6), 1792–1793.

Fukumizu, M., Kaga, M., Kohyama, J., & Hayes, M. J. (2005). Sleep-related nighttime crying (yonaki) in Japan. A community based study. *Pediatrics, 115,* 217–224.

Gender Equality Bureau, Cabinet Office. (2006). *Steps toward gender equality in Japan.* Retrieved November 4, 2006, from http://www.gender.go.jp/english_contents/Pamphlet2006.pdf

Ishihara, J., Sobue, T., Yamamoto, S., Sasaki, S., Akabane, M., & Tsugane, S. (2001). Validity and reproducibility of a self-administered questionnaire to determine dietary supplement users among Japanese. *European Journal of Clinical Nutrition, 55*(5), 360–365.

Ito, M., & Sharts-Hopko, N. (2002). Japanese women's experience of childbirth in the United States. *Health Care for Women International, 23*(6–7), 666–677.

Japan Media Review. (2006). *Publishers push the return of the E-book.* Retrieved November 19, 2006, from http://ojr.org/japan/media/1082135229.php

Japan Red Cross. (2006). *About us.* Retrieved December 11, 2006, from http://www.jrc.or.jp/english/index.html

Kanazumi, F. (1997). Interview. In S. Buckley (Ed.), *Broken silence: Voices of Japanese feminism* (pp. 70–81). Berkeley: University of California Press.

Kashiwazaki, C., & Akaha, T. (2005). *Japanese immigration policy: Responding to conflicting pressures.* Retrieved November 19, 2006 from http://www.migrationinformation.org/Profiles/display.cfm?ID=487

Keene, D. (1983). Ise. In D. Richie (Ed.), *Discover Japan: Vol. 2. Words, customs and concepts* (pp. 196–197). Tokyo: Kodansha International, Ltd.

Kinjo, K., Sato, H., Nakatani, D., Mizuno, H., Shimizu, M., Hishida, E., Ezumi, A., Hoshida, S., Koretsune, Y., & Hori, M. (2004). Predictors of length of hospital stay after myocardial infarction in Japan. *Circulation Journal, 68*(9), 809–815.

Leonardsen, D. (2004). *Japan as a low-crime nation.* New York: Palgrave Macmillan.

Levy, R. A. (1993). Ethnic and racial differences in response to medicines: Preserving individualized therapy in managed pharmaceutical programmes. *Pharmaceutical Medicine, 7,* 139–165.

Longevity Japan. (2006). *The spread of corporate measures to support child care and family care. One dimension of action in response to the declining birth rate in Japan.* Retrieved December 1, 2006, from http://longevity.ilc-japan.org/f_issues/060706.html

Makino, M., Hashizume, M., Yasushi, M., Tsuboi, K., & Dennerstein, L. (2006). Factors associated with abnormal eating attitudes among female college students in Japan. *Archives of Women's Mental Health, 9*(4), 203–208.

Ministry of Health, Labour and Welfare. (2006). *Vital statistics tables 2005.* Retrieved January 26, 2007, from Ministry of Health, Labour and Welfare Homepage http://www.mhlw.go.jp/

Ministry of Internal Affairs and Communications. (2006). *Statistical handbook of Japan.* Retrieved November 30, 2006, from http://www.stat.go.jp/English/data/handbook/c02cont.htm#cha2_4

Miyoshi, Y., Teraoka, J. K., Date, E. S., Kim, M. J., Nguyen, R. T., & Miyoshi, S. (2005). Changes in stroke rehabilitation outcomes after the implementation of Japan's long term care insurance system: A hospital based study. *American Journal of Physical Medical Rehabilitation, 84*(8), 613–619.

Morita, T., Tsunoda, J., Inoue, S., & Chihara, D. (2000). Pain and symptom management. Terminal sedation for existential distress. *American Journal of Hospice and Palliative Care, 17*(3), 189–195.

Nakao, M., & Takeuchi, T. (2006). The suicide epidemic in Japan and strategies of depression screening for its prevention. *Bulletin of the World Health Organization, 84*(6), 492–493.

Ohwaki, K., Yano, E., Shirouzu, M., Kobayashi, A., Nakagomi, T., & Tamura, A. (2006). Factors associated with attitude and hypothetical behaviour regarding brain death and organ transplantation: Comparison between medical and other university students. *Clinical Transplantation, 20*(4), 416–422.

Orenstein, P. (2002, April 21). Mourning my miscarriage. *New York Times.* Retrieved from http://www.NYTimes.com

Reischauer, E. O., & Jansen, M. (1995). *The Japanese today.* New York. Longitude Books.

Sato, R., & Iwasawa, M. (2006). Contraceptive use and induced abortion in Japan: How is it so unique among developed countries? *The Japanese Journal of Population, 4*(1), 33–54.

Sharts Engel, N. (1989). An American experience of pregnancy and childbirth in Japan. *Birth, 16*(2), 81–86.

Shinto Online Network Association. (2006). Retrieved December 11, 2006, from http://www.jinja.or.jp/english

Takakura, M., & Sakihara, S. (2000). Gender differences in the association between psychosocial factors and depressive symptoms in Japanese junior high school students. *Journal of Epidemiology, 10*(6), 383–391.

Tamura, T., & Lau, A. (1992). Connectedness versus separateness: Applicability of familty therapy to Japanese families. *Family Process,* (4), 319.

Teramoto, S. (2000). Doctors' attitudes to complementary medicine. *The Lancet, 355,* 501–502.

Tierney, M. J., & Tierney, L. M. (1994). Nursing in Japan. *Nursing Outlook, 42*(5), 210–213.

Tsuchiya, K. J., & Takei, N. (2004). Mental health care in Japan: An overview. *The British Journal of Psychiatry,* (184), 88–92.

UNAIDS. (2006). *Country progress report: Japan 2005/2006.* Retrieved December 8, 2006, from http://data.unaids.org/pub/Report/2006/2006_country_progress_report_japan_en.pdf

UN Secretariat. (2005). *Possibilities and limitations of Japanese migration policy in the context of economic partnership in Asia.* New York: UN Department of Economic and Social Information Affairs.

U.S. Commercial Service. (2006). *Japanese tourism marketing opportunities.* Retrieved November 20, 2006, from http://www.buyusa.gov/japan/en/tourism06.html

U.S. Department of State. (2006). *Background note—Japan.* Updated June 2006. Retrieved November 30, 2006, from http://www.state.gov/r/pa/bgn/4142.htm

Wang, Y., & Lobstein, T. (2006). Worldwide trends in childhood overweight and obesity. *International Journal of Pediatric Obesity, 1*(1), 11–25.

Woss, F. (1992). When blossoms fall: Japanese attitudes towards death and the other world: Opinion polls 1953–1987. In R. Goodman & K. Refsing (Eds.), *Ideology and practice in modern Japan* (pp. 72–100). New York: Routledge.

Yanagisako, S. J. (1985). *Transforming the past: Tradition and kinship among Japanese Americans.* Stanford, CA: Stanford University Press.

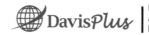

Chapter *16*

People of Jewish Heritage

LARRY D. PURNELL and JANICE SELEKMAN

Overview, Inhabited Localities, and Topography

OVERVIEW

Being **Jewish** refers to both a people and a religion, not a race. Throughout history, the terms *Hebrew, Israelite*, and *Jew* have been used interchangeably. In the Bible, Abraham's grandson, Jacob, was renamed Israel. His 12 sons and their descendants became known as the **children of Israel**. The term **Jew** is derived from Judah, one of Jacob's sons. **Hebrew** is the official language of the state of Israel and is used for religious prayers by all Jews wherever they live. "Thus today, the people are called Jewish, their faith Judaism, their language Hebrew, and their land Israel" (Donin, 1972, p. 7).

Judaism is both a religion and a culture. The religion is practiced along a wide continuum that ranges from liberal **Reform**, 31 percent; to **Conservative**, 33 percent; to strict **Orthodox**; 8 percent; to **Reconstructionism**, 2 percent. Only 53 percent belong to a synogague (American Jewish Committee, 2006). Although **Reform** Jews might not engage in any special daily practices, they still observe holidays, religious rites, and selected dietary or cultural customs. The traditional **Orthodox** Jew attempts to adhere to most of the religious laws. **Ultra-Orthodox** groups also exist. No caste system or social hierarchy exists within the Jewish community. However, instances occur within the ultra-Orthodox communities when individuals cannot make decisions without consulting their rabbis.

A significant issue within Orthodox communities in Israel, frequently debated in America is, "Who is a Jew?" A child born to a Jewish mother is Jewish. As mixed marriages have increased, the debate over patrilineal descent has ensued. A child born from the union of a Jewish father and a non-Jewish mother is recognized as Jewish by those in the Reform movement but not by those in the Orthodox movement. Although Judaism does not actively proselytize, the vast majority welcome converts as full members of their community. Clergy offer preconversion classes for adults and perform conversions.

Whereas the goal of this chapter is to provide an understanding of all Jewish Americans, the focus is on the needs of the more-traditional religious individuals and their families. These descriptions may vary somewhat for Jewish people according to the primary and secondary characteristics of culture (see Chapter 1) and the other parts of the world in which they inhabit.

HERITAGE AND RESIDENCE

The initial group of 23 Jews in North America arrrived in 1624, having fled the Office of the Inquisition in Brazil. Their numbers grew as a result of European immigrations to between 1000 and 2500 individuals by the time of the American Revolution, when many fought for the colonial army (Haim Solomon, a banker, raised significant funds in Europe and the colonies and dedicated all his personal resources and finances to George Washington's army). Their numbers reached aproximately 250,000 by the 1880s, close to 6 million a century later, and finally stabilized by 2002. Greater than half currently live in the Northeast, primarily in New York and New Jersey, and the Southeast, mainly in Florida (Wertheimer, 2002). Although many prefer to live in or within reach of large Jewish communities in order to have access to specific services, Jews make their homes in rural as well as urban centers in the United States.

REASONS FOR MIGRATION AND ASSOCIATED ECONOMIC FACTORS

Migration of Jews from Europe began to increase in the mid-1800s, often because of the fear of religious persecution. However, the greatest influx of immigrants occurred between 1880 and 1920. Many of these immigrants came from Russia and Eastern Europe after a wave of **pogroms**, anti-Jewish riots and murders (Jewish American Committee, 2006). Once in America, acculturation became their motivation to live safely and practice their religion.

Most Jewish families in America today are descendants of these Eastern European and Russian immigrants. They are referred to as **Ashkenazi** Jews. Ashkenazi Jews make up 82 percent of the world's Jewish population (Haumann, 2002). Many American Jews of Ashkenazi descent have stories of how some members of their families escaped to America, whereas others had relatives who were part of more than the six million Jews killed in the pogroms and the Holocaust. **Sephardic** Jews, conversely, are originally from Spain, Portugal, the Mediterranean area, and North Africa. They represent a more diverse group. A *Sabra* is a Jew who was born in Israel.

In the 1980s and 1990s, a significant increase occurred in the number of Jewish immigrants from Russia. Because the practice of religion was illegal there for over half a century, these Jews often have a relatively relaxed connection to religious and cultural practices. The same was true of the Falasha Jewish community in 1984. These black Jews from Ethiopia participated in a mass exodus to Israel, and subsequently, a small number continued on to America.

EDUCATIONAL STATUS AND OCCUPATIONS

Despite bias against Jews in every century, they have made major contributions to society, across the arts and professions, including the fine arts, sciences, and health care. Throughout their history, they have placed a major emphasis on education and social justice through social action.

Continued learning is one of the most respected values of the Jewish people, who are often called the *People of the Book* (Robinson, 2000). Whereas this usually refers to the study of **Torah**, it includes both Jewish and secular learning. Formal education is highly valued, and advanced degrees are respected. Overall, this population is well educated. Jews have won 39 percent of the Nobel Prizes in the life sciences, 11 percent in chemistry, and 41 percent in physics (Haumann, 2002). Well-known composers of Jewish ancestry include George Gershwin and Aaron Copland; the American theater counts Arthur Miller as one of its most celebrated of playwrights. The 20th century finally saw the first Jewish Supreme Court Justices in Louis Brandeis and, most recently, Ruth Ginzberg.

Because of their emphasis on education, a high percentage of Jewish Americans have succeeded in science, medicine, law, and dentistry. Thirty-nine percent of Jewish men and over 36 percent of Jewish women list their occupation as professional, compared with only 15 percent of the American white population. With respect to higher education, over 10 percent of professors in American colleges and universities are Jewish (Jewish American Committee, 2006). Their traditional values of study and preserving life have contributed to directing many into the life sciences, medicine, and research.

Throughout their history, Jews were repeatedly forbidden to own land, and the Christian Church barred its members from moneylending. As a result, since the early Middle Ages, Jews frequently became moneylenders, peddlers, and tailors because these were the only options available to them. The early Jews in America were businessmen and craftsmen (Center for Jewish History, 2007). They became well respected for their expertise in trade and commerce. Today, one-quarter of Jewish men are in retail sales.

Their emphasis on social action, volunteerism, and involvement in helping others are common vocations or avocations. The term *tzedakah* (justice) is used to indicate charity, a central concept to Judaism. Jewish children are raised with the concept of giving *tzedakah* by sharing with others who have less than they do.

Communication

DOMINANT LANGUAGE AND DIALECTS

English is the primary language of Jewish Americans. Although Hebrew is the official language of Israel and is used for prayers, it is generally not used for conversation in the United States.

Many older Ashkenazi Jews who immigrated early in the 20th century or who are first-generation Americans speak **Yiddish**, a Judeo-German dialect. Many Yiddish terms have worked their way into the English language, including *kvetch* (to complain); *chutzpah* (clever audacity); *bagel* (a boiled roll with a hole in the middle); *challah* (a rich, braided white bread); *knish* (a dumpling with filling); *nosh* (a [or to] snack); *zaftig* (plump); *tush, tushie,* or *tuchus* (buttocks); *ghetto* (a restricted area in which certain groups live); *klutz* (a clumsy person); *mentsch* or *mensh* (a respected person with dignity); *shlep* (to drag or carry); *kosher* (legal or okay); and *oy* or *oy vey* (oh my), and *oy veys mier* (woe is me).

Common Hebrew expressions include *l'chaim* (to life), which is said after blessing wine; *shalom alechem* (peace be with you) a traditional salutation; *mazel tov* (congratulations) and *shabbat shalom* (a good and peaceful Sabbath) which are said from Friday evening at sunset until Saturday at sunset.

CULTURAL COMMUNICATION PATTERNS

No religious ban or ethnic characteristics prevent Jews from openly expressing their feelings. Communication practices are more related to their American upbringing than to their religious practices.

Humor is frequently used as a coping mechanism and as a way to communicate with others. However, jokes are considered to be insensitive when they reinforce mainstream stereotypes about Jews, such as implying that Jews are cheap or pampered (e.g., Jewish American Princess). Any jokes that refer to the Holocaust or concentration camps are also inappropriate. Jewish self-criticism through humor is acceptable, but is usually expressed "in-house."

Modesty is a primary value in Orthodox Judaism. It is seen in the style of dress and in all behavior. Modesty involves humility. Jews are encouraged not to "show off" or try to impress others.

Hasidic Jewish men are not permitted to touch a woman other than their wives. They often keep their hands in their pockets to avoid touch. They do not shake hands with women, and their failure to do so when one's hand is extended should not be interpreted as a sign of rudeness. Because women are considered seductive, Hasidic men may not engage in idle talk with them nor look directly at their faces. Non-Hasidic Jews may be much more informal and may use touch and short spatial distance when communicating. Health-care providers should touch Hasidic men only when providing direct care. "Therapeutic touch" is not appropriate with these clients.

TEMPORAL RELATIONSHIPS

Jews live with regard for and in the present, conscious of being a part of a long historical tradition, and with both hope and a wary eye to the future. The last 2 millenia have seen a sucession of struggles to survive external pressures, yet the tradition affirms their belief in survival and a better time to come. They are raised with stories of their past, including the relatively recent Holocaust. They are warned to "never forget," lest history be repeated. Therefore, their time orientation is simultaneously to the past, the present, and the future.

The Jewish calendar is based on both a lunar and a solar year, with each month beginning with the appearance of the new moon. The festivals and holidays are based on lunar phases, whereas the seasons are based on the solar year, which is 11 days longer than the lunar year. Therefore, an extra month is periodically added.

FORMAT FOR NAMES

For secular use, the Jewish format for names follows the Western tradition. The given name comes first, followed by the family surname. Only the given name is used with friends and in informal situations. In more formal situations, the surname is preceded by the appropriate title of Mr., Miss, Ms., Mrs., and the like.

Babies may be named after someone who has died, to keep their memory alive, or after a living person, to honor them. The format chosen largely depends on whether the family is of Ashkenazi or Sephardic heritage. In ultra-Orthodox circles, children are not referred to by their names until after the *bris* or *brit milah* (circumcision). The biblical traditions are preserved for religious occasions. Infants are given a Hebrew name that is used when they are older and are called to read from the Torah. An example would be Josef ben Ezra (Joseph, son of Ezra). Although one's Hebrew name may be the same as one's birth certificate "official" name, parents may choose a non-Hebrew, main-culture name for the birth certificate that is entirely different or one that preserves the initial letter (i.e., *Ezra* could become *Edward*).

Family Roles and Organization

HEAD OF HOUSEHOLD AND GENDER ROLES

The family is the core of Jewish society, and whereas the man is traditionally considered the breadwinner for the household, and the woman is recognized for running the home and being responsible for the children, in recent times, there is more flexibility for gender roles, even in very observant homes. According to Jewish law, the father has the legal obligation to educate his children in Judaism, to teach them right from wrong, to teach them to swim, and to teach his sons a trade (Robinson, 2000). He must provide his daughters with the means to make them marriageable. With acculturation, little difference is seen today between Jewish and non-Jewish white families with regard to gender roles. In most Jewish families, both parents share the responsibilities for supporting the home and raising the children.

According to the Talmud, Jewish husbands are required to provide their wives with food, clothing, medical care, and conjugal relations, in addition to meeting other needs. They are prohibited from "beating their wives, forcing them to have sex, or restricting their free movement" (Robinson, 2000, p. 161).

Although traditional Jewish law is clearly male-oriented, Jewish women have been at the forefront of activities to demand and protect all human rights, especially those of women. They were prominent in movements to gain women's suffrage, reproductive health-care rights, and equal rights for all segments of society. Women are now expected to achieve an optimal level of education and to seek gainful employment if they so desire. Both sexes are expected to give service to their community.

PRESCRIPTIVE, RESTRICTIVE, AND TABOO BEHAVIORS FOR CHILDREN AND ADOLESCENTS

Children are the most valued treasure of the Jewish people. They are considered a blessing and are to be treated with respect and provided with love. Jewish children are to be afforded an education, not only in studies that help them progress in society but also in studies that transmit their Jewish heritage and the laws. Jewish school-age children typically attend Hebrew school as least two afternoons a week after public school throughout the school year. Children are welcomed and incorporated into most holiday celebrations and services.

Respecting and honoring one's parents is the fifth of the Ten Commandments. Children should be forever grateful to their parents for giving them the gift of life. Jewish parents are expected to be consistent and fair to all their children, avoiding favoritism. In addition, parents should not promise something to their children that they cannot deliver. They must be flexible and yet caring and attentive to discipline. The individuality of each child's special traits should be recognized (Amsel, 1994).

In Judaism, the age of religious majority is 13 years for a boy and 12 years for a girl. At this age, children are deemed capable of differentiating right from wrong and capable of committing themselves to performing the commandments (Amsel, 1994). Recognition of religious adulthood and assumption of its responsibilities occurs during a religious ceremony called a *bar* or *bat mitzvah* (son or daughter of the commandment). In America, this rite of passage is usually accompanied by a family celebration. However, because sons and daughters are still teenagers living at home, it is recognized that they are still the responsibility of their parents.

FAMILY GOALS AND PRIORITIES

The goal of the Orthodox family is to live their lives as prescribed by *halakhah*, which emphasizes maintaining health, promoting education, and helping others. In addition, "each person must find those qualities and characteristics that make him or her unique and then he or she must attempt to maximize potential by fully developing those qualities" (Amsel, 1994, p. 234). The family is central to Jewish life and essential to the continuation of Judaism from one generation to the next.

Marriage is considered the ideal human state for adults. The Bible states that man should not be alone. The two goals of this union are to procreate and provide companionship (Kolatch, 2000), allowing an individual to focus on another person. Marriages are monogamous, and limitations on whom one may marry exclude close blood relatives.

Sexuality is a right of both men and women. In addition to procreation requirements, conjugal rights for women exist. Nonprocreative intercourse is required for married women who may be pregnant or are unable to conceive, and this is not considered as "wasting seed" (Kolatch, 2000). Sexual intercourse is viewed as a pure and holy act when performed mutually within the relationship of marriage. With some exceptions, a husband's refusal to have sex with his wife is grounds for a divorce (Robinson, 2000). However, the act of sex, if performed in the wrong context, is considered disgusting and against Jewish values (Amsel, 1994). Premarital sex is not condoned.

Among the ultra-observant, women must physically separate themselves from all men during their menstrual periods and for 7 days after (Robinson, 2000). No man may touch a woman nor sit where she sat until she has been to the *mikveh*, a ritual bath, after her period is over. Sexual contact for this group may, therefore, occur only during 2 weeks of each month.

Judaism supports the need for sex education. The Jewish community sees this as its responsibility. This belief has been re-emphasized during the AIDS epidemic, with the goals of protecting the next generation and providing them with accurate information so they can make informed choices.

Whereas it is recognized that the later years are a time of physical decline, older people receive respect, especially for the wisdom they have to share. The Talmud defines older people as those who have reached their 61st birthday (Robinson, 2000). Old age is a state of mind rather than a chronological age; one may continue to "give" to society in a variety of ways other than employment. In addition, one may never "retire" from practicing the commandments.

Honoring one's parents is a lifelong endeavor and includes maintaining their dignity by feeding, clothing, and sheltering them, even if they suffer from senility. Respect for older people is essential even when their actions are irrational. The care of an older family member is the responsibility of the family; when the family is unable to provide care owing to physical, psychological, or financial reasons, the responsibility falls to the community. This role has always been a hallmark of Jewish communal life (Robinson, 2000). A number of older Jewish people move to Florida or other warm states after retirement because the weather there is more conducive to maintaining their health and safety. Of noninstitutionalized older adults, one-third live alone.

Few Jewish American families now have three generations living together. Older immigrants who experienced imprisonment in concentration camps during the Holocaust in the 1940s, or those more recently incarcerated in Russia, may refuse to enter long-term-care facilities for fear of returning to an institutional environment that robs them of their freedom (Martha Braverman, personal communication, February 4, 2007).

ALTERNATIVE LIFESTYLES

The Jewish view on homosexuality varies with the branch of Judaism. As might be expected, the Orthodox are largely unanimous in scripture-based (Lev. 18:22) nonacceptance of same-sex unions. The Bible, especially as interpreted by the Orthodox, prohibits homosexual intercourse (Kolatch, 2000); it says nothing specifically about sex between lesbians (Dorff, 1998). Some of the objections to gay and lesbian lifestyles include the inability of these unions to fulfill the commandment of procreation and the possibility that acting on the recognition of one's homosexuality could ruin a marriage. The official position of the Conservative movement had sided with the Orthodox until as recently as 2006, when it revised its position to increase inclusivity of views within Jewish philosophy. This implies allowing ordination of gay and lesbian clergy, although not recognizing same-sex marriage. The liberal movement within Judaism, however, supports "full legal and social equality for homosexuals" (Washofsky, 2000, p. 320).

Workforce Issues

VIGNETTE 16.1

Lisa H., a registered nurse, has worked triage in the Emergency Department in a regional midwestern hospital for 12 years. Originally from New Jersey, she was a nonpracticing Jew until her late 20s. Now, approaching 40, she has become increasingly committed to religious observance. She keeps kosher at home, bringing her own food to staff lunch meetings. She has been able to use vacation time for the major High Holy Days, but would like to be **shomer shabbos** (follow strict sabbath observance) and has requested a permanent schedule change from her supervisor, with a written explanation attached, to reflect her need to not work any Friday afternoon through

Saturday evening. The supervisor refused her, saying it would not be fair to the other nurses, that Lisa should also try to "fit in more—be part of the team," as the others perceived her as "standoffish." When Lisa said it was a religious requirement for her, the supervisor said maybe she should ". . . consider going back to New York where she'd be more comfortable."

1. How do you feel about Lisa's request?
2. How might this request be honored?
3. Was the supervisor culturally competent in this situation?
4. If Lisa were to discuss the issue at a team meeting, how could she present her concerns?

CULTURE IN THE WORKPLACE

Specific workforce issues may occur, especially with Sabbath observance. Jews who observe the Sabbath must have Friday evening and Saturday off. They may work on Sundays. Supervisors must be sensitive to the needs of Jewish staff and recognize the holiness of the Sabbath. Jewish staff should be allowed to request time off for the major Jewish holidays. Remembering that all holidays begin the evening before, they must have off the evening shift before and the following day. Staff should not be penalized by having to use this time off as unpaid holidays or vacation time, but they should have the option to exchange for the Christmas and Easter holidays, time usually afforded to Christian staff.

Jewish health-care providers are fully acculturated into the American workforce. Judaism's beliefs are congruent with the values American society places on the individual and family. As English is the primary language for Jewish Americans, no language barriers to communicating in the workplace exist. For some newer Jewish immigrants (e.g., those from Russia), English may pose a challenge.

ISSUES RELATED TO AUTONOMY

Jewish nurses have begun to speak out on their needs in the workplace. With the recent emphasis on cultural competence, including cultural sensitivity, many are now addressing this long-ignored area. In 1990, a National Nurses Council was established through Hadassah, the Zionist women's organization (Benson, 1994). This group promotes solidarity and empowerment to enhance sensitivity within the health-care community. Still proportionally under-represented among American nurses, Jewish nurses have a disproportionate percentage of advanced degrees and positions in management, education, and research (Benson, 2001). Ways in which the professional nursing community demonstrates its insensitivity to Jewish nurses are by scheduling major nursing conferences during the High Holy Days in the fall or during Passover in the spring or by serving pork products during catered affairs.

Biocultural Ecology

SKIN COLOR AND OTHER BIOLOGICAL VARIATIONS

Ashkenazi Jews have the same skin coloring as white Americans. They may range from fair skin and blonde hair to darker skin and brunette hair. Sephardic Jews have slightly darker skin tones and hair coloring, similar to those from the Mediterranean area and those who lived for centuries in nearby regions such as Yemen. There are also Jewish groups throughout Africa who are black, most notably, the Jews originally from Ethiopia, known as *Falasha*.

DISEASES AND HEALTH CONDITIONS

Because Jews are integrated throughout the United States, no specific risk factors are based on topography. Genetic risk factors vary based on whether the family immigrated from Ashkenazi or Sephardic areas. There is a greater incidence of some genetic disorders among individuals of Jewish descent, especially those who are Ashkenazi. Most of these disorders are autosomal recessive, meaning that both parents carry the affected gene. Although the best known is Tay-Sachs disease, Gaucher's disease is more prevalent. Others include Canavan's disease, familial dysautonomia, torsion dystonia, Niemann-Pick disease, Bloom syndrome, Fanconi's anemia, and mucolipidosis IV (Center for Jewish Genetic Diseases, 2007).

Gaucher's disease is the most common genetic disease affecting Ashkenazi Jews, with 1 in 10 carrying the gene (Center for Jewish Genetic Diseases, 2007). Gaucher's disease is a lipid-storage disorder. This inborn error of metabolism results in a defective enzyme that normally breaks down glucocerebroside, a lipid by-product of erythrocytes. The glucocerebroside accumulates in the body, resulting in weakening and fracturing of the bones owing to infarctions, anemia, and platelet deficiencies. There are 34 different genetic mutations of the disease; 4 of them account for 95 percent of cases in Ashkenazi Jews. The disorder can be detected by a blood test for both those affected and carriers. Gene therapy treatments are now being tested (National Gaucher Foundation, 2001).

The gene for Tay-Sachs disease (also called *infantile cerebromacular degeneration*) is carried by 1 in 27 Ashkenazi Jews and 1 in 250 Jews of Sephardic origin. This autosomal recessive condition is a lysosomal sphingolipid storage disorder caused by an absence of hexosaminidase A, resulting in an accumulation of a lipid called *GM2 ganglioside* in the neural cells. The onset of mental and developmental retardation begins in the middle of the first year of life, with progressive deterioration, increasing seizure activity, and death by approximately age 5 (Center for Jewish Genetic Diseases, 2007). Because of the ease of testing for carriers as well as testing the fetus during pregnancy, and because of a concerted effort among the Jewish American community to provide testing, the incidence of Tay-Sachs disease has decreased significantly since the early 1980s. Because the ultra-Orthodox are opposed to abortion, this group recommends the testing only before marriage (Washofsky, 2000). It should be noted that because there are 50 different mutations, testing can identify 95 percent of carriers with a Jewish background and 60 percent of non-Jewish individuals (Center for Jewish Genetic Diseases, 2007).

Canavan's disease is a rare, fatal, degenerative brain disease caused by a defective gene that impairs the formation of myelin. Approximately 1 in 40 Ashkenazi Jews carry the gene. The resulting symptoms begin in midinfancy and include developmental delay, loss of vision, and a loss of reflexes resulting in death by the age of 10 years (Center for Jewish Genetic Diseases, 2007).

Familial dysautonomia, or Riley-Day syndrome, is also an autosomal recessive genetic disease, with the gene located on chromosome 9q31. It causes dysfunction of the autonomic and peripheral sensory nervous systems. Affected children have decreased myelinated fibers on nerves that lead to afferent impulses but maintain a normal intelligence. Symptoms include a decrease in the number of taste buds; altered pain sensation; increased salivation and sweating; abnormal sucking or swallowing difficulties and vomiting, resulting in failure to thrive; decreased tears, resulting in increased risk of corneal ulceration; and temperature and blood pressure fluctuations. Fifty percent live to the age of 30. One in 30 Ashkenazi Jews is a carrier (Center for Jewish Genetic Diseases, 2007).

Other autosomal recessive conditions also have a higher incidence among Ashkenazi Jews. The gene for torsion dystonia is carried by 1 in 70 Ashkenazi Jews in the United States. The disease leads to rapid progression in loss of motor control and twisting spasms of the limbs. Affected individuals lead a full life and have a normal intelligence. Niemann-Pick disease type A is a severe neurodegenerative disorder that starts at 6 months of age. It involves an abnormal storage of sphingomyelin and cholesterol in organs caused by an enzyme deficiency and leads to central nervous system degeneration. Whereas those with type A usually die by age 3, those with type B survive into their 50s and have a milder presentation, with the sphingomyelin building up in their liver, spleen, lymph nodes, and brain.

Bloom syndrome, a rare genetic condition, involves increased risk of respiratory and gastrointestinal infections, erythema, telangiectasia, photosensitivity, and dwarfism. Whereas the intelligence of those affected is usually normal, they face an increased risk of infertility, malignancy, and diabetes. Fanconi's anemia results in pancytopenia and an increased risk of cancer. Many die before early adulthood. Type C is found more frequently among Ashkenazi Jews; 1 in 89 are carriers. Mucolipidosis IV is found in 1 of 100 Ashkenazi Jews. This lipid-storage disease results in central nervous system deterioration during the first year with motor and mental retardation as well as various eye disorders. The prognosis varies (Center for Jewish Genetic Diseases, 2007).

Orthodox rabbis usually do not support genetic testing because it might cause couples to "refrain from marrying or having children, thus preventing them from fulfilling the *mitzvah* of procreation" (Washofsky, 2000, p. 266). The Reform movement supports a couple's right to make the decision as to whether or not to have the testing done. "If we have the means by which to discover this information, so vital to the emotional and psychological well-being of a couple, then we must use them; failure to do so cannot be morally justified" (Washofsky, 2000, p. 267).

Other conditions occur with increased incidence in the Jewish population. Inflammatory bowel disease (ulcerative colitis and Crohn's disease) is seen four to five times more often in white Jews than in other white groups. Colorectal cancer appears to be seen with increased frequency in Ashkenazi Jews (6 percent) (American Cancer Society, 2001). Although the incidence of breast cancer among Jews is similar to that in other Caucasians, "three distinct mutations in the BRCA1 and BRCA2 genes, found in one out of every 40 Jewish women of Ashkenazic background, increase a woman's odds of getting breast and ovarian cancers" (Wyce, 2001, p. 20).

VARIATIONS IN DRUG METABOLISM

One of the few drugs found to have a higher rate of side effects in people of Ashkenazic ancestry is clozapine, used to treat schizophrenia. Twenty percent of Jewish clients taking this drug developed agranulocytosis, compared with about 1 percent of non-Jewish clients. A specific genetic haplotype has been identified to account for this finding (Levy, 1993). Thus, health-care providers must order testing for agranulocytosis when Jewish clients are prescribed clozapine.

High-Risk Behaviors

According to Jewish law, individuals may not intentionally damage their bodies or place themselves in danger. The basic philosophy is that the body must be protected from harm. To the religious, the body is viewed as belonging to God; therefore, it must be returned to Him intact when death occurs. Consequently, any substance or act that harms the body is not allowed. This includes smoking, suicide, taking nonprescription or illegal medications, and permanent tattooing (Washofsky, 2000).

Alcohol, especially wine, is an essential part of religious holidays and festive occasions and is a traditional symbol of joy. The Jewish attitude toward wine is ambivalent. The Bible speaks of the undesirable effects of wine on the person, as well as its positive use as a medicine. Consequently, wine is appropriate and acceptable as long as it is used in moderation.

HEALTH-CARE PRACTICES

Because of the respect afforded physicians and the emphasis on keeping the body and mind healthy, Jewish Americans are health conscious. In general, they practice preventive health care, with routine physical, dental, and vision screening. This is also a well-immunized population. Although the older generation is still more likely to defer to medical authority, Jewish adults tend to want to participate in health-care decision-making.

Nutrition

MEANING OF FOOD

Eating is important to Jews on many levels. Besides satisfying hunger and sustaining life, it also teaches discipline and reverence for life. For those who follow the dietary laws, a tremendous amount of attention is given to the slaughter, preparation, and consumption of food. In addition, the family dinner table is often the site for religious holiday celebrations and services, especially the Sabbath, Passover, Rosh Hashanah (Jewish New Year), and breaking the fast for Yom Kippur (Day of Atonement). Jewish dietary practices serve as a spiritually refining act of self-discipline and are a unifying factor in ethnic identity.

COMMON FOODS AND FOOD RITUALS

VIGNETTE 16.2

Anna Novack, a 90-year-old widow and Holocaust survivor from Poland, came to New York City after WW II; she worked in the garment district, marrying another survivor and raising a family in a strictly kosher household. Her diagnosis of "dementia" has progressed such that her youngest son, who lives nearby, has had to place her in the Alzheimer's unit of a long-term-care facility. She does not recognize him or anyone else during his weekly visits. Her son was shocked and angry today when he looked for her in the dining hall and found her eating breakfast sausage and drinking a carton of milk. Although the nursing home did not have a kosher kitchen, Mr. Novack had been assured by the staff that his mother's traditions would be respected. Deeply upset, he demanded an explanation. The health-care technician and nurse explained that, although her cultural preferences were known to the staff and they were aware of what she was eating, there were several factors that lead them to look the other way, especially in the last 6 months as her condition deteriorated. They reminded him that she seemed unable to distinguish kosher from nonkosher anymore. In addition, she had been slowly losing weight, so they were glad she was willing to eat.

1. What does it mean to be kosher?
2. What in Mrs. Kovack's meal violated kosher dietary laws?
3. Why was Mr. Novack so upset?
4. Did the staff act in the best interest of the patient?
5. Short of relocating Anna, what could be done by her son and the staff to remedy the situation?
6. Where might the long-term-care facility get kosher meals?

Perhaps the food identified as "Jewish" that receives the most attention is chicken soup. This has frequently been referred to as *Jewish penicillin*, and is often served with *knaidle balls* (dumplings made of matzoh meal). Although it has no intrinsic meaning or religious value, it is a staple in religious homes, especially on Friday evenings to usher in the Sabbath and during times of illness. It is frequently associated with a mother's warmth and love.

Other common foods include gefilte fish (ground freshwater fish molded into oblong balls, steamed, then served cold with horseradish), challah (a rich, braided white bread), kugel (noodle pudding), blintzes (crepes filled with a sweet cottage cheese), chopped liver (served cold), hamentashen (a triangular pastry with different types of filling), and lox or nova (cold smoked salmon) served with cream cheese and salad vegetables, on a bagel.

The laws regarding food are found in Leviticus and Deuteronomy. They are commonly referred to as the laws of **kashrut**, or the laws that dictate which foods are permissible under religious law. The term **kosher** means "fit to eat"; it is not a brand or form of cooking. Whereas some believe that the mandatory statutes were developed and implemented for health reasons, religious scholars dispute this view, claiming that the only reason for following the laws is that they are mandatory commandments of God. Therefore, the laws are followed as a personal attachment to the religion and as a belief that God has mandated them (Kolatch, 2000). The laws' promotion of health is only a secondary gain. Kashruth issues may be a significant part of an in-patient stay, making it helpful to know what is and is not acceptable.

Foods are divided into those considered kosher (permitted or clean) and those considered **treyf** (forbidden or unclean). A permitted animal may become *treyf*, or forbidden, if it is not slaughtered, cooked, or served properly. Because life is sacred and animal cruelty is forbidden, kosher slaughter of animals must be done in a way that prevents undue cruelty to the animal and ensures the animal's health for the consumer. The jugular vein, carotid arteries, and vagus nerve must be severed in a single quick stroke with a sharp, smooth knife, causing the animal to die instantly. No sawing motion and no second stroke are permitted (Robinson, 2000). This also allows the maximal amount of blood to leave the body. Care must be taken that all blood is drained from the animal before it is eaten. Drinking of blood is prohibited. An animal that dies from old age or disease may not be eaten, nor may it be eaten if it meets a violent death or is killed by another animal. In addition, flesh cut from a live creature may not be eaten.

Milk and meat may not be mixed together in cooking, serving, or eating in order to respect the sensitivity of living creatures (You must not boil a calf in its mother's milk [Deut. 14:20]). To avoid mixing foods, utensils and plates used to serve them are separated. Religious Jews who follow the dietary laws have two sets of dishes, pots, and utensils: one set for milk products (*milchig* in Yiddish) and the other for meat (*fleishig*). Because glass is not absorbent, it can be used for either meat or milk products, although religious households still usually have two sets (Kolatch, 2000). Therefore, cheeseburgers, lasagna made with meat, and grated cheese on meatballs and spaghetti are unacceptable. Milk cannot be used in coffee if it is served with a meat meal. Nondairy creamers can be used instead, as long as they do not contain sodium caseinate, which is derived from milk.

A number of foods are considered *parve* (neutral) and may be used with either dairy or meat dishes. These include fish, eggs, anything grown in the soil (vegetables, fruits, coffee, sugar, and spices), and chemically produced goods (Robinson, 2000). A "U" with a circle around it is the seal of the Union of Orthodox Jewish Congregations of America and is used on food products to indicate that they are kosher. A circled "K" and other symbols may also be found on packaging to indicate that a product is kosher.

When working in a Jewish person's home, the health-care provider should not bring food into the house without knowing whether or not the client adheres to kosher standards. If the client keeps a kosher home, do not use any cooking items, dishes, or silverware without knowing which are used for meat and which for dairy products. Health-care providers must fully understand the dietary laws so they do not offend the client, can advocate for kosher meals if they are requested, and can plan medication times accordingly.

Mammals are considered clean if they meet the other requirements for their slaughter and consumption and have split (cloven) hooves and chew their cud. These animals include buffalo, cattle, goat, deer, and sheep. The pig is an example of an animal that does not meet these criteria. Although liberal Jews decide for themselves which dietary laws they will follow, many still avoid pork and pork products out of a sense of tradition and symbolism. Serving pork products to a Jewish client, unless specifically requested, is insensitive.

Birds of prey are considered "unclean" and unacceptable because they grab their food with their claws. Acceptable poultry includes chicken, one of the most frequently consumed forms of protein, turkey, goose, and duck. Fish can be eaten if it has both fins and scales. Nothing that crawls on its belly is allowed, including clams, lobsters and other shellfish, tortoises, and frogs (Robinson, 2000).

In religious homes, meat is prepared for cooking by soaking and salting to drain all the blood from the flesh. As increased residual salt may result, clients with sodium restrictions may need counseling to assist them in making dietary adjustments. Broiling is acceptable, especially for liver, because it drains the blood (Robinson, 2000). Care must be taken in serving cheese to ensure that no animal substances are served at the same time. Breads and cakes made with lard are *treyf*, and breads made with milk or milk by-products (e.g., casein) cannot be served with meat meals. Eggs from nonkosher birds, milk from nonkosher animals, and oil from nonkosher fish are not permitted. Butter substitutes are used with meat meals. Honey is allowed.

Kosher meals are available in most hospitals. They arrive on paper plates and with sealed plastic utensils. Health-care providers should not unwrap the utensils or change the foodstuffs to another serving dish. Frozen kosher meals are available on a commercial basis. Help may be needed for a patient to choose from a facility's menu options. Neither a carton of milk nor one of yogurt should be included on a tray with meat, nor may butter accompany the bread. Even salad dressing needs to be made without dairy ingredients. If health-care providers have difficulty locating a supplier, they should contact a local rabbi. Determining a client's dietary preferences and practices regarding dietary laws should be done during the admission assessment.

DIETARY PRACTICES FOR HEALTH PROMOTION

As mentioned previously, although many Jewish dietary practices afford the secondary gain of preventing disease, their intention is not for health promotion, but rather for observance of a commandment. Many Jews understand the dietary laws as a guide to raising the act of eating to a spiritual level, which is also true of the practice of washing one's hands and praying before and after eating.

NUTRITIONAL DEFICIENCIES AND FOOD LIMITATIONS

No nutritional deficiencies are common to individuals of Jewish descent. As with any ethnic group, nutritional deficiencies may occur in individuals in lower socioeconomic groups because of the expense of certain foods.

In addition to the dietary laws discussed previously, other dietary laws are followed at specified times. For example, during the week of Passover, no bread or product with yeast may be eaten. Matzoh (unleavened bread) is eaten instead. Any product that is fermented or can cause fermentation may not be eaten (Kolatch, 2000). Rather than attend synagogue, the family conducts the service (*seder*) around the dinner table during the first 2 nights and incorporates dinner into a service that includes all participants in study, singing, and retelling the story of Moses and the Exodus from Egypt.

The Jewish calendar has a number of fast days. The most observed is the holiest day of the year, Yom Kippur. On this Day of Atonement, Jews abstain from food and drink as they pray to God for forgiveness for the sins they have committed during the past year. They eat an early dinner on the evening before the holiday begins, then fast until after sunset the following day. Ill people, older people, the young, pregnant or lactating mothers, and the physically incapacitated are absolved from fasting and may need to be reminded of this exception to Jewish law. Maintaining an ill person's health supersedes the act of fasting. If concerns arise, a consultation with the client's rabbi may be necessary.

Pregnancy and Childbearing Practices

FERTILITY PRACTICES AND VIEWS TOWARD PREGNANCY

God's first commandment to humanity is, "Be fruitful and multiply." Children are considered a gift and a duty, with men considered more important by the ultra-Orthodox because they can say **kaddish** (the prayer for the dead) for their parents. In other branches of Judaism, both sexes may recite the *kaddish*. Families are encouraged to have at least two children (Kolatch, 2000).

Couples who are unable to conceive should try all possible means to have children. This includes infertility counseling and interventions, comprising egg and sperm donation. "Orthodox opinion is virtually unanimous in prohibiting . . . artificial insemination when the semen donor is a man other than the woman's husband" (Washofsky, 2000, p. 234). Some Orthodox Jews view this as adultery, whereas others argue that it cannot be considered adultery if no sexual intercourse has occurred. When all natural attempts have been made, adoption may be pursued. Having children allows religious parents to fulfill many of the commandments.

The lower number of pregnancies occurring among Jewish Americans and the high intermarriage rate have resulted in a decreased Jewish population. By age 45, Jewish women averaged 1.6 children compared with 2.1

children born to non-Jewish white women in the same age range. Because one-third of all Jews were killed during the Holocaust, some believe that today's Jews "have a special moral obligation to bring one more child into the world than they would have normally" (Amsel, 1994, p. 314).

Prevention of pregnancy in the more Orthodox view implies deferring the commandment to be fruitful and multiply. Unless pregnancy jeopardizes the life or health of the mother, contraception is not looked on favorably among the ultra-Orthodox. Liberal Judaism recognizes that children have the right to be wanted and that they should be born into homes in which their needs can be met. Therefore, the use of temporary birth control may be acceptable. Condom use is supported, especially if unprotected sexual intercourse would pose a medical risk to either spouse.

To the Orthodox, it is important to know the mechanism of action of the birth control. Coitus interruptus and masturbation are not acceptable because they result in the needless expenditure of semen, although most Jews consider the former practice a normal, healthy activity (Kolatch, 2000). Barrier techniques are not acceptable because they interfere with the full mobility of the sperm in its natural course. The birth control pill does not result in any permanent sterilization, nor does it prevent semen from traveling its normal route. Therefore, use of this method is the least objectionable to most branches of Judaism. "Today, almost all rabbinic authorities permit the use of contraceptive devices . . . in cases where pregnancy may imperil the life of the mother or where it is certain that the newborn might be afflicted with a serious congenital disease or abnormality" (Kolatch, 2000, p. 153). Sterilization implies permanence, and Orthodox Jews generally oppose this practice, unless the life of the mother is in danger. Reform Judaism leaves the choice of what to use and whether to use contraceptives up to the parents.

Recognizing that Judaism's primary focus is the sanctity of life, it is important to identify when life begins. The fetus is not considered a living soul or person until it has been born. Birth is determined when the head or "greater part" is born (Robinson, 2000). Until that time, it is merely part of the mother's body and has no independent identity.

The mother and her health are paramount. If her physical or mental health is endangered by the fetus, all branches of Judaism see the fetus as an aggressor and require an abortion (Kolatch, 2000). Whereas saving the mother's life is certainly grounds for abortion, random abortion is not permitted by the Orthodox branch because the fetus is part of the mother's body and one must not do harm to one's body.

Reform Judaism believes that a woman maintains control over her own body and it is up to her whether to abort a fetus. Although no connotation of sin is attached to abortion, the decision is not to be made without serious deliberation. Most Jews favor a woman's right to choose regarding abortion.

PRESCRIPTIVE, RESTRICTIVE, AND TABOO PRACTICES IN THE CHILDBEARING FAMILY

A Hasidic husband may not touch his wife during labor and may choose not to attend the delivery, because by Jewish law he is not permitted to view his wife's genitals.

These behaviors should never be interpreted as insensitivity on the part of the husband. During the delivery of a child to an ultra-Orthodox family, these interventions should be initiated: The mother should be given hospital gowns that cover her in the front and back to the greatest extent possible. She may prefer to wear a surgical cap so that her hair remains covered. The father should be given the opportunity to leave during procedures and during the birth, or if he chooses to stay, the mother can be draped so that the husband may sit by his wife without viewing her perineum, including by way of mirrors, in order to protect her dignity. Because he is not permitted to touch his wife, he may offer only verbal support. The female nurse may need to provide all of the physical care. Pain medication during delivery is acceptable.

For male infants, circumcision, which is both a medical procedure and a religious rite, is performed. The origin of this ritual dates back to Abraham and Isaac in the Book of Genesis. A *brit milah* (sometimes referred to as a *bris*) symbolizes the covenant made between the Jewish people and God (Lau, 1997). The procedure itself and the accompanying ceremony are performed on the 8th day of life by person called a *mohel*, an individual trained in the circumcision procedure, asepsis, and the religious ceremony. Although a rabbi is not necessary, it is also possible to have the procedure done by a physician with a rabbi present to say the blessings. Jewish parents who are not very observant and/or are unaffiliated may still opt for medical circumcision, illustrating how the power of this ritual endures over thousands of years.

Attending a *brit milah* is the only mitzvah for which religious Jews must violate the Sabbath, so that the *brit* can be completed at the proper time (Robinson, 2000). The *brit milah* is a family festivity, and many relatives are invited. In most cases today, the ceremony is performed in the home; however, if the child is still in the hospital, it is important for the hospital to provide a room for a small private party to celebrate. Whereas the medical community sometimes debates the practice of circumcision, to even suggest to Jewish parents that the practice is "barbaric" is insensitive.

A circumcision may be delayed for medical reasons, including unstable condition owing to prematurity, life-threatening concerns during the early weeks after birth, bleeding problems, or a defect of the penis, which may require later surgery. At birth, a child is free of all sin; failure to circumcise carries no eternal consequences should the child die.

Although there is no rule against designating godparents for a newborn, it is considered local, not traditional, custom.

Death Rituals

VIGNETTE 16.3

Mercedes Colon, RN, came from a small city in Colombia. Two months into her new career at a large pediatric hospital, she continues adjusting to life and work in the United States.

Although her English comprehension is good, she still has trouble expressing herself. Mercedes has felt very close to the Kaplans, whose only child, 3-year-old David, is being treated for acute lymphocytic leukemia. The staff was optimistic, based on his excellent response so far. David's mother said just yesterday that she "... used to hope he'd become a doctor or university professor, but now I'm just happy for him to grow into a happy, healthy adult." Unfortunately, just as Mercedes came on shift this morning, the child coded and died. Mercedes' manager told her to stay with the Kaplans until the pastoral care department could send someone, and to "prepare them" as they might be asked to sign for an autopsy. Mercedes looks in to see the Kaplans sitting on opposite sides of David's bed, staring without expression. Mercedes doesn't know what to do.

1. What could Mercedes do and say to help the parents?
2. When should she begin asking them questions?
3. Mercedes was recently oriented on autopsy protocol for Jews. How might she relay this information to the Kaplans?
4. What resources might this nurse use to help the family?

DEATH RITUALS AND EXPECTATIONS

Death is an expected part of the life cycle. Yet, each day is to be appreciated and lived as fully as possible. Religious Jews start each day with a prayer of appreciation for having lived another day. The goal is to appreciate things and people while one still has them. Brain death as a criteria for organ donation remains controversial, with some sects agreeing to this criteria while others do not (Beitowitz, 2006). Many also accept a flat electroencephalogram (EEG) as determining death. Traditional Judaism believes in an afterlife in which the soul continues to flourish, although many dispute this interpretation because it is not mentioned in the Torah (Beitowitz, 2006). Most Jews do not dwell much on life after death and are unconcerned about it; their focus is on how to conduct one's present life.

Active euthanasia, in which something is given or done to result in death, is forbidden for religious Jews. One of the Ten Commandments is "Thou shalt not kill," and euthanasia is considered murder. A dying person is considered a living person in all respects. Sufficient pain control should be provided, even if it decreases the person's level of consciousness (Beitowitz, 2006). Withholding food from a deformed child to speed its death is considered active euthanasia and is forbidden.

Passive euthanasia may be allowed, depending on its interpretation. Nothing may be used or initiated that prevents a person from dying naturally or that prolongs the dying process. Therefore, anything that artificially prevents death (e.g., cardiopulmonary resuscitation, use of ventilators) may possibly be withheld, depending on the wishes of the patient and his or her religious views. Regardless of the decisions made, pain control must be maintained.

Taking one's own life is prohibited and is viewed as a criminal act and morally wrong because it is forbidden to harm any human being, including oneself. To the ultra-religious, suicide removes all possibility of repentance.

Adult Jews who commit suicide, who are not insane or depressed, and who belong to ultra-religious factions of Judaism are not afforded full burial honors. They are buried on the periphery of the Jewish cemetery and mourning rites are not observed, unless the individual was not mentally competent. However, the more-liberal view is to emphasize the needs of the survivors, and all burial and mourning activities proceed according to the usual traditional rites and wishes of the family. Children are never considered to have intentionally killed themselves and are afforded all burial rights.

The dying person should not be left alone. It is considered respectful to stay with a dying person, unless the visitor is physically ill or their emotions are out of control (Lamm, 2000). Judaism does not have any ceremony similar to the Catholic sacrament of the sick. Any Jew may ask God's forgiveness for her or his sins; no confessor is needed. However, it is not commonly known that Jews have a personal confession called **Viddui**, which is recited when death is imminent. It may be said by the dying person or by somebody for her or him. Some Jews feel solace in saying the *Shema* in Hebrew or English. This prayer confirms one's belief in one God. At the time of death, the nearest relative can gently close the eyes and mouth; the face is covered with a sheet. The body is treated with respect and revered for the function it once filled. Health-care providers may need to ask the closest relative of the deceased specifically about the practices to follow after death. Health-care providers who have acquired some familiarity with Jewish attitudes and practices associated with death go a long way toward helping their patients and families. They are performing *mitzvot* (good deeds) with their informed presence that will continue to benefit all involved as the long process of integrating loss into their lives continues.

Ultra-Orthodox Jews follow a ritual that is not conducive to hospital protocols and is more commonly observed for those who die at home. After the body is wrapped, it is briefly placed on the floor with the feet pointing toward the door. A candle may be placed near the head. However, this does not occur on the Sabbath or holy days. The dead body is not left alone before the funeral, so as not to leave it defenseless.

Autopsy is usually not permitted among religious Jews because it results in desecration of the body, and it is important that the body be interred whole. Allowing an autopsy might also delay the burial, something that is not recommended. Conversely, autopsy is allowed if its results would save the life of another patient. Many branches of Judaism currently allow an autopsy if (1) it is required by law; (2) the deceased person has willed it; or (3) it saves the life of another, especially an offspring (Dorff, 1998). The body must be treated with respect during the autopsy.

Any attempt to hasten or retard decomposition of the body is discouraged. Cremation is prohibited because it unnaturally speeds the disposal of the dead body. Embalming is prohibited because it preserves the dead (Lamm, 2000). However, in circumstances in which the funeral must be delayed, some embalming may be approved. Cosmetic restoration for the funeral is discouraged.

Jewish funerals and burials follow certain practices; they usually occur within 24 to 48 hours after the death.

The funeral service is directed at honoring the departed by speaking only well of him or her. Flowers either at the funeral or at the cemetery are not the usual; this was a Christian custom used to offset the odor of decaying bodies. The casket should be made of wood with no ornamentation. The body may be wrapped only in a shroud to ensure that the body and casket decay at the same rate. A wake or viewing is not part of a Jewish funeral. The prayer said for the dead, *kaddish*, is usually not said alone, but is recited in and with the company of others. The prayer says nothing about death, but rather, it praises God and reaffirms one's own faith. A funeral according to *halachah* (Jewish law) emphasizes that death is death. Realism and simplicity are the characteristics of the Jewish burial.

After the funeral, mourners are welcomed at the home of the closest relative. Water to wash one's hands before entering is outside the front door, symbolic of cleansing the impurities associated with contact with the dead. The water is not passed from person to person, just as it is hoped that the tragedy is not passed. At the home, a meal is served to all the guests. This "meal of condolence" or "meal of consolation" is traditionally provided by the neighbors and friends; it frequently includes hard-boiled eggs.

Shiva (Hebrew for "seven") is the 7-day period that begins with the burial. *Shiva* helps the surviving individuals face the actuality of the death of the loved one. During this period when the mourners are "sitting *shiva*," they do not work. When health-care providers are the ones experiencing the loss, it is important for supervisors to understand the mourning customs. In some homes, mirrors are covered to decrease the focus on one's appearance; no activity is permitted to divert attention from thinking about the deceased; and evening and morning services may be conducted in the closest relative's home. Condolence calls and the giving of consolation are appropriate during this time.

After *shiva*, the mourning period varies based on who has died. Mourning for a relative lasts 30 days, and for a parent, 1 year. Judaism does not support prolonged mourning. A tombstone is erected within 1 year of the death, at which time, a graveside service is held. This is called an *unveiling*. According to the Jewish calendar, the anniversary of the death is called *yahrzeit*, and at this time, candles are lit and the *kaddish* is said.

Understanding some specific practices related to death and dying may have an impact on other aspects of health care, including the death of premature infants and the care of amputated limbs. Mourning is not required for a fetus that is miscarried or stillborn. This is also true of any premature infant who dies within 30 days of birth. However, parents are required to mourn for full-term infants who die at birth or shortly thereafter (Washofsky, 2000). Although the baby should be named, not all of the traditional burial customs are followed.

Within Orthodoxy, when a limb is amputated before death, the amputated limb and blood-soaked clothing are buried in the person's future gravesite. This custom might not be practiced by recent Russian immigrant Jews because they were not allowed to practice their faith under Communism and, therefore, lost many of the traditional practices. Because the blood and limb were part of the person, they are buried with the person. No mourning rites are required. In the case of an amputation, the health-care provider may need to assist with arrangement for burial of the body part.

RESPONSES TO DEATH AND GRIEF

The period following a death has discrete segments to assist mourners in their adjustment to the loss. The period of time between the death and the burial is short, and is the time for the emotional reaction to the death. The burial may be delayed only if required by law, if relatives must travel great distances, or if it is the Sabbath or a holy day. Mourners are absolved from praying during this time. Crying, anger, and talking about the deceased person's life are acceptable. A common sign of grief is the tearing of the garment that one is wearing before the funeral service. In liberal congregations, a black ribbon with a tear in it is a symbolic representation of mourning. During *shiva*, the mourner sets the tone and initiates the conversation. Because there are such discrete periods of mourning, Judaism tells the mourner that it is wrong to mourn more than 30 days for a relative and 1 year for parents.

Spirituality

DOMINANT RELIGION AND USE OF PRAYER

Judaism is over 3000 years old. Its early history and laws are chronicled in the **Torah**, called the *Old Testament* by Christians. Jews consider only the Torah as their Bible. They have a history of being singled out as a people and have often been persecuted; expelled from countries; forbidden to practice their religion; "black-balled" from jobs, housing, and admission to college; rounded up and killed; and mass-exterminated.

Judaism is a monotheistic faith that believes in one God as the Creator of the universe. The watchword of the faith is found in Deuteronomy (6:4), "Hear O Israel, the Lord is our God, the Lord is One." No physical qualities are attributed to God, and making and praying to statues or graven images are forbidden by the second commandment.

Many Jews in America have immediate family members who were killed in the pogroms in Russia in the early 1900s and in the Holocaust in Eastern Europe. Yet, throughout this persecution, Judaism has lived and flourished. The spiritual leader is the **rabbi** (teacher). He (or she, in liberal branches) is the interpreter of Jewish law. Rabbis are not considered to be any closer to God than common people are. All Jews pray directly to God. They do not need the rabbi to intercede, to hear confession, or to grant atonement. Some of the major principles that guide Judaic bioethics are

- Man's purpose on earth is to live according to certain God-given guidelines.

- Life possesses enormous intrinsic value, and its preservation is of great moral significance.

- All human lives are equal.

- Our lives are not our own exclusive private possessions (Perlin, 2006).

The first five books of the Bible, also known as the *five books of Moses*, are handwritten in Hebrew on parchment scrolls called *Torah*. These scrolls are kept in the "Holy Ark" within each synagogue under an "eternal light." The Torah directs Jews on how they should live their lives; it provides guidance on every aspect of human life. The rest of the Bible includes sacred writings and teachings of the prophets.

The 613 commandments within the Torah (also called *Mitzvot*) and the oral law derived from the biblical statutes determine Jewish law, or *halakhah*. These commandments ask for a commitment in behavior and also address ethical concerns. Thus, the commandments reflect the will of God, and religious Jews feel it is their duty to carry them out to fulfill their covenant with God. This makes Judaism not only a religion but also a way of life.

The current practice of Judaism in America spans a wide spectrum. Whereas there is only one religion, there are three main branches or denominations of Judaism. The Orthodox are the most traditional. They adhere most strictly to the *halakhah* (Code of Jewish Law) of traditional Judaism and try to follow as many of the laws as possible while fitting into American society. They observe the Sabbath by attending the synagogue on Friday evening and Saturday morning and by abstaining from work, spending money, and driving on the Sabbath. Orthodox Jews observe the Jewish dietary laws; men wear a *yarmulke* or *kippah* (head covering) at all times in reverence to God, whereas women usually wear long sleeves and modest dress. In many Orthodox synagogues, the services are primarily in Hebrew, and men and women sit separately.

Orthodox Jews and some Conservative men and women use the *tefillin*, or phylacteries, during morning prayer services. These are two small black boxes, with parchment containing biblical passages, that are connected to long leather straps. These are wrapped around the arms and forehead as reminders of the laws of the Torah. The *tallis* (or *tallit*) is a rectangular prayer shawl with fringes. This is also used only during prayer but is frequently used by both Conservative and Orthodox Jews. Ultra-Orthodox men wear a special garment under their shirts year-round; the *tzitzit* has long fringes as a reminder of the laws of the Torah.

A *mezuzah* is a small container with scripture inside. Its origin was a sign ensuring God's protection; it serves as a reminder of the presence of God, His commandments, and a Jew's duties to Him. Jewish homes have a *mezuzah* on the doorframe of the house. A number of individuals also wear a *mezuzah* as a necklace. Other religious symbols include the *Star of David*, a six-pointed star that has been a symbol of the Jewish community since the 1350s, and the *menorah* (candelabrum).

The Conservative branch is not quite as strict in its tradition. Whereas Conservative Jews observe most of the *halakhah*, they do make concessions to modern society. Many drive to the synagogue on the Sabbath, and men and women sit together. Many keep a kosher home, but they may or may not follow all of the dietary laws outside the home. Women are ordained as rabbis and are counted in a *minyan*, the minimum number of 10 required for communal prayer. (These practices are unacceptable to

the Orthodox.) Whereas a yarmulke is required in the synagogue, it is optional outside of that environment.

The liberal or progressive movement is called *Reform*. Reform Jews claim that postbiblical law was only for the people of that time, and only the moral laws of the Torah are binding. They practice fewer rituals, although they frequently have a *mezuzah* for their homes, celebrate the holidays, and have a strong ethnic identity. They consider education and ethics of paramount importance in one's personal life and try to link Jewish religious values with American political liberalism. They may or may not follow the Jewish dietary laws, but they may have specific unacceptable foods (e.g., pork), which they abstain from eating. Men and women share full equality, and they engage in many social-action activities.

Of the many small groups of ultra-Orthodox fundamentalists; the **Hasidic** (or **Chasidic**) Jews are perhaps the most recognizable. They usually live, work, and study within a segregated area. They are visually identifiable by their full beards, uncut hair around the ears (*pais*), black hats or fur *streimels*, dark clothing, and no exposed extremities. Women, especially those who are married, also keep their extremities covered and may have shaved heads covered by a wig and often a hat as well.

A relatively new denomination, **Reconstructionism** is a mosaic of the three main branches. It views Judaism as an evolving religion of the Jewish people and seeks to adapt Jewish beliefs and practices to the needs of the contemporary world. Many Jews do not indicate any affiliation.

The Jewish house of prayer is called a **synagogue**, **temple**, or **shul**. It is never referred to as a *church*. However, Jews may pray alone or as a group anywhere that 10 Jews over the age of 13 who have had their *bar mitzvah* are gathered together for prayer. This group is called a *minyan*. Orthodox Jews pray three times a day: morning, late afternoon, and evening. They wash their hands and say a prayer on awakening in the morning and before meals.

Religious clients in hospitals may want their prayer items (*yarmulke* or *kippah, tallit, tzitzit, tefillin*) and may request a minyan. Hospital policies regarding the number of visitors in the sick person's room may have to be ignored in such instances.

One of the most common religious practices related to patients involves "visiting the sick" (*bikkur cholim*). This commandment is one of the social obligations of Judaism and ensures that Jews look after the physical, emotional, psychological, and social well-being of others and provides hope as well as companionship. Moreover, one must consider the patient's welfare and not stay too long, tire the patient, or come only to satisfy one's own needs.

MEANING OF LIFE AND INDIVIDUAL SOURCES OF STRENGTH

The preservation of life is one of Judaism's greatest priorities. Even the laws that govern the Sabbath may be broken if one can help save a life. Each individual is considered special, and the individuality of the human experience is one of the precepts of the faith. Good health is considered an asset. In this regard, individuals who are ill must *not* fast during Yom Kippur (Robinson, 2000).

SPIRITUAL BELIEFS AND HEALTH-CARE PRACTICES

The second of the Ten Commandments is to remember the Sabbath day and keep it holy. The Sabbath begins 18 minutes before sunset on Friday. Lighting candles, saying prayers over challah and wine, and participating in a festive Sabbath meal usher in this weekly holy day. It ends 42 minutes after sunset (or when three stars can be seen) on Saturday, with a service called *Havdalah*. The Sabbath serves as a release from weekday concerns and pressures. During this time, religious Jews engage in congregational study and do no manner of work, including answering the telephone, operating any electrical appliance, driving, or operating a call bell from a hospital bed.

If an Orthodox client's condition is not life-threatening, medical and surgical procedures should not be performed on the Sabbath or holy days. However, extenuating circumstances such as illness or foul weather are legitimate reasons for not attending the services. Although the Sabbath is holy, matters involving human life take precedence over it (Robinson, 2000). Therefore, a gravely ill person and the work of those who need to save her or him are exempted from following the commandments regarding the Sabbath.

In addition to the Sabbath, a number of Jewish holidays are celebrated with special traditions. Rosh Hashanah (Jewish New Year) and Yom Kippur (Day of Atonement) are called the *High Holy Days*, and usually occur in September or early October. They mark a 10-day period of self-examination and repentance. Rosh Hashanah is started by eating apples and honey to wish for a sweet year, and on Yom Kippur, one fasts for a day to cleanse and purify oneself. Fasting for Yom Kippur may be broken for reasons of critical illness or labor and delivery or for children under the age of 12. The holiday includes the blowing of the *shofar* (a ram's horn) and the greeting, "May you be inscribed in the book of life for a good year."

Other major holidays include Passover, the Feast of the Unleavened Bread, which lasts 8 days and celebrates the Exodus from Egypt and freedom from slavery; Sukkot, a festival of the harvest in which individuals may live in temporary huts built outside their homes or synagogues for a week; and Shavuot, which celebrates the giving of the Ten Commandments. Minor holidays include Chanukah, an 8-day holiday, and Purim, both of which celebrate religious freedom. Table 16–1 provides a list of Jewish holidays for the years 2006 through 2010.

Health-Care Practices

HEALTH-SEEKING BELIEFS AND BEHAVIORS

According to those who interpret Jewish law, all people have a duty to keep themselves in good health. This encompasses physical and mental well-being and includes not only early treatment for illness but also prevention of illness. Judaism teaches its members to "choose life." "To refuse lifesaving medical treatment is to commit suicide, to choose death over life" (Washofsky, 2000, p. 223). All denominations recognize that religious requirements may be laid aside if a life is at stake or if an individual has a life-threatening illness. However, once it is clear that an individual is dying and that medical treatment is no longer working, individuals may choose not to interfere with death. Hospice care is fully consonant with Jewish beliefs.

In ultra-Orthodox denominations of Judaism, taking medication that is not necessary to preserve life on the Sabbath may be viewed as "work" (i.e., an action performed with the intention of bringing about a change in existing conditions) and is unacceptable. This belief may result in some people with conditions such as asthma not recognizing the severity of their condition; they may also be unaware of the laws that allow them to take their necessary medications. These patients need to be taught about the potential life-threatening sequelae of their condition as well as the exceptions to Jewish law that permit them to take their medications.

In the Jewish faith, all individuals have value regardless of their condition. This includes individuals with developmental disabilities and AIDS. The Jewish AIDS Network (2006) has been established with a mission of opposing discrimination against people with physical, mental, and developmental conditions.

RESPONSIBILITY FOR HEALTH CARE

Although it is the responsibility of health-care providers to heal, individuals must seek the services of the physician to ensure a healthy body. Once individuals have the knowledge necessary to effect their healing, it is their obligation to do so. To abstain from healing would be equivalent to murder. Jews believe that God provides human beings with wisdom, and it is up to them to use

TABLE 16.1 *Jewish Holidays: 2006–2010**

Holiday	2006–2007 (5767)[†]	2007–2008 (5768)[†]	2008–2009 (5769)[†]	2009–2010 (5770)[†]
Rosh Hashanah	9/23–24	9/13–14	9/30–10/1	9/19–20
Yom Kippur	10/2	9/22	10/9	9/28
Sukkot	10/7–12	9/27–10/2	10/14–19	10/3–8
Chanukah	12/16–23	12/5–12	12/22–29	12/12–19
Purim	3/4	3/21	3/10	2/28
Passover	4/3–10	4/20–27	4/9–16	3/30–4/6
Shavuot	5/23–24	6/9–10	5/29–30	5/19–20

*Jewish holidays always begin at sundown the evening before the date recorded on this type of calendar; holidays end at sundown on the date shown.
[†]Dates on the Jewish calendar.

that wisdom to create a better world. This includes the discovery of new medications and treatments to eliminate or modify disease and suffering. Jews also believe that God gives humans freedom of choice.

Because the preservation of life is paramount, all ritual commandments are waived when danger to life exists. Physical and mental illnesses are legitimate reasons for not fulfilling some of the commandments. Because adult Jews are often well read, they may be interested in trying the newest available treatments. This could have both positive and negative consequences. The literature reveals no studies regarding Jews' self-medicating practices.

FOLK AND TRADITIONAL PRACTICES

Jewish folk practices are historically and biblically based. Jews have adopted and adapted to customs from the cultures and countries they have lived in during the centuries of diaspora. Specific practices are explained in the sections of this chapter on Nutrition and Spiritual Beliefs and Health-Care Practices.

BARRIERS TO HEALTH CARE

Aside from the unavailability of health insurance for some people, or being underinsured secondary to economic situations, no major barriers to health care for Jews in contemporary America exist. The Jewish community helps those in need, including new immigrants, and assists fellow Jews in becoming self-sufficient. Community organizations that include programs to help the needy are ubiquitous today wherever Jews live in the United States.

CULTURAL RESPONSES TO HEALTH AND ILLNESS

The verbalization of pain is acceptable and common. Individuals want to know the reason for the pain, which they consider just as important as obtaining relief from it. The sick role for Jews is highly individualized and may vary among individuals according to the severity of symptoms. As prescribed in the *halakhah*, the family is central to Jewish life; therefore, family members share the emphasis on maintaining health and assisting with individual responsibilities during times of illness.

Many Jews have become physicians, psychoanalysts, psychiatrists, and psychologists. In addition, many of their clients are Jewish. The maintenance of one's mental health is considered just as important as the maintenance of one's physical health. This designation includes psychiatric conditions. However, requirements for those who are rational but have cognitive deficiencies are decided on an individual basis.

According to Jewish law, individuals must be taught the Torah regardless of their age or level of disability. This speaks to the unique value of each individual.

BLOOD TRANSFUSIONS AND ORGAN DONATION

Jewish law views organ transplants from four perspectives: the recipient, the living donor, the cadaver donor,

and the dying donor. Because life is sacred, if the recipient's life can be prolonged without considerable risk, then transplant is favorably viewed. For a living donor to be approved, the risk to the life of the donor must be considered. One is not obligated to donate a body part unless the risk is small. Examples include kidney and bone marrow donations (Lamm, 2000). The action of donating an organ to save another is considered a great *mitzvah*.

Conservative and Reform Judaism approve using the flat EEG as the determination of death so that organs, such as the heart, can be viable for transplant. Burial may be delayed if organ harvesting is the cause of the delay. However, among other groups, this definition of death remains controversial (Beitowitz, 2006). Health-care providers may need to assist Jewish clients to obtain a rabbi when they are making a decision regarding organ donation or transplant.

The use of a cadaver for transplant is generally approved if it is to save a life. No one may derive economic benefit from the corpse. Although desecration of the dead body is considered purposeless mutilation, this does not apply to the removal of organs for transplant. Use of skin for burns is also acceptable.

Health-Care Practitioners

The ancient Hebrews are credited with promoting hygiene and sanitation practices and basic principles for public health care. From the practice of visiting the sick and the desire to initiate measures to prevent the spread of disease, Lillian Wald, a well-known Jewish nurse, developed the Henry Street Settlement as a prototype of public health nursing for those in need.

STATUS OF HEALTH-CARE PROVIDERS

Physicians are held in high regard. Whereas physicians must do everything in their power to preserve life, they are prohibited from initiating measures that prolong the act of dying (Rosner, 1993). Once standard therapy has failed, or if additional treatments are unavailable, "the physician's role changes from that of curer to that of carer. Only supportive care is required for that state and includes care such as food and water, good nursing care, and optimal psychosocial support" (Rosner, 1993, p. 10).

REFERENCES

American Cancer Society. (2001). Retrieved September 16, 2007, from http://www.Cancer.org/eprise/main/ docroot/cri/cri_2_3x

American Jewish Committee. (2006). Retrieved February 4, 2007, from www.ujc.org

Amsel, N. (1994). *The Jewish encyclopedia of moral and ethical issues.* Northvale, NJ: Jason Aronson.

Beitowitz, Y. A. (2006). Brain death controversy in Jewish Law. Retrieved February 4, 2007, from http://www.jlaw.com/Articles/brain.html

Benson, E. (1994). Jewish nurses: A multicultural perspective. *Journal of the New York State Nurses Association, 25*(2), 8–10.

Benson, E. (2001). *As we see ourselves: Jewish women in nursing.* Indianapolis, IN: Center Nursing Publishing.

Center for Jewish Genetic Diseases. (2007). Retrieved February 4, 2007, from http://www.mssm.edu/jewish_genetics/genetic_diseases.shtml

Center for Jewish History. (2007). Retrieved February 4, 2007, from http://www.cjh.org/

Donin, H. (1972). *To be a Jew: A guide to Jewish observance in contemporary life*. New York: Basic Books.

Dorff, E. (1998). *Matters of life and death: A Jewish approach to modern medical ethics*. Philadelphia: The Jewish Publication Society.

Haumann, H. (2002): *A history of East European Jews*. Central European University Press.

The Jewish AIDS Network. (2006). Retrieved February 4, 2007, from http://www.jewishaidsnetwork.org/

Kolatch, A. (2000). *The second Jewish book of why*. Middle Village, NY: Jonathan David.

Lamm, M. (2000). *The Jewish way in death and in mourning*. Middle Village, NY: Jonathan David.

Lau, I. (1997). *Practical Judaism*. Jerusalem: Feldheim.

Levy, R. (1993). Ethnic and racial differences in response to medicines: Preserving individualized therapy in managed pharmaceutical programmes. *Pharmaceutical Medicine, 7*, 139–165.

National Gaucher Foundation. (2001). Retrieved September 16, 2007, from http://www.gaucherdisease.org

Perlin, E. (2006). Jewish bioethics and medical genetics. *Journal of Religion and Health, 33*(4), 333–340.

Robinson, G. (2000). *Essential Judaism: A complete guide to beliefs, customs, and rituals*. New York: Pocket Books.

Rosner, F. (1993, July/August). Hospice, medical ethics, and Jewish customs. *American Journal of Hospice and Palliative Care*, 6–10.

Washofsky, M. (2000). *Jewish living: A guide to contemporary reform practice*. New York: UAHC (Union of American Hebrew Congregations) Press.

Wertheimer, J. (2002). *American Jewish yearbook*. New York: The American Jewish Committee.

Wyce, M. (2001, Summer). *Genetic profiling: Who will be seen as damaged goods? Inside*, 18–22.

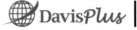

For case studies, review questions, and additional information, go to http://davisplus.fadavis.com

Chapter 17

People of Korean Heritage

EUN-OK IM

Overview, Inhabited Localities, and Topography

OVERVIEW

This chapter focuses on the commonalities among people of Korean heritage, with historical reference to the mother country, South Korea. The word *Korea* limitedly refers to the Republic of Korea. Because some information may not be pertinent to every Korean, this chapter serves as a guide for health-care providers rather than as a mandate of facts. Differences in beliefs and practices among Koreans in Korea, the United States, and other countries vary according to the primary and secondary characteristics of culture as presented in Chapter 1. An understanding of Korean culture and history gives health professionals the insight needed to perform culturally appropriate assessments, plan effective care and follow-up, and work effectively with Koreans in the workforce.

South Korea is a peninsula separated by North Korea to the north at the 38th parallel and surrounded by the former Soviet Union to the northeast, the Yellow Sea to the west, and the Sea of Japan to the east. South Korea has a landmass of 98,480 square kilometers (38,031 square miles), which is about the size of the state of Indiana, and a population of 48 million (CIA, 2007). South Korea has 1 percent of the landmass of the United States, but has one-sixth as many people, making it 16 times more densely populated than the United States (Kohls, 2001). The mega-modern metropolitan area of Seoul, the capital, has a population of 10.3 million people (Asianinfo, 2007a). A new international state-of-the art airport is located in Incheon, 60 kilometers from the center of Seoul. Other large cities are Busan (Pusan) and Daegu (Taegu). Planes, trains, and buses link all South Korean major cities, making travel easy and efficient. With the recent increase in the number of automobiles and the construction of highways, motorways are becoming more congested. Major industries are electronics, telecommunications, automobile production, chemicals, shipbuilding, and steel (CIA, 2007). South Korea is now well known as riding on the "*hallyu* movement" or the "Korean wave," which is the globalization of Korean dramas throughout Singapore, Malaysia, Japan, China, and the United States. Since the 1990s, the entertainment industry of South Korea has grown explosively, producing Asia-wide successes in music, television, and film.

The continental and monsoon climate of Korea is fairly consistent throughout the peninsula, except during the winter months. North Korea has cold, snowy winters, with an average temperature in January of 17°F. South Korea is milder, with an average January temperature of 23°F. During the summer months, the monsoon winds create an average temperature of 80°F, with high humidity throughout the peninsula. Precipitation occurs mostly during the summer months and is heavier in the south. The peninsula is mountainous; only 20 percent of the terrain is located in lowlands. Such topography encourages the development of concentrated living areas. Most cities and residential areas are located along the coastal plains and the inland valleys opening to the west coast.

HERITAGE AND RESIDENCE

Korea is one of the two oldest continuous civilizations in the world, second only to China. Koreans trace their heritage to 2333 B.C. In the 1st century A.D., tribes from central and northern Asia banded together to form this "Hermit Kingdom," littering the countryside with palaces, pagodas, and gardens. Over the ensuing centuries, Mongols, Japanese, and Chinese invaded the Korean peninsula. Japan forcibly annexed Korea in the early 20th century, ruling it harshly and leaving ill will that persists to this day. As a result of the Potsdam Conference after World War II, the United States took over the occupation of South Korea, with the USSR occupying North Korea. By 1948, Korea's new government was recognized by the United Nations, only to be followed by the North Korean Communist forces invading South Korea in 1950. The result was the Korean War, which lasted until 1953 and caused mass devastation, from which the country has made a remarkable recovery. Open aggression between North and South Korea again occurred in 1998 and 1999. In 2000, the two Koreas signed a vague, yet hopeful, agreement that the two countries would be reunited. However, North Korea's recent resumption of its nuclear weapons program has set its neighbors and much of the rest of the world on edge (CNN, 2007).

In 1988, the year Seoul hosted the Olympic Games, elections were held, and relations were re-established with China and the Soviet Union. Intermittent corruption among political officials has continued to surface, threatening internal relationships and the economy. In 1997, South Korea's economy tumbled dramatically, resulting in economic and democratic reforms. With unwavering persistence, Koreans have rebuilt their major world economy, reflecting a 4 percent annual growth rate with moderate inflation (CIA, 2007). The United States continues to maintain a strong military presence throughout South Korea (Fig. 17–1).

REASONS FOR MIGRATION AND ASSOCIATED ECONOMIC FACTORS

Koreans are one of the most rapidly increasing immigrant groups in the United States (Korean American Coalition, 2003). The first major immigration from Korea to the United States occurred between 1903 and 1905, when the Korean government prohibited further emigration: About 10,000 Koreans had entered Hawaii and 1000 reached the U.S. mainland. The U.S. Immigration Act of 1924 practically closed the door to Japanese and Koreans. During the civil rights movements of the 1950s and 1960s, new immigration laws repealed the earlier limitations on Asian immigration. Koreans continue to immigrate to America to pursue the American dream, to increase socioeconomic opportunities, and to attend colleges and

universities. In addition, many Koreans and Americans marry, making both Korea and America their homes. Korea ranks fourth in the number of Asian immigrants to the United States, with 1.3 million, closely following the Philippines, China, and Vietnam (Shin & Shin, 1999). According to the *2003 Statistical Yearbook* of the Immigration and Naturalization Service, 12,512 Koreans were admitted to the United States in 2003 (U.S. Department of Homeland Security, 2004).

EDUCATIONAL STATUS AND OCCUPATIONS

Most of the population pursues higher education, and South Korea has more citizens with PhDs per capita than any other country in the world. Owing to Confucian cultural influence, education is emphasized as a virtue of human beings (all human beings should be educated) and is highly valued in the Korean culture (Im, 2002).

Before the late 19th century, education was primarily for those who could afford it. State schools educated the youth from the **yangban** (upper class), focusing on Chinese classics in the belief that these contained the tools of Confucian morality and philosophy that also apply in politics. In the late 1800s, the state schools were opened to all citizens. Early Christian missionary work introduced the Western style of modern education to Korea. Initially, many Koreans were skeptical of the radical curriculum and instruction for females, but the popularity of this style grew rapidly.

After the takeover of Korea by the Japanese in 1910, two types of schools emerged, one for Japanese and another for Koreans. The Korean schools focused on vocational training, which prepared Koreans for only lower-level positions. Japanese colonial education was designed to keep Koreans subordinate to ethnic Japanese in all ways (Sorensen, 1994). In 1949, South Korea allowed for the implementation of a educational system similar to that of the United States. This 6–3–3–4 ladder (6 years in elementary school, 3 years in junior high, 3 years in high school, and 4 years in college) continues today in contemporary South Korea. Anti-Communism and morality are taught throughout elementary and secondary schools.

In the United States, many Koreans own their own small businesses, which vary from mom-and-pop stores and gas stations to grocery stores and real estate agencies to retail shops. Their reputation for hard work, independence, and self-motivation has given them the reputation of the "model minority." However, this has caused a backlash in some communities, such as Washington, DC, where they have been compared with other minority groups. The message has become: "If the Koreans can do it, why not other groups?" The turmoil and riots that took place in Los Angeles in April 1992 between the African American community and the Korean American merchants is another example of conflicts that arise from such labeling.

Many Korean small businesses are located in African American neighborhoods because of low capital investment requirements and limited resources of the owners. Korean merchants begin dealing in inexpensive consumer goods as a practical way to start a business in a capitalistic society. Koreans often assist each other in establishing

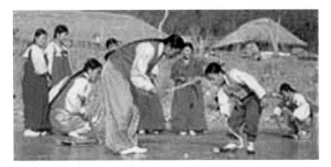

FIGURE 17–1 Traditional Korean dancers.

businesses by pooling their money and taking turns with rotating credit associations to provide each family with the opportunity for financial success.

Communication

VIGNETTE 17.1

Ho Park and Ok Park, ages 58 and 57 years, immigrated to New York from South Korea in 1984. They arrived with their four children and lived with Ok's sister and her family for 2 years. They saved their money and eventually moved into a small two-bedroom apartment where they lived for 10 years. Later, they moved into a three-bedroom house in New Jersey where they have now lived for the past 12 years. Ho is a college graduate from one of the top universities in South Korea, and Ok is a graduate from a prestigious women's college in South Korea. Despite their college degrees, they have been working as housekeepers in a hospital.

The three sons and one daughter have matured without any problem. The daughter, Teresha, is a nurse and works in Michigan. The oldest son, Eugene, is a military officer and lives with his wife in Maryland. The third son, Phyllip, is a graduate student in biology at the University of Minnesota. However, their second son, David, is not doing well. Since he graduated from high school, 3 years ago, he has lived with Ho and Ok without getting a job. He sits on the couch and spends most of his time watching TV or playing computer games and gaining weight. Ho and Ok are concerned about him, but are unsure how to help him.

Ok has developed allergies and has difficulty breathing when exposed to chemicals used in her cleaning job at the hospital. In addition, she is having serious backaches that she links to using heavy equipment. However, she can not quit her job because her husband's salary will not meet their financial needs, which include university tuition for Phyllip and a home mortgage. Despite her health problems, Ok takes full responsibility for household tasks such as cooking, dishwashing, and laundry.

With Ok's health problems and David's unemployment, Ho is thinking about opening a small Korean grocery store. However, he has heard many strories of Koreans who opened small businesses and went bankrupt or got killed by robbers. Considering that he is not a friendly person who easily smiles or welcomes customers, he believes that he would not be good at operating a Korean grocery store. Even thinking about the new business makes him smoke more than usual: He has smoked a pack of cigarettes daily for the past 30 years, and now smokes more than a pack a day. Recently, he is experiencing frequent coughing and shortness of breath.

1. How does the Park family fit the "model minority" culture and work ethic?
2. Identify three health concerns for the Park family and describe culturally congruent strategies for resolving them.
3. Identify how Korean traditional gender roles are affecting Ok's health problems and family dynamics.
4. Describe Koreans' traditional attitudes toward smoking and discuss interventions for Ho's smoking.

DOMINANT LANGUAGE AND DIALECTS

The dominant language in Korea is *Korean*, or *han'gul*, which originated in the 15th century with King Se Jong, and is believed to be the first phonetic alphabet in East Asia. The Korean language belongs to the Ural-Altaic language family, which includes Turkic, Mongolian, and Tungusic as major branches (Comrie, Matthews, & Polinsky, 1996). Dialects do not exist in Korean, but slang terminology is characteristic of specific age groups and regions.

Korean language has four levels of speech that are determined based on the degree of intimacy between speakers. These varying levels reflect inequalities in social status based on gender, age, and social positions. Use of an inappropriate sociolinguistic level of speech is unacceptable and is normally interpreted as intended formality to, disrespect for, or contempt to a social superior.

Chinese and Japanese have influenced the Korean language, which has 14 consonants and 10 vowels. During their annexation in the early 20th century, the Japanese forbade public use of the Korean language, requiring the use of the Japanese written and spoken language.

Most Koreans in the United States can speak, read, write, and understand English to some degree. However, some Americans may have difficulty understanding the English spoken by Koreans, especially those who learned English from Koreans who spoke with their native intonations and pronunciations.

CULTURAL COMMUNICATION PATTERNS

The sharing of thoughts, feelings, and ideas is very much based on age, gender, and status in Korean society. Traditionally, the Korean community values the group over the individual, men over women, and age over youth. Those holding the dominant position are the decision-makers who share thoughts and ideas on issues.

Koreans prefer indirect communication because they perceive direct communication as an indication of intention or opinions as rude. Moreover, Koreans may agree with the health-care provider in order to avoid conflict or hurting someone's feelings, even if something is impossible (Im, 2002). Thus, it is important to read between the lines when working with these families and remember those growing up in the United States may adopt the dominant American communication style.

Koreans tend to avoid eye contact especially with older people, perceived authorities (e.g., health-care providers), and strangers. Avoiding direct eye contact with older people and perceived authorities indicates respect, and women's avoiding direct eye contact with men shows modesty. Younger generations of Koreans educated in the United States may adopt the dominant communication style of eye contact. Koreans are usually comfortable with silence owing to Confucian teaching, "silence is golden." Silence was traditionally emphasized as a virtue of educated people. Even among Korean Americans, people who are silent, especially men, are viewed as humble and well-educated. However, the social fabric and cultural norms of Koreans are changing as they interact with Western societies and culture. Younger generations of Koreans, even in South Korea, are noted as being very sociable and kind to visitors (Asianinfo, 2007b).

Close personal space (less than a foot) is shared with family members and close friends, but it is inappropriate for strangers to step into "intimate space" unless needed for health care (Im, 2002). Visitors from America may be uncomfortable with Koreans' spatial distancing in public spaces. Koreans stand close to one another and do not excuse themselves if they bump into someone on the street. This may be due to the high population density in the metropolitan areas of South Korea (1274 per square mile) and Koreans' cultural attitudes toward strangers (e.g., they usually do not speak with strangers). Among family members and close friends, touching, friendly pushing, and hugging are accepted. However, among strangers, touching is considered disrespectful unless needed for care. Also, touching among friends and social equals of the same sex is common and does not carry a homosexual connotation as it might in Western societies. However, more social etiquette rules apply when it comes to touching older family members or those of higher social status. Hugging and kissing recently have become common among parents and young children as well as among young children and aunts or uncles.

Feelings are infrequently communicated in facial expressions. Smiling a lot shows a lack of intellect and disrespect. One would not smile to a stranger on the street nor try to joke during a serious conversation. Joking and amusement have their designated times. In Korea, men frequent bars after work and may express their sense of humor in this setting. Men and women alike appreciate and encourage jokes and laughter in appropriate settings. Koreans generally do not express their emotions directly or in public; expressing emotions in front of others, including family members, is regarded as shameful, especially among men (Im, 2002). A common Korean belief related to men's emotions is that men should cry only three times in their lives: (1) When they are born, (2) when their parents die, and (3) when their country perishes (Im, 2002). Given these cultural communication patterns, health-care providers should not interpret these nonverbal behaviors as meaning that Korean clients are not interested in, or do not care about, information presented during health teaching and health promotion interventions.

TEMPORAL RELATIONSHIPS

Traditional Koreans are past-oriented. Much attention is paid to the ancestry of a family. Yearly, during the Harvest Moon in Korea, *chusok* (respect) is paid to ancestors by bringing fresh fruits from the autumn harvest, dry fish, and rice wine to gravesites. However, the younger and more-educated generation is more futuristic and achievement oriented.

In Korea, palm readers are visited to determine the best home to purchase, the date for having a wedding, and when new businesses should open. The busiest time of the year for the palm reader is just before the Chinese New Year. Koreans are eager to know their fortune for the coming year. Many believe that misfortunes occur because ancestors are unhappy. During these times, families show

respect to ancestors by more frequent visits to their gravesites in the hope of appeasing the spirits. Shamans are also used in Korea to rid homes and new places of business from spirits, and they may be used by Koreans of all socioeconomic levels.

The Korean conception of time depends on the circumstances. Koreans embrace the Western respect for time for important appointments, transportation connections, and working hours, all of which are recognized as situations in which punctuality is necessary. Yet, socially, Korean Americans arrive at parties and visit family and friends within 1 to 2 hours later than the agreed-upon time. This is socially acceptable when the person or family is waiting at home. If the social meeting is being held in a public setting, a half-hour time span for arrival at the meeting place can be expected.

FORMAT FOR NAMES

The number of surnames in Korea is limited, with the most common ones being Kim, Lee, Park, Rhee or Yi, Choi or Choe, and Chung or Jung. Korean names contain two Chinese characters, one of which describes the generation and the other the person's given name. The surname comes first; however, because this may be confusing to many Americans, some Koreans in the United States follow the Western tradition of using the given name first, followed by the surname. Adults are not addressed by their given names unless they are on friendly terms; individuals should be addressed by their surname with the title Mr., Mrs., Ms., Dr., or Minister.

Given the diversity and acculturation of Korean Americans, health-care providers need to determine the Korean clients' language ability, comfort level with silence, and spatial-distancing characteristics. In addition, Koreans should be addressed formally until they indicate otherwise.

Family Roles and Organization

VIGNETTE 17.2

Kay and Sook Lim, ages 55 and 57 years, immigrated from Korea in 1988 at the invitation of Kay's brother who lived in Chicago. They came to Chicago with only $200 and began working as clerks in a Korean laundry. Owing to Kay's excellent management skills and Sook's diligent work ethic, they have been able to establish a real estate business. They now live in a prestigious home and regularly donate money to their church. Their fellow church members frequently tell them that they are role models for the many Korean immigrants in the area.

The Lims have two children: one daughter and one son. Their daughter, Grace, of whom they were very proud, was one of the top students in her high school and entered Cornell University, a special honor for them. However, she married a white man, became pregnant, and abandoned her studies. Kay and Sook had to accept her marriage because of her pregnancy, but they did not let other relatives and friends know about her marriage. Grace moved to Los Angeles with her husband and does not want to see her parents again because they do not heartily approve of her marriage and pregnancy.

Their son, John, has recently been a family concern. Until Kay and Sook received a telephone call from a policeman, they did not know that he had been skipping classes. In addition, they were unaware that he was coming home very late at night because they also came home late at night. John was involved in a gang fight in which a victim was badly hurt, necessitating additional expenses for an attorney.

Because of the circumstances of both children, Kay became very depressed and could not go to work. Moreover, they could not get help from a health-care provider or emotional support from relatives or church friends because they did not want others to know about these unfortunate occurrences with their children. Furthermore, whenever John comes home late at night, he and Sook quarrel, which frequently results in physical altercations. Thus Kay becomes more depressed and separates herself from others.

1. What cultural strategies can a public-health case manager employ for Kay's depression?
2. If the Lim family were to seek health care, what type of care provider would they most likely seek?
3. What cultural barriers exist for the Lim family in seeking mental-health counseling and obtaining social support?
4. Discuss traditional Korean prescriptive, restrictive, and taboo practices for adolescents and young adults. How does the Kim family vary from these traditional practices and values?

HEAD OF HOUSEHOLD AND GENDER ROLES

Fundamental ideas about morality and the proper ordering of human relationships among Koreans are closely associated with kinship values derived mainly from Confucian concepts of filial piety, ancestor worship, funerary rites, position of women, the institution of marriage, kinship groups, social status and rank, and respect for scholars and political officials. Although constitutional law in South Korea declares equality for all citizens, not all aspects of society have accepted this. Korean culture is largely based on patriarchal and Confucian norms that subordinate women (Im, 2002). In Confucian traditional Korean families, the father was always the head of the family; he had power to control the family, and the family had to obey any order from the father. Wives did not share household tasks with their husbands, so they tended to be physically overloaded and psychologically distressed. Wives' exploitation was hidden under Confucian norms that praised women who sacrifice themselves for their families and nation (Im & Meleis, 2001). Also, the wife was confined to the home and bore the major responsibility for household tasks; the husband was the breadwinner.

Among Korean immigrants in the United States, women hold the family together and play a vital role in building an economic base for the family and community, often sacrificing themselves in the immigration process. The Korean immigrant woman may have started as a cleaning woman or seamstress, then worked at a fast food restaurant, and then in a small shop owned with her husband. However, the women's financial contributions to the family usually do not change the gender roles: Their husbands still occupy center stage, exercise the authority, and make the major family decisions (Im & Meleis, 2001).

PRESCRIPTIVE, RESTRICTIVE, AND TABOO BEHAVIORS FOR CHILDREN AND ADOLESCENTS

In contrast to the Western culture, in which mothering is individually fashioned and relies on the expertise of health-care providers, in the highly ritualistic Korean culture, mothering is molded by societal rules and information is less frequently sought from health-care providers. In this context, mothers tend to view infants as passive and dependent, and they seek guidance from folklore and the extended family (Choi, 1995). In Korea, children over the age of 5 years are expected to be well behaved because the whole family is disgraced if a child acts in an embarrassing manner. Most children are not encouraged to state their opinions. Parents usually make the decisions.

Korean families have high standards and expectations for their children, and "giving a whip to a beloved child" is the basis for discipline of children (Im, 2002). Thus, the pressure of high performance in school and entering a highly ranked university is prevalent among Korean children and adolescents (Im, 2002). Usually, Koreans are not happy with very masculine girls or very feminine boys (Im, 2002).

"Teaching to the test" is also common in Korea, but the role of teachers is also to encourage self-study. The future of Korean students is determined by their teachers' recommendations, and this pressure can be extremely intense for students who are not doing well. The teaching style is one in which students listen and learn what is being taught. Regardless of private doubts, a student rarely questions a teacher's authority. Korean children in America must be taught the teaching style in American schools, in which questioning is positive and is valued as class participation. Even if Korean American students understand the style of teaching, it can be difficult to know the appropriate timing for asking questions.

The pressure of doing well in school and attending a university of high quality leaves Korean adolescents little room for social interactions. Activities that interfere with one's education are considered taboo for adolescents. In Korea, students frequently attend study groups after school or special tutoring sessions paid for by their families in preparation for examinations to enter a university. Short coffee breaks or snacks at local coffee shops or noodle houses are permissible, but then it is "back to the books."

Dating is uncommon among high school students in Korea, although it is allowed. Adolescent girls are usually not allowed to spend the night at their friends' houses, virginity is emphasized, and sexual activities and pregnancy at puberty stigmatize the family across social classes. Although talking about sexuality, contraception, or pregnancy in public is taboo, close girlfriends or boyfriends exchange information on these topics or get their information from women's magazines. Neither the school system nor the family assumes responsibility for sex education. Girls in elementary school are given a class regarding their menstrual cycle, but no information is given about sexual relations.

Once young adults have entered a university, they receive their freedom and are then permitted to make their own decisions about personal and study time. Group outings are common for meeting the opposite sex. Dating may occur from these group meetings and consists of movies, dinner, and walks in the park.

Issues arise between the first-generation Korean immigrant parents and the second-generation children in relation to conflicting values and communication. With rapid acculturation, the second generation often takes on the values of the dominant society or culture. Thus, parents who are of the first generation in most cases are challenged when their second-generation children do not accept traditional values and ideals that they may still hold dear. The different cultures between the first-generation parents and the second-generation children are sometimes the cause of domestic violence. Most of the first generation of Korean immigrants were educated in Korea, and they have a strong stereotype of Korean patriarchal culture. However, because the second generation is educated in the United States (some of them never visited Korea), most second-generation individuals feel a spirit of insubordination and often quarrel. For some, physical abuse might be involved if they do not follow orders (Kim, Cain, & McGubbin, 2006; Kim & Chung, 2003; Park, 2001).

FAMILY GOALS AND PRIORITIES

In Korea, the family is described as "corporate," in which family members have specific rights and duties within their family. A Korean cannot belong to more than one corporate family, and a family member replaces the roles of another family member who dies. This traditional corporate family is dissolving among both Koreans and Korean Americans. Usually, both parents work to provide every opportunity possible for their family. As each family member learns to adjust to the changing roles, conflict can result. Children adapt most easily to the new culture and may even take on the dominant culture's values.

Lee and Lee (1990) studied the adjustment of Korean immigrant families in the United States in relation to roles, values, and living conditions between husbands and wives and parents and children. The findings showed a transition from an independent family structure, in which the woman had little knowledge of the man's activities outside the home, to a joint family structure. Many activities were carried out together with an interchange of roles at home. Conflict centered on undefined role expectations. In Korea, the roles of men and women were very clear. However, upon immigrating to the United States, men and women were faced with conflicting roles in the new culture and had to struggle to redefine them. Other conflict areas were the couple's ability to speak English, the woman's inability to drive, the degree of acculturation, the limited social contact, and the stressors of living in a new culture.

In Korea, education is a family priority. The outcome of having a highly educated child was a secure old age for the parents. Because of the dependent relationship between parents and their children, parents were more willing to make drastic sacrifices for the advancement of their children's education. Today, status is achieved rather than inherited in Korea. Education in Korea is a determinant of status, independent of its contribution to economic success.

Traditionally in Korea, parents expected their children to care for them in old age. *Hyo* (filial piety), which is the obligation to respect and obey parents, care for them in old age, give them a good funeral, and worship them after death, was a core value of Korean ethics. The obligation to care for one's parents is written into civil code in Korea. The burden was on the eldest son, who was obliged to reside with his parents and carry on the family line. Such an arrangement made the generations dependent on each other. The son felt obligated to care for his parents because of the sacrifices they made for him. Similarly, he made the same sacrifices for his children and expected them to provide for him and his wife in their old age. Many of these traditions in Korea have changed. Some of the eldest children emigrated, leaving the responsibility for their parents to the siblings who remained in Korea.

Some older Koreans were brought to the United States without their friends and with minimal or no English skills. They often felt obligated to assist the family in any way possible by preparing meals or taking care of the children when the parents were not home. Decision-making for older people was hampered in their new culture. Korean older people were frequently consulted on important family matters as a sign of respect for their life experiences. Older people's roles as decision-makers in the United States have shifted with the younger generation of Korean Americans wanting the final decision-making authority in their young families.

Traditionally, Koreans give great respect to their older people. Old age begins when one reaches the age of 60 years, with an impressive celebration prepared for the occasion. The historical significance of this celebration is related to the Chinese lunar calendar. The lunar calendar has 60 cycles, each with a different name. At the age of 60, the person is starting the calendar cycle over again. This is called **hwangap**. This celebration was more significant in the past when life expectancy in Korea was much lower than it is today. Despite a change in the direct role of older people in their families, older Koreans are socially well respected in Korea. In public, an older woman is called *Halmoni* (grandmother), and those who are not blood relatives call an older man *Harabuji* (grandfather). Older people are offered seats on buses out of respect and honor.

Traditionally, the extended Korean family played an important role in supporting its members throughout the life span. With the break up of the extended family, Korean Americans support each other through secondary organizations such as the church. The church assists new immigrants with the transition to life in the United States. The church is a resource for information about child care, language classes, and social activities (Im & Yang, 2006; Tritto, 2004). Korean Americans without family support may seek other Korean Americans who live in the area. With Korean Americans dispersed throughout the United States; however, this task can be difficult.

Whereas some Koreans inherit social status, many have the ability to change their status through their education and professions. Traditional Korean culture espouses respect not only for older people but also for those of valued professions. In modern Korea, professors, bureaucrats, business executives, physicians, and attorneys receive a high level of respect. Historically, those with the highest education were handsomely paid. Even though the salary differences between university professors and other professions have narrowed significantly in recent years in Korea, the status of the intellectual remains high. Similarly, the bureaucratic officer has a high social status, wielding much respect and influence.

ALTERNATIVE LIFESTYLES

Alternative lifestyles are usually frowned upon in Korean culture. Women who divorce suffer social stigma, the degree of which depends on the situation. However, recent changes in the Family Law in South Korea now permit women to head a household, recognize a wife's right to a portion of the couple's property, and allow a woman to maintain greater contact with her children after a divorce (U.S. Department of State, 2006). Partially owing to the law change, South Korea now has one of the highest divorce rates in the world, with 47.4 percent of marriages ending in divorce (U.S. Department of State, 2006). Yet, the stigma of divorce remains strong among Koreans in both South Korea and the United States, and there is little government or private assistance for divorced women (U.S. Department of State, 2006). Mixed marriages, between a Korean and a non-Korean, are highly disregarded by some, and the Korean government makes it very difficult for these marriages to occur. Korean women who have married American servicemen are often the objects of Korean jokes and are ridiculed by some.

Living together before marriage is not customary in Korea. If pregnancy occurs outside marriage, it may be taken care of quietly and without family and friends being aware of the situation. In the United States, pregnancy outside of marriage may not carry such a great stigma among the more acculturated.

As in other Asian cultures, homosexuality has not been accepted in Korean culture (Kimmel & Yi, 2004). Also, Korean's understanding and knowledge of homosexuality are ambigous and limited (Kim & Hahn, 2006): Koreans think that homosexuality is an abnormal and impure modern phenomenon. Despite the recent coming out of several Korean homosexual entertainers in South Korea, those who have relations with a person of the same sex still remain "in the closet." Personal disclosure to friends and family usually jeopardizes the family name and may lead to ostracism. The community may stigmatize both the family and the individual, making it difficult to conduct their personal lives.

Workforce Issues

CULTURE IN THE WORKPLACE

Korean Americans come from a culture that places a high value on education. Many Korean immigrants are college educated and held white-collar jobs in Korea. Moreover, it

is difficult for Korean immigrants to obtain work in the United States commensurate with their experience because of language difficulties, restricted access to corporate America, and unfamiliarity with American culture (Im & Meleis, 2001). The skills and work experiences they had in Korea are often not accepted by American businesses, forcing them to take jobs in which they may be overskilled while they save money to start their own businesses. Korean American women frequently need to find jobs to assist the family financially, which may cause role conflicts between more traditional husbands and wives.

Korean Americans have a strong work ethic. They work long hours each week for the advancement of family opportunities. Family is the priority for Korean Americans, but on the surface, this may not always be apparent when long hours are devoted to work. The goal is to save money for education and other opportunities, so the family can provide for their children in the future.

The number of Korean medical personnel working in the American health-care system is unknown. Significant numbers of Korean nurses and physicians are practicing in the United States and Canada; many have received part or all of their education in the United States. Yi and Jezewski's study (2000) of 12 Korean nurses' adjustment to hospitals in the United States identified five phases of adjustment. The first three phases, relieving psychological stress, overcoming language barriers, and accepting American nursing practice, take 2 to 3 years. The remaining two phases, adopting the styles of American problem-solving strategies and adopting the styles of American interpersonal relationships, take an additional 5 to 10 years. Accordingly, orientation programs need to address language skills, practice differences, and communication and interpersonal relationships to help Koreans adjust to the American workforce. These same phases may occur with other Korean health professionals.

ISSUES RELATED TO AUTONOMY

Those in supervisory positions need to recognize the roles and relationships that exist between Koreans and their employers. A supervisor is treated with much respect in work and in social settings. Informalities and small talk may be difficult for Korean immigrants. For an employee to refuse an employer's request is unacceptable, even if the employee does not want or feel qualified to complete the request. Supervisors should make an effort to promote open conversation and the expression of ideas among Korean Americans. Asking Korean employees to demonstrate procedures is better than asking them whether they know how to perform them. Those who have adjusted to the American business style may be more assertive in their positions, but an understanding of this work role gives supervisors the tools to more readily use Korean Americans' skills and knowledge.

As with any new language, it is often difficult to understand American slang and colloquial language. Employers and other employees should be clear in their communication style and be understanding of miscommunications. Ethnic biases are often directed at Korean Americans who speak English with an accent. Employers' and coworkers' preconceived notions of immigrants can also be a deterrent to Korean Americans in the workforce.

Biocultural Ecology

SKIN COLOR AND OTHER BIOLOGICAL VARIATIONS

Koreans are an ethnically homogeneous Mongoloid people who have shared a common history, language, and culture since the 7th century A.D. when the peninsula was first united. Common physical characteristics include dark hair and dark eyes, with variations in skin color and degree of hair darkness. Skin color ranges from fair to light brown, with those residing in the southern part of South Korea being darker. Epicanthal skin folds create the distinctive appearance of Asian eyes.

DISEASES AND HEALTH CONDITIONS

Schistosomiasis and other parasitic diseases are endemic to certain regions of Korea. Therefore, health-care providers should consider parasite screening with Korean immigrants, when appropriate. South Korea continues to manufacture and use asbestos-containing products and has not taken the precautions necessary to adequately protect employees and meet international standards. Thus, Koreans emigrating to the United States need to be assessed for asbestos-related health problems (Johanning, Goldberg, & Kim, 1994).

The high prevalences of stomach and liver cancer, tuberculosis, hepatitis, and hypertension in South Korea predispose recent immigrants to these conditions. High rates of hypertension lead to an increase in cardiovascular accidents and renal failure. The high incidence of stomach cancer is associated with environmental risks, such as diet and infection (*Helicobacter pylori*), and in some cases, genetic predisposition (Kim, 2003). As with other Asians, a high occurrence of lactose intolerance exists among people of Korean ancestry. Dental hygiene and preventive dentistry have recently been emphasized in health promotion in South Korea. Because of the high incidence of gum disease and oral problems, however, these conditions deserve attention.

VARIATIONS IN DRUG METABOLISM

Growing research in the field of pharmacogenetics has found variations in drug metabolism among ethnic groups. Studies suggest that Asian populations require lower dosages of psychotropic drugs (Levy, 1993). Other studies have shown variations in drug metabolism and interaction with propranolol, isoniazid, and diazepam among Asians in comparison with those of European Americans and other ethnic groups (Meyer, 1992). Although these studies primarily focus on people of Chinese and Japanese heritage, health-care professionals should be aware and attentive to the possibility of drug metabolism variations among Korean Americans (Munoz & Hilgenberg, 2005).

High-Risk Behaviors

Because Koreans place great emphasis on education, many subject their children to intense pressure to do well in school. A survey conducted among middle and high school students in Korea demonstrated such pressures. Three-quarters of the students reported having considered running away or committing suicide because of their lack of success in school (Sorensen, 1994). Another study conducted at Seoul National University, the apex of universities in South Korea, reported that 14 percent of the students admitted to the class of 1980 experienced nervous disorders, character blocks, or nervous breakdowns (Sorensen, 1994). Similar pressures have been seen in the United States, where suicide has occurred in Korean high school and college students because of intense pressure to do well in school.

Korea has a high incidence of alcohol consumption, up from 7.0 L in 1980 to 8.1 L per adult per capita, which is similar to that of the United States and Ireland at 7.8 L per adult per capita. However, among adult men in Korea, consumption is 18.4 L per capita, one of the highest rates of alcohol consumption in the world (Park, Oh, & Lee, 1998). Korean business transactions commonly occur after the decision-makers have had several drinks. Koreans believe that people let their masks down when they drink and that they truly get to know someone after they have had a few drinks. Socioeconomic changes in Korea have resulted in differences in alcohol-related social and health problems, with a change from drinking mild fermented beverages with meals to drinking distilled liquors without meals. In the United States, 62 percent of Korean American men and 39 percent of Korean American women drink alcoholic beverages, with beer the alcoholic beverage most commonly consumed (Yu, 1990b).

In Korea, women drink far less than men. Sons' drinking patterns are similar to their fathers' patterns. A substantial generational difference exists among females, with daughters abstaining from alcohol less frequently than their mothers and drinking more, and more often, than their mothers (Weatherspoon, Park, & Johnson, 2001). In the United States and Korea, drinking and vehicular accidents among Koreans and Korean Americans are a cause for concern.

One-third of Korean Americans living in the Los Angeles area smoke, and Korean American men (37 percent) smoke more than Korean American women (20 percent) (Yu, 1990b). In their study, Lee, Sobal, and Frongillo (2000) found that bicultural Korean men were least likely to smoke, whereas acculturated and bicultural women were more likely than traditional women to smoke. In Korea, a few women do smoke, and for those who do, smoking in public, such as on the street, is considered taboo.

Cho and Faulkner (1993) studied the cultural conceptions of alcoholism among Korean and American university students. Students had to decide whether the person described in a vignette was an alcoholic or not and why. The results showed that American-born students tended to define alcoholism in terms of social and interpersonal problems related to drinking, whereas Korean-born students defined alcoholism in terms of physical degeneration and physiological addiction. The authors cautioned against the misuse of American concepts and diagnostic scales in the cross-cultural arena. Cultural factors should be examined closely in relation to the study, diagnosis, and treatment of alcohol problems.

HEALTH-CARE PRACTICES

Seat belts are infrequently worn in South Korea, although there has been recent pressure to use them. Korean Americans understand the legal mandates in the United States and comply with seat-belt and child-restraint laws.

Hobbies such as hiking and golf are enjoyed in South Korea. Korean Americans do not identify hiking as a frequent pastime, either because of environmental constraints or because of living situations. Golf remains a significant activity among those Korean Americans who are financially able to play the sport.

Nutrition

MEANING OF FOOD

Food takes on a significant meaning when one has been without food. Many Koreans over the age of 50 who fought in the Korean War experienced a time when their next meal was not guaranteed. Because of a devastated economy and agricultural base, barley and *kimchee*, a spicy pickled cabbage, were dietary staples during the war.

COMMON FOODS AND FOOD RITUALS

Korean food is flavorful and spicy. Rice is served with 5 to 20 small side dishes of mostly vegetables and some fish and meats. The variety of seasonings in Korean cooking includes red and black pepper, garlic, green onion, ginger, soy sauce, and sesame seed oil. The traditional Korean diet includes steamed rice; hot soup; *kimchee*; and side dishes of fish, meat, or vegetables served in some variation for breakfast, lunch, and dinner. Breakfast is traditionally considered the most important meal.

Kimchee is made from a variety of vegetables but is primarily made from a Chinese, or Napa, cabbage (Fig. 17–2). Spices and herbs are added to the previously salted cabbage, which is allowed to ferment over time and is served with every meal in a variety of forms. Some common Korean American dishes:

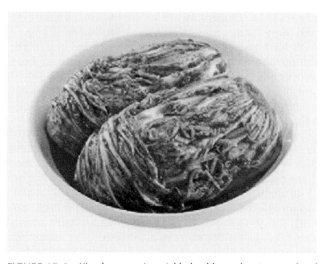

FIGURE 17–2 Kimchee, a spicy pickled cabbage that is a staple of the Korean diet.

Beebimbap is a combination of rice, finely chopped mixed vegetables, and a fried egg served in a hot pottery bowl. Hot pepper paste is usually added.

Bulgolgi is thinly sliced pieces of beef marinated in soy sauce, sesame oil, green onions, garlic, and sugar, which is then barbecued.

Chopchae are clear noodles mixed with lightly stir-fried vegetables and meats.

Rice is usually served in individual bowls, set to the left of the diner. Soup is served in another bowl, placed to the right of the rice. Chopsticks and large soupspoons are used at all meals. Korean Americans may use forks and knives, depending on their degree of assimilation into American culture. Meals are frequently eaten in silence, using this opportunity to enjoy the food. When Koreans migrate to the United States, they increase their consumption of beef, dairy products, coffee, soda, and bread as well as decrease their intake of fish, rice, and other grains. However, incorporating a larger quantity of Western foods does not make a less-healthy diet. They consume diets consistent with their traditional Korean food patterns, with 60 percent of calories coming from carbohydrates and 16 percent of calories from fat (Kim, Yu, Chen, Cross, & Kim, 2000). To increase compliance with dietary prescriptions, health teaching should be geared to the unique Korean American food choices and practices.

Understanding the ritual offering of food and drink to guests is important. Koreans offer a guest a drink on first arriving at their home. The guest declines courteously. The host offers the drink again and the guest again declines. This ritual can occur three to five times before the guest accepts the offer. This interaction is done out of respect for the hosts and their generosity to share with their guest and to express an unwillingness to impose on the hosts. Accepting an offer when first asked is considered rude and selfish.

DIETARY PRACTICES FOR HEALTH PROMOTION

Most dietary practices for health promotion apply to pregnancy, discussed later in this chapter. Someone suffering from the common cold is served soup made from bean sprouts. Dried anchovies, garlic, and other hot spices are added to the hot soup, which assists in clearing a congested nose.

NUTRITIONAL DEFICIENCIES AND FOOD LIMITATIONS

Kim, Yu, Liu, Kim, and Kohrs (1993) examined the nutritional status of older Chinese, Korean, and Japanese Americans. Along with a dietary interview and anthropometric measurements, a 24-hour recall technique was used to obtain dietary data. The results of the study showed that older Korean Americans had the poorest diets, particularly with regard to inadequate amounts of vitamins A and C. Korean American women had a low intake of protein. The results also suggested that older Asian Americans are at high risk for calcium deficiencies. The authors concluded that a large-scale national nutritional survey is needed for Asian Americans to plan health programs based on the specific needs of selected populations.

A study by Park, Murphy, Sharma, and Kolonel (2005) indicated that the proportion of overweight or obesity was 31.4 percent in U.S.-born Korean women and 9.4 percent in Korean-born Korean women. They also reported that U.S.-born Korean women had higher intakes of total fat and fat as a percentage of energy and lower intakes of sodium, vitamin C, beta-carotene, and carbohydrate as a percentage of energy than Korean-born women. In addition, Cho and Juon (2006) reported that of 492 Korean American respondents, 38 percent were overweight and 8 percent were obsese according to the World Health Organization for Asian populations. These findings suggest that acculturation of Korean immigrants affects dietary intakes in ways that may alter their risks of several chronic diseases.

Korean Americans, as with most other Asians, are at a high risk for lactose intolerance. Thus, milk and other dairy products are not part of the traditional Korean diet, emphasizing the need to assess them for calcium deficiencies.

Korean Americans living in or near large metropolitan cities have access to Korean markets and restaurants. When no Korean stores are available, Chinese or Japanese markets may contain some of the foods Koreans enjoy. When no Asian markets are available, the American grocery store suffices.

Pregnancy and Childbearing Practices

VIGNETTE 17.3

Jay and Sue Kim, ages 29 and 26 years and married for 2 years, immigrated from South Korea and settled in Los Angeles. They have lived in a small one-bedroom apartment since their arrival. Both of them graduated from the same Korean university with baccalaureate degrees in English literature. They have one child, Joseph, age 1 year.

When they arrived in the United States, Jay was unable to find a job because of his poor proficiency in English, despite his major in English Literature. He eventually obtained a job with a moving company through a church friend. Sue is not working because of their son. Although the Kims did not attend a church before immigration, they are now regularly attending a Korean Protestant church in their neighborhood.

Sue is pregnant again, determined by a home pregnancy kit, with their second child and concerned about the medical costs. They did not use any contraceptives because she was breastfeeding. Because of financal limitations, Sue did not initially have prenatal care with her first pregnancy. However, she did keep up with the Korean traditional prenatal practice, tae-kyo. Eventually, she received help from her church and delivered a healthy son. She is not sure whether she can get financial help from her church again but is confident that her second child will be healthy if she follows the Korean traditional prenatal practices.

Jay is concerened about job security because he recently heard from colleagues that the moving company might soon go bankrupt. Although Jay has not been satisfied with his current job (he thinks that he is overqualified), this news is still a cause for concern. Moreover, Sue's recent pregnancy has made Jay more stressed, and he has started drinking alcohol.

Joseph cannot stand up by himself and still wants to be breastfed. Although Sue has tried to give foods such as oranges, apples, steamed rice, and milk (because she is now pregnant), Joseph refuses to eat them and cries for breastfeeding. Joseph's weight is low normal for same-age babies.

1. How might Jay have improved his English language skills to increase his opportunities to obtain a position for which his education qualifies him?
2. Describe the Korean cultural practice tae-kyo. Is this practice congruent with allopathic recommendations for prenatal care?
3. How do food choices among Koreans differ with pregnancy and postpartum?
4. Describe cultural attitudes toward drinking among Koreans.
5. Identify two or three culturally congruent strategies for addressing Jay's drinking.

FERTILITY PRACTICES AND VIEWS TOWARD PREGNANCY

To curtail population growth in Korea, the government promotes the concept of two children per household. The government supported the use of contraception when a 10-year family planning program was adopted in the early 1960s, resulting in a mass public education program on contraception. When contraceptive devices became easily available in Korea, fertility control spread widely among married women. Contraceptive devices are covered by the present national health insurance of Korea. Recently, South Korea's fertility rate fell to a new record low in 2005 as more women engaged in economic activities and got married at older ages (Hankyoreh, 2007). The average number of babies per woman of child-bearing age was 1.08 in 2005, down from 1.16 in 2004, and the number of newborn babies fell by 38,000, or 7.9 percent, to 438,000 (Hankyoreh, 2007). As part of efforts to address those issues, the South Korean government is to spend a total of 30.5 trillion won (U.S. $432.8 billion) over the next 5 years to strengthen the country's social safety net and boost its record-low birth rate (Hankyoreh, 2007).

Before the 1950s, abortion was illegal in Korea, although induced abortions were performed widely. Today, abortion is legal and is widely used in Korea. Abortion is not highly publicized in Korea, yet there is an unspoken acceptance of the practice. The government keeps a hands-off policy, which has not met with major opposition. Women are not expected to get their husband's consent, nor are underage youth required to have their parents' acknowledgment. The government does not pay for abortions; rather, patients pay a set price from personal funds.

Pritham and Sammons (1993) investigated Korean women's attitudes toward pregnancy and prenatal care with regard to their beliefs and interactions with healthcare professionals from the United States. The survey was conducted of 40 unemployed Korean women between the ages of 18 and 35 at an American military medical-care facility in a major metropolitan area of Korea.

Attitudes toward childbearing practices and relationships with health-care providers were elicited. The results indicated that these women were happy about their pregnancies. Only one-third of the respondents agreed with the traditional preference for a male child. About 40 percent of the women reinforced strong food taboos and restrictions and acknowledged the need to avoid certain foods during pregnancy. Twenty percent disagreed with the use of prenatal vitamins, and 25 percent indicated needing only a 10- to 15-lb weight gain in pregnancy. The women generally had sound health habits in relation to physical activity and recognized the harm of smoking while pregnant. The study sample was homogeneous and small, limiting the ability to generalize about the findings.

Pregnancy in the Korean culture is traditionally a highly protected time for women. Both the pregnancy and the postpartum period have been ritualized by the culture. A pregnancy begins with the **tae-mong**, a dream of the conception of pregnancy. Once a woman is pregnant, she starts practicing **tae-kyo**, which literally means "fetus education." The objective of *tae-kyo* is to promote the health and well-being of the fetus and the mother by having the mother focus on art and beautiful objects. If the pregnant woman handles unclean objects or kills a living creature, a difficult birth can ensue (Howard & Barbiglia, 1997). Some women wear tight abdominal binders beginning at 20 weeks' gestation or work physically hard toward the end of the pregnancy to increase the chances of having a small baby (Howard & Barbiglia, 1997). In addition, expectant mothers should avoid duck, chicken, fish with scales, squid, or crab because eating these foods may affect the child's appearance. For example, eating duck may cause the baby to be born with webbed feet (Howard & Barbiglia, 1997).

Kendall's study (1987) in Honolulu supported the belief that Korean women attribute a variety of complaints to *naeng* (chill), a cold imbalance of the womb that brings on a heavy vaginal discharge and can make women who experience it sterile. The researcher emphasized that an intimate condition such as *naeng* may be lost in translation in non-Korean contexts.

PRESCRIPTIVE, RESTRICTIVE, AND TABOO PRACTICES IN THE CHILDBEARING FAMILY

Ludman, Kang, and Lynn's study (1992) explored the food beliefs and diets of 200 pregnant Korean American women. The food items most frequently consumed were *kimchee* (82.5 percent), rice or noodles (81.5 percent), and fresh fruit (79 percent). Foods avoided during pregnancy included coffee (19.8 percent), spicy foods (9.9 percent), chicken (6.9 percent), and crab (6.9 percent). A list of 20 food items was then given to the women, who were asked to respond whether they consumed the food or not and, if not, to indicate their reasons. A number of respondents indicated that they did not eat rabbit (91.5 percent), sparrow (91.5 percent), duck (89.5 percent), goat (84 percent), or blemished fruit (63 percent) because of dislike or lack of availability. The reason most frequently given for not eating blemished fruit was that it might produce a skin disease on the infant or cause an unpleasant face. The study showed that, although many Korean American women were aware of traditionally taboo foods, they did not avoid consuming them. An awareness of these beliefs can give health professionals a basis for nutritional education for Korean American women.

Birthing practices among both Koreans and Korean Americans are highly influenced by Western methods. Women commonly labor and deliver in the supine position. After the delivery, women are traditionally served seaweed soup, a rich source of iron, which is believed to facilitate lactation and to promote healing of the mother. Bed rest is encouraged after pregnancy for 7 to 90 days. Women are also encouraged to keep warm by avoiding showers, baths, and cold fluids or foods.

The postpartum period is seen as the time when women undergo profound physiological, psychological, and sociological changes; this period is known as the *Sanhujori* belief system. In this dynamic process, postpartum women should care for their bodies by augmenting heat and avoiding cold, resting without working, eating well, protecting the body from harmful strains, and keeping clean (Howard & Barbiglia, 1997). In Western society in which they may lack extended family members from whom to seek assistance, Korean women may be faced with a cultural dilemma.

Park and Peterson (1991) studied Korean American women's health beliefs, practices, and experiences in relation to childbirth. Using structured questions, they interviewed in Korean a nonrandom sample of 20 female volunteers. Those interviewed subscribed to a holistic view, which emphasized both emotional and physical health. Only one-half of the women interviewed rated themselves healthy. The authors related this to the stresses of immigration and pregnancy. Preventive practices were not found among members of this group. Only one woman regularly received Pap smears and did breast self-examinations. A common finding was that most women participated in a significant rest period during puerperium. Those who did not rest lacked help for the home. All the women ate brown seaweed soup and steamed rice for about 20 days after childbirth to cleanse the blood and to assist in milk production. Because pregnancy is a hot condition and heat is lost during labor and delivery, some women avoided cold foods and water after childbirth to prevent chronic illnesses such as arthritis. The baby should be wrapped in warm blankets to prevent harm from cold winds. Herbal medicines are also used during puerperium to promote healing and health (Howard & Barbiglia, 1997).

Health-care professionals can improve the health of Korean American women by providing factual information about Pap smears and teaching breast self-examination. Pregnant Korean American women should be asked about their use of herbal medicine during pregnancy so that harmless practices can be incorporated into biomedical care. Recommendations for improving postpartum care among Korean American women include (1) developing an assessment tool that health-care providers can use to identify traditional beliefs early in a pregnancy, (2) developing a bilingual dictionary of common foods, (3) developing pamphlets with medical terms used in the U.S. health-care system, and (4) providing time for practicing English skills (Park & Peterson, 1991).

Death Rituals

DEATH RITUALS AND EXPECTATIONS

Traditionally, in Korea, it was important for Koreans to die at home. Bringing a dead body home if the person died in the hospital is considered bad luck. Consequently, viewing of the deceased occurred at home if the individual died at home and at the hospital if the person died at the hospital. Several days or more were set aside for the viewing, depending on the status of the deceased. The eldest son was expected to sit by the body of the parent during the viewing (Martinson, 1998). Friends and relatives paid their respects by bowing to a photograph of the deceased placed in the same room in which the body rested. The guests were then offered the favorite foods of the deceased. Today, most Korean Americans are not accustomed to viewing the body of the deceased. More commonly, relatives and friends come to pay their respect by viewing photographs of the deceased.

Although Korean Americans view life support more positively than European Americans, the majority in one study did not want such technology (Blackhall et al., 1999). In addition, they were less likely to have made a prior decision about life support. Older and more educated Koreans were less likely to favor truth telling, believing that patients should not be told that they have a terminal illness.

An ancestral burial ceremony follows, with the body being placed in the ground facing south or north. Both the place and the position of the deceased are important for the future fortune of the living relatives. Koreans believe that if the spirit is content, good fortune will be awarded to the family. Unlike Western graves, a mound of dirt covers the gravesite of the deceased in Korea.

Cremation is an individual and family choice and is practiced more commonly in Korea for those who have no family or die at a young age. For example, when unmarried people die without any children to perform ancestral ceremonies, they are often cremated and their ashes scattered over a body of water.

Rice wine is traditionally sprinkled around the grave. Korean families bow two to four times in respect at the gravesite, and then the men, in descending order from the eldest to the youngest, drink rice wine. Some Korean Americans dedicate a corner of their home to honor their ancestors because they cannot go to the gravesite.

Circumstances in which "do not resuscitate" orders are an issue need to be addressed cautiously. Families trust physicians and may not question other options. Because death and dying are fairly well accepted in the Korean culture, prolonging life may not be highly regarded in the face of modern technology. Korean hospitals focus on acute care. Families are expected to stay with family members to assist in feeding and personal care around the clock. Thus, many Korean Americans may expect to care for their hospitalized family members in health-care facilities.

RESPONSES TO DEATH AND GRIEF

Mourning rituals, with crying and open displays of grief, are commonly practiced and socially accepted at funerals, and they signify the utmost respect for the dead. The eldest son or male family member who sits by the deceased sometimes holds a cane and makes a moaning noise to display his grief. The cane is a symbol of needing support. Health-care personnel may need to provide a private setting for Korean Americans to be able to grieve in culturally congruent ways.

Spirituality

DOMINANT RELIGION AND USE OF PRAYER

Confucianism was the official religion of Korea from the 14th to the 20th century. Buddhism, Confucianism, Christianity, shamanism, and **Chondo-Kyo** are practiced in Korea today. *Chondo-Kyo* (religion of the Heavenly Way) is a nationalistic religion founded in the 19th century that combines Confucianism, Buddhism, and Daoism. Among Korean Americans, the most recent estimates of organized religions include no affiliation, 46 percent; Christianity, 26 percent; Buddhism, 26 percent; Confucionism, 1 percent; and other, 1 percent, of which the majority are *Chondo-Kyo* (CIA, 2007). In the United States, the church acts as a powerful social support group for Korean immigrants (Im & Yang, 2006). Yu (1990a) speculated that with the growth of other organizations that facilitate the transition for Korean immigrants, they might have less need for churches as the major source of emotional support and practical information on life in the United States.

Kim (1990) studied Korean Christian churches in the Pacific Northwest in an attempt to prove the importance of the structure and function of the church as a secondary association for Korean immigrants in the United States. Many of the churches were young in terms of both years of operation and age of the membership. Most had been in operation between 5 and 10 years. Most of the churches were hierarchically organized, and only a couple of the churches reported having female pastors. A variety of services other than prayer meetings were offered, such as English and Korean language programs, income tax seminars, health education including AIDS prevention, information on U.S. citizenship and laws, driver's licenses, job searches, and assistance with older family members. Kim reinforced the role of churches in preserving Korean culture and, consequently, ethnic identity. Kim also stressed the importance of retaining one's ethnic identity in the Korean culture. Korean immigrants experience a dramatic transition and are frequently faced with the forces of racism and individualism.

Koreans in America might not pray in the same fashion as Westerners, but for many people, the spirits demand homage. Korean churches often have prayer meetings several times a week, some with early-morning prayers. Buddhist temples have spirit rooms attached to them. Although Buddhists believe the spirit enters a new life, the beliefs of the shamans are so strong that the Buddhist church incorporated an area of their church for those who believe that ancestral spirits need honoring and homage. With such a variety of spiritual beliefs, caregivers must assess each Korean client individually for religious beliefs and prayer practices.

MEANING OF LIFE AND INDIVIDUAL SOURCES OF STRENGTH

Family and education are central themes that give meaning to life for Korean Americans. The nuclear and extended families are primary sources of strength for Korean Americans in their daily lives. These concepts were previously covered under Family Roles and Organization and Educational Status and Occupations.

SPIRITUAL BELIEFS AND HEALTH-CARE PRACTICES

Shamanism is a powerful belief in natural spirits. All parts of nature contain spirits: rivers, animals, and even inanimate objects. The many religions of Koreans create numerous ideologies about what happens with the spirits of the deceased. Christians believe the spirit goes to heaven; Buddhists believe the spirit starts a new life as a person or an animal; and Shamanists believe the spirit stays with the family to watch over them and guide their actions and fortunes. Such a variety of faith systems provides a great diversity in beliefs of the Korean people. Given this diversity of spiritual beliefs among Koreans, each client needs an individual assessment with regard to spiritual and health-care practices.

Health-Care Practices

HEALTH-SEEKING BELIEFS AND BEHAVIORS

Beliefs that influence health-care practices include religious beliefs (see Dominant Religion and Use of Prayer) and dietary practices (see Nutrition). Health-care providers need to be aware that the theme dominating these beliefs is a holistic approach, which emphasizes both emotional and physical health.

Health-care practices among Koreans in America are primarily focused on curative rather than preventive measures. Health promotion in Korea is a relatively new public-health focus. In Korea, education on dental hygiene, sanitation, environmental issues, and other preventive health measures is being encouraged. Visits to the physician for an annual physical examination, Pap smears, and breast self-examination are uncommon. Among Koreans, traditional patterns of health promotion include harmony with nature and the universe, activity and rest, diet, sexual life, covetousness, temperament, and apprehension (Lee, 1993).

RESPONSIBILITY FOR HEALTH CARE

One American study reported that only 13.5 percent of Korean American men and 11.3 percent of Korean American women had a digital rectal examination (DRE) for occult blood. Regression analysis indicated that gender, education, knowledge of the warning signs of cancer, and length of residence in the United States were significantly related to having undergone DRE. The researchers determined that this group of Korean Americans did not see health-care providers or health brochures as valuable sources of information, and to target this group, efforts should be coordinated with church and community leaders and enhanced by developing brochures in the Korean language (Kim, Yu, Chen, Kim, & Britnall, 1998).

Because of women's modesty during physical examinations and their preferences that women perform intimate examinations, many Korean women defer having Pap tests or breast cancer screening tests (Lee, Fogg, & Sadler, 2006; Wismer et al., 1998). A recent study among Korean immigrant women reported that 78 percent of the participants had had a mammogram at some point and that 38.6 percent had had one in the previous year (Lee et al., 2006). This reluctance for undergoing Pap tests directly relates to cervical cancer's rating as the number-one female cancer diagnosed among women in Korea (Lee, 2000). Modesty has also been associated with low rates of mammography among Korean Americans (Maxwell, Bastani, & Warda, 1998) as well as limited knowledge about breast self-examination and causes of breast cancer (Han, Williams, & Harrison, 2000).

Recent Korean immigrants come from a country in which universal health insurance was implemented in the late 1980s. A government mandate established employer-based health insurance for medium and large firms. Regional health insurance systems, subsidized by the government, were later established for small firms, farmers, and the self-employed. Yu (1990a) found that 55 percent of the Koreans surveyed in Los Angeles and Orange counties have medical insurance; however, the rates vary according to income, with higher rates among the high-income group and lower rates among the low-income group.

The use and availability of over-the-counter medications vary tremendously between the United States and Korea. Many prescription drugs in the United States such as antibiotics, anti-inflammatory and cardiac medications, and certain pain control medications can be purchased over-the-counter in Korea at any *yak bang* (pharmacy). For example, when feeling "tired" or "fatigued," older people in Korea may perform home infusions of dextrose and water or albumin.

Self-medication with herbal remedies is also practiced. Ginseng is a root used for anything from a remedy for the common cold to an aphrodisiac. Seaweed soup is used as a medicine. Chinese herbs are used to control the degree of "wind" that may be in the body. Other herbal medications are taken for preventive or restorative purposes, For example, *haigefen* (clamshell powder) has high levels of lead, which can cause abdominal colic, muscle pain, and fatigue (Markowitz, Nunez, Klitzman, & Munshi, 1994). Accordingly, health-care professionals should query their patients about their use of traditional Korean medicine and must be aware that herbal medicine may be used in conjunction with Western biomedicine.

FOLK AND TRADITIONAL PRACTICES

Hanyak, traditional herbal medicine used for creating harmony between oneself and the larger cosmology, is a healing method for the body and soul. **Hanbang**, the traditional Korean medical-care system, works on the principle of a disturbed state of **ki**, cosmological vital energy. Symptoms are often interpreted in terms of a psychological base. Treatments include acupuncture, acumassage, acupressure, herbal medicines, and moxibustion therapy. The therapeutic relationship between **hanui** (oriental medicine doctors) and their clients is genuine, spontaneous, and harmonious. Clients who use both Western and traditional Korean practitioners may experience conflicts because of the lack of cooperation between *hanui* and biomedical practitioners (Pang, 1989). In 1993 in Korea, a pharmaceutical act supported pharmacists in prescribing and dispensing herbal drugs, creating a lucrative business and increasing conflicts among *hanui* physicians and pharmacists (Cho, 2000).

Shamans are used in healing rituals to ward off restless spirits. Shamans originated with the religious belief of **shamanism**, the belief that all things possess spirits. A shaman, **mundang**, is usually a woman who has special abilities for communicating with spirits. The shaman is used to treat illnesses after other means of treatment are exhausted. The shaman performs a **kut**, a shamanistic ceremony to eliminate the evil spirits causing the illness. Such a ceremony may take place when a young person dies to prevent his or her spirit from staying tied to the earth. Others believe a shaman can eliminate evil spirits that may be causing difficulty with financial transactions. Although shamans have been around for many years, Koreans consider them part of the lowest class. Health-care providers need to determine whether Koreans in America are using folk therapies and should include nonharmful practices with biomedical therapies and prescriptions.

BARRIERS TO HEALTH CARE

Because many Korean Americans use various options for healing, Western medical practices may be used in conjunction with acupressure, acupuncture, and herbal medicine. Barriers for Koreans in America may result from the expense of non-Western therapies, because insurance companies often do not cover alternative therapies.

As for many other American residents, the lack of insurance creates barriers to health care. Paying for health care out-of-pocket is expensive and not feasible for many Korean American families. Language, modesty, cultural attitudes toward certain illnesses, and communication problems also serve as impediments for access to health care.

CULTURAL RESPONSES TO HEALTH AND ILLNESS

Perceptions of pain vary widely among Koreans. Some Koreans are stoic and are slow to express emotional distress from pain. Others are expressive and discuss their smallest discomforts. Family and friends are useful resources for learning some of the historical coping mechanisms of sick individuals. Nonverbal cues and facial expressions must be monitored for those who are stoic rather than expressive. Pain assessments should be conducted regularly, and patient education may be necessary for stoic individuals.

Mental illness is stigmatized in the Korean culture. Kim and Grant (1997) conducted a study of Korean American women and their reluctance to use mental-health professionals in the United States. Their study concluded that these women experienced gender-role disruption, evidence

of depressive symptoms, and subsequent risk of substance abuse, suicide, battering, loss of employment, deficits in parenting, and low use of mental-health professionals. A study in Korea of 3711 respondents showed that 23.1 percent of men and 27.4 percent of women were at risk for depression, which is a higher rate than in the United States and other Western countries. In this study, female gender, less than 13 years of education, and disrupted marriage were significant predictors of severe, definitive symptoms of depression (Cho, Nam, & Suh, 1998). Pang (1990) explored the cultural construction of **hwa-byung** among a group of Korean immigrant women in the United States, using a convenience sample. *Hwa-byung*, a traditional Korean illness, results from the suppression of anger or other emotions (Donnelly, 2001). *Hwa* means "fire and anger," and *byung* means "illness." All the women in the study knew the meaning of *hwa-byung*, and 80 percent reported having experienced it. The emotions they reported suppressing were sadness, depression, worry, anger, fright, and fear. Most of the emotions described were related to conflicts with close relatives or family, such as sons and daughters or significant others. These were expressed as physical complaints, ranging from headaches and poor appetites to insomnia and lack of energy. The complaints were chronic in nature, and a variety of remedies were used to alleviate the symptoms. Most of the women suggested that *hwa-byung* was difficult to cure and accepted the symptoms as inevitable. For these older Korean women, *hwa-byung* was a mode for constructing illness as a personal, social, and cultural adaptive response (Pang, 1990). These women expressed life's hardships by channeling their emotional illnesses into physical symptoms.

A community study of Korean Americans addressed the prevalence, clinical significance, and meaning of *hwa-byung* (Lin, Lau, Yamamoto, Zheng, & Kim, 1992). The results indicated a high percentage of Korean Americans (11.9 percent) who identified themselves as suffering from *hwa-byung*. A strong association was shown between *hwa-byung* and major depressive disorders. Although *hwa-byung* is found predominantly among older Korean women with little education, this study's findings did not support this conclusion. The ability to generalize these findings, however, is limited because assignment to the study groups was not completely random and because the sample size was small.

Historically, the area of special education has not been well studied or researched in Korea. Families who have children with mental or physical disabilities often question what they have done wrong to make their ancestors angry. Families feel stigmatized for such a misfortune and cannot accept their children's disfigurement or low intellect. Korea lacks social support to assist families in caring for children with mental or physical disabilities. Some families abandon these children in their desperate need for support with long-term care and expenses. Other children are kept from the public eye in the hope of saving the family from stigmatization.

Seo, Oakland, Han, and Hu (1992) explored the historical and future needs of special education in South Korea. Korea is faced with high teacher-pupil ratios, a reliance on self-contained programs, negative attitudes toward the disabled, and lack of advocacy for them. Of the 600,000 children aged 6 to 17 years who were disabled, only 15 percent received service in special private or public schools or classes. Negative attitudes toward the disabled influence the idea of mainstreaming mildly disabled students in South Korea. Korean Americans may hold these same views regarding the mentally and physically disabled and need special support in obtaining assistance.

In Korea, once hospitalized people are physically stable, they are discharged to their homes to be with the family. Bowel training and physical therapy activities are not the responsibility of the hospital. The families must care for family members at home with the support of other family members. Long-term care for chronic problems or for rehabilitation is rare in Korea. Thus, Korean Americans are familiar with the concept of family home care. Depending on their adaptation to the American health-care system, and families' contact with American health-care professionals, some Korean Americans adjust their ideologies on the sick role.

BLOOD TRANSFUSIONS AND ORGAN DONATION

No beliefs held by Korean Americans prevent the acceptance of blood transfusions. Organ donation and organ transplantation are rare, reflecting traditional attitudes toward integrity and purity. These issues need to be approached sensitively with Korean Americans because they may be influenced by the individual's religious beliefs.

Health-Care Practitioners

TRADITIONAL VERSUS BIOMEDICAL PRACTITIONERS

In general, no taboos exist that prevent health-care practitioners from delivering care to the opposite gender. Female physicians are definitely preferred for maternity care and female problems because women feel more comfortable discussing gynecological and obstetric issues with female physicians. However, more-traditional Koreans frequently prefer health-care providers who speak Korean, are older, and are of the same gender, although many will seek health care from others who do not meet these requirements if their preferred care provider is not available. Miller (1990) studied the use of traditional health practitioners, acupuncturists, and herbalists among a group of 102 Korean immigrants. The findings indicated that Korean immigrants with higher incomes were more likely to use traditional Korean practitioners.

The area of social work is new in Korea. The hospitals have no positions for such a role. A few educational programs exist in Korea for social workers, but much development is needed in the area of social support. Because these roles may be new to many Koreans, health-care providers may need to encourage Korean Americans to use these services.

STATUS OF HEALTH-CARE PROVIDERS

Because traditional Korean culture accords high respect to men, older people, and physicians, the ideal physician is an older man with gray hair. This shows that he has experience and wisdom and is able to make the best decisions. With such a high status in Korea, physicians expect respect from all other health professionals. Usually, nurses are expected to carry out physicians' orders explicitly. This is not to say that the nurse cannot question orders, but great time and effort are spent consulting other nurses before questioning physicians in the most respectful way. However, as nurses are becoming more educated in Korea, they are becoming more assertive and more closely mirror Western practice patterns.

With an emphasis on increasing the educational level of nurses, they too are gaining stature and respect in Korean culture. Baccalaureate, masters, and doctoral programs are available for nurses in Korea. Although exact numbers are not available, Korea has approximately 600 doctorally prepared nurses as of 2001.

REFERENCES

Asianinfo. (2007a). *General information—Seoul*. Retrieved January 7, 2007, from http://www.asianinfo.org/asianinfo/seoul/general_information.htm

Asianinfo. (2007b). *Korean drama*. Retrieved January 7, 2007, from http://www.asianinfo.org/asianinfo/korea/korean_drama.htm

Blackhall, L., Frank, G., Murphy, S., Michel, V., Palmer, J., Azen, S., et al. (1999). Ethnicity and attitudes toward life sustaining technology. *Social Science Medicine, 48*(12), 1779–1789.

Cho, B. (2000). The politics of herbal drugs in Korea. *Social Science Medicine, 51*(4), 505–509.

Cho, J., & Juon, H. S. (2006). Assessing overweight and obesity risk among Korean Americans in California using World Health Organization body mass index criteria for Asians. *Prevention of Chronic Disease, 3*(3), A79.

Cho, Y. I., & Faulkner, W. R. (1993). Conception of alcoholism among Koreans and Americans. *International Journal of the Addictions, 28*(8), 681–694.

Cho, M., Nam, J., & Suh, G. (1998). Prevalence of symptoms of depression in a nationwide sample of Korean adults. *Psychiatric Residence, 81*(3), 341–352.

Choi, E. (1995). A contrast of mothering behaviors in women from Korea and the United States. *Journal of Obstetric, Gynecologic, and Neonatal Nursing, 24*(4), 363–369.

CIA. (2007). *World FactBook: Korea*. Retrieved March 29, 2007, from https://www.cia.gov/cia/publications/factbook/geos/ks.html

Comrie, B., Matthews, S., & Polinsky, M. (1996). *The atlas of languages*. London: Quarto Publishing, Inc.

CNN. (2007). *Special report. North Korea nuclear tension*. Retrieved March 29, 2007 from http://edition.cnn.com/SPECIALS/2003/nkorea/

Donnelly, P. L. (2001). Korean American family experiences of caregiving for their mentally ill adult children: An interpretative study. *Journal of Transcultural Nursing, 12*(4), 292–301.

Han, Y., Williams, R., & Harrison, R. (2000). Breast cancer screening knowledge, attitudes, and practices among Korean-American women. *Oncology Nursing Forum, 27*(10), 1589–1591.

Hankyoreh (2007). *S. Korea's fertility rate falls to new record low*. Retrieved January 6, 2007, from http://english.hani.co.kr/arti/english_edition/e_national/121634.html

Howard, J., & Barbiglia, V. (1997). Caring for childbearing Korean women. *Journal of Obstetric, Gynecologic, and Neonatal Nursing, 26*(6), 665–671.

Im, E. O. (2002). Korean culture. In P. S. St. Hill, J. Lipson, & A. I. Meleis (Eds.), *Caring for women cross-culturally: A portable guide*. Philadelphia: F.A. Davis Company.

Im, E. O., & Meleis, A. I. (2001). Women's work and symptoms during menopausal transition: Korean immigrant women. *Women and Health, 33*(1/2), 83–103.

Im, E. O., & Yang, K. (2006). Theories on immigrant women's health. *Health Care Women International, 27*(8), 666–681.

Johanning, E., Goldberg, M., & Kim, R. (1994). Asbestos hazard evaluation in South Korean textile production. *International Journal of Health Services, 24*(1), 131–144.

Kendall, L. (1987). Cold wombs in balmy Honolulu: Ethnography among Korean immigrants. *Social Science Medicine, 25*(4), 367–376.

Kim, E., Cain, K., & McCubbin, M. (2006). Maternal and paternal parenting, acculturation, and young adolescents' psychological adjustment in Korean American families. *Journal of Child Adolescent Psychiatric Nursing, 19*(3), 112–129.

Kim, H. (1990). Korean Christian churches in the Pacific Northwest: Resources for Korean ethnic identity? In H. C. Kim & E. H. Lee (Eds.), *Koreans in America: Dreams and realities* (pp. 177–192). Seoul: Institute of Korean Studies.

Kim, H., & Chung, R. H. (2003). Relationship of recalled parenting style to self-perception in Korean American college students. *Journal of Genetic Psychology, 164*(4), 481-492.

Kim, K., Yu, E. S., Chen, E. H., Kim, J., & Britnall, R. A. (1998). Colorectal cancer screening: Knowledge and practices among Korean Americans. *Cancer Practices, 6*(3), 167–175.

Kim, K. E. (2003). Gastric cancer in Korean Americans: Risks and reductions. *Korean American Studies Bulletin, 13*(1/2), 84–90.

Kim, K. K., Yu, E. S., Chen, E. H., Cross, N., & Kim, J. (2000). Nutritional status of Korean Americans: Implications for cancer risk. *Oncology Nursing Forum, 27*(10), 1573–1583.

Kim, K. K., Yu, E. S., Liu, W. T., Kim, J., & Kohrs, M. B. (1993). Nutritional status of Chinese-, Korean-, and Japanese-American elderly. *Journal of the American Dietetic Association, 93*(12), 1416–1422.

Kim, Y., & Grant, D. (1997). Immigration patterns, social support, and adaptation among Korean immigrant women and Korean American women. *Cultural Diversity in Mental Health, 3*(4), 235–245.

Kim, Y. G., & Hahn, S. J. (2006). Homosexuality in ancient and modern Korea. *Culture Health and Sex, 8*(1), 59-65.

Kimmel, D. C., & Yi, H. (2004). Characteristics of gay, lesbian, and bisexual Asians, Asian Americans, and immigrants from Asia to the U.S.A. *Journal of Homosexuality, 47*(2), 143–172.

Kohls, R. L. (2001). *Learning to think Korean.* Yarmouth, ME: Intercultural Press.

Korean American Coalition. (2003). Retrieved January 7, 2007, from www.kacdc.org/data/VIP%20Handbook.doc

Lee, D. C., & Lee, E. H. (1990). Korean immigrant families in America: Role and value conflicts. In H. C. Kim & E. H. Lee (Eds.), *Koreans in America: Dreams and realities* (pp. 165–177). Seoul: Institute of Korean Studies.

Lee, E. E., Fogg, L. F., & Sadler, G. R. (2006). Factors of breast cancer screening among Korean immigrants in the United States. *Journal of Immigrant and Minority Health, 8*(3), 223–233.

Lee, M. (2000). Knowledge, barriers, and motivators related to cervical cancer screening among Korean-American women. A focus group approach. *Cancer Nursing, 23*(3), 168–175.

Lee, S., Sobal, J., & Frongillo, E. (2000). Acculturation and health in Korean Americans. *Social Science Medicine, 51*(2), 159–173.

Lee, Y. (1993). Health promotion: Patterns of traditional health promotion in Korea. *Kanhohak Tamgu, 2*(2), 21–36.

Levy, R. (1993). Ethnic and racial differences in response to medicines: Preserving individualized therapy in managed pharmaceutical programmes. *Pharmaceutical Medicine, 7,* 139–165.

Lin, K., Lau, J. K., Yamamoto, J., Zheng, Y. P., & Kim, K. H. (1992). Hwa-Byung: A community study of Korean Americans. *Journal of Nervous and Mental Disease, 180*(6), 386–391.

Ludman, E. K., Kang, K. J., & Lynn, L. L. (1992). Food beliefs and diets of pregnant Korean American women. *Journal of the American Dietetic Association, 92*(12), 1519–1520.

Markowitz, S., Nunez, C. M., Klitzman, S., & Munshi, A. A. (1994). Lead poisoning due to haigefen. The porphyrin content of individual erythrocytes. *Journal of the American Medical Association, 271*(12), 932–934.

Martinson, I. M. (1998). Funeral rituals in Taiwan and Korea. *Oncology Nursing Forum, 25*(10), 1756–1760.

Maxwell, A., Bastani, R., & Warda, U. (1998). Misconceptions and mammography use among Filipino- and Korean-American women. *Ethnic Diversity, 8*(3), 377–384.

Meyer, U. (1992). Drugs in special patient groups: Clinical importance of genetics in drug effects. In M. Melmon & T. Morrelli (Eds.), *Clinical pharmacology: Basic principles in therapeutics* (8th ed., pp. 62–83). New York: Pergamon Press.

Miller, J. (1990). Use of traditional Korean health care by Korean immigrants to the United States. *Sociology and Social Research, 75*(1), 38–48.

Munoz, C., & Hilgenberg, C. (2005). Ethnopharmacology. *American Journal of Nursing, 105*(8), 40–49.

Pang, K. Y. (1989). The practice of traditional Korean medicine in Washington, DC. *Social Science Medicine, 28*(8), 857–884.

Pang, K. Y. (1990). Hwa-Byung: The construction of a Korean popular illness among Korean elderly immigrant women in the United States. *Culture, Medicine, and Psychiatry, 14,* 495–512.

Park, K. Y., & Peterson, L. M. (1991). Beliefs, practices, and experiences of Korean women in relation to childbirth. *Health Care for Women International, 12*(2), 261–269.

Park, M. S. (2001). The factors of child physical abuse in Korean immigrant families. *Child Abuse Neglect, 25*(7), 945–958.

Park, S., Oh, S., & Lee, M. (1998). Korean Status of alcoholics and alcohol-related health problems. *Alcohol and Clinical Expression Research, 22*(3, Suppl), 170S–172S.

Park, S. Y., Murphy, S. P., Sharma, S., & Kolonel, L. N. (2005). Dietary intakes and health-related behaviours of Korean American women born in the USA and Korea: The multiethnic cohort study. *Public Health Nutrition, 8*(7), 904–911.

Pritham, U. A., & Sammons, L. N. (1993). Korean women's attitudes toward pregnancy and prenatal care. *Health Care for Women International, 14,* 145–153.

Seo, G., Oakland, T., Han, H. S., & Hu, S. (1992). Special education in South Korea. *Exceptional Children, 2,* 213–218.

Shin, K., & Shin, C. (1999). The lived experience of Korean immigrant women acculturating into the United States. *Health Care for Women International, 20*(6), 603–617.

Sorensen, C. W. (1994). Success and education in South Korea. *Comparative Education Review, 38*(1), 10–35.

Tritto, T. (2004). Faith organizations and ethnically diverse elders: A community action model. *Journal of Religious Gerontology, 18*(1–2), 1573–1578.

U.S. Department of Homeland Security, Office of Immigration Statistics. (2004). *2003 yearbook of immigration statistics.* Pittsburgh, PA: Author.

U.S. Department of State. (2006). Retrieved January 8, 2007, from http://travel.state.gov/family/family_issues/divorce/divorce_592.html

Weatherspoon, A., Park, J., & Johnson, R. (2001). A family study of homeland Korean alcohol use. *Addictive Behavior, 26*(1), 101–113.

Wismer, B., Moskowitz, J. M., Chen, A. M., Kang, S. H., Novotny, T. E., Min, K., & Lew, R. (1998). Rates and independent correlates of Pap smear testing among Korean American women. *American Journal of Public Health, 88*(4), 656–660.

Yi, M., & Jezewski, M. (2000). Korean nurses' adjustment to hospitals in the United States of America. *Journal of Advanced Nursing, 32*(3), 721–729.

Yu, E. Y. (1990a). Korean American community in 1989: Issues and prospects. In H. C. Kim & E. H. Lee (Eds.), *Koreans in America: Dreams and realities* (pp. 112–126). Seoul: Institute of Korean Studies.

Yu, E. Y. (1990b). Korean community profile: Life and consumer patterns. *Korea Times,* p. 3.

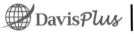

For case studies, review questions, and additional information, go to http://davisplus.fadavis.com

Chapter *18*

People of Mexican Heritage

RICK ZOUCHA and CECILIA A. ZAMARRIPA

Overview, Inhabited Localities, and Topography

OVERVIEW

People of Mexican heritage are a very diverse group geographically, historically, and culturally and are not easy to describe. Although no specific set of characteristics can fully describe people of Mexican heritage, some commonalities distinguish them as an ethnic group, with many regional variations that reflect subcultures in Mexico and in the United States. A common term used to describe Spanish-speaking populations in the United States, including people of Mexican heritage, is **Hispanic**. However, the term can be misleading and can encompass many different people clustered together owing to a common heritage and lineage from Spain. Many Hispanic people prefer to be identified by descriptors more specific to their cultural heritage, such as Mexican, Mexican American, Latin American, Spanish American, **Chicano**, **Latino**, or **Ladino**. Therefore, when referring to Mexican Americans, use that phrase instead of Hispanic or Latino (Vázquez, 2001). As a broad ethnic group, people of Mexican heritage often refer to themselves as **la raza**, which means "the race." The Spanish word for race has a different meaning than the American interpretation of race. The concept of *la raza* has brought people together from separate worlds to make families and is about inclusion (Vázquez, 2000).

HERITAGE AND RESIDENCE

Mexico, with a population of 107,449,525 (CIA, 2007), is a blend of Spanish white and Indian, Native American,

Middle Eastern, and African. Mexican Americans are descendants of Spanish and other European whites; Aztec, Mayan, and other Central American Indians; and Inca and other South American Indians as well as people from Africa (Schmal & Madrer, 2007). Some individuals can trace their heritage to North American Indian tribes in the southwestern part of the United States.

Mexico City, one of the largest cities in the world, has a population of over 20 million. Mexico is undergoing rapid changes in business and health-care practices. Undoubtedly, these changes have accelerated and will continue to accelerate with the passage of the North American Free Trade Agreement as people are more able to move across the border to seek employment and educational opportunities.

Historically, people of Mexican heritage lived on the land that is now known as the southwestern United States for generations, long before the first white settlers came to the territory. By 1853, approximately 80,000 Spanish-speaking settlers lived in the area lost by Mexico during the Texas Rebellion, the Mexican War, and the Gadsden Purchase. After the northern part of Mexico was annexed to the United States, the settlers were not officially considered immigrants but were often viewed as foreigners by incoming white Americans. By 1900, Mexican Americans numbered approximately 200,000. However, during the "Great Migration" between 1900 and 1930, an additional 1 million Mexicans entered the United States. This may have been the greatest immigration of people in the history of humanity (Library of Congress, 2005).

Hispanics, the fastest growing ethnic population in the United States, include over 35.3 million people, or 13.2 percent of the population. Fifty-eight percent are of Mexican heritage, with an increase from 13.5 million in

309

1990 to 20.6 million in 2000 (U.S. Bureau of the Census, 2001). Mexican Americans reside predominantly in California, Texas, Illinois, Arizona, Florida, New Mexico, and Colorado. However, the major concentration of Mexican Americans, totaling over 18 million, are found in the southern and western portions of the United States (U.S. Bureau of the Census, 2001). Ninety percent of Mexican Americans live in urban areas such as San Diego, Los Angeles, New York City, Chicago, and Houston, whereas less than 10 percent reside in rural areas.

REASONS FOR MIGRATION AND ASSOCIATED ECONOMIC FACTORS

Historically, many Mexicans left Mexico during the Mexican Revolution to seek political, religious, and economic freedoms (Congress, 2005). Following the Mexican Revolution, strict limits were placed on the Catholic Church, and until recently, clerics were not allowed to wear their church garb in public. For many, this restricted the expression of faith and was a minor factor in their immigration north to the United States (Meyer & Beezley, 2000). Since the "Great Migration," limited employment opportunities in Mexico, especially in rural areas, has encouraged Mexicans to migrate to the United States as sojourners or immigrants or with undocumented status; the latter are often derogatorily referred to as *wetbacks* (*majodos*) by the white and Mexican American populations.

Of undocumented immigrants in the United States, an estimated 6 million are from Mexico (Van Hook, Bean, & Passel, 2005). Before the Immigration Reform and Control Act of 1986, hundreds of thousands of Mexicans crossed the border, found jobs, and settled in the United States. Although the numbers have decreased since 1986, border towns in Texas and California still experience large influxes of Mexicans seeking improved employment and educational opportunities. The tide of illegal immigration to the United States has increased, as evidenced by the apprehension of Mexicans attempting to enter the United States annually, with estimates of 250,000 to 300,000 people entering illegally (Passel, 2004).

Even though the economy of Mexico has grown, the buying power of the peso has decreased and inflation rates have increased faster than wages; thus, 43 percent of the population continues to live in poverty (CIA, 2007). Recent Mexican immigrants are more likely to live in poverty, more pessimistic about their future, and less educated than previous immigrants. Many Mexicans are among the very poor, with little hope of improving their economic status. Between the years 1999 and 2000 in the United States, the poverty rate for Hispanics was 22.6 percent (U.S. Bureau of the Census, 2001).

EDUCATIONAL STATUS AND OCCUPATIONS

Many second- and third-generation Mexican Americans have significant job skills and education. By contrast, many, especially newer immigrants from rural areas, have poor educational backgrounds and may place little value on education because it is not needed to

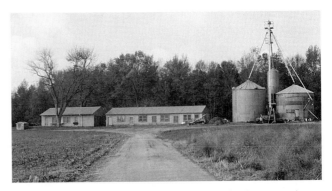

FIGURE 18–1 A migrant worker camp on Maryland's eastern shore. The Sanchez family (discussed in the Case Study on line) lives in such a camp, as do many Mexican American farm workers in the United States.

obtain jobs in Mexico. Once in the United States, they initially find work similar to that which they did in their native land, including farming, ranching, mining, oil production, construction, landscaping, and domestic jobs in homes, restaurants, and hotels and motels. Economic and educational opportunities in the United States are attainable, which allows immigrants to pursue the great American dream of a perceived better life (Kemp, 2001). Many Mexicans and Mexican Americans work as seasonal migrant workers, who may relocate several times each year as they "follow the sun." Sometimes, their unwillingness or inability to learn English is related to their intent to return to Mexico; however, this may hinder their ability to obtain better paying jobs (Fig. 18–1).

The mean educational level in Mexico is 5 years. Until 1992, Mexican children were required to attend school through the sixth grade, but since the Mexican School Reform Act of 1992, a ninth-grade education is required. However, great strides have been made in educational standards in Mexico, which now reports a 92 percent literacy rate among its population (CIA, 2007). A common practice among parents in poor rural villages is to educate their children in what they need to know. This group often finds immigration to the United States to be their most attractive option. For many Mexicans, high school and a university education is unavailable and, in many cases, unattainable.

Hispanics are the most undereducated ethnic group in the United States, with only 57 percent aged 25 years or older having a high school education, compared with 88.4 percent for non-Hispanic whites. However, that number increased from 43 percent to 57 percent completing high school from 1993 to 2000 (U.S. Bureau of the Census, 2001). Some migrant worker camps have free or low-cost bilingual educational programs to assist Mexican Americans in learning to read and write in both languages. Only 10.6 percent of Mexican Americans aged 25 years or older have a college degree. However, the number of Hispanics who completed 4 years of college doubled between 1990 and 2000 (U.S. Bureau of the Census, 2001).

Communication

DOMINANT LANGUAGE AND DIALECTS

Mexico is one of the largest Spanish-speaking countries in the world, with over 80 million speaking the language. The dominant language of Mexicans and Mexican Americans is Spanish. However, Mexico has 54 indigenous languages and more than 500 different dialects (Spanish Language, 2007). Knowing the region from which a Mexican American originates may help to identify the language or dialect the individual speaks. For example, major indigenous languages besides Spanish include Nahuatl and Otami, spoken in central Mexico; Mayan, in the Yucatan peninsula; Maya-Quiche, in the state of Chiapas; Zapotec and Mixtec, in the valley of Oaxaca; Tarascan, in the state of Michoacan; and Totonaco, in the state of Veracruz. Many of the Spanish dialects spoken by Mexican Americans have similar word meanings. However, the dialects of Spanish spoken by other groups may not have the same meanings. Because of the rural isolationist nature of many ethnic groups and the influence of native Indian languages, the dialects are so diverse in selected regions that it may be difficult to understand the language, regardless of the degree of fluency in Spanish.

Radio and television programs broadcasting in Spanish in both the United States and Mexico have helped to standardize Spanish. For the most part, public broadcast communication is primarily derived from Castilian Spanish. This standardization reduces the difficulties experienced by subcultures with multiple dialects. When speaking in a nonnative language, health-care providers must select words that have relatively pure meanings in the language and avoid the use of regional slang.

Contextual speech patterns among Mexican Americans may include a high-pitched, loud voice and a rate that seems extremely fast to the untrained ear. The language uses **apocopation**, which accounts for this rapid speech pattern. An apocopation occurs when one word ends with a vowel and the next word begins with a vowel. This creates a tendency to drop the vowel ending of the first word and results in an abbreviated, rapid-sounding form. For example, in the Spanish phrase for How are you?, ¿Cómo está usted? may become ¿Comestusted?. The last word, usted, is frequently dropped. Some may find this fast speech difficult to understand. However, if one asks the individual to enunciate slowly, the effect of the apocopation or truncation is less pronounced.

To help bridge potential communication gaps, health-care providers need to watch the client for cues, paraphrase words with multiple meanings, use simple sentences, repeat phrases for clarity, avoid the use of regional idiomatic phrases and expressions, and ask the client to repeat instructions to ensure accuracy. Approaching the Mexican American client with respect and *personalismo* (being friendlike) and directing questions to the dominant member of a group (usually the man) may help to facilitate more open communication. Zoucha and Husted (2002) found that becoming personal with the client or family is essential to building confidence and promoting health. The concept of *personalismo* may be difficult for some health-care professionals because they are socialized to form rigid boundaries between the caregiver and the client and family.

CULTURAL COMMUNICATION PATTERNS

Whereas some topics such as income, salary, or investments are taboo, Mexican Americans generally like to express their inner beliefs, feelings, and emotions once they get to know and trust a person. Meaningful conversations are important, often become loud, and seem disorganized. To the outsider, the situation may seem stressful or hostile, but this intense emotion means the conversants are having a good time and enjoying each other's company. Within the context of *personalismo* and **respeto**, respect, health-care providers can encourage open communication and sharing and develop the client's sense of trust by inquiring about family members before proceeding with the usual business. It is important for health-care providers to engage in "small talk" before addressing the actual health-care concern with the client and family (Zoucha & Reeves, 1999).

Mexican Americans place great value on closeness and togetherness, including when they are in an in-patient facility. They frequently touch and embrace and like to see relatives and significant others. Touch between men and women, between men, and between women is acceptable. To demonstrate respect, compassion, and understanding, health-care providers should greet the Mexican American client with a handshake. Once rapport is established, providers may further demonstrate approval and respect through backslapping, smiling, and affirmatively nodding the head. Given the diversity of dialects and the nuances of language, culturally congruent use of humor is difficult to accomplish and, therefore, should be avoided unless health-care providers are absolutely sure there is no chance of misinterpretation. Otherwise, inappropriate humor may jeopardize the therapeutic relationship and opportunities for health teaching and health promotion.

Mexican Americans consider sustained eye contact when speaking directly to an older person to be rude. Direct eye contact with teachers or superiors may be interpreted as insolence. Avoiding direct eye contact with superiors is a sign of respect. This practice may or may not be seen with second- or third-generation Mexican Americans. Health-care providers must take cues from the client and family.

TEMPORAL RELATIONSHIPS

Many Mexican Americans, especially those from lower socioeconomic groups, are necessarily present oriented. Many individuals do not consider it important or have the income to plan ahead financially. The trend is to live in the "more important" here and now, because *mañana* (tomorrow) cannot be predicted. With this emphasis on living in the present, preventive health care and immunizations may not be a priority. *Mañana* may or may not really mean tomorrow; it often means "not today" or "later."

Some Mexicans and Mexican Americans perceive time as relative rather than categorically imperative. Deadlines and commitments are flexible, not firm. Punctuality is generally relaxed, especially in social situations. This concept of time is innate in the Spanish language. For example, one cannot be late for an appointment; one can only arrive late! In addition, a few immigrants from rural environments in which adhering to a strict time clock is unimportant may not own a clock or even be able to tell time.

Because of their more relaxed concept of time, Mexican Americans may arrive late for appointments, although the current trend is toward greater punctuality. Health-care facilities that use an appointment system for clients may need to make special provisions to see clients whenever they arrive. Health-care providers must carefully listen for clues when discussing appointments. Disagreeing with health-care providers who set the appointment may be viewed as rude or impolite. Therefore, some Mexican Americans will not tell you directly that they cannot make the appointment. In the context of the discussion, they may say something like "my husband goes to work at 8:00 a.m. and the children are off to school, then I have to do the dishes . . . ." The health-care professional should ask: "Is 8:30 a.m. on Thursday okay for you?" The person might say yes but the health-care professional must still intently listen to the conversation and then possibly negotiate a new time for the appointment. In the conversation, the client may give clues that they will not arrive at the intended time, because it is important to save face and avoid being rude by saying they will not arrive on time.

FORMAT FOR NAMES

Names in most Spanish-speaking populations seem complex to those unfamiliar with the culture. A typical name is La Señorita Olga Gaborra de Rodriguez. Gaborra is the name of her father, and Rodriguez is her mother's surname. When she marries a man with the surname Guiterrez, she becomes La Señora (denotes a married woman) Olga Guiterrez de Gaborra y Rodriguez. The word de is used to express possession, and the father's name, which is considered more important than the mother's, comes first. However, this full name is rarely used except on formal documents and for recording the name in the family Bible. Out of respect, most Mexican Americans are more formal when addressing nonfamily members. Thus, the best way to address Olga is not by her first name but rather as Señora Guiterrez. Titles such as Don and Doña for older respected members of the community and family are also common. If using English while communicating with people older than the nurse or health-care provider, use titles such as Mr., Ms., Miss, or Mrs., as a sign of respect.

Health-care providers must understand the role of older people when providing care to people of Mexican heritage. To develop confidence and personalismo, an element of formality must exist between health-care providers and older people. Becoming overly familiar by using physical touch or addressing them by first names may not be appreciated early in a relationship (Kemp, 2001). As the health-care professional develops confidence in the relationship, becoming familiar may be less of a concern. However, using the first name of an older client may never be appropriate (Zoucha & Husted, 2000).

Family Roles and Organization

HEAD OF HOUSEHOLD AND GENDER ROLES

The typical family dominance pattern in traditional Mexican American families is patriarchal, with evidence of slow change toward a more egalitarian pattern in recent years (Grothaus, 1996). Change to a more egalitarian decision-making pattern is primarily identified with more educated and higher socioeconomic families. **Machismo** in the Mexican culture sees men as having strength, valor, and self-confidence, which is a valued trait among many. Men are seen as wiser, braver, stronger, and more knowledgeable regarding sexual matters. The female takes responsibility for decisions within the home and for maintaining the family's health. *Machismo* assists in sustaining and maintaining health not only for the man but also with implications for the health and well-being of the family (Sobralske, 2006).

PRESCRIPTIVE, RESTRICTIVE, AND TABOO BEHAVIORS FOR CHILDREN AND ADOLESCENTS

Children are highly valued because they ensure the continuation of the family and cultural values (Locke, 1999). They are closely protected and not encouraged to leave home. Even *compadres* (godparents) are included in the care of the young. Each child must have godparents in case something interferes with the parents' ability to fulfill their child-rearing responsibilities. Children are taught at an early age to respect parents and older family members, especially grandparents. Physical punishment is often used as a way of maintaining discipline and is sometimes considered child abuse in the United States. Using children as interpreters in the health-care setting is discouraged owing to the restrictive nature of discussing gender-specific health assessments.

FAMILY GOALS AND PRIORITIES

VIGNETTE 18.1

Mr. Perez is a 76-year-old Mexican American who was recently diagnosed with a slow heartbeat requiring an implanted pacemaker. Mr. Perez has been married for 51 years and has 6 adult children (three daughters aged 50, 48, and 42; three sons aged 47, 45, and 36), 11 grandchildren; and 2 great grandchildren. The youngest boy lives three houses down from Mr. and Mrs. Perez. The other children, except the second-oldest daughter, live within 3 to 10 miles from their parents. The second-oldest daughter is a registered nurse and lives out of state. All members of the family except for Mr. Perez were born in the United States. He was born in Monterrey, Mexico, and immigrated to the United States at the age of 18 in order to work and send money back to the family in Mexico. Mr. Perez has returned to Mexico throughout the years to visit and has lived in Texas ever since. Mr. Perez is retired from work in a machine shop. Mr. Perez has one living older brother who lives within 5 miles. All members of the family speak Spanish and English fluently.

The Perez family is Catholic, as evidenced by the religious items hanging on the wall and prayer books and rosary on the coffee table. Statues of St. Jude and Our Lady of Guadalupe are on the living room table. Mr. and Mrs. Perez have made many *mandas* (bequests) to pray for the health of the family, including one to thank God for the healthy birth of all the children, especially after the doctor had discouraged them from having any children after the complicated birth of their first child. The family attends Mass together every Sunday morning and then meets for breakfast *chorizo* at a local restaurant frequented by many of their church's other parishioner families. Mr. Perez believes his health and the health of his family are in the hands of God.

The Perez family lives in a modest four-bedroom ranch home that they bought 22 years ago. The home is located in a predominantly Mexican American neighborhood located in *La Loma* section of town. Mr. and Mrs. Perez are active in the church and neighborhood community. The Perez home is usually occupied by many people and has always been the gathering place for the family.

During his years of employment, Mr. Perez was the sole provider for the family and now receives social security checks and a pension. Mrs. Perez is also retired and receives a small pension for a short work period as a teacher's aide. Mr. and Mrs. Perez count on their nurse daughter to guide them and advise on their health care. Mr. Perez visits a *curandero* for medicinal folk remedies. Mrs. Perez is the provider of spiritual, physical, and emotional care for the family. In addition, their nurse daughter is always present during any major surgeries or procedures. Mrs. Perez and her daughter the nurse will be caring for Mr. Perez during his procedure for a pacemaker.

1. Explain the significance of family and kinship for the Perez family.
2. Describe the importance of religion and God for the Perez family.
3. Identify two stereotypes about Mexican Americans that were dispelled in this case with the Perez family.
4. What is the role of Mrs. Perez in this family?

The concept of *familism* is an all-encompassing value among Mexicans, for whom the traditional family is still the foundation of society. Family takes precedence over work and all other aspects of life. In many Mexican families, it is often said "God first, then family." The dominant Western health-care culture stresses including the client and family in the plan of care. Mexicans are strong proponents of this family care concept, which includes the extended family. By including all family members, health-care providers can build greater trust and confidence and, in turn, increase compliance with health-care regimens and prescriptions (Wells, Cagle, & Bradley, 2006).

Blended communal families are almost the norm in lower socioeconomic groups and in migrant-worker camps. Single, divorced, and never-married male and female children usually live with their parents or extended families, regardless of economics. Extended kinship is common through *padrinos*, godparents who may be close friends are usually considered family members (Zoucha & Zamarripa, 1997). Thus, the words brother, sister, aunt, and uncle do not necessarily mean that they are related by blood. For many men, having children is evidence of their virility and a sign of *machismo*.

When grandparents and older parents are unable to live on their own, they generally move in with their children. The extended family structure and the Mexicans' obligation to visit sick friends and relatives encourage large numbers to visit hospitalized family members and friends. This practice may necessitate that health-care providers relax strict visiting policies in health-care facilities.

Social status is highly valued among Mexican Americans, and a person who holds an academic degree or position with an impressive title commands great respect and admiration from family, friends, and the community. Good manners, a family, and family lineage, as indicated by extensive family names, also confer high status for Mexicans.

ALTERNATIVE LIFESTYLES

Twenty-six percent of Mexican families in the United States live in poverty, and many are headed by a single female parent. This percentage is lower than that for other minority groups in the United States (U.S. Bureau of the Census, 2001). Because the Hispanic cultural norm is for a pregnant woman to marry, Mexicans are more likely to marry at a young age. Yet, common law marriages (*unidos*) are frequently practiced and readily accepted, with many couples living together their entire lives.

Although homosexual behavior occurs in every society, The Williams Project reported that five states (California, Texas, New York, Florida, and Illinios) have the highest number of same-sex Latino couples, totaling 100,796, living together in the United States (Gates, Lau, & Sears, 2006). Newspapers from Houston, Texas; Washington, D.C.; and Chicago, Illinois, report on the efforts of Hispanic lesbian and gay organizations in the areas of HIV and AIDS (*La SIDA* in Spanish) and life partner benefits. In Mexico, antihate groups raised serious concerns about killings of homosexual men, causing many to remain closeted (Redding, 1999). In Mexico, *machismo* plays a large part in the phobic attitudes toward gay behavior. Larger cities in the United States may have *Ellas*, a support group for Latina Lesbians; El Hotline of Hola Gay, which provides referrals and information in Spanish; or Dignity, for gay Catholics. Health-care providers who wish to refer gay and lesbian clients to a support group may use such agencies.

Workforce Issues

CULTURE IN THE WORKPLACE

In the United States, Hispanics are the most underrepresented minority group in the health-care workforce.

Although over 13 percent of the American population is of Hispanic origin, only 1.8 percent of registered nurses are from Hispanic heritage (National Sample Survey of Registered Nurses, 2004). Cultural differences that influence workforce issues include values regarding family, pedagogical approach to education, emotional sensitivity, views toward status, aesthetics, ethics, balance of work and leisure, attitudes toward direction and delegation, sense of control, views about competition, and time.

People educated in Mexico are likely to have been exposed to pedagogical approaches that include rote memorization and an emphasis on theory with little practical application taught within a rigid, broad curriculum. American educational systems usually emphasize an analytical approach, practical applications, and a narrow, in-depth specialization. Thus, additional training may be needed for some Mexicans when they come to the United States.

Because family is a first priority for most Mexicans, activities that involve family members usually take priority over work issues. Putting up a tough business front may be seen as a weakness in the Mexican culture. Because of this separation of work from emotions in American culture, most Mexican Americans tend to shun confrontation for fear of losing face. Many are very sensitive to differences of opinion, which are perceived as disrupting harmony in the workplace. People of Mexican heritage find it important to keep peace in relationships in the workplace.

For many Mexicans, truth is tempered by diplomacy and tact. When a service is promised for tomorrow, even when they know the service will not be completed tomorrow, it is promised to please, not to deceive. Thus, for many Mexicans, truth is seen as a relative concept, whereas for most European Americans, truth is an absolute value and people are expected to give direct yes and no answers. These conflicting perspectives about truth can complicate treatment regimens and commitment to the completion of work assignments. Intentions must be clarified and, at times, altered to meet the needs of the changing and multicultural workforce.

For most Mexicans, work is viewed as a necessity for survival and may not be highly valued in itself, whereas money is for enjoying life. Most Mexican Americans place a higher value on other life activities. Material objects are usually necessities and not ends in themselves. The concept of responsibility is based on values related to attending to the immediate needs of family and friends rather than on the work ethic. For most Mexicans, titles and positions may be more important than money.

Many Mexicans believe that time is relative and elastic, with flexible deadlines, rather than stressing punctuality and timeliness. In Mexico, shop hours may be posted but not rigidly respected. A business that is supposed to open at 8:00 a.m. opens when the owner arrives; a posted time of 8:00 a.m. may mean the business will open at 8:30 a.m., later, or not at all. The same attitude toward time is evidenced in reporting to work and in keeping social engagements and medical appointments. If people believe that an exact time is truly important, such as the time an airplane leaves, then they may keep to a schedule. The real challenge for employers is to stress the importance and necessity of work schedules and punctuality in the American workforce.

ISSUES RELATED TO AUTONOMY

Many Mexican Americans respond to direction and delegation differently from European Americans. Many newer immigrants are used to having traditional autocratic managers who assign tasks but not authority, although this practice is beginning to change with more American-managed companies relocating to Mexico. A Mexican worker who is not accustomed to responsibility may have difficulty assuming accountability for decisions. The individual may be sensitive to the American practice of checking on employees' work.

Mexicans who were born and educated in the United States usually have no difficulty communicating with others in the workplace. When better-educated Mexican immigrants arrive in the United States, they usually speak some English. Newer immigrants from lower socioeconomic groups have the most difficulty acculturating in the workplace and may have greater difficulty with the English language.

Biocultural Ecology

SKIN COLOR AND OTHER BIOLOGICAL VARIATIONS

Because Mexican Americans draw their heritage from Spanish and French peoples and various North American and Central American Indian tribes and Africans, few physical characteristics give this group a distinct identity. Some individuals with a predominant Spanish background might have light-colored skin, blond hair, and blue eyes, whereas people from indigenous Indian backgrounds may have black hair, dark eyes, and cinnamon-colored skin. Intermarriages among these groups have created a diverse gene pool and have not produced a typical-appearing Mexican.

Cyanosis and decreased hemoglobin levels are more difficult to detect in dark-skinned people, whose skin appears ashen instead of the bluish color seen in light-skinned people. To observe for these conditions in dark-skinned Mexicans, the practitioner must examine the sclera, conjunctiva, buccal mucosa, tongue, lips, nailbeds, palms of the hands, and soles of the feet. Jaundice, likewise, is more difficult to detect in darker-skinned people. Thus, the practitioner needs to observe the conjunctiva and the buccal mucosa for patches of bilirubin pigment in dark-skinned Mexicans.

DISEASES AND HEALTH CONDITIONS

Common health problems most consistently documented in the literature for both people from Mexico and Mexican Americans are difficulty in assessing and utilizing health care, malnutrition, malaria (in some places), cancer, alcoholism, drug abuse, obesity, hypertension, diabetes, heart disease, adolescent pregnancy, dental disease, and HIV and AIDS (Kemp, 2001). In Mexican American migrant-worker populations, infectious, communicable, and parasitic diseases continue to be major health risks. Substandard housing conditions and employment in low-paying jobs have perpetuated higher rates of tuberculosis in Mexican Americans. Intestinal parasitosis, amoebic dysentery, and bacterial diarrhea (*Shigella*) are common among Mexican immigrants (Kim-Godwin, Alexander, Felton, Mackey, & Kasakoff, 2006).

Newer Mexican immigrants from coastal lowland swamp areas and from some mountainous areas where mosquitoes are more prevalent may also have a higher incidence of malaria. People from high mountain terrains may have increased red blood cell counts on immigration to the United States (Centers for Disease Control and Prevention [CDC], 2006). Health-care providers must take these topographic factors into consideration when performing health screening for symptoms of anemia, lassitude, failure to thrive, and weight loss among Mexican immigrants.

Cardiovascular disease is the leading cause of death and disability in minority populations, including Mexican Americans (Kurian & Cardarelli, 2007). However, current research shows that despite the adverse cardiovascular risk profile, including the incidence of obesity, diabetes, and untreated hypertension, Mexican Americans have a lower rate of coronary heart disease mortality than nonwhite Hispanics (Pandey, Labarthe, Goff, Chan, & Nichaman, 2001). Cardiovascular risk factors are influenced by behavioral, cultural, and social factors. Mexican Americans have the highest prevalence of no leisure time physical activity (Kurian & Cardarelli, 2007). In addition, poor health, low social support, lack of educational and occupational opportunities, low access to health care, and discrimination contribute to the risk factors associated with cardiovascular disease (Kemp, 2001).

Mexican Americans have five times the rate of diabetes mellitus, with an increased incidence of related complications, as that in European American cohort groups. In addition, health-care professionals working with Mexican immigrants and Mexican Americans should offer screening and teach clients preventive measures regarding pesticides and communicable and infectious diseases because many of these people work with chemicals and live in crowded housing conditions.

VARIATIONS IN DRUG METABOLISM

Because of the mixed heritage of many Mexican Americans, it may be more difficult to determine a therapeutic dose of selected drugs. Several studies report differences in absorption, distribution, metabolism, and excretion of drugs, including alcohol, in some Hispanic populations. The mixed heritage of Mexican Americans makes it more difficult to generalize drug metabolism. Few studies include only one subgroup of Hispanics; therefore, health-care providers need to consider some notable differences when prescribing medications. Hispanics require lower doses of antidepressants and experience greater side effects than non-Hispanic whites.

High-Risk Behaviors

Alcohol plays an important part in the Mexican culture. Many of this group's colorful lifestyle celebrations include alcohol consumption. Men overall drink in greater proportion than women, but this trend is changing owing to acculturation. Mexican American women are consuming more alcohol than their mothers or grandmothers (Collins & McNair, 2002).

Because of these drinking patterns, alcoholism represents a crucial health problem for many Mexicans. More-acculturated Hispanics consume more alcoholic beverages than non-Hispanic whites, possibly expecting alcohol to make them more socially acceptable and extroverted. Low acculturation and distorted self-image problems have special implications for nursing and health care.

Marijuana is the number-two drug used by Mexican Americans because it is readily available in their native land and easily accessible from people who work in farming and ranching occupations. Some adults who can afford drugs use cocaine and heroin, and the younger population uses inhalants (Eden & Aguilar, 1989).

The trend toward decreasing cigarette smoking in the United States is extending to the Mexican American culture, in which cigarette smoking rates have steadily declined for both men and women between 1990 and 2004 (CDC, 2007). However, the reported decrease in cigarette smoking rates for Mexican American men and women should not promote a sense of complacency for nurses and health-care professionals.

HEALTH-CARE PRACTICES

Responsibility for health promotion and safety may be a major threat for those of Mexican heritage accustomed to depending on the family unit and traditional means of providing health care. Continuing disparities in health and health-seeking behaviors have been reported in several studies. Lower socioeconomic conditions and acculturation are responsible for Latina women being overweight, exhibiting hypertension, experiencing high cholesterol levels, and having increased smoking behaviors (Kemp, 2001). Latino men are less likely to have cancer screening or physical examinations than their non-Latino white counterparts. High-risk health behaviors such as drinking and driving, cigarette smoking, sedentary lifestyle, and nonuse of seat belts increase with fewer years of educational attainment. Through educational programs and enforcement of state laws, more Mexicans are beginning to use seat belts; however, it is still common to see their children traveling unrestrained in automobiles.

Nutrition

MEANING OF FOOD

As in many other ethnic groups, Mexicans and Mexican Americans celebrate with food. Mexican foods are rich in color, flavor, texture, and spiciness. Any occasion—births, birthdays, Sundays, religious holidays, official and unofficial holidays, and anniversaries of deaths—is seen as a time to celebrate with food and enjoy the companionship of family and friends. Because food is a primary form of socialization in the Mexican culture, Mexican Americans may have difficulty adhering to a prescribed diet for illnesses such as diabetes mellitus and cardiovascular disease. Health-care professionals must seek creative alternatives and negotiate types of foods consumed with individuals and families in relation to these concerns.

COMMON FOODS AND FOOD RITUALS

The Mexican American diet is extremely varied and may depend on the individual's region of origin in Mexico. Thus, one needs to ask the individual specifically about his or her dietary habits. The staples of the Mexican American diet are rice (*arroz*), beans, and tortillas, which are made from corn (*maíz*) treated with calcium carbonate. However, in many parts of the United States, only flour tortillas are available. Even though the diet is low in calcium derived from milk and milk products, tortillas treated with calcium carbonate provide essential dietary calcium. Popular Mexican American foods are eggs (*huevos*), pork (*puerco*), chicken (*pollo*), sausage (*chorizo*); lard (*lardo*), mint (*menta*), chili peppers (*chile*), onions (*cebollas*), tomatoes (*tomates*), squash (*calabaza*), canned fruit (*fruta de lata*), mint tea (*hierbabuena*), chamomile tea (*té de camomile* or *manzanilla*), carbonated beverages (*bebidas de gaseosa*), beer (*cerveza*), cola-flavored soft drinks, sweetened packaged drink mixes (*agua fresa*) that are high in sugar (*azucar*), sweetened breakfast cereals (*cereales de desayuno*); potatoes (*papas*), bread (*pan*), corn (*maíz*), gelatin (*gelatina*), custard (*flan*), and other sweets (*dulces*). Other common dishes include chili, enchiladas, tamales, tostadas, chicken mole, arroz con pollo, refried beans, tacos, tripe soup (*Menudo*) and other soups (*caldos*). Soups (*caldos*) are varied in nature and may include chicken, beef, and pork with vegetables.

Mealtimes vary among different subgroups of Mexican Americans. Whereas many individuals adopt North American schedules and eating habits, many continue their native practices, especially those in rural settings and migrant-worker camps. For these groups, breakfast is usually fruit, perhaps cheese, or bread alone or in some combination. A snack may be taken in midmorning before the main meal of the day, which is eaten from 2 to 3 p.m. and, in rural areas especially, may last for 2 hours or more. Mealtime is an occasion for socialization and keeping family members informed about each other. The evening meal is usually late and is taken between 9 and 9:30 p.m. Health-care providers must consider Mexican Americans' mealtimes when teaching clients about medication and dietary regimens related to diabetes mellitus and other illnesses.

DIETARY PRACTICES FOR HEALTH PROMOTION

A dominant health-care practice for Mexicans and many Mexican Americans is the hot-and-cold theory of food selection. This theory is a major aspect of health promotion and illness and disease prevention and treatment. According to this theory, illness or trauma may require adjustments in the hot-and-cold balance of foods to restore body equilibrium. The hot-and-cold theory of foods is described under Health-Care Practices, later in this chapter.

NUTRITIONAL DEFICIENCIES AND FOOD LIMITATIONS

In lower socioeconomic groups, wide-scale vitamin A deficiency and iron deficiency anemia exist (Mendoza, Ventura, Saldivar, Baisden, & Martorell, 1992). Some Mexican and Mexican Americans have lactose intolerance, which may cause problems for schools and health-care organizations that provide milk in the diet because of its high calcium content.

Because major Mexican foods and their ingredients are available throughout the United States, native food practices may not change much when Mexicans immigrate. Of course, Mexican foods are extremely popular throughout the United States and are eaten by many Americans because of the strong flavors, spiciness, and color. Table 18–1 lists the Mexican names of popular foods, their description, and ingredients. Individual adaptations to these preparations commonly occur.

Pregnancy and Childbearing Practices

FERTILITY PRACTICES AND VIEWS TOWARD PREGNANCY

Mexican American birth rates were 24.9 or 677,621 live births in 2004; the numbers of births have continued to rise every year since 1989 (National Vital Statistics Report, 2004). Multiple births are common, especially in the economically disadvantaged groups. Men view a large number of children as proof of their virility. The optimal childbearing age for Mexican women is between 19 and 24 years. Fertility practices of Mexican Americans are connected with their predominantly Catholic religious beliefs and their tendency to be modest. Some women practice the belief that prolonged infant breastfeeding is a method of birth control. Abortion in many communities is considered morally wrong and is practiced (theoretically) only in extreme circumstances to keep the mother's life intact. However, legal and illegal abortions are common in some parts of Mexico and the United States. Despite the strong influence of the Catholic Church over fertility practices, being Catholic does not prevent some Mexican American women from using contraceptives, sterilization, or abortion for unwanted pregnancies.

Diaphragms, foams, and creams are not commonly used for birth control practice, mostly because they are not approved by Catholic doctrine and partly because of the belief that women are not supposed to touch their genitals. Birth control pills are unacceptable because they are an artificial means of birth control. Physicians' offices and clinics that see large numbers of migrant workers on the Delmarva Peninsula on the U.S. east coast report that many younger female clients are using Norplant (levonorgestrel; a long-term contraceptive system) for birth control. Men are reluctant to use condoms because they are associated with prostitutes and because of the belief

T A B L E 18.1 *Mexican Foods*

Common Name	Description	Ingredients
Arroz con pollo	Chicken with rice	Chicken baked, boiled, or fried and served over boiled or fried rice
Chili	Chili	Same as the United States but tends to be more spicy
Chili con carne	Chili with meat	Chili with beef or pork
Chili con salsa	Chili with sauce	Chili with a sauce that contains no meat
Dulces	Sweets	Candy and desserts usually high in sugar, lard, and eggs
Enchiladas	Enchiladas	Tortilla rolled and stuffed with meat or cheese and a spicy sauce
Papas fritas	Fried potatoes	Potatoes usually fried in lard
Flan	Flan	Popular dessert made of egg custard; may be filled with fruit or cheese
Gelatina	Gelatin	Popular dessert made with sugar, eggs, and jelly
Pollo con molé	Chicken molé	Chicken with a sauce made of hot spices, chocolate, and chili
Salchica or *chorizo*	Sausage	Sausage almost always made with pork and spices
Tacos	Tacos	Tortilla folded around meat or cheese
Tamales	Tamales	Fried or boiled chopped meat, peppers, cornmeal, and hot spices
Tortilla	Tortilla	A thin unleavened bread made with cornmeal and treated with lime (calcium carbonate)
Tostadas	Tostadas	Toast that may have a spicy sauce

that they should be used only for disease control. A woman may reject the use of a condom and find it offensive because it means that she is "dirty." Family planning is one area in which health-care providers can help the family to identify more realistic outcomes consistent with current economic resources and family goals.

Foreign-born Mexicans are less likely to give birth to low-birth-weight babies than U.S.-born Mexican women, even though U.S.-born mothers are usually of higher socioeconomic status and receive more prenatal care. Research suggests that better nutritional intake and lower prevalence of smoking and alcohol use are some reasons for these protective outcomes (American Public Health Association, 2002).

Because pregnancy among Mexican Americans is viewed as natural and desirable, many women do not seek prenatal evaluations. In addition, because prenatal care is not available to every woman in Mexico, some women do not know about the need for prenatal care. With the extended family network and the woman's role of maintaining the health status of family members, many pregnant women seek family advice before seeking medical care. Thus, *familism* may deter and hinder early prenatal check-ups. To encourage prenatal check-ups, health-care providers can encourage female relatives and husbands to accompany the pregnant woman for health screening and incorporate advice from family members into health teaching and preventive care services. Using videos with Spanish-speaking Mexican Americans is one culturally effective way for incorporating health education, especially for those clients who have a limited understanding of English. In addition, incorporating cultural brokers known to the Mexican American family may help to empower clients and reduce conflict for Mexicans and Mexican Americans.

PRESCRIPTIVE, RESTRICTIVE, AND TABOO PRACTICES IN THE CHILDBEARING FAMILY

Beliefs related to the hot-and-cold theory of disease prevention and health maintenance influence conception, pregnancy, and postpartum rituals. For instance, during pregnancy, a woman is more likely to favor hot foods, which are believed to provide warmth for the fetus and enable the baby to be born into a warm and loving environment (Eggenberger, Grassley, & Restrepo, 2006). Cold foods and environments are preferred during the menstrual cycle and in the immediate postdelivery period. Many pregnant women sleep on their backs to protect the infant from harm, keep the vaginal canal well lubricated by having frequent intercourse to facilitate an easier birth, and keep active to ensure a smaller baby and to prevent a decrease in the amount of amniotic fluid (Burk, Wieser, & Keegan, 1995). An important activity restriction is that pregnant women should not walk in the moonlight because it might cause a birth deformity. To prevent birth deformities, pregnant women may wear a safety pin, metal key, or some other metal object on their abdomen (Villarruel & Ortiz de Montellano, 1992). Other beliefs include avoiding cold air, not reaching over the head in order to prevent the baby's cord from wrapping around its neck, and avoiding lunar eclipses because they may result in deformities.

In more traditional Mexican families, the father is not included in the delivery experience and should not see the mother or baby until after both have been cleaned and dressed. This practice is based on the fear that harm may come to the mother, baby, or both. Integrating men into the birthing of a child is a process that requires changing social habits in relation to cultural aspects of life and gender roles. For many, the presence of men during delivery is considered an uninvited intrusion into the Mexican culture. Among less-traditional and more-acculturated Mexican Americans, men participate in prenatal classes and assist in the delivery room. However, based on personal experiences, men who provide support during delivery may receive friendly gibing from their male counterparts for taking the role of the wife's mother (personal communication, Larry Purnell, June 2007). In any event, health-care providers must respect Mexicans' decision to not have men in the delivery room.

During labor, traditional Mexican women may be quite vocal and are taught to avoid breathing air in through the mouth because it can cause the uterus to rise up. Immediately after birth, they may place their legs together to prevent air from entering the womb (Olds, London, & Ladewig, 2000). Health-care providers can help the Mexican pregnant woman have a better delivery by encouraging attendance at prenatal classes.

The postpartum preference for a warm environment may restrict postpartum women from bathing or washing their hair for up to 40 days. Although postpartum women may not take showers or sit in a bathtub, this does not mean that they do not bathe. They take sitz baths, wash their hair with a washcloth, and take sponge baths. Other postpartum practices include wearing a heavy cotton abdominal binder, cord, or girdle to prevent air from entering the uterus; covering one's ears, head, shoulders, and feet to prevent blindness, mastitis, frigidity, or sterility; and avoiding acidic foods to protect the baby from harm (Olds, London, & Ladewig, 2000).

When the baby is born, special attention is given to the umbilicus; the mother may place a belt around the umbilicus (*ombliguero*) to prevent the naval from popping out when the child cries. Cutting the baby's nails in the first 3 months is thought to cause blindness and deafness.

Health-care providers need to make special provisions to provide culturally congruent health teaching for lactating women who work with or are exposed to pesticides, such as dichlorodiphenyldichlorothene (DDE), the most stable derivative from the pesticide DDT. High DDE levels among lactating women have a direct correlation with a decrease in lactation and increase in breast cancer, especially in women who have had more than one pregnancy and previous lactation (Gladen & Rogan, 1995). Education level and degree of acculturation are key issues when developing health education and interventions for risk reduction.

Death Rituals

DEATH RITUALS AND EXPECTATIONS

Mexicans often have a stoic acceptance of the way things are and view death as a natural part of life and the will of God (Eggenberger et al., 2006). Death practices are primarily an adaptation of their religion. Family members may arrive in large numbers at the hospital or home in times of illness or an approaching death. In more-traditional families, family members may take turns sitting vigil over the sick or dying person. Autopsy is acceptable as long as the body is treated with respect. Burial is the common practice; cremation is an individual choice.

RESPONSES TO DEATH AND GRIEF

When a person dies, the word travels rapidly, and family and friends travel from long distances to get to the funeral. They may gather for a **velorio**, a festive watch over the body of the deceased person before burial. Some

Mexican Americans bury the body within 24 hours, which is required by law in Mexico.

More-traditional grieving families may engage in protection of the dying and bereaved such as small children who have difficulty dealing with the death (Andrews & Boyle, 2003). Mexican Americans encourage expressions of feeling during the grieving process. In these cases, health-care providers can assist the person by providing support and privacy during the bereavement.

Spirituality

DOMINANT RELIGION AND USE OF PRAYER

The predominant religion of most Mexicans and Mexican Americans is Catholicism. The major religions in Mexico are Roman Catholic, 89 percent; Protestant, 6 percent; and other, 5 percent of the population. Since the mid-1980s, other religious groups such as Mormons, Jehovah's Witnesses, Seventh Day Adventists, Presbyterians, and Baptists have been gaining in popularity in Mexico (CIA, 2007). Although many Mexicans and Mexican Americans may not appear to be practicing their faith on a daily basis, they may still consider themselves devout Catholics, and their religion has a major influence on health-care practices and beliefs. For many, Catholic religious practices are influenced by indigenous Indian practices.

Newer immigrant Mexican Americans may continue their traditional practice of having two marriage ceremonies, especially in lower socioeconomic groups. A civil ceremony is performed whenever two people decide to make a union. When the family gets enough money for a religious ceremony, they schedule an elaborate celebration within the church. Common practice, especially in rural Mexican villages and some rural villages in the southwestern United States, is to post a handwritten sign on the local church announcing the marriage, with an invitation for all to attend.

Frequency of prayer is highly individualized for most Mexican Americans. Even though some do not attend church on a regular basis, they may have an altar in their homes and say prayers several times each day, a practice more common among rural isolationists.

MEANING OF LIFE AND INDIVIDUAL SOURCES OF STRENGTH

The family is foremost to most Mexicans, and individuals get strength from family ties and relationships. Individuals may speak in terms of a person's soul or spirit (*alma or espiritu*) when they refer to one's inner qualities. These inner qualities represent the person's dignity and must be protected at all costs in times of both wellness and illness. In addition, Mexicans derive great pride and strength from their nationality, which embraces a long and rich history of traditions.

Leisure is considered essential for a full life, and work is a necessity to make money for enjoying life. Mexican

Americans pride themselves on good manners, etiquette, and grooming as signs of respect. Because the overall outlook for many Mexicans is one of fatalism, pride may be taken in stoic acceptance of life's adversities.

SPIRITUAL BELIEFS AND HEALTH-CARE PRACTICES

VIGNETTE 18.2

Mrs. Lopez is a 65-year-old Mexican American recently diagnosed with breast cancer who will undergo a radical mastectomy and chemotherapy. Mrs. Lopez is recently widowed and is grieving for her husband of 50 years. Mrs. Lopez has 7 children (3 daughters aged 49, 44, and 41; 4 sons aged 47, 45, 43, and 39), 8 grandchildren, and 20 great grandchildren. The youngest son lives at home with his mother along with his wife and four children. The other children live within 10 blocks. Mrs. Lopez spends a lot of time helping to care for the grandchildren while her children work. The five youngest members of the family were born in the United States, and the rest of the family was born in Vera Cruz, Mexico. Mrs. Perez has never worked outside of the home and receives survivor benefits from her husband's pension. The only job she has ever done is baby-sitting for neighbors, nieces, and nephews. Mrs. Lopez has one living brother who lives 5 miles away and a sister who died of breast cancer 7 years ago.

The Lopez family members are Catholics. Mrs. Lopez is a very devout Catholic and attends Mass daily at the church two blocks away. The children attend Mass with the family on occasional Sundays. Mrs. Lopez prays the rosary and novenas so that God will take care of her and her family. Mrs. Lopez is a good cook and prepares dinner every evening for her son and his family. The daughter-in-law helps cook the meals even after a full day of work. Mrs. Lopez and her family live in a three-bedroom wood frame house. The home is located in a Mexican American neighborhood 2 miles from the Mexican border in San Juan, Texas.

Mrs. Lopez does not have any work experience and is grateful her husband left a small but substantial life insurance policy. Mrs. Lopez receives help with shopping and rides to the doctor from her youngest daughter and many comadres. One of her comadres is a *curandera* who has been offering Mrs. Lopez herbs and teas to help healing. Mrs. Lopez enjoys making tamales in her kitchen along with her family and comadres. All of the Lopez children and comadres have committed to help Mrs. Lopez during and after her surgery.

1. When the home health nurse comes to assess Mrs. Lopez's incision and teaches about Jackson Pratt drain care, who should be included in the teaching and why?
2. Explain the importance of familism to the Lopez family.
3. Mrs. Lopez has been offered herbal tea by the *curandera* while the home nurse is making a visit. Should the nurse intervene to stop this practice? Please provide rationale for your answer.
4. The nurse is making a visit when the family is praying the rosary together for the health of Mrs. Lopez. The nurse is invited to join. What should the nurse do in this situation?

Most Mexicans enjoy talking about their soul or spirit, especially in times of illness, whereas many health-care providers may feel uncomfortable talking about spirituality. This tendency may communicate to Mexicans that the health-care provider has suspect intentions, is insensitive, and is not really interested in them as individuals. It may be common for a person needing care in the home or hospital to have a statue of a patron saint or a candle with a picture of the saint. Rosaries may be present, and at times, the family may pray as a group. Depending on the confidence maintained with the family and client, a health-care professional may be asked to join in the prayer. If time permits, it is very appropriate to pray with the family even if only for a few minutes. This action promotes confidence in the relationship and can have a positive impact on the health and well-being of the client and family (Zoucha, 2007).

Health-Care Practices

VIGNETTE 18.3

Juan Diaz is a 26-year-old Mexican man who was recently diagnosed with a herniated lumbar disc after a work-related injury. An emergency room physician has recommended back surgery and physical therapy. Juan is unmarried and is a recent immigrant from Oaxaca, Mexico. Juan is an undocumented worker and has been working for a construction company doing roofing and bricklaying. Juan's family resides in Mexico. His parents, maternal grandparents, five sisters, and two brothers live in a small two-bedroom stone home in Oaxaca. Juan is the oldest of the children and has come to the United States to work and send money back to the family. Juan's dad is being treated for tuberculosis and needs money to pay for health care. Juan is also trying to earn enough money to bring his dad to the United States for tuberculosis treatment. Juan speaks mainly Spanish with limited ability in English.

Juan is a devout Catholic who attends Mass weekly and prays the rosary to La Virgen de Guadalupe daily. Juan often blesses himself with holy water he brought from San Juan de Los Lagos. Juan believes that God will heal him and that his health is in the hands of God.

Juan is sharing the rent on a three-bedroom apartment with five other migrant workers from Mexico. The apartment is located 10 miles from his job where new homes are being built outside the city. Juan usually takes two buses to work. One of the migrant workers has an uncle who helped secure the jobs for them. Juan and his coworkers cook and eat dinner together most evenings and enjoy drinking *cervezas* (beer) on the weekends.

Juan has saved money from working over the past 11 months but is worried about health-care coverage. He usually goes to a local clinic for his health-care needs. His friends suggested that he should visit a *bruja* because he might have had a spell cast upon him. He and his friends believe that the *bruja* can rid him of the spell and heal him. Juan's friends are able to help take care of him on weekends only because of their weekday 12-hour work schedules. Juan has an uncle from Mexico who is trying to get money together for a trip up to help Juan as he recovers. Juan will require home physical therapy and nursing care after his surgery.

1. The home care case manager, a registered nurse, is sending a physical therapist to the home. What should the nurse consider?
2. What does the nurse need to know about where Juan and his family are from in Mexico?
3. Identify potential communication needs of Juan, his friends, and his visiting family.
4. Juan is concerned about letting his boss down because of his illness. Why is Juan concerned about this with his boss?

HEALTH-SEEKING BELIEFS AND BEHAVIORS

The family is the most credible source of health information and the most significant impediment to positive health-seeking behavior. Mexican Americans' fatalistic worldview and external locus of control are closely tied to health-seeking behaviors. Because expressions of negative feelings are considered impolite, Mexicans may be reluctant to complain about health problems or to place blame on the individual for poor health. If a person becomes seriously ill, that is just the way things are; all events are acts of God (Eggenberger et al., 2006). This belief system may impair the dominant view of communications and hinder health teaching, health promotion, and disease prevention practices. Therefore, it is imperative for health-care professionals to plan health promoting activities and teaching that are consistent with this belief but encourage health. For instance, if a person believes that the illness is due to a punishment from God, it may be possible to ask to be forgiven by God, thereby restoring health. This may be an opportune time to call a priest or minister for official recognition of forgiveness.

RESPONSIBILITY FOR HEALTH CARE

To many Mexicans, good health may mean the ability to keep working and have a general feeing of well-being (Zoucha, 1998). Illness may occur when the person can no longer work or take care of the family. Therefore, many Mexicans may not seek health care until they are incapacitated and unable to go about the activities of daily living. Unfortunately, many people of Mexican heritage may not know and understand the occupational dangers inherent in their daily work. Migrant workers are often unaware of the dangers of pesticides and the potentially dangerous agricultural machinery. Health-care professionals must serve as advocates for these people regarding occupational safety. Often, the companies do not tell the workers of the dangers of the work, or the workers may not understand owing to the inability of the company officials to speak the language of the workers.

The use of over-the-counter medicine may pose a significant health problem related to self-care for many Mexican Americans. In part, this is a carryover from Mexico's practice of allowing over-the-counter purchases of antibiotics, intramuscular injections, intravenous fluids, birth control pills, and other medications that require a prescription in the United States. Often, Mexican immigrants bring these medications across the border and share them with friends. In addition, friends and relatives in Mexico send drugs through the mail. To protect clients from contradictory or potentiating effects of prescribed treatments, health-care providers need to ask clients about prescription and nonprescription medications they may be taking.

FOLK AND TRADITIONAL PRACTICES

Mexican Americans engage in folk medicine practices and use a variety of prayers, herbal teas, and poultices to treat illnesses. Many of these practices are regionally specific and vary between and among families. The Mexican *Ministerio de Salud Publica y Asistencia Social* (Ministry of Public Health and Social Assistance) publishes an extensive manual on herbal medicines that are readily available in Mexico. Lower socioeconomic groups and well-educated upper and middle socioeconomic Mexicans to some degree practice traditional and folk medicine. Many of these practices are harmless, but some may contradict or potentiate therapeutic interventions. Thus, as with the use of other prescription and nonprescription drugs discussed earlier, it is essential for health-care providers to be aware of these practices and to take them into consideration when providing treatments (Rivera, Anaya, & Meza, 2003). The provider must ask the Mexican American client specifically whether she or he is using folk medicine.

To provide culturally competent care, health-care practitioners must be aware of the hot-and-cold theory of disease when prescribing treatment modalities and when providing health teaching. According to this theory, many diseases are caused by a disruption in the hot-and-cold balance of the body. Thus, eating foods of the opposite variety may either cure or prevent specific hot-and-cold illnesses and conditions. Physical or mental illness may be attributed to an imbalance between the person and the environment. Influences include emotional, spiritual, and social state, as well as physical factors such as humoral imbalance expressed as either too much hot or cold. As health-care providers, it is important to understand that if people of Mexican heritage believe in the hot-and-cold theory, it means that they do not believe or use professional Western practices (Spector, 2004). Unless a level of trust and confidence is maintained, Mexicans who follow these beliefs may not express them to health professionals (Zoucha & Husted, 2000).

Hot and **cold** are viewed as specific properties of various substances and conditions, and sometimes opinions differ about what is hot and what is cold in the Mexican community. In general, cold diseases or conditions are characterized by vasoconstriction and a lower metabolic rate. **Cold diseases or conditions** include menstrual cramps, *frio de la matriz*, rhinitis (*coryza*), pneumonia, *empacho*, cancer, malaria, earaches, arthritis, pneumonia and other pulmonary conditions, headaches, and musculoskeletal conditions and colic. Common hot foods used to treat cold diseases and conditions include cheeses, liquor, beef, pork, spicy foods, eggs, grains other than barley, vitamins, tobacco, and onions (Kemp, 2001).

Hot diseases and conditions may be characterized by vasodilation and a higher metabolic rate. Pregnancy, hypertension, diabetes, acid indigestion, *susto, mal de ojo* (bad eye or evil eye), *bilis* (imbalance of bile, which runs into the blood stream), infection, diarrhea, sore throats, stomach ulcers, liver conditions, kidney problems, and fever may be examples of hot conditions. Common cold foods used to treat hot diseases and conditions include fresh fruits and vegetables, dairy products (even though fresh fruits and dairy products may cause diarrhea), barley water, fish, chicken, goat meat, and dried fruits (Neff, 1998).

Folk practitioners are consulted for several notable conditions. *Mal de ojo* is a folk illness that occurs when one person (usually older) looks at another (usually a child) in an admiring fashion. Another example of *mal de ojo* is if a person admires something about a baby or child, such as beautiful eyes or hair. Such eye contact can be either voluntary or involuntary. Symptoms are numerous, ranging from fever, anorexia, and vomiting to irritability. The spell can be broken if the person doing the admiring touches the person admired while it is happening. Children are more susceptible to this condition than women, and women are more susceptible than men. To prevent *mal de ojo*, the child wears a bracelet with a seed (*ojo de venado*) or a bag of seeds pinned to the clothes (Kemp, 2001).

Another childhood condition often treated by folk practitioners is *caida de la mollera* (fallen fontanel). The condition has numerous causes, which may include removing the nursing infant too harshly from the nipple or handling an infant too roughly. Symptoms range from irritability to failure to thrive. To cure the condition, the child is held upside down by the legs.

Susto (magical fright or soul loss) is associated with epilepsy, tuberculosis, and other infectious diseases and is caused by the loss of spirit from the body. The illness is also believed to be caused by a fright or by the soul being frightened out of the person. This culture-bound disorder may be psychological, physical, or physiological in nature. Symptoms may include anxiety, depression, loss of appetite, excessive sleep, bad dreams, feelings of sadness, and lack of motivation. Treatment sometimes includes elaborate ceremonies at a crossroads with herbs and holy water to return the spirit to the body (R. Zamarripa, personal communication, April 2006).

Empacho (blocked intestines) may result from an incorrect balance of hot and cold foods, causing a lump of food to stick in the gastrointestinal tract. To make the diagnosis, the healer may place a fresh egg on the abdomen. If the egg appears to stick to a particular area, this confirms the diagnosis. Older women usually treat the condition in children by massaging their stomach and back to dislodge the food bolus and to promote its continued passage through the body.

Health-care practitioners are cautioned against diagnosing psychiatric illnesses too readily in the Mexican population. The syndromes *mal ojo* and *susto* are culture bound and are potential sources of diagnostic bias. The potential culture-bound mental illness must be understood in the context of the culture and the unique symptoms that accompany each illness.

BARRIERS TO HEALTH CARE

Thirty-two percent of Mexican Americans, compared with 14 percent of the U.S. population in general, do not have health insurance (U.S. Bureau of the Census, 2001). A number of factors may account for this high percentage of uninsured individuals. First, many Mexican Americans constitute the working poor and are unable to purchase insurance. Second, many are migratory and do not qualify for Medicaid. Third, many have an undocumented status and are afraid to apply for health insurance. Fourth, even though insurance is available in their native homeland, it is very expensive and not part of the culture.

Whereas wealthier Mexican Americans have little difficulty accessing health care in the United States, lower socioeconomic groups may experience significant barriers, including inadequate financial resources, lack of insurance and transportation, limited knowledge regarding available services, language difficulties, and the culture of health-care organizations. Like many other immigrant groups who lack a primary provider, Mexican Americans may use emergency rooms for minor illnesses. Health-care providers have the opportunity to improve the care of Mexican Americans by explaining the health-care system, incorporating a primary-care provider whenever possible, using an interpreter of the same gender, securing a cultural broker, and assisting clients in locating culturally specific mental health programs (Zoucha & Husted, 2000).

CULTURAL RESPONSES TO HEALTH AND ILLNESS

Good health to many Mexican Americans is to be free of pain, able to work, and spend time with the family. In addition, good health is a gift from God and from living a good life (Zoucha, 1998).

Mexicans and Mexican Americans tend to perceive pain as a necessary part of life, and enduring the pain is often viewed as a sign of strength. Men commonly tolerate pain until it becomes extreme (Luckmann, 1999). Often, pain is viewed as the will of God and is tolerated as long as the person can work and care for the family. These attitudes toward pain delay seeking treatment; many hope that the pain will simply go away. Research has shown that many Mexican Americans experience more pain than other ethnic groups, but that they report the occurrence of pain less frequently and endure pain longer (Sobralske & Katz, 2005). Six themes have emerged that describe culturally specific attributes of Mexican Americans experiencing pain:

Mexicans accept and anticipate pain as a necessary part of life.

They are obligated to endure pain in the performance of duties.

The ability to endure pain and to suffer stoically is valued.

The type and amount of pain a person experiences is divinely predetermined.

Pain and suffering are a consequence of immoral behavior.

Methods to alleviate pain are directed toward maintaining balance within the person and the surrounding environment (Villarruel & Ortiz de Montellano, 1992).

By using these themes, health-care providers can evaluate Mexicans experiencing pain within their cultural framework and provide culturally specific interventions.

Because long-term-care facilities in Mexico are rare and tend to be crowded, understaffed, and expensive, many Mexican Americans may not consider long-term care as a viable option for a family member. In addition, because of the importance of extended family, Mexican Americans may prefer to care for their family members with mental illness, physical handicaps, and extended physical illnesses at home. In Mexican American culture, someone with a mental illness is not looked on with scorn or blamed for their condition because mental illness, like physical illness, is viewed as God's will. It is common to accept those with mental illness and care for them in the context of the family until the illness is so bad that they cannot be managed in the home (Zoucha & Husted, 2000).

Mexicans can readily enter the sick role without personal feelings of inadequacy or blame. A person can enter the sick role with any acceptable excuse and be relieved of life's responsibilities. Other family members willingly take over the sick person's obligations during his or her time of illness.

BLOOD TRANSFUSIONS AND ORGAN DONATION

Extraordinary means to preserve life are frowned on in the Mexican and Mexican American cultures, and ordinary means are commonly used to preserve life. Extraordinary means are defined and determined by the individual, taking into account such factors as finances, education, and availability of services.

Blood transfusions are acceptable if the individual and the family agree that the transfusion is necessary. Organ donation, although not deemed morally wrong, is not a common practice and is usually restricted to cadaver donations, because donating an organ while the person is still alive means that the body is not whole. Acceptance of organ transplant as a treatment option is seen primarily among more-educated people. One reason that organ transplant is unacceptable to some groups is the belief that *mal aire* (bad air) enters the body if it is left open too long during surgery and increases the potential for the development of cancer.

Health-Care Practitioners

TRADITIONAL VERSUS BIOMEDICAL PRACTITIONERS

Educated physicians and nurses are often seen as outsiders, especially among newer immigrants. However, health-care professionals are viewed as knowledgeable and respected because of their education (Zoucha & Husted, 2002). To overcome this initial awkwardness, health-care providers should attempt to get to know the client on a more personal level and gain confidence before initiating treatment regimens. Engaging in small talk unrelated to the health-care encounter before obtaining a health history or providing health education is advised. Health-care providers must respect this cultural practice to achieve an optimal outcome from the encounter.

Folk practitioners, who are usually well known by the family, are usually consulted before and during biomedical treatment. Numerous illnesses and conditions are caused by witchcraft. Specific rituals are carried out to eliminate the evils from the body. Lower socioeconomic and newer immigrants are more likely to use folk practitioners, but well-educated upper- and middle-class people also visit folk practitioners and *brujas* (witches) on a regular basis (Torres, 2001). Although often no contradictions or contraindications to folk remedies exist, health-care providers must always consider clients' use of these practitioners to prevent conflicting treatment regimens.

Even though the Catholic Church preaches against some types of folk practitioners, they are common and meet yearly for several days in Catemaco, Veracruz. Folk practitioners include the *curandero*, who may receive their talents from God or serve an apprenticeship with an established practitioner. The *curandero* has great respect from the community, accepts no monetary payment (but may accept gifts), is usually a member of the extended family, and treats many traditional illnesses. A *curandero* does not usually treat illnesses caused by witchcraft.

The *yerbero* (also spelled *jerbero*) is a folk healer with specialized training in growing herbs, teas, and roots and who prescribes these remedies for prevention and cure of illnesses. A *yerbero* may suggest that the person go to a *botanica* (herb shop) for specific herbs. In addition, these folk practitioners frequently prescribe the use of laxatives.

A *sobador* subscribes to treatment methods similar to those of a Western chiropractor. The *sobador* treats illnesses, primarily affecting the joints and musculoskeletal system, with massage and manipulation.

Even though Mexicans like closeness and touch within the context of family, most tend to be modest in other settings. Women are not supposed to expose their bodies to men or even to other women. Female clients may experience embarrassment when it is necessary to touch their genitals or may refuse to have pelvic examinations as a routine part of a health assessment. Men may have strong feelings about modesty as well, especially in front of women, and may be reluctant to disrobe completely for an examination. Mexican Americans often desire that members of the same gender provide intimate care (C. Zamarripa, personal communication, March 2002). Health-care providers must keep in mind clients' need for modesty when disrobing or being examined. Thus, only the body part being examined should be exposed, and direct care should be provided in private. Whenever possible, a same-gender caregiver should be assigned to Mexican Americans.

STATUS OF HEALTH-CARE PROVIDERS

Mexican American clients have great respect for health-care providers because of their training and experience.

They expect health-care providers to project a professional image and be well groomed and dressed in attire that reflects their professional status (Zoucha, 2002). Whereas they have great respect for health-care providers, some Mexican Americans may distrust them out of fear that they will disclose their undocumented status. Health-care practitioners who incorporate folk practitioners, the concept of *personalismo*, and respect into their approaches to care of Mexican American clients will gain their clients' confidence and be able to obtain more thorough assessments.

Health-care providers can demonstrate respect for Mexican American clients by greeting the client with a handshake, touching the client, or holding the client's hand, all of which help to build trust in the therapeutic relationship. Providing information and involving the family in decisions regarding health; listening to the individual's concerns; and treating the individual with *personalismo*, which stresses warmth and personal relationships, also fosters trust.

REFERENCES

American Public Health Association. (2002). *Maternal health risks of immigrant women from Latin America*. Retrieved March 2, 2007, from http://www.apha.org

Andrews, M., & Boyle, J. (2003). *Transcultural concepts in nursing care* (4th ed.). Philadelphia: Lippincott.

Burk, M. E., Wieser, P. C., & Keegan, L. (1995). Cultural beliefs and health behaviors of pregnant Mexican-American women: Implications for primary care. *Advances in Nursing Science, 17*(4), 37–52.

Centers for Disease Control and Prevention (CDC). (2006). *Regional malaria information*. Retrieved February 20, 2007, from http://www.cdc.gov/travel/regionalmalaria/camerica.htm

Centers for Disease Control and Prevention (CDC). (2007). *Health of Mexican American population*. Retrieved September 25, 2007, from http://www.cdc.gov/nchs/fastats/mexican_health.htm

CIA. (2007). Retrieved September 25, 2007, from http://www.cia.gov

Collins, R. L., & McNair, L. D. (2002). Minority women and alcohol use. *Alcohol Research and Health, 26*(4), 251–256.

Congress. (2005). *Mexico: Revolution and 20th century*. Retrieved September 25, 2007, from http://www.casahistoria.net

Eden, S., & Aguilar, R. (1989). The Hispanic chemically dependent client: Considerations for diagnosis and treatment. In G. Lawson & A. Lawson (Eds.), *Alcoholism and substance abuse in special populations* (pp. 291–295). Rockville, MD: Aspen.

Eggenberger, S. K., Grassley, J., & Restrepo, E. (2006). Culturally competent nursing care: Listening to the voices of Mexican-American women. *Online Journal of Issues in Nursing, 11*(3), 7.

Gates, G., Lau, H., & Sears, B. (2006). *Race and ethnicity of same-sex couples in California*: The Williams Project on Sexual Orientation Law and Public Policy UCLA School of Law. Los Angeles: UCLA.

Gladen, B., & Rogan, W. (1995). DDE and shortened duration of lactation in a northern Mexican town. *American Journal of Public Health, 85*(4), 504–508.

Grothaus, K. L. (1996). Family dynamics and family therapy with Mexican Americans. *Journal of Psychosocial Nursing and Mental Health Services, 34*(2), 31–37.

Kemp, C. (2001). Hispanic health beliefs and practices: Mexican and Mexican-Americans (clinical notes) [Electronic version]. Retrieved May 23, 2003, from http://www3.baylor.edu/~Charles_Kemp/hispanic_health.htm

Kim-Godwin, Y. S., Alexander, J. W., Felton, G., Mackey, M. C., & Kasakoff, A. (2006). Prerequisites to providing culturally competent care to Mexican migrant farmworkers: A Delphi study. *Journal of Cultural Diversity, 13*(1), 27–33.

Kurian, A. K., & Cardarelli, K. M. (2007). Racial and ethnic differences in cardiovascular disease risk factors: A systematic review. *Ethnic Diseases, 17*(1), 143–152.

Library of Congress. (2005). *Mexican immigration*. Retrieved March 2, 2007, from http://memory.loc.gov/learn/features/immig/mexican.html

Locke, D. (1999). *Increasing multicultural understanding: A comprehensive model* (2nd ed.). Newbury Park, CA: Sage.

Luckmann, J. (1999). *Transcultural communication in nursing*. Albany, NY: Delmar.

Mendoza, F. S., Ventura S., Saldivar L., Baisden K., & Martorell R. (1992). In A. Furino (Ed.), *Health policy and the Hispanic* (pp. 97–115). Boulder, CO: Westview Press.

Meyer, M., & Beezley, W. (2000). *The Oxford history of Mexico*. Oxford: Oxford University Press.

National Sample Survey of Registered Nurses. (2004). Retrieved March 2, 2007, from http://bhpr.hrsa.gov/healthworkforce/reports/rnpopulation/preliminaryfindings.htm

National Vital Statistics Report. (2004). Retrieved September 25, 2007, from http://www.cdc.gov/nchs/data

Neff, N. (1998). *Folk medicine in Hispanics in the Southwestern United States*. Retrieved March 2, 2007, from http://www.riceinfo.edu/projects/Hispanichealth/Courses/mod7/mid7.html

Olds, S., London, M., & Ladewig, P. (2000). *Maternal newborn nursing: A family-centered approach* (5th ed.) Redwood City, CA: Addison Wesley.

Pandey, D. K., Labarthe, D. R., Goff, D. C., Chan, W., & Nichaman, M. Z. (2001). Community-wide coronary heart disease mortality in Mexican Americans equals or exceeds that in non-Hispanic whites: The Corpus Christi Heart Project. *American Journal of Medicine, 110*(2), 81–87.

Passel, J. (2004). Mexican immigration to the US: The latest estimates [Electronic version]. *Migration Information Source*. Retrieved February 13, 2007, from http://www.migrationinformation.org/usfocus/display.cfm?ID=208

Redding, A. (1999). *Mexico: Update on treatment of homosexuals*. Resource Center of the Immigration and Naturalization Service, U.S. Department of Justice. Retrieved March 9, 2002, from http://world-policy.org/Americas/sexorient/mexgay-99.html

Rivera, J. O., Anaya, J. P., & Meza, A. (2003). Herbal product use in Mexican-Americans. *American Journal of Health-System Pharmacy, 60*(12), 1281–1282.

Schmal, J., & Madrer, J. (2007). Ethnic diversity in Mexico [Electronic version]. *Mexico Connect*. Retrieved January 17, 2007, from http://www.mexconnect.com/mex_/feature/ethnic/ethnicindex.html#imm

Sobralske, M. (2006). Machismo sustains health and illness beliefs of Mexican American men. *Journal of American Academy of Nurse Practitioners, 18*(8), 348–350.

Sobralske, M., & Katz, J. (2005). Culturally competent care of patients with acute chest pain. *Journal of American Academy of Nurse Practitioners, 17*(9), 342–349.

Spanish Language. (2007). *Fact, figures and statistics about Spanish*. Retrieved February 15, 2007, from http://spanish.about.com/library/weekly/aa070300a.htm

Spector, R. (2004). *Cultural diversity in health and illness* (6th ed.). Upper Saddle River, NJ: Pearson.

Torres, E. (2001). *The folk healer: The Mexican American tradition of curanderismo*. Albuquerque, NM: Nieves Press.

U.S. Bureau of the Census. (2001). *Census 2000 briefs and special reports*. Retrieved February 10, 2007, from http://www.census.gov/population/www/cen2000/briefs.html

Van Hook, J., Bean, F., & Passel, J. (2005). Unauthorized migrants living in the United States: A mid-decade portrait [Electronic version]. *Migration Information Source*. Retrieved February 12, 2007, from http://www.migrationinformation.org/Feature/display.cfm?ID=329

Vázquez, R. (2000). Is the phrase "La raza" racist? [Electronic version]. *Las Culturas*. Retrieved January 17, 2007, from http://www.lasculturas.com/aa/aa031200a.htm

Vázquez, R. (2001). ¿Hispanic or Latino [Electronic version]. *Las culturas*. Retrieved February 7, 2007, from http://www.lasculturas.com/aa/aa070501a.htm

Villarruel, A. M., & Ortiz de Montellano, B. (1992). Culture and pain: A Mesoamerican perspective. *Advances in Nursing Science, 15*(1), 21–32.

Wells, J. N., Cagle, C. S., & Bradley, P. J. (2006). Building on Mexican-American cultural values. *Nursing, 36*(7), 20–21.

Zoucha, R. (2007). Understanding *confianza* (confidence) in the nursing relationship with Mexican Americans. Pittsburgh: Duquesne University School of Nursing.

Zoucha, R., & Husted, G. L. (2000). The ethical dimensions of delivering culturally congruent nursing and health care. *Issues in Mental Health Nursing, 21*(3), 325–340.

Zoucha, R., & Husted, G. L. (2002). The ethical dimensions of delivering culturally congruent nursing and health care. *Review Series in Psychiatry, 3*, 10–11.

Zoucha, R., & Zamarripa, C. (1997). The significance of culture in the care of the client with an ostomy. *Journal of Wound, Ostomy, and Continence Nursing, 24*(5), 270–276.

Zoucha, R. D. (1998). The experience of Mexican Americans receiving professional nursing care: An ethnonursing study. *Journal of Transcultural Nursing, 9*(2), 34–44.

Zoucha, R. D., Reeves, J. (1999). A view of professional caring as personal for Mexican Americans. *International Journal for Human Caring, 3*(3), 14–20.

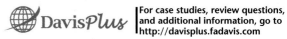

For case studies, review questions, and additional information, go to http://davisplus.fadavis.com

Chapter *19*

People of Russian Heritage

LINDA S. SMITH

Overview, Inhabited Localities, and Topography

OVERVIEW

Russians are blessed with a rich and beautiful language and culture. **Russia**, also known as the *Russian Federation*, is nearly twice the size of the United States, covers 11 time zones, and is a democratic federation of 89 republics. The climate ranges from temperate and humid to arctic in the polar north. With 6.9 million square miles, it is the largest country in the world. Ethnically, 80 percent of those living in Russia are **Russian**, 3.8 percent are **Tatars**, 2 percent are **Ukrainian**, and 14.4 percent are other smaller groups. Owing to over 7 decades of religious suppression under communist rule, a large number of Russians are either nonreligious or nonpracticing. Between 15 and 20 percent of Russians are **Russian Orthodox**, 10 to 15 percent are **Muslim**, and 2 percent belong to other Christian groups. Only about 500,000 Russians are **Jews**. Russia enjoys one of the highest literacy rates in the world at 99.6 percent, with men and women equally literate. The population of Russia at 143 million is declining with 1.5 deaths for each birth (CIA, 2006). This high death rate is related to high-risk behaviors such as sexual promiscuity, smoking, and alcoholism plus traffic accidents and heart disease. The life expectancy of Russian men is 58 years, and of Russian women, 73. Adding to this population decline is a low fertility rate of 1.1 (replacement level is considered to be 2.1 children per woman of reproductive age) (CIA, 2006; Library of Congress, 2005; Marquez, 2005). The two largest cities—Moscow, Russia's capital, and St. Petersburg—have 10 million and 4.5 million people, respectively. Although major cities are heavily populated, 27 percent of Russians live in very rural areas (Library of Congress, 2005).

In 1917, the imperial Czar was overthrown and Vladimir Lenin took power, followed by Josef Stalin. The overthrow was partly due to the horrific defeat of the Russian armies during World War I and resulted in rioting and discontent. After Lenin left power, Stalin further strengthened and unified Communist rule over the Soviet Union, which comprised 15 republics, the largest of which was the Republic of Russia. These 15 republics are ethnically and culturally diverse. On August 24, 1991, Russia gained independence when the Soviet Union collapsed. Each of the 15 republics of the Soviet Union developed into independent nations. Russia adopted a constitution in 1993. Unfortunately, Russia's poverty rate is 17.8 percent with an 11.5 percent inflation rate (CIA, 2006), with a large number of adults unemployed (7.6 percent) or underemployed. In January 2007, one Russian ruble was worth 3.7 cents (US$0.0037) (OANDA, 2007). By contrast, in 1989, 1 Ruble was worth US$6.

Economically, Russia has some of the most abundant natural resources, including rich deposits of oil, natural gas, coal, timber, and minerals such as diamonds, nickel, aluminum, and platinum. Russia has over 20 percent of the world's forests. Regrettably, during the Soviet rule under Stalin and others, water, land, and air pollution prevailed (Energy Information Administration [EIA], 2004). In addition, after 1991, economic and social reform was plagued by high crime rates (police have low pay, low status, and high corruption) and political bribery and corruption. At present, there are three branches of government, the executive, the legislative, and the judiciary, but Russia's president has formidable powers and has used these powers to turn back some of the important democratic reforms made in the 1990s.

HERITAGE AND RESIDENCE

During the Soviet rule between 1917 and 1991, Soviet citizens moved between and among republics, often leaving their own culture and birthplace. Since the fall of the Soviet empire, a return migration to the republic and culture of birth has been occurring (Aroian, 2003).

Russians have also left their homelands and settled in the United States. Russian Americans are one of the fastest-growing ethnic groups in the United States. According to the U.S. Bureau of the Census (2000), over 2.6 million Russians live in the United States. Between 1996 and 2000, the average number of new Russian immigrants to the United States was 15,411 per year (U.S. Department of Homeland Security, 2005b). The Russian-speaking population in the United States increased 254 percent between 1990 and 1998. During the year 2005, 4652 Russian children were adopted by U.S. citizens (U.S. Department of Homeland Security, 2005c).

Of the 18,083 Russians who came to the United States in 2005, the largest number (2786) relocated in New York state, followed by California, Illinois, Florida, and the Pacific Northwest (U.S. Department of Homeland Security, 2005a). Almost 90 percent of Russian Americans live in urban areas such as New York City and the Tri-State area (24 percent), Boston, Philadelphia, Baltimore, Miami, Atlanta, Cleveland, Chicago, Detroit, Denver, Houston, Los Angeles, San Diego, San Francisco, Seattle, and Portland, Oregon (Allied Media Corp., 2006). In Canada, Russians primarily live in Toronto, Vancouver, and Montreal (Aroian, 2003).

REASONS FOR MIGRATION AND ASSOCIATED ECONOMIC FACTORS

Since 1917, four major waves of migration from Russia to the United States have occurred. Three of these comprised ethnic and national minority groups, the largest from Russia being the Soviet Jews. This emigration was primarily due to the persecution experienced as well as their refugee status (Aroian, 2003). Soviet Jews were one of the few groups allowed, and in some cases encouraged, to leave Russia under Communist rule. The last wave of Russian immigrants has occurred since 1993 and has resulted from much more freedom to immigrate, harsh economic conditions, political turmoil, and greater overtly expressed Russian nationalism and anti-Semitism. U.S. immigration rules such as quotas, job requirements, and sponsorships apply (Aroian, 2003). During and after the transition from Communism to a free-market system, teachers, scientists, and physicians were the hardest hit. Salaries were fixed and well below poverty levels, causing a desperate migration in hopes of an improved quality of life for themselves and their children (Wikipedia, 2006).

Prior to 1991, people who came to the United States from Russia were unhappy with the oppression of free thought imposed by the Communist regime. Ethnic minorities were often tortured for their beliefs. More recently, however, Russians came to the United States to reunite with families and loved ones (Bistrevsky, 2005).

EDUCATIONAL STATUS AND OCCUPATIONS

⊙— VIGNETTE 19.1

Vera (34 years old) and Alexander Sarkisova (38 years old) are ethnic Russians living in Chicago, Illinois. They were both born in Moscow, Russia, and immigrated to the United States 4½ years ago. Vera and Sasha (short for Alexander) came to Chicago to be with Alexander's parents and two brothers. As they prepared for their relocation to the United States and awaited their visas, Vera and Alexander took a year of English language classes at Moscow State University. In Russia, Vera was trained as an optometrist and Alexander was an electrical engineer. Even though they knew some English upon arrival, both were dismayed by their lack of ability to understand spoken English. Vera and Sasha work in Chicago—Vera cleans offices at night and Alexander drives a taxi cab. They live in the basement of the home of Alexander's brother. Fortunately, they both have health insurance through Alexander's employment but this insurance covers only a portion of the real health-care costs.

1. How does this couple's immigration profile compare with other Russian immigrants over the last 100 years?
2. What health risks can be identified for Vera and Alexander Sarkisova considering their immigration experience?
3. What barriers might this couple experience in securing health-care services?
4. Name four nonverbal behaviors that might offend the Sarkisovas?
5. How should Russian Americans be addressed?

The average age for U.S. Russian immigrants is 42 years, with nearly one-fourth of the total U.S. Russian population being 65 years of age or older. Of adults over age 25, one million have at least a bachelor's degree, and this high level of education is reflected in the median household income of $59,950 (U.S. Bureau of the Census, 2000). Nearly 64 percent are married, with 1.6 children per couple. They are ambitious professionals and over 18 percent have graduate degrees. Thus, the average adult Russian in the United States works in a professional area, is well educated, and has a better-than-average income (Allied Media Corp, 2006).

Education is highly valued and strongly promoted for both genders. Russian extended families frequently pool their financial resources, and even work additional hours, to provide a good education for their children. Good grades are an expectation. Men look for well-educated wives who are intelligent, critical thinkers. Women are an important part of the workforce in Russia, although the roles of mother and homemaker are also valued. Even though Russian women pursue education and careers, the expectation remains that they fulfill home and child-care responsibilities (Aroian, 2003).

Teaching/learning systems in Russia are rigid, compared with U.S. standards. Until recently, however, learning English was not a priority in Soviet schools, which presents a very real language barrier for Russian immigrants, especially older people, who came to the United

States during the first three immigrant waves. Recently, English has grown more popular in Russia owing to media, film, music, and Western advertising.

Not all Russian immigrants are financially secure. Sixty percent of those receiving public assistance in one California area had an annual household income of less than $10,000, and 28 percent of the families had an income between $10,000 and $30,000. Importantly, most Russians receiving public assistance have a college education (Hobbs, 2002).

Employed Russians receiving public assistance work half time in areas such as computer hardware and software, retail, elder and child care, and education. In Russia, these individuals all worked—and were employed in fields such as engineering, math, medicine, computer science, education, and other professions. Unfortunately, these positions are not often open to them in the United States owing to language, licensing, and credentialing problems. Over half (58 percent) of the employed Russians receiving assistance report that their jobs come without medical benefits, sick leave, or retirement plans. When Russian Americans start their own small businesses, the biggest barriers are language, unfamiliar legal regulations, and unfamiliar start-up processes such as securing business loans (Hobbs, 2002). In contrast, more recent Russian immigrants tend to be less well educated and more likely to pursue technical and service occupations (Minnesota Department of Employment and Economic Development [MDEED], 2006).

Communications

DOMINANT LANGUAGE AND DIALECTS

Russian is a uniquely rich, expressive, and beautiful living language. The primary language for over 150 million people, it is one of the world's major languages (Rendaxa Software, 2007; Wikipedia, 2007) and the most pervasive of all Slavic languages. Russian is one of the six official languages of the United Nations. Russian, official language of the Russian Empire, unified the 15 Soviet republics and the Soviet-controlled satellite nations, although each had its own language and culture. School children in these satellite countries were required to take many years of Russian language courses.

Importantly, not all Russian speakers in the United States are ethnic Russians. Prior to the Soviet collapse in 1991, most Russian speakers in North America were Russian-speaking Jews (Wikipedia, 2007). Therefore, for these families, languages of **Yiddish** and **Ladino** (the Spanish dialect spoken by some Sephardic Jews but written in Hebrew script) may be spoken in the home; however, younger Russian Jews, although they may understand spoken Yiddish, may not be fluent in the language (MDEED, 2006). According to the U.S. Bureau of the Census (2003), 706,242 persons over age 5 spoke Russian at home. Of these, only 43 percent reported speaking English very well, 29 percent spoke English well, 21 percent spoke English "not well," and 6 percent could not speak English at all. Often of limited English proficiency, Russian immigrants can read and write English better than speak it, and most Russians, with the exception of Russian older people, learn and become proficient in English. Many large urban centers of Russian speakers have their own newspapers and self-maintained communities, especially when these communities primarily include Russian immigrants who arrived prior to 1991. Therefore, immigrants from the former Soviet Union speak both Russian and their own native languages (e.g., Ukrainian, Georgian), but may have very limited English proficiency.

Two main Russian dialects, **Northern** and **Southern**, have distinct tone, pronunciations, and even grammar characteristics. **Standard Russian**, based in Moscow, has characteristics of both Southern and Northern dialects (Culture tips, 2000). Written Russian uses the Cyrillic alphabet, derived from but not the same as the Greek alphabet. Russian is considered phonetic, and even children as young as 5 years of age can read the classics. Russian language includes five vowels and numerous consonants that are considered hard or soft. Russian language experts have identified 350,000 to 500,000 words (Wikipedia, 2007). Interestingly, Russian does not include articles (e.g., "the") and is often called a *house green* language ("the" and "is" are omitted).

CULTURAL COMMUNICATION PATTERNS

Russians enjoy intellectual conversations that focus on political, economic, cultural, and social issues. Word of mouth among Russian speakers is a strong influencing factor for Russians making decisions regarding health care and major purchases (Allied Media Corp, 2006). Russians seek emotional support from their spouses, relatives, and friends and report not being free to trust religious advisors, teachers, social services workers, or community leaders. They did report a willingness to talk with physicians and other health-care workers, especially when these workers are able to speak Russian (Hobbs, 2002).

Russians tend to speak loudly, even during socially pleasant communications (MDEED, 2006). They have great insight into their own and another's feelings and may communicate on an emotional level. Russians make eye contact, nod their head in a gesture of affirmation or approval, and are, mostly, respectful in their verbal and nonverbal behaviors toward older people and persons of perceived rank or authority (Culture tips, 2000; MDEED, 2006).

Between men, Russians appreciate a firm handshake, and this symbol of agreement is considered more binding than paper documents. Shaking hands with a female stranger is not appropriate, unless the woman is a health-care professional. The doorway of the home of a Russian is considered the center of the house spirit, and it is a bad omen to shake hands over the threshold. Remove shoes prior to entering the home (MDEED, 2006).

Behavior in public must be respectful. Russians do not appreciate gestures such as standing with hands inserted into pockets or arms crossed over the chest; neither do they appreciate slouching postures when being interviewed or seeing the soles of shoes when sitting across from someone who is crossing their legs. Russians also do not appreciate the crossing and stretching of arms behind the head. Making the nonverbal sign for "OK" may be considered an obscene gesture. Shaking a fist shows anger or disagreement, and pointing with the index finger is considered rude (Hobbs, 2002; MDEED, 2006).

Russians freely touch friends and family members. Greetings that include kisses on each cheek, with close friends, are common. Furthermore, Russians often require less personal space than most other North Americans. Russians are social diplomats and will "bend" the truth for the sake of politeness or for the purpose of softening bad news (Birch, 2006).

Russians perceive themselves as spontaneous and emotional, able to be extremely empathetic toward the suffering of others. They are emotionally strong and have a long and distinguished history of enduring great hardship and adversity. Thus, Russians may present a pervasive attitude of endurance with comments such as "we have overcome many troubles and we can overcome these troubles because we are strong . . . we are Russians." They look to others for the same level of respect and recognition of social order as they give. Thus, Russians have a sense of duty, self-sacrifice, and genuine caring toward others (Culture tips, 2000).

TEMPORAL RELATIONSHIPS

Russians who have immigrated to other countries tend to be both present and future oriented. This is not the case, however, among nonimmigrants. Russians living in Russia have shared their need to live within the present, "because we have no future."

Russians are punctual and value this attribute. For appointments, Russians will arrive either early or right on time.

FORMAT FOR NAMES

Russians use titles such as Mr., Mrs., Dr., Professor, aunt, and grandfather to show the appropriate respect (Culture tips, 2000; Hobbs, 2002). Even when friendships are established, they often ask to be addressed by their first name plus their patronymic. The patronymic is the first name of their father with either a feminine or a masculine ending, depending on the person's gender. An example of a preferred name format might be Oleg Vasiliovitch (Oleg, son of Vaslav).

Family Roles and Organization

HEAD OF HOUSEHOLD AND GENDER ROLES

In Russia, younger adults and youth lean and depend on the wisdom of their parents and grandparents whenever important decisions need to be made. In the United States, especially owing to the English language barrier, older Russians tend to depend on their children and grandchildren to guide decision-making. This is especially true when older Russians live within Russian-language communities, purchasing food and supplies from Russian retailers. Such communities provide little incentive to learn English. Importantly, Russians will be reluctant to

sign consent forms and other documents without first consulting their family members (Keefe, 2006). In addition, family members will often attend health-care appointments in order to provide cognitive as well as affective support (Aroian, 2003). Different from other immigrant groups, Russian immigrants arrived in the United States in multigenerational family units. Thus, older Russians may not have left their Russian homes completely by choice.

PRESCRIPTIVE, RESTRICTIVE, AND TABOO BEHAVIORS FOR CHILDREN AND ADOLESCENTS

Russian children are taught to obey their parents and older people, as well as to achieve high grades in school and complete a university education. The expectation of children is to care for family members who are ill and in need of care (Culture tips, 2000). Older people are expected to raise their grandchildren, especially if both parents are employed.

Sexual topics such as contraception and sex education are not thought to be appropriate public discussion topics. Sexual activity outside of marriage is not sanctioned, and if teen girls get pregnant, abortion is the primary intervention (Aroian, 2003). Older Russian immigrants tend to be more modest (Aroian, 2003) and loathe public displays of affection.

FAMILY GOALS AND PRIORITIES

Russians have great cultural pride and sense of family; they have a strong family and group focus, and the family or group is more important than the person. Thus, they depend upon and trust the influence of a network of family, neighbors, friends, and colleagues. Historically, collectivism was part of Russian society for centuries, with the communal good holding higher value than individual needs. Russians have great love for their extended family members and a strong and cohesive sense of the importance of family. Therefore, during crises, Russians pull together with their family, seeking their love and support. Consequently, Russians report amazement with the American value for individualism and independence. Spouses consult each other (Culture tips, 2000), and to a Russian, friends are considered close and important. Most Americans reserve those close, intimate ties for immediate family members.

Russian young people are expected to have and complete household chores, which are gender specific, with girls doing tasks such as cooking and cleaning and boys doing more physical labor—except for grocery shopping, which is a task for both boys and girls. Although education and a good job are considered important for Russian women, finding a good husband is even more important and being an "old maid" is socially frowned upon (Aroian, 2003).

Domestic violence is a rising concern in Russia. Therefore, for Russian immigrants, especially women, who may not trust police and social/mental health services, domestic violence is seldom reported (Aroian, 2003). Moreover, Russian women will only rarely admit to and report being raped.

ALTERNATIVE LIFESTYLES

Divorce rates in Russia are high, and small families are also typical owing to economic hardships. Russian immigrants have small families and high divorce rates, perhaps because Russian American women grow more independent as they acculturate, stress increases owing to immigration, and Russian women wait to reach their new country prior to ending an unhappy marriage (Aroian, 2003). Recent Russian immigrants tend not to be religious owing to the influence and antireligion dogma of Communism. Therefore, among Russian immigrants, divorce does not negatively affect social status. Divorced men in Russia are never awarded child custody, and although they pay child support, they do not remain active in their children's lives (Aroian, 2003). This tendency is also noted with Russian immigrants.

Although Russian women are expected to marry by age 25 and have children, they are also expected to continue to pursue education and career paths. This is possible because the mothers and grandmothers become primary caregivers for young children; men are seldom expected to fulfill child-care responsibilities. Importantly, Russian women with fertility problems are not considered desirable spouses (Aroian, 2003).

Following a survey in Russia that reflected answers to questions related to the Russian culture (Russians who, 2005), 65 percent of Russians favor the death penalty and 56 percent oppose adoption of Russian children by foreigners. They also believed that Russian women who married foreigners should forfeit their citizenship. These strong beliefs are likely due to the resurgence of a strong Russian identity separate from Western influences.

Public displays of affection between same-sex couples are extremely rare in Russia. Overtly expressed antigay graffiti is commonly seen on the streets and buildings of downtown Moscow. Homosexuality is no longer a crime with the new Russian Penal Code effective on January 1, 1997. The age of consent is set at 16 years, regardless of sexual orientation. In July 1997, the first gay and lesbian pride festival occurred in Moscow. However, alternative lifestyle choices are still stigmatized by a large part of the population (News about gay Russia, N.D.). Traditional Russian Americans may not accept same-sex relationships; therefore, gay and lesbian Russians in the United States are likely to remain closeted unless significant trust is developed with their health-care providers. Same-sex behavior should not be disclosed to family members or friends.

Workforce Issues

CULTURE IN THE WORKPLACE

The concept of employed persons with disabilities may be difficult for Russians to grasp. Russians believe that disabilities and negative health events are caused by something the person did not do and should have or did do and should not have. For example, Russians agree that eating well and keeping warm are important for good health (MDEED, 2006).

Russians believe that members of health-care professions should work hard to create membership that reflects the diversity of the communities in which they work. With an ever-increasing Russian immigrant population in North America, it is essential that Russian-trained health-care providers, with their values for holistic health care, earn credentials in their new countries.

Russian immigrant nurses work hard and have as their practice motto the relief of suffering. With nurses and physicians in short supply in the United States, the skills of Russian-trained nurses and physicians are greatly needed. However, the concept of teamwork is new to Russian nurses, as are critical thinking and sensitive care giving. In addition, the idea of lifelong learning is difficult in an authoritarian work environment (Alaniz, 2001). Russian nursing education has been likened to that of the American Licensed Practical Nurses (Alaniz, 2001).

When communicating in the workplace, Russians have a very different value system. For example, Russians will perform and promote the value of positive politeness. **Positive politeness** is a technique that employs rules of positive social communication. The employee using positive politeness will say nice things that show that the person is accepted, while simultaneously providing support and empathy and avoiding negative discourse with coworkers. When negotiating compromise, Russians express more emotion and invest more time and effort into supporting decisions and requests. With colleagues and friends, Russians communicate directly, which is considered to be a sign of sincerity. Russians expect to be specifically asked for information (Bergelson, 2003).

ISSUES RELATED TO AUTONOMY

In the United States, nurses and physicians work as a unit, as a team, yet each member maintains independence. In Russia, the physician makes the decisions and performs the problem-solving processes. Thus, the nursing profession carries limited status and respect from the Russian-speaking public (Alaniz, 2001). One Russian immigrant explained, "What do we expect from nurse? We don't expect anything—we only expect something from doctor. Nurse is just someone who obeys" (Smith, 1996).

Biocultural Ecology

SKIN COLOR AND OTHER BIOLOGICAL VARIATIONS

Ethnic Russians are primarily Caucasians. Cultural assimilation is considered easier when the immigrants' skin color is the same as or similar to the majority group. Stature and skin color for ethnic Russians are similar to other North American groups, with the exception of high rates of obesity among Russian immigrants. Researchers Dubrova, Kurbatova, Kholod, and Prokhorovskaya (1995) retrospectively reviewed documents from a Moscow maternity hospital over a 40-year time period. Between 1930 and 1949, they found the age of menarche decreased at a rate of 12 months per decade, with a parallel increase in maternal height by 1.8 cm per decade—significantly greater gains than those for women in Western European countries. These increases ended during the second half of the study. The infants' weight, length, and head and chest circumferences showed changes—assumed to be related to increases in the mother's stature.

DISEASES AND HEALTH CONDITIONS

Common health disorders seen in Russian immigrants include hypertension, coronary disease, gastrointestinal disorders, and diabetes. Common disabilities include the results of diabetes (sensory impairment), alcoholism, chronic health disorders, hypertension, psychosocial disorders, arthritis, lung diseases such as asthma and chronic obstructive pulmonary disease (COPD), and cancer (Keefe, 2006; MDEED, 2006; Shpilko, 2006). Alcoholism is far less prevalent among Russian Jews and women (Aroian, 2003).

Russian Jews who immigrated to Israel between 1989 and 1992 reported, from a list of 11 disease states, an average of 3.5 chronic diseases—a much higher rate than that reported among immigrants from other countries. The highest age-specific disease prevalence rates were in musculoskeletal diseases, ischemic heart diseases, gastrointestinal diseases, and high blood pressure. Women in this study reported higher rates than men for all disease states. The researchers suggest that health-care facilities need to be aware of and prepared for higher rates of disease and disability among this immigrant group (Rennert, Luz, Tamir, & Peterburg, 2002).

Many Russians prefer to somatize psychological disorders, especially depression, rather than to admit to them. For example, clinical depression is a very real concern for many older Russian immigrants, but these individuals present with vague complaints of skeletal or gastrointestinal problems.

Depression among Russian immigrants was studied by Tran, Khatutsky, Aroian, Balsam, and Conway (2000). Health status among older Russian-speaking immigrants was also studied. These researchers found that when Russian older people lived alone, they were more likely to experience a much greater level of depression than when they lived with family or friends. In addition, those older Russians with better English skills had better health and less depression. Older Russian immigrants who spoke limited or no English exhibited a poorer health status and more depression. These researchers recommended supportive health services for this immigrant group as well as sensitivity to the living arrangements and family circumstances of older Russian immigrants.

In a study by Vadlamani et al. (2001), Russian-speaking Jewish immigrants had a much higher than average rate of polyps. Therefore, these researchers suggest more aggressive colorectal cancer screening for this patient population. Perhaps related to these findings are those of Mehler, Scott, Pines, Gifford, Bigerstaff, and Hiatt (2001) in their study of the incidence of cardiovascular risk factors among Russian immigrants. In their study ($N = 204$), Russian immigrants had a greater incidence of hyperlipidemia and hypertension (56 percent). Nearly half of their study participants had two or more cardiovascular risk factors. Most were overweight, but surprisingly few reported alcohol or tobacco use, probably owing to the influence of religion (Jew and Pentecostal Christians) on these practices. Different from the findings of other studies on Russian immigrants, Mehler et al. did not note increased rates of diabetes.

VARIATIONS IN DRUG METABOLISM

Gaikovitch (2003) extensively investigated drug metabolism properties that make medications more water-soluble and thereby more readily excreted in the urine. She examined genetic polymorphism variations in the metabolism of many drugs. She writes that, "the frequency of functionally important mutations and alleles of genes coding for xenoobiotic metabolizing enzymes shows a wide ethnic variation . . . " (para. 1). Her purpose in doing the research was to provide a foundational pharmacogenetic information databank for Russians, the largest Slavic group. Gaikovitch found that the allele distribution of ". . . important drug and xenobiotic metabolizing enzymes among Russians shows that the allele frequency is similar to that of other Caucasians. Therefore, it may be expected that drug side effects and efficacy problems due to an individual's genetic background are similar when compared to those in other European populations" (para. 1).

The metabolism of alcohol may be the exception. According to Gabriel (2005), Russians inherited, via the Mongolian invaders to their country, a genetic characteristic that prevents the processing of ethanol derived from fruit or potatoes. He believes that this genetic trait makes Russians more susceptible to alcoholism, especially when the preferred alcoholic beverage is cognac or vodka.

High-Risk Behaviors

Russians' reluctance to immunize may be considered a high-risk behavior. In Russia, immunizations are available but have been and continue to be of poor quality. Furthermore, reports of hepatitis- and HIV-positive–contaminated immunization needles have created fear and distrust among Russian parents. Therefore, Russians do not immunize their children in order to avoid these risks. Another high-risk behavior is the common practice Russian immigrants have of sharing left-over medications with family and friends (Aroian, 2003).

Russia has an alcohol problem. Russians drink hard liquor, mostly vodka and cognac at family gatherings and celebrations. Worthy of note, the typical Russian toast translates as "to your health" (Culture tips, 2000). Heavy alcohol consumption is a part of daily life for this population, partly owing to the sustained indifference to address the problem by Russian authorities. Russian statisticians estimate that over 30 percent of deaths in Russia are directly related to alcohol (Nemtsov, 2005; Nicholson, Bobak, Murphy, Rose, & Marmot, 2005).

Smoking is also prevalent; Russia is one of the few countries that currently do little or nothing to curb tobacco use. Nearly 63 percent of Russian men and 15 percent of Russian women smoke, and this number increases by about 2 percent per year. Although 60 percent of current smokers want to quit, no state-supported programs exist to help them do so. For this and other reasons, the male life expectancy in Russia is just above 58 years (Parfitt, 2006). Although Russian immigrants do not demonstrate the same level of smoking and drinking behaviors as their native counterparts, more recent Russian immigrants engage in these behaviors at higher rates than previous groups (Hasin et al., 2002).

High-risk sexual behaviors among Russia immigrant adolescent girls were investigated by Jeltova, Fish, and Revenson (2005). The results highlight the importance of maintaining emotional ties with the traditional Russian culture. They found that the more acculturated to the American culture the girl is, the greater the incidence of risky sexual behavior.

HEALTH-CARE PRACTICES

Russians define health as the absence of illness. Importantly, Russian immigrants generally adhere to health-care appointments, treatment regimens, and medication use (Aroian, 2003). Russians may, however, distrust physicians and choose to combine the prescribed treatments with homeopathic remedies. Mental illnesses are considered a disgrace in Russia; so Russian immigrants may not provide answers to questions regarding any family or personal history of mental illness (University of Michigan Health System, 2007).

When Russian-speaking immigrant women of all ages were asked about their U.S. health-care practices and utilization, the women asserted that they preferred female physicians but believed male doctors to be more skilled and competent (Ivanov & Buck, 2002). They wanted always to be able to see their own physicians and expressed frustration when that was not possible. These Russian women also expressed dissatisfaction with family physicians owing to their perceived lack of professionalism. They were dissatisfied with the general appearance of health-care professionals and how difficult it is to distinguish between the nurse and the janitor. Not surprisingly, they stated that language, in addition to cost, was a major barrier to health care and, therefore, chose to receive their health information from their mothers and grandmothers. These Russian women valued massage and herbal remedies and would access medical care when these remedies were ineffective. However, access to care was primarily only for illness, not for preventive care such as Pap smears and mammograms. They want the physician to refer them for preventive services and to inform them about everything they need to know to stay well (Ivanov & Buck, 2002).

Russians often self-diagnose and therefore seek out and read Russian-language health articles related to their disorders. One important method of receiving health-care information is through the mass media and Internet. Through a website called *RussianDoctor.com*, users can access a list of Russian-speaking dentists and physicians by specialty and location (city/state). *Rulist.com* is a search engine that provides a kind of Russian yellow pages with information on health and wellness. Russian immigrants may also subscribe to the Russian health magazine. The publishers of this magazine profess a strong commitment to increase the medical awareness of Russian speaking people in the United States.

Nutrition

MEANING OF FOOD

For Russians, and most especially for Russian Jews, food and nutritional practices are considered essential ingredients for health and healing (University of Washington Medical Center, 2005). Food also carries ritual and ceremony. When entertaining, Russians often use food as a demonstration of their love and respect for their visitors. They often spend days purchasing and preparing food for their most-treasured guests.

Russian immigrants eat three meals a day, with their largest meal at noon. Russians enjoy snacks and tea, water, and fruit juices without ice. Russian Jews do not eat pork or shellfish (Hobbs, 2002). Russian immigrants have reported little interest in American food.

COMMON FOODS AND FOOD RITUALS

Nutritional issues are believed to be a major contributing factor toward the chronic diseases experienced by Russian immigrants. Heart disease, diabetes, and hypertension are related to nutritional habits such as high-salt, carbohydrate, and fat intake (Keefe, 2006).

DIETARY PRACTICES FOR HEALTH PROMOTION

When Russians are ill, they love soup and broths, bland foods, chicken, potatoes, fruit and vegetables, and yogurt. Tea with honey and milk is considered medicinal (Hobbs, 2002).

NUTRITIONAL DEFICIENCIES AND FOOD LIMITATIONS

Russian diets contain high levels of saturated fat (and hydrogenated vegetable fats), salt, and carbohydrate (Keefe, 2006). This contributes to the over 60 percent of Russian adults with high blood cholesterol as well as the high rates of obesity and hypertension (Marquez, 2005). Although fresh fruits and vegetables are not routinely consumed in Russia owing to limited availability and high cost, Russians enjoy eating them and Russian immigrants enjoy them with their meals whenever possible.

Pregnancy and Childbearing Practices

VIGNETTE 19.2

Vera and Sasha Sarkisova want to have at least two children but Vera has had great difficulty sustaining the last two pregnancies. Eight years ago in Moscow, Vera had an abortion, which resulted in a painful infection that took months to clear. Joyfully, Vera believes she is now, once again, 3 months' pregnant. Upon the advice of an American coworker, she reluctantly visits the women's health clinic and is seen by a nurse practitioner specializing in women's care. Vera tells her about the unusual drainage she's been having. Vera is examined vaginally by the nurse practitioner, after which she receives two prescriptions, one for vitamins and the second for her "morning sickness."

That night, Vera experiences yet another miscarriage. She blames the miscarriage on the examination performed by the nurse as well as on the medication she took for nausea. Vera feels confused and alone. Sasha wants children and has threatened to leave her if she is unable to fulfill his wishes. Vera and Sasha are not religious but believe in the strong spiritual bonds of family; therefore, having children is essential to them both.

1. What would a culturally competent health-care provider do to help Vera during this time of crisis?
2. How might typical Russian beliefs regarding the role of the nurse affect Vera's perceptions of the etiology of her miscarriage?
3. Why might Vera be susceptible to fertility problems?
4. Where might the nurse or social worker get assistance for Vera?

FERTILITY PRACTICES AND VIEWS TOWARD PREGNANCY

Russians delay marriage and childbearing until age 20. Childbearing and child rearing are expectations, and infertility is perceived by Russians as a health problem, disappointment, and even punishment for some feminine wrongdoing (Aroian, 2003).

Contraception for Russian women is allowed without sanctions or taboos. Even so, many Russian immigrants are afraid of birth control pills and refuse to take them. One possible reason for this reluctance was the poor quality and the high dosage of oral contraceptives in Russia. To compound this problem, condoms in Russia were poorly made, and many jokes have evolved about the routine breakage of Russian-made condoms. Furthermore, Russian men believe that condoms hinder sexual pleasure and, therefore, refuse to wear them. Most Russian men also refuse vasectomies (Aroian, 2003). Consequently, abortion was and is one of the most common forms of birth control in Russia. Russia has the world's highest abortion rate, with the average woman having three or more abortions in her lifetime; self-induced abortions are not uncommon. In 1990, there were 1972 abortions per 1000 live births. In 2002, this number dropped to 1276 (World Health Organization [WHO], 2005). Thus, Russian immigrant women have high rates of infertility, and these infertility issues may lead to marital discord and divorce.

Russian women are responsible for contraception and often make contraception decisions without consulting their male partners. These decisions often relate to access and cost. Young Russian women are discouraged from strenuous exercise, including swimming, while menstruating (Aroian, 2003).

PRESCRIPTIVE, RESTRICTIVE, AND TABOO PRACTICES IN THE CHILDBEARING FAMILY

Pregnant Russian women do not engage in heavy lifting and often commit to bed rest if it is prescribed. Russian women who are pregnant receive more respect. When born, boys are dressed in blue and girls in pink (Aroian, 2003). Breastfeeding is encouraged, and nursing women are told to drink tea with milk and eat nuts to improve their milk supply (Aroian, 2003).

Owing to religious beliefs, Russian Jews circumcise their male infants. Ethnic Russians do not circumcise their newborn boys.

Death Rituals

DEATH RITUALS AND EXPECTATIONS

Flowers are used to beautify caskets and funeral services, and even Russian Jews have open caskets. Food and beverages are usually served during wakes and funerals. Friends and family come to pay their respects for 7 days postmortem, but the expected total period of official mourning is 1 full year, after which time, a surviving spouse may remarry. Close relatives of the deceased dress in black. Russians do not hesitate to cry and sob at funerals (Aroian, 2003), but overt wailing is often confined to the home of the deceased.

Family will hold vigil day and night if their loved one is dying. All relatives and friends are expected to visit a dying patient and often sit with the person for hours. If a part of their religious practices, the placing of hands on the ill person's forehead may be noted, as a kind of ritual blessing gesture. In addition, religious symbols may be placed at the ill person's bedside, and at the time of death, a spiritual advisor should be present. Also at the time of death, all mirrors may be covered with black fabric and the dead person's mouth and eyes closed (University of Washington Medical Center, 2005).

If the patient and family are Russian Orthodox, cremation is unlikely (University of Washington Medical Center, 2005). Spiritual leaders from the Russian Orthodox religion institute a special prayer vigil, called *panikhida*, over the deceased. This is a special time that includes chants, prayers, singing of hymns, and gospel readings (Yehieli, Lutz, & Grey, 2005).

Russian Jews bury the dead within 24 hours except during holidays, on Saturday, or if awaiting the arrival of additional friends and family (University of Washington Medical Center, 2005). For Russian immigrants, cremation is far less common than burial. However, Russian immigrants may chose cremation so that the deceased's ashes can be shipped back to "Mother" Russia (Yehieli et al., 2005).

RESPONSES TO DEATH AND GRIEF

Russian Orthodox followers believe that life and death are connected and that they will, if they live and worship appropriately, enjoy eternal life in heaven (Yehieli et al., 2005). Therefore, the death of a loved one is a family affair whereby large numbers of extended family members pay vigil to the terminally ill and deceased person. They connect in prayer and ask the heavens to show mercy on the soul of their deceased loved one (Yehieli et al., 2005).

Perhaps as a mechanism of diplomacy, Russians are loathe to disclose to patients the critical nature of their terminal illness (Birch, 2006; MDEED, 2006; Norman, 1996) and tend to be cheery and happy in the presence of a dying person. Norman (1996) found that the rationale for this reluctance was due to the belief that the stress of such bad news would cause increased morbidity and even death. Moreover, the dying person would lose hope and succumb to the illness, the physicians could be making an incorrect diagnosis, and the family, responsible for the care of their members, needed to do everything that was possible to protect that person from psychological turmoil. Russians and some Russian Americans believe that talking about death is a bad omen. Therefore, it is important to carefully and diplomatically talk with the family first, prior to disclosure of bad news to the patient (MDEED, 2006).

Related to their sense of community and family, Russians believe that a problem for one family member is a problem for the entire family. In addition, the physician needs to identify the lead family spokesperson and work with him or her. Family members generally do not openly grieve in front of a sick or dying loved one, but the dying person is allowed to express her or his own sadness and grief. However, taking morphine or other analgesia may be perceived as a last resort in a hopeless situation. Administration of potent narcotics is also perceived as patient abandonment (University of Washington Medical Center, 2005). Requests for Living Wills or Durable Powers of Attorney, as well as consents for withholding or withdrawing treatment, are usually declined by Russian patients and family members (University of Washington Medical Center, 2005).

Spirituality

RELIGIOUS PRACTICES AND USE OF PRAYER

Preferred religious practices for Russian immigrants vary, depending upon the chosen spiritual beliefs. Some Russians, having lived within the antireligious confines of the former Soviet Union, will deny religious affiliations. Conversely, Russian Jews and those who are Russian Orthodox will practice accordingly. Prior to the overthrow of Czarist Russia, ethnic Russians were predominantly Russian Orthodox. During the Soviet era, however, religious practices of all types were condemned and, in many cases, severely punished. With the resurgence of Russian nationalism, the Russian Orthodox Church has again taken a major role in the life and politics of Russian people. As evidence of this renewed emphasis, once crumbling, decaying Russian Orthodox Churches are now being carefully restored, perhaps symbolic of the restoration of the Russian Orthodox faith and practices.

MEANING OF LIFE AND INDIVIDUAL SOURCES OF STRENGTH

Ethnic Russians may not believe in an afterlife, but self-professed atheism has had a dramatic decline since 1991.

Russian immigrants gain spiritual strength, stability, and meaning through their associations with family and friends.

SPIRITUAL BELIEFS AND HEALTH-CARE PRACTICES

Seriously ill patients and family members who are religious (e.g., Russian Orthodox, Russian Jew) consider prayer as an essential and powerful tool toward health and healing (University of Washington Medical Center, 2005). Members of the Russian Orthodox faith believe in the heavenly position of saints as well as religious miracles.

Health-Care Practices

VIGNETTE 19.3

Sasha Sarkisova smokes two packages of cigarettes a day, loves high-fat food, and drinks "occasionally." He has been diagnosed with hypertension and is going to a traditional healer for "Russian" medicine and massage treatments. His allopathic physician has prescribed three medications for his cholesterol and hypertension.

1. How should Alexander's medical case manager approach the long-term nature of his hypertension?
2. How might the health-care professional utilize this couple's sense of family to improve health outcomes?
3. What interventions might improve medication adherence and health-care utilization for Alexander?
4. What specific food choices would you expect from Sasha? How might these food choices be altered in a culturally congruent manner?

HEALTH-SEEKING BELIEFS AND BEHAVIORS

Among Russian immigrants, health is defined as the absence of disease. They feel alienated from the American health-care system and, therefore, may fail to seek the health care needed. Older Russian immigrants do not adhere well to preventive health practices (Benisovich & King, 2003).

Homeopathic and traditional herbal remedies, however, are used and valued by Russian immigrants. Russians historically have known and implemented homeopathic remedies for centuries, and often, as in Russia, these remedies are used simultaneously with those of Western medical science. Russians, and especially Russian older people, may use herbal teas, tinctures, (Yehieli et al., 2005), mud baths, massage (with and without oils), saunas, and other alternative medicines and healing practices. Russians want to know the cause of their health problems and will expect their health-care providers to holistically diagnose the etiology of any health concerns. Many believe that Western medicine places too much emphasis on medications and laboratory results and not enough on clinical diagnosis and holistic care.

Many Russian immigrants believe that ill health may be the direct result of family and economic stress.

Although they avoid being chilled and seek warmth when ill, they firmly believe in the value of fresh air, sunlight, and good nutritious food.

Although Russian immigrants believe in the value of good food, some have a very different view of obesity when compared with the dominant U.S. culture. Stevens et al. (1997) compared attitudes and behaviors related to body size and other parameters among black, white, and Russian adolescents. Russian teen girls were found to be less likely than black and white adolescent girls to identify obese and overweight status as a concern.

RESPONSIBILITY FOR HEALTH CARE

Regardless of age, most Russians take an active role in their health and health care, and using alternative and homeopathic remedies; they commit to self-care. Russian immigrants may even bring health kits with them to the clinics and hospitals. Health kits contain a variety of remedies for the treatment of indigestion, headache, and infection (Yehieli et al., 2005). These medicines are available for direct purchase at Russian pharmacies.

During focused interviews with Russian immigrants, Ivanov and Buck (2002) learned that these women believed the physician to be responsible for any and all preventive information and referrals. The expectation is that they would be told exactly what to do and how to do it to get or stay well.

FOLK AND TRADITIONAL PRACTICES

Russian immigrants may implement the treatment called "cupping," a technique whereby the inside of a glass "cup," a *bonzuk*, is heated and then placed on a person's back, shoulder, or chest in order to remove sickness and evil. Cupping practices are especially popular when patients have respiratory problems such as bronchitis and asthma. In Russia, physicians and nurses go to patients' homes to perform cupping. In addition to cupping, home and folklore illness remedies include rubbing of oils and ointments, enemas, saunas and whirlpools, mineral water (for soaking as well as drinking), herbal teas, hot and cold soups, liquors, and mud plasters (Bistrevsky, 2005).

BARRIERS TO HEALTH CARE

Awareness and Attitudes

Respect and trust focused on health-care professionals must be earned. Russians do not appreciate being spoken to with disrespect, and they expect their health-care providers to look and act professional. Russian immigrants also expect health-care professionals to respect the self-treatments they have used prior to seeking medical care. Russians are also very involved with the care of their family members, most particularly children, and will not appreciate the patient-only individual approach of some providers. Owing to social and political sanctions against psychiatric illness in Russia, Russian immigrants may also be reluctant to disclose mental health issues and family histories of mental disorders. Therefore, providers need to approach the subject carefully and with full assurances of confidentiality.

In addition, Russians are unaccustomed to the concept of "gatekeeper." They want direct access to the health-care specialist of their choice, and when this is not possible, they believe the additional step to be expensive, wasteful, and unhealthy. Recent Russian immigrants may also be unfamiliar with concepts such as defensive health care and medical malpractice.

Affordability

In the former Soviet Union, health care was free. Therefore, concepts of private pay, co-pay, and insurance premiums are difficult to understand. Russian immigrants need help and support in their efforts to comprehend U.S. health-care systems, including Medicaid and Medicare programs. During Ivanov and Buck's (2002) focus interviews with Russian immigrants, they learned that although most of the interviewees had some form of health insurance, they still believed that health-care costs were a major health-care barrier and, therefore, preferred to use home remedies and Russian-made medications. Russian participants mentioned that after paying for food and other household essentials, little or no money was left for medicines and physician services.

About 85 percent of Russian immigrants carry some kind of health insurance coverage including employer-based private insurance as well as government plans such as Medicaid, Medicare, and Tri-Care (military) (Ethnic population, 2003). Even so, health care is perceived as far too expensive. An additional confusion may be that Russians are egalitarian and believe in an equal distribution of health-care benefits (Culture tips, 2000).

Language Proficiency

Although English-competent family members agree to step in as interpreters, the use of relatives for interpretive services is ill advised. Russian immigrants strongly prefer Russian-speaking health-care professionals and will actively look for them. Unfortunately, many Russian-trained physicians and nurses are not appropriately credentialed in the United States, yet they choose to diagnose and treat without licensure, using medications and treatments sent from Russia.

Related to language is also lack of relevant health-care information, which has also been identified as a barrier (Shpilko, 2006). Not surprisingly, Russians with only limited English proficiency report feeling isolated and alone and experience greater morbidity and mortality.

Accessibility

When Benisovich and King (2003) asked older Russian immigrants about health-care barriers, they stated that health care needed to be convenient and transportation to and from their appointments needed to be provided for them. Transportation is also perceived as being too expensive.

CULTURAL RESPONSES TO HEALTH AND ILLNESS

In a study of Russian children and the prevalence of mental health disorders as measured with reliable and valid assessment tools, Goodman, Slobodskaya, and Knyazev (2005) found that psychiatric disorders were nearly 70 percent higher in this population compared with those in Great Britain. The two most common categories were emotional and behavioral disorders. The most predictive factors in this study were the child's school performance, the mother's mental health, a close relative with alcohol addiction, and the witnessing of domestic violence. Obviously, Russian children are at risk.

Long-term case management may be a difficult concept for Russian immigrants. Russians are unaccustomed to the role of primary-care providers in the United States and may have an unrealistic, cure-oriented expectation of U.S. health-care professionals.

When one physician is unable to meet the Russian immigrant's expectations, it is likely the patient will seek the services of others. Prescribed treatments may not be disclosed to other care providers, and therefore, concerns over polypharmacy may surface (Aroian, 2003). Furthermore, Russians are accustomed to health-care professionals placing a greater emphasis on treatment than prevention. Being familiar with long in-patient hospitalizations, Russian immigrants are quite dismayed by the very short hospital stays in the United States.

BLOOD TRANSFUSION AND ORGAN DONATION

Requests for organ donations are usually declined (University of Washington Medical Center, 2005). Most Russians believe that the human body is sacred and are thus reluctant to allow organ donations and autopsies (Hobbs, 2002). Owing to contaminated blood supplies in Russia and the former Soviet Union, health-care professionals may have a difficult time convincing Russian immigrants to consent to giving or receiving human blood products.

Health-Care Practitioners

TRADITIONAL VERSUS BIOMEDICAL CARE

In Russia, the majority of physicians are female. However, male physicians are more likely to hold positions of authority. Therefore, Russian women generally do not hold preference regarding the physician's gender but believe male physicians to be more skilled and competent. For women, this lack of gender bias seems to also hold true for other health-care professionals (Ivanov & Buck, 2002).

STATUS OF HEALTH-CARE PROVIDERS

Of all health-care professionals, physicians are considered to be the most knowledgeable and "in charge" of any health teaching or service. In Russia, for every 1000 people, there are 4.25 physicians, 0.32 dentists, and 8 nurses. When comparing these numbers with the United States (2.56,

1.63, and 9.37, respectively) (WHO, 2006), Russian immigrants may perceive U.S. health-care professionals as being far less accessible. Russian traditional healers are afforded respect by Russian immigrants using their services.

Importantly, the Russian American Medical Association (RAMA) and the Russian American Dental Association have been established. RAMA was founded in 2002 and is based in Willoughby, Ohio. Dr. Nikolay Vasilyev is editor-in-chief of their peer-reviewed journal. They also have a website with information relevant to all Russian-speaking health-care professionals. For example, their website contains a link with an important description of all levels of nursing in the United States. The site also contains links for members, programs, RAMA Journal, job search, practice, and students/residents (RAMA, 2007).

REFERENCES

Alaniz, J. (2001, September 11). Crossing cultures: Russian nurses navigate the unfamiliar US health care system, finding career advantages and obstacles. *NurseWeek*. Retrieved January 28, 2007, from www.nurseweek.com/news/features/01-09/cultures_print.html

Allied Media Corp. (2006). Television for Russian Americans RTVI. (Author). *Multicultural communication*. Retrieved January 21, 2007, from www.allied-media.com/RussianMarket/rtvi.htm

Aroian, K. J. (2003). Russians (former Soviets). In P. St. Hill, J. Lipson, & A. I. Meleis, (Eds.), *Caring for women cross-culturally* (pp. 249–263). Philadelphia: F. A. Davis.

Benisovich, S. V., & King, A. C. (2003). Meaning and knowledge of health among older adult immigrants from Russia: A phenomenological study. *Health Education Research, 18*(2), 135–144.

Bergelson, M. B. (2003). *Russian cultural values and workplace communication. III International RCA Conference–2006 "communication and (re) making social worlds."* Retrieved January 28, 2007, from www.russ-comm.ru/eng/rca_biblio/b/bergelson03_eng.shtml

Birch, D. (2006, August 27). In Russia, the truth is optional [Electronic version]. *The Baltimore Sun*, opinion section.

Bistrevsky, T. (2005, Summer). Insight into Spokane's Russian families. *ABCD and ABCDE Newsletter*. Spokane Regional Health District. Retrieved January 28, 2007, from www.SRHD.org

CIA. (2006). *World FactBook: Russia*. Retrieved April 12, 2007, from www.cia.gov/cia/publications/factbook/geos/rs.html

Culture tips: Understanding the Russian culture and individual. (2000). *Cross Cultural Connection, 5*(4), 3–4.

Dubrova, Y. E., Kurbatova, O. L., Kholod, O. N., & Prokhorovskaya, V. D. (1995). Secular growth trend in two generations of the Russian population. *Human Biology, 67*(5), 755–767.

Energy Information Administration [EIA]. (2004, May). *Russia: Environmental issues*. Retrieved June 25, 2006, from www.eia.doe.gov/emeu/cabs/russenv.html

Ethnic Population. (2003, July 30). *Russian market in USA*. Retrieved January 21, 2007, from www.inforeklama.com/market.htm

Gabriel, R. (2005, March). A commentary on pharmacogenomics: What can it do? *Medical Laboratory Observer*. Nelson Publishing/Gale Group. Retrieved January 28, 2007, from http://findarticles.com/p/articles/

Gaikovich, E. A. (2003, July 14). *Genotyping of the polymorphic drug metabolizing enzymes cytochrome P450 2D6 and 1A1, and N-acetyltransferase 2 in a Russian sample*. Dissertation, Humbolt University, Berlin, Germany. Retrieved January 28, 2007 from http://edoc.hu-berlin.de/dissertationen/gaikovitch-elena-a-2003

Goodman, R., Slobodskaya, H., & Knyazev, G. (2005). Russian child mental health: A cross-sectional study of prevalence and risk factors. *European Child and Adolescent Psychiatry, 14*, 28–33.

Hasin, D., Aharonovich, E., Liu, X., Mamman, Z., Matseoane, K., Carr, L., & Li, T-K. (2002). Alcohol and ADH2 in Israel: Ashkenazis, Sephardics, and recent Russian immigrants. *American Journal of Psychiatry, 159*(8), 1432–1434.

Hobbs, R. (2002, July 16). *Knowledge of immigrant nationalities: Russia*. Retrieved January 22, 2007, from www.immigrantinfo.org/kin/russia.htm

Ivanov, L. L., & Buck, K. (2002). Health care utilization patterns of Russian-speaking immigrant women across age groups. *Journal of Immigrant Health, 4*(1), 17–27.

Jeltova, I., Fish, M. C., & Revenson, T. A. (2005). Risky sexual behaviors in immigrant adolescent girls from the former Soviet Union: Role of natal and host culture. *Journal of School Psychology, 43*(1), 3–22.

Keefe, S. (2006, August 21). Russian-speaking home care nurses help bridge language and cultural barriers among Brooklyn's Russian immigrants. *ADVANCE* Newsmagazines: Merion Publications. Retrieved January 22, 2007, from http://nursing.advanceweb.com/common/editorial

Library of Congress. (2005, August). *Country profile: Russia.* Library of Congress—Federal Research Division, Library of Congress call number: DK510.23.R883 1998. Retrieved June 24, 2006, from http://memory.loc.gov/frd/cs/rutoc.html

Marquez, P. V. (2005). *Dying too young: Addressing premature mortality and ill health due to non-communicable diseases and injuries in the Russian Federation.* Washington, DC: World Bank.

Mehler, P. S., Scott, J. Y., Pines, I., Gifford, N., Biggerstaff, S., & Hiatt, W. R. (2001). Russian immigrant cardiovascular risk assessment. *Journal of Health Care for the Poor and Underserved, 12*(2), 224–235.

Minnesota Department of Employment and Economic Development [MDEED]. (2006). *Russian immigrants in Minnesota.* Minnesota State Services for the Blind. Retrieved January 21, 2007, from www.mnssb.org/rcb/moc/russian.htm

Nemtsov, A. (2005). Russia: Alcohol yesterday and today. *Addiction, 100,* 146–149.

News about gay Russia. (N.D.). Retrieved January 31, 2007, from http://russia.bi.org/news.html

Nicholson, A., Bobak, M., Murphy, M., Rose, R., & Marmot, M. (2005). Alcohol consumption and increased mortality in Russian men and women: A cohort study based on the mortality of relatives. *Bulletin of the World Health Organization, 83*(11), 812–819.

Norman, C. (1996). Breaking bad news: Consultations with ethnic communities. *Australian Family Physician, 25*(10), 1583–1587.

OANDA Corporation. (2007). *FXConverter results: Currency converter for 164 currencies.* US dollar to Russian ruble. Retrieved January 21, 2007, from www.oanda.com/convert/classic

Parfitt, T. (2006). Campaigners fight to bring down Russia's tobacco toll. *The Lancet, 368,* 633–634.

Rendaxa Software. (2007). *Study Russian and the Russian language history!* HomeWorkLang. Retrieved January 28, 2007, from www.homeworklang.com/russian-language-history.htm

Rennert, G., Luz, N., Tamir, A., & Peterburg, Y. (2002). Chronic disease prevalence in immigrants to Israel from the former USSR. *Journal of Immigrant Health, 4*(1), 29–33.

Russian American Medical Association [RAMA]. (2007). Retrieved January 29, 2007, from www.russiandoctors.org/

Russians who. (2005). *Russian Life, 48*(5), 10.

Shpilko, I. (2006). Russian-American health care: Bridging the communication gap between physicians and patients. *Patient Education and Counseling, 64,* 331–341.

Smith, L. S. (1996). New Russian immigrants: Health problems, practices, and values. *Journal of Cultural Diversity, 3*(3), 68–73.

Stevens, J., Alexandrov, A. A., Smirnova, S. G., Deev, A. D., Gershunskaya, Y. B., Davis, C. E., & Thomas, R. (1997). Comparison of attitudes and behaviors related to nutrition, body size, dieting, and hunger in Russian, black-American, and white-American adolescents. *Obesity Research, 5,* 227–236.

Tran, T. V., Khatutsky, G., Aroian, K., Balsam, A., & Conway, K. (2000). Living arrangements, depression, and health status among elderly Russian-speaking immigrants. *Journal of Gerontological Social Work, 33*(2), 63–77.

U.S. Bureau of the Census. (2000). *Fact sheet: United States. Census 2000 demographic profile highlights: Selected population group: Russian* (pp. 148–151). Summary file 4(SF4). Retrieved June 25, 2006, from http://factfinder.census.gov

U.S. Bureau of the Census. (2003). *Language use and English-speaking ability: 2000. Census 2000 brief. Table 1: 20 Languages most frequently spoken at home by English ability for the population 5 years and over: 1990–2000.* Washington, DC: U.S. Department of Commerce, Economics and Statistics Administration, U.S. Bureau of the Census.

U.S. Department of Homeland Security. (2005a). *Supplemental Table 2: Legal permanent resident flow by leading core-based statistical areas (CBSAs) of residence and region and country of birth: Fiscal year 2005.* Retrieved June 25, 2006, from www.uscis.gov/graphics/shared/statistics/yearbook/LPRO5.htm

U.S. Department of Homeland Security. (2005b). *Table 3: Legal permanent resident flow by region and country of birth: Fiscal years 1995 to 2005.* Retrieved June 25, 2006, from www.uscis.gov/graphics/shared/statistics/yearbook/LPRO5.htm

U.S. Department of Homeland Security. (2005c). *Table 12: Immigrant orphans adopted by US citizens by gender, age, and region and country of birth: Fiscal year 2005.* Retrieved June 25, 2006, from www.uscis.gov/graphics/shared/statistics/yearbook/LPRO5.htm

University of Michigan Health System. (2007). *Cultural competency.* Patient Education. Ann Arbor. Retrieved January 28, 2007, from www.med.umich.edu/pteducation/cultcomm2.htm

University of Washington Medical Center. (2005, April). *Communicating with your Russian patient.* Culture clues: Staff Development Workgroup, Patient and Family Education Committee. Seattle. Retrieved July 26, 2006, from http://depts.washington.edu/pfes/cultureclues. html

Vadlamani, A., Maher, J. F., Shaete, M., Smirnoff, A., Cameron, D. G., Winkelmann, J. C., & Goldberg, S. J. (2001). Colorectal cancer in Russian-speaking Jewish émigrés: Community-based screening. *American Journal of Gastroenterology, 96*(9), 2755–2760.

Wikipedia, The Free Encyclopedia. (2006, May). *Economy of Russia.* Wikimedia Foundation, Inc. Retrieved June 24, 2006, from http://en.wikipedia.org/wiki/Economy_of_Russia

Wikipedia, The Free Encyclopedia. (2007, January 26). *Russian language.* Wikimedia Foundation, Inc. Retrieved January 28, 2007, from http://en.wikipedia.org/wiki/Russian_language

World Health Organization [WHO]. (2005, January 14). *Country profile.* WHO Regional Office for Europe. Retrieved January 16, 2005, from http://hfadb.who.dk/HFA

World Health Organization [WHO]. (2006). *Health workers: A global profile. The world health report 2006: Working together for health.* Annex table 4, pp. 197–199. Retrieved September 26, 2007, from http://www.who.int/whr/2006/en/

Yehieli, M., Lutz, G., & Grey, M. (Eds.). (2005, November). Russians and other immigrants from the former Soviet Union. *Health disparity factsheets.* Cedar Falls, IA: Center for Health Disparities, University of Northern Iowa.

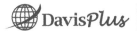 **DavisPlus**

For case studies, review questions, and additional information, go to http://davisplus.fadavis.com

Chapter *20*

People of Polish Heritage

HENRY M. PLAWECKI, LAWRENCE H. PLAWECKI,
JUDITH A. PLAWECKI, and MARTIN H. PLAWECKI

Overview, Inhabited Localities, and Topography

OVERVIEW

Over 9 million people in the United States and 800,000 people in Canada* identify their ancestry as Polish (Statistics Canada, 2001; U.S. Bureau of the Census, 2004). **Poland**, officially the *Republic of Poland*, occupies 312,683 square kilometers, or roughly 120,727 square miles. Poland is approximately the size of New Mexico (121,599 square miles) (New Mexico Tourism Department, 2006). Poland has its capital in Warsaw. Located in Central Europe, Poland, with a population of about 38,111,000 in 2003, was the eighth largest country in Europe, accounting for 5.3 percent of the entire European population (Republic of Poland, 2003). In 2001, females were 51.4 percent of Poland's total population and males were 48.6 percent. Consequently, there were 106 women for every 100 men in Poland. There were more females than males in both its urban and its rural populations; however, the disporportion of females to males was larger in the towns. Women accounted for over 52 percent of the urban population, and nearly 48 percent were men. Thus, there were about 110 women for every 100 men in the urban areas. In the rural areas, 50.1 percent were female and 49.9 percent male, reflecting 100.4 women for every 100 men (Republic of Poland, 2002f). The life expectancy in Poland has been increasing. By 2025, the life expectancy is projected to continue to increase for men from 69 to 74 years and for women from 78 to 81 years. The average Pole is nearly 35 years of age—37 years for women and 33 years for men. Over 56 percent of

Poles are below the age of 40, 27 percent are between 40 and 59 years of age, nearly 17 percent are above 60, and 2 percent are 80 or above (Republic of Poland, 2002a).

Poland shares its western border with Germany. To the south, Poland is bordered by Slovakia and the Czech Republic. Ukraine, Belarus, Lithuania, and Russia all share eastern and northeastern borders with Poland. The Baltic Sea borders the majority of the northernmost part of the country. Poland is a relatively low-lying country, with nearly 92 percent of its land mass situated at an altitude of less than 300 meters below sea level (Republic of Poland, 2002h). Most of the country is a plain without any natural boundaries except the Carpathian Mountains in the south and the Oder and Neisse rivers in the west (Republic of Poland, 2002b).

The year A.D. 966 marks Poland's origin as an independent, Christian, centralized state. Over the centuries, Poland survived a difficult and tumultous history of frequent invasions, division, and rule by others. Through a series of agreements made between 1772 and 1795, Russia, Prussia, and Austria partitioned Poland among themselves. From 1795 to 1918, Poland ceased to exist as an independent country and its land was divided among Prussia, Russia, and Austria (Library of Congress, 1992a; Republic of Poland, 2002c). The nonexistence of Poland and its re-emergence after 120 years demonstrated the Polish people's strong ties to its culture, language, and religion. Throughout this period, the people's tenacity, determination, and dedication to the Catholic Church played a significant role in enabling the Poles to maintain their language, culture, and heritage. After World War I (WW I), between 1920 and early 1939, Poland once again existed as a separate, self-governing country (Library of

Congress, 1992b). In 1939, Hitler's Nazi forces invaded Poland. Displaying fierce patriotism, courage, and determination to resist another occupation, Poland was the only country to combat Germany from the first day of the Nazi invasion until the end of the war in Europe (Library of Congress, 1992c). Between the 1939 Nazi invasion and the end of World War II (WW II) in 1945, nearly six million Poles, over 15 percent of Poland's total population, perished. This number included many Polish Jews who were exterminated by the Nazis in the Holocaust, prisoners killed in concentration or forced labor camps, soldiers, and civilians (Library of Congress, 1992d). After WW II, Stalin, Churchill, and Roosevelt determined Poland's future borders at the Peace Conferences in Yalta and Potsdam. The decisions made at these conferences resulted in Poland losing 10,000 square miles to the east and 50,000 square miles to the west. In total, Poland lost some 20 percent of its pre–WW II territory (Republic of Poland, 2002e). However, it did remain a separate, identifiable country, although it became a satellite of the United Soviet Socialist Republic (USSR).

In 1947, elections officially brought the Communist Party to power. The Stalinist model was implemented until 1956. After Stalin's death, Polish Communism vacillated between repression and liberalization until about 1970. Poland's resistance to Communist rule began in 1970 with the emergence of Lech Walesa, the leader of a strike in the Gdansk shipyards. Walesa headed Solidarnosc (Solidarity), the first free trade union in Eastern Europe. *Solidarnosc* was created because of the Communists' violent repression of the workmen of Radom in 1976 and a second strike at the Gdansk shipyards in 1980, the result of the government's raising food prices (Centreurope.org, 2006).

In addition to the events cited previously, the 1978 election of the Polish Cardinal, Karol Wojtyla, as Pope John Paul II, led to unprecedented social and political changes in Poland. The 1980 emergence of Solidarity and the election of the Polish Pope rekindled a religious rebirth in the Poles, an increased sense of self, social identity, and the realization of their collective strength. Solidarity became a major social movement and phenomenon unheard of within the Soviet bloc's political system. Despite negotiations, confrontations, and ultimately, repressive military operations by the ruling Polish Communist Party, the Solidarity movement survived as its influential unofficial opposition. Ultimately, the Polish Communist Party recognized that the people's massive opposition reduced their ability to govern. In 1988, formal negotiations between the Polish Communist Party leaders and the unofficial opposition, called the *Round Table talks*, resulted in partially free Parlimentary elections. Solidarity won a landslide victory in the June 1989 elections. In July 1989, the newly elected Parliament changed the country's name and constitution, establishing the Third Republic of Poland and a democratic system of government (Republic of Poland, Ministry of Foreign Affairs, 2002g; von Geldern & Siegelbaum, 2003).

Polish immigrants and their descendants who immigrated to America for many generations have maintained their ethnic heritage by promoting their culture, attending Catholic churches, attending parades and festivals, maintaining ethnic food traditions, speaking the Polish language, and promoting interest in their home country through media events as well as economic and political channels. For newer immigrant Poles, maintaining ethnic heritage meant learning English and obtaining a good job (Erdmans, 1998). Newer immigrants are less concerned with raising consciousness over Polish American issues than they are with financially helping families who remained in Poland and raising concerns over the political and economic climate in their homeland.

HERITAGE AND RESIDENCE

The first contribution of the Poles to the development of American democracy occurred during the American Revolutionary War. Benjamin Franklin, an American statesman, went to Europe and recruited experienced Polish leaders and soldiers. Two prominent Poles recruited to assist the colonists in their fight for independence were Count Kazimierz (Casimir) Pulaski and Tadeusz Kosciusko. General Pulaski, a valiant cavalryman, led soldiers by courage and example. His many heroic actions on behalf of the colonists lead to naming him the *Father of the American Cavalry* (Polish American Center, 1997). In 1929, recognizing his contributions to the American Revolution, Congress designated October 11th as *Pulaski Day* and authorized the U.S. Postal Service to issue a commemorative stamp in his honor. General Kosciusko served the American Revolution as both an engineer and a field commander. Kosciusko developed the defenses used in the major battles at Saratoga and West Point, New York, and then organized the blockade of Charleston, South Carolina, which led to the end of the South's resistance. After the defeat of the British in 1784, Kosciusko was promoted to the rank of Brigadier General, given American citizenship, and presented the Cincinnati Order Medal by George Washington (Wilde, 2001). Both Pulaski and Kosciusko contributed significantly to the colonists' victory and were recognized as heroes of the new republic. Many American towns, counties, parks, and other memorials bear the names of these Polish heroes.

The Poles' dedication to the welfare of the United States was summarized by the motto of the first Polish American political club, the *Kosciuszko Club*, established in 1871, which states "A good Pole is a good American citizen" (Jarczak, N.D.). Immigrants, regardless of their country of origin, leave their homeland for a variety of reasons that include avoiding ethnic, religious, and political persecution; seeking a better lifestyle; and/or providing a means of support for family and relatives who remained in the homeland. Once in the United States, they may be incapable, unprepared, or unwilling to drastically change their homeland's culturally influenced patterns of behavior. Like any other group that perceives themselves as unaccepted, displaced, and different, the Polish immigrants established a geographically and socially segregated area called a **Polonia**, the medieval name for Poland. Polonia allowed members of the immigrant group to experience social comfort, speak their native language, and openly practice the customs of their homeland.

The initial migration of about 2000 Polish immigrants occurred between 1800 and 1860. This group consisted of intellectuals and nobles who were motivated by political insurrections. The first substantive Polish settlement in America was founded in 1854 by Father Leopold Moczygemba and 100 Polish immigrant families in Panna Maria, Texas (Panna Maria, 2006). Even though most Poles preferred living in agrarian communities, they gravitated to cities where work for laborers was plentiful.

Between the early 1800s and the beginning of WW II, over 5 million Polish immigrants came to the United States. Many of these immigrants perceived America only as a temporary home. This first major immigrant group was called *za chlebem* or "for-bread" immigrants. These immigrants came to earn money and then return to Poland. Polish immigration to America continues today. A new generation of immigrants recently freed from foreign domination are now coming to the United States seeking better lives (Library of Congress, 2004).

The predominant residence for Polish immigrants in the United States is north of Ohio and east of the Mississippi River. The states of New York, Illinois, Michigan, Pennsylvania, New Jersey, and Wisconsin have the largest numbers of self-reported Poles and Polish Americans (U.S. Bureau of the Census, 2004). However, Polish communities with retirees and new immigrants are growing in Florida, Texas, and California.

At the peak of Polish migration, Chicago was considered the most well-developed Polish community in the United States (Pacyga, 2004). The first Polish immigrants to Chicago were primarily nobles who fled Poland after the Polish-Russian war of 1830 to 1831. They came with plans of establishing a "New Poland" in Illinois (Pacyga, 2004). Chicago's Polish community grew rapidly after 1850. By the beginning of the Civil War, approximately 500 Poles had established a small enclave on Chicago's northwest side. Peter Kiolbassa, who served as a captain in the Sixth Colored Cavalry during the Civil War, emerged as a local leader. Kiolbassa organized the first Polish Society of St. Stanislaus Kostka in 1864. This organization prepared the community for the development of the city's first Polish Roman Catholic parish. Located along the north branch of the Chicago River, the residents of Polonia initally attended a German parish church. Facing hostility from some of the Germans, who discouraged their priest from ministering to the Polish religious needs, the Polish community established its own Roman Catholic parish, St. Stanislaus Kostka. The parish was central to the creation of Polonia, because the establishment of ethnic Catholic parishes provided the community with a stable institutional base and served as a status symbol for the new immigrant colony. St. Stanislaus Kostka parish became the first of approximately 60 Polish parishes in the Chicago archdiocese.

The traditional Polish community in Chicago, a highly organized ethnic settlement that developed after the Civil War, matured and reached almost-complete institutional self-sufficiency before WW I. This community published major Polish-language newspapers, established the foundation for a parochial school system, and provided a layer of ethnically based social service insititutions, such as St. Joseph's Home for the Aged, St. Hedwig's Orphanage, the Polish Welfare Association, and St. Adalbert Cemetery, as well as a well-developed business enterprise (Pacyga,

2004). In addition, a thriving Polish and Eastern European Jewish business community developed in these neighborhoods.

The Polish community's development allowed them to actively participate in the labor movement, which along with their involvement with fraternal groups, led to the development of neighborhood organizations. By 1980, Hispanics and African Americans had largely replaced Poles in the inner-city core neighborhoods. Polish Chicagoans left the old neighborhoods, moving to the suburbs. Chicago's Polonia played a crucial role in the political, religious, educational, business, institutional, and cultural life of Chicago. Pulaski Street, Solidarity Drive, the Copernicus Center, and a number of other landmarks bear Polish names symbolizing Chicago's Polish heritage (Pacyga, 2004).

More than one million Poles live in the Chicago metropolitean area, northwestern Indiana, and suburban Illinois. This number represents the largest Polish community outside of the home country; only Warsaw has a larger Polish community (Bolzen, 2006). The city of Chicago and its suburbs is home to more Polish immigrants and their extended families than any other city outside of Poland (USA Weekend.com, 2005).

Polonia was also the name given to Polish communities found in northeastern and midwestern cities after 1945 (Best, 2004). Members of these communities kept Polish nationalism alive by speaking their native language, preserving customs, and attending the local Catholic Church run by Polish clergy and the Felician Sisters. Because Poland was partitioned until 1919, Poles coming to America during the 1800s and early 1900s were unable to report Poland as their emigrating country, but they tenaciously worked to ensure the survival of the Polish culture. Over time, the 120-year partition of Poland and its absence from the world map significantly reduced the number of immigrants who could identify Poland as their emigrating country. Therefore, the partition ultimately led to an undercount of the actual number of Americans with Polish ancestry.

Polonias were very well organized. Establishing residence in a Polonia isolated the immigrants and allowed them to avoid dealing with unfamiliar written and spoken languages and different cultural perspectives. For many older Poles, the neighborhood is their community. Polonias, especially in urban ethnic communities, provide a sense of belonging, reduce alienation, and enhance the people's ability to solve problems and maintain the motivation to address modern-day frustrations. "The assumption of voluntary Americanization continues to exist in spite of the behaviors of past generations who resisted the assimilation process and have, in fact, reestablished their pre-immigration cultures in multiple voluntarily segregated ethnic enclaves/communities" (Plawecki, 2000, p. 7). Many Eastern European immigrants, such as the Poles, have the same demographic characteristics as the majority of Americans. As a consequence, their unique cultural perspectives have been ignored by both society and those responsible for providing health care. Immigrants from Eastern European cultures, including those from Poland, need to have their cultural beliefs, attitudes, and values considered if health-care providers are to provide sensitive, appropriate, and acceptable health care.

Culture has generally been defined as a socially transmitted behavior pattern that is based upon the acceptance of the beliefs, attitudes, language, and practices that are typical of a community of individuals at a given time. The geographic, economic, and social segregation of any ethnic or racial group reinforces the culturally influenced behavior patterns. Consequently, the segregated group develops communication styles, cultural beliefs, and interactive behaviors that are socially accepted within their community but are different than those expected by the general populace (Plawecki, 1992, p. 4).

The Polish immigrants established religious and voluntary organizations dedicated to the support of schools, organized trade, established banks, and initiated political and social activities designed to mirror those in Poland. Many of these Polish organizations still exist today and have used their influence to name monuments, statues, historical sites, major roadways, and bridges dedicated to Polish Americans and Polish nationals. These symbols of Poland's contribution to America can be found in many towns and cities settled by Polish immigrants.

Poles are a heterogeneous group. As such, they were slow to assimilate into multicultural America. Much of the variation within this ethnic group is due to the primary and secondary characteristics of culture (see Chapter 1).

Polish Americans were well represented in the WW II war effort of the United States. Significant numbers of Polish Americans, both native and immigrant, joined the U.S. military. Thousands of Polish Americans were killed defending America. Even after displaying that sense of duty, honor, and patriotism, Polish Americans often experienced discrimination during and after the war. Poles were passed over for jobs because they had difficulties speaking English and their names were difficult to pronounce or spell. As a reaction to this discrimination, name changes became common for upwardly mobile Polish Americans. The shortening and changing of names were intended to decrease discrimination and promote greater acceptability in the job market as well as increase social acceptance. Many Polish Americans still experience discrimination and ridicule through ethnic Polish jokes, which are similar in scope to those about Irish, Italian, and Mexican Americans. However, the attitudes toward the Poles have improved since the Solidarity movement in the 1970s and 1980s, the election and activities of Pope John Paul II (the first Polish pope and the first non-Italian pope since 1523), Poland's 1999 admission to the North Atlantic Treaty Organization (NATO), its 2004 entry into the European Union, and its leadership and involvement with the United States in Iraq as well as with Euro-Atlantic countries in antiterrorist activities (Republic of Poland, 2004).

VIGNETTE 20.1

Cylka and Marcin Majda, both 90-year-old first-generation Polish Americans, painstakingly decorate their home with symbols of Catholicism, patriotic statues, an American flag, and related memoriabilia on the 4th of July and September 11th. As the September 11th anniversary approached, Mrs. Majda asked her grandson, Larry, to accompany them to the memorial services at St. Adalbert's parish. Puzzled by his grandparents' activities related to September 11th, Larry asked them about their reasons for observing this anniversary. Mrs. Majda responded that her only brother, Anthony, died for this country when he was killed in World War II. She stated that when she was a little girl living in Chicago's Polonia, her parents taught her that she was "an American first, a Pole second, and a Catholic third."

Upon arrival at the Church, the choir was singing "God Bless America." The priest ordered the choir to stop singing "God Bless America." Although nothing was said at the time, Mr. and Mrs. Majda were furious.

1. Why did Mr. and Mrs. Majda become furious?
2. What cultural values are Mr. and Mrs. Majda demonstrating?
3. Why would the priest act in such a manner?
4. What priorities will determine the actions taken by the Majdas?

REASONS FOR MIGRATION AND ASSOCIATED ECONOMIC FACTORS

Polish immigration to the United States occurred in three major waves. The first wave of immigrants, arriving in the early 1800s through 1914, came to America primarily for economic, political, and religious reasons. Many immigrants were illiterate, peasants, or unskilled laborers (Grocholska, 1999). They took low-paying jobs and lived in crowded dwellings just to make a meager living.

The second major wave of immigration occurred after WW II. During the war, Poland lost over 6 million of its 35 million people (Brogan, 1990). Proportionally, Poland lost more people than any other nation during WW II. The country's infrastructure was devastated, resulting in unbearable living conditions in post–WW II Poland. The nearly complete destruction of Poland prompted the post–WW II wave of Polish immigrants to come to America. This group primarily included political prisoners, dissidents, and intellectuals from refugee camps all over Europe. These immigrants, who both were educated and had a basic knowledge of English, assimilated more easily into American culture than those from the first wave. They consciously separated from Polonia and aligned themselves with other middle-class and professional groups in America. The upwardly mobile and middle-class aspirations of this group differed from the working-class orientation of the first- and second-generation descendants of the first wave (Grocholska, 1999).

The current third wave of immigrants, often called the *Solidarity immigrants*, began arriving in 1978 (Grocholska, 1999). These Solidarity immigrants reflect the ideologies of the first two waves—that is, they want to work and to speak freely about political and intellectual issues. Two types of third-wave immigrants came to America. The first came to work without any initial interest in permanently relocating. They entered this country on a visitor's visa and left their families in Poland. These immigrants frequently lived in low-income housing, shared rooms with other immigrants, and worked hard to send money to their families in Poland. Networking with other Poles was their primary source of job contacts. They quickly took any job available, particularly as laborers, domestics, and unskilled farm workers. Because many of these immigrants were sending money to their families in Poland, they often overstayed their visitor visas. In 2006, illegal immigration became a serious political issue in the United States, attributed primarily to the vast number of illegal immigrants from Mexico. In addition to those individuals, it has been estimated that Polish immigrants account for a large segment (once estimated at the ninth largest) of illegal immigrants in the United States.

Immigrants save money on food by eating nutritionally inadequate diets and seek care only when a health problem becomes serious. Because many of these immigrants have been abused and taken advantage of by unscrupulous Poles and others, they distrust strangers, bureaucrats, and even health-care providers whom they fear may report them and, ultimately, cause their deportation. When Polish immigrants are deported, they must wait at least 7 years before they can apply for another visa to return to America.

The second type of third-wave Polish immigrants chose to come to America for political and economic reasons. This group typically consists of well-educated professionals and small-business owners. They consciously decided to leave Poland forever and bring their families with them. This group epitomizes the Polish characteristics of hard work, determination, and frugality. Although many in this group are underemployed, they actively use English and integrate into their new country, recognizing that this may be a necessary first step to assimilation.

Many second- and third-wave immigrants avoid Polish communities because they believe that American ethnic Polonias are different from those in Poland. The concerns and issues of political representation and discrimination of established immigrants living in America are irrelevant to this wave of immigrant Poles. In addition, many older Polonias are located in diverse, changing inner-city neighborhoods, and the upwardly mobile Polish Americans, like other successful groups, have begun to leave the cities for the suburbs.

EDUCATIONAL STATUS AND OCCUPATIONS

Educational priorities and their desire to assimilate into American culture vary widely among Polish immigrants. The educational status, socioeconomic levels, and cultural philosophy often depend upon the time frame when the family emigrated from Poland.

In 1999, Poland initiated a reform of the educational system designed to raise educational levels and adapt to current labor market requirements. Since 2002, at least 90 percent of the students have completed their upper secondary education. Only about 46 percent of those aged 25 to 64 have attained at least upper secondary education (Organization for Economic Cooperation and Development [OECD], 2005). In 2003, 99.8 percent of the total population aged 15 and over was able to read and write (CIA, 2006).

Until Poland's decision to reform education in 1999, most Poles generally had limited education. In the mid-1990s, nearly 34 percent of the Polish population had completed only primary education, whereas almost 7 percent had either incomplete or no primary education. In addition, slightly over 50 percent of the Poles completed secondary education, whereas fewer than 10 percent attained post-secondary or higher education (Republic of Poland, 2002d). Since 2002, following the educational reform, at least 90 percent of Poland's younger generation has completed upper secondary education.

Until the 1950s and 1960s, many Polish families were slow to recognize the value of education for their children. Before WW II, most Polish children went to Catholic schools, where they learned about their culture, its language, and Catholicism. After WW II, parents felt an acute responsibility to have their children learn English. Subsequently, the Polish language was eliminated from the curriculum of many schools, and its use was restricted to the home.

For first-wave immigrants, work was more important than education. The value of hard work and material goods was easily understood. Illiterate first-wave Poles initially had difficulty with unionized labor; however, once they understood what was at stake, they became staunch union supporters. A family's "union" loyalty influenced many children to follow in their fathers' footsteps by working in similar jobs. They worked in meat-packing houses in Chicago, steel mills and oil refineries in northwestern Indiana, assembly lines in Detroit, and coal mines in Pennsylvania. Because young Poles followed in their parents' occupational footsteps, upward mobility was slower for Poles than for some other ethnic minorities (Lopata, 1994).

The second wave of Polish immigrants placed a high value on education and culture. Educated, cultured Poles were expected to read widely and speak several languages. Cultured Poles have great pride and respect for Poland's most famous people, such as composer Frederic Chopin, two-time Nobel laureate scientist Marie Curie, novelist Joseph Conrad, astronomer Nicolaus Copernicus, and Karol Wojtyla, better known as Pope John Paul II. Poles are known for epic works in prose and poetry. Major themes in Polish literature are nationality, freedom, exile, and oppression.

In the 1950s, the Polish communities in America had a renewed interest in scholarly and cultural endeavors. The Polish Institute of Arts and Sciences began publishing *The Polish Review*, a scholarly journal, devoted to the works of Polish scholars. The Kosciusko Foundation encourages cultural exchanges between Poland and America and provides scholarships to Polish American students. Once the Polish community recognized the value of education for their children, Poles became one of the highest represented ethnic groups in institutions of higher learning. "The proportion of young people who finished college was more than double that of older Polish Americans, and the proportion of young people who attended college was at least triple" (Lopata, 1994, p. 149).

After WW II, many Polish Catholics were blue-collar workers who perceived hard work as honorable. Many feared that education and its resultant mobility were a threat to their family, religious, and community life. For women, education was seen as even less necessary because of the value placed upon their staying at home and raising their children. Television helped change the character of ethnic communities forever as it brought the outside world into both the community and the home. The descendants of immigrants who did go to college valued obedience and self-control, respected authority, and exhibited determination (Bukowczyk, 1987). Young Poles tend to study and work, become preoccupied with their careers, run their own businesses, and appear to increasingly postpone marriage and starting families (Republic of Poland, 2002a).

Communication

DOMINANT LANGUAGE AND DIALECTS

The Polish language was influenced by the countries surrounding Poland and by the Latin of 11th- and 12th-century kings. Depending on the regional and cultural background of the speaker, Polish may sound German, Russian, or French. The Polish language has a lyrical quality that is pleasant to the ear, even if one has difficulty understanding the words. Poles are an animated group, and facial expressions generally convey the tone of the conversation.

The dominant language of people living in Poland is **Polish**, although there are some regional dialects and differences. Generally, most Polish-speaking people can communicate with one another. Recently, a resurgence of interest in learning to speak the Polish language has occurred among Polish Americans. Both adults and children are learning Polish in church-affiliated language schools, cultural centers, and colleges. Polish radio stations help keep an ongoing interest in the language, music, and culture.

CULTURAL COMMUNICATION PATTERNS

Poles use touch as a form of personal expression of caring. Touch is common among family members and friends, but Poles may be quite formal with strangers and health-care providers. Handshaking is considered polite. In fact, failing to shake hands with everyone present may be considered rude. Most Poles feel comfortable with close personal space, but distances increase when interacting with strangers.

First-generation Poles and other people from Eastern European countries commonly kiss "Polish style," that is, once on each cheek and then once again. For Poles, kissing the hand is considered appropriate if the woman extends it. Two women may walk together arm in arm, or two men may greet each other with an embrace, a hug, and a kiss on both cheeks.

To Poles, love is expressed through covert actions and displayed easily in the form of tenderness to children. However, loving phrases are uncommon among adult Polish Americans. Poles praise each others' deeds and good work, but they may be reluctant to acknowledge how they feel about one another. These behavioral variations may have persevered through generations of assimilated Poles.

Acknowledging the hostess is important when Poles visit each other's homes; bringing flowers or candy is always in good taste. Normally, guests are discouraged from assisting the hostess in the kitchen or with cleanup after meals. After the event, thank-you letters and greeting cards should be sent to demonstrate an appreciation for the host's hospitality.

Many Polish Americans consider the use of spoken second-person familiarity rude. Polish people speak in the third person. For example, they might ask, "Would Martin like some coffee?" rather than "Would you like some coffee?" Although the first expression might sound awkward, the latter expression may be considered impolite and too informal, especially if the person being asked is older.

A health-care provider is *Pani Doktor*, literally translated as "Lady Doctor" instead of "Doctor." Many Polish names are difficult to pronounce. Even though a name may be mispronounced, a high value is placed on the attempt to pronounce it correctly.

When interacting with others, Poles consider age, gender, and title. For example, when a group is walking through a door, an unspoken hierarchy requires the person of lower standing to hold the door for a woman or those of a higher title. To many Americans, this behavior may seem excessive, but for Poles, it shows respect and courtesy. Polish Americans also use direct eye contact when interacting with others. Many Americans may feel uncomfortable with this sustained eye contact and feel it is quite close to staring, but to Poles, it is considered ordinary.

Most Poles enjoy a robust conversation and have a keen sense of humor. Polish humor sometimes has an openness and bawdiness that may be unnerving to those unaccustomed to it. Cultural nuances may make it difficult to understand the underlying meaning of some transactions or exchanges. Because Poles in Poland have been censored for centuries, they have raised satire and political savvy to an art form.

Poles, as a group, tend to share thoughts and ideas freely, particularly as part of their hospitality. A guest in a Polish home is warmly welcomed and may be overwhelmed by the outpouring of generosity. Americans talk of sports while Poles speak of their personal life, their jobs, families, spouse, aspirations, and misfortunes.

TEMPORAL RELATIONSHIPS

Punctuality is important to Polish Americans. To be late is a sign of bad manners. Depending upon the status of the person for whom they are waiting, Poles may be intolerant of lateness. Even in social situations, people are expected to arrive on time and stay late.

Polish Americans are both past and future oriented. The past is very much a part of Polish culture, with the families passing on their memories of WW II, which still haunt them in some way. A strong work ethic encourages Poles to plan for the future. Polish parents very much want their children to have a better life than the one they have experienced.

FORMAT FOR NAMES

Many Polish peasants did not have surnames until the 1600s. The use of surnames appeared in the first half of the 18th century. After 1850, the practice of creating surnames had ended.

Traditional Polish names are often a description of a person (e.g., John Wysocki, meaning "John the tailor"), a profession (e.g., the surname Recznik, meaning "butcher"), a place (e.g., Sokolowski, meaning "one came from a town named Sokoly or Sokolka"), or even a thing. Many factors caused this rather logical process to become somewhat confusing. Historical, linguistic, and political factors also directly affected the structure of Polish surnames. First of all, the partition of Poland for almost 120 years made it impossible for any emigrant at that time to claim Poland as their homeland. Consequently, names may have been "adjusted" to sound more like those of the dominant ethnic group (e.g., Russian, Prussian, or Austrian) controlling that part of Poland at the time. Second, changes in surnames may have been made during the country's record-keeping process or during the immigration processing on Ellis Island. The transfer of information from emigrant to official records was highly dependent on the pronunciation, spelling, and writing skills of both the recorder and the applicant (Generations Network, 2007).

Some examples of common Polish names include *Kowal* meaning "blacksmith." Numerous suffixes, such as "icz," "czyk," "iak," and "czak," which mean "son of," can be added. One of the most common suffixes is "ski," which originally was added to many names because it was associated with nobility. Over time, it was retranslated to mean "son of." The suffix "cki" became the phonetic version of "ski." Surnames ending in "y," "ow," "owo," and "owa" are usually derived from names of places. The "ak" suffix is typical of western Poland, whereas "uk" is found in the east.

Family Roles and Organization

HEAD OF HOUSEHOLD AND GENDER ROLES

Life in the Polish culture centers on family. Each family member has a certain position, role, and related responsibilities. All members are expected to work, make contributions, and strive to enhance the entire family's reputation and social and economic position. Individual concerns and personal fulfillment are afforded little consideration, and sacrifices for the betterment of the family are expected. The family structure is interwoven with strong beliefs and traditions. In the United States, the Polish family has maintained itself as a strong economic unit.

In most Polish families, the father is perceived as the head of the household. Depending on the degree of assimilation, the father may rule with absolute authority in first-, second-, and even third-generation Polish American families. Depending on circumstances, only the Church may have greater authority than the father. For example, if a child wants to leave home and attend college, the priest may help in convincing the family that it is an appropriate thing to do. However, among some third- and fourth-generation Polish Americans and second- and third-wave immigrants, more-egalitarian gender roles are becoming the norm. In addition, the father, as head of the house, worked as many hours a day in a mine or a factory as was permitted. He assumed responsibility of finding jobs for both offspring and newly immigrated friends and relatives.

Historically, large families were expected and commonplace among Poles. Polish women who followed the Church's teachings had many children, often experiencing between 5 and 10 pregnancies. Although women were pregnant a good deal of their early married lives, the wife began the workday well before dawn, and her responsibilities included cooking, caring for the children, laundering the clothes, and cleaning the house. If necessary, the wife also worked outside the home for additional income. Although the husband was the final authority in most matters, it was the woman who ran the house, disciplined the children, and cared for elderly family members.

In the early 1990s, Polish women married at the age of 22, whereas in the mid-1990s, the age of marriage was closer to 23, and in 2002, it was 24. Currently, most women become mothers between the ages of 25 and 29, whereas in the early 1990s, motherhood came between 20 and 24. The better the women are educated, the more frequently they postpone having children until their late 20s. The number of unmarried women is also increasing. Unmarried women represent about 20 percent of the population, as compared with 5 percent in the early 1990s. Although the most common family model found remains 2 + 2 (2 parents and 2 children), it is becoming increasingly common for couples to have only one child (Republic of Poland, 2002a).

In 2001, Szaflarski used the data from the 1994 Polish General Social Survey to estimate the structural and psychosocial effects on self-reported health, risk behaviors, and social participation between the genders. Employment status was identified as improving the health of men, whereas marital happiness increased the probability of better health for women. Marital status was identified to influence social interactions. Married women were found to socialize less than unmarried women, whereas marital status had no effect on men's socialization. Smoking was found to decline with the educational level among men but not among women, whereas excessive drinking increased for unhappily married men. Religiosity was determined to enhance and protect the health of both men and women (Szaflarski, 2001).

PRESCRIPTIVE, RESTRICTIVE, AND TABOO BEHAVIORS FOR CHILDREN AND ADOLESCENTS

The most valued behavior for Polish American children is obedience. Taboo child behaviors include anything that undermines parental authority. Parents are quite demonstrative with young children, but they resist showing much affection toward them once they are older than toddler age. This is the parents' way of teaching children to be strong and resilient. Many parents praise children for self-control and completing chores. Little sympathy is wasted on failure, but doing well is openly praised. Children are taught to resist feelings of helplessness, fragility, or dependence.

FAMILY GOALS AND PRIORITIES

Traditional family values and loyalty are strong in most Polish households. Children are valued in the Polish American family. For many first-wave immigrants, marriage is an institution of respect and economic solidarity and may not necessarily include romance. In the past, husbands owed their wives loyalty, fidelity, and financial support; whereas wives owed their husbands fidelity and obedience. Children owed their parents emotional and financial support before and after marriage. An important family priority for many is to maintain the honor of the family in the larger society, have a good job, and be a good Catholic.

The elderly are highly respected in most Polish families. They attend church regularly and carry on Polish traditions. The Polish ethic of contributing to the family and enhancing its status extends to the aged as well. The elderly play an active role in helping grandchildren learn Polish customs and in assisting adult children in their daily routine with families. For some families, one of the worst disgraces, as seen through the eyes of the Polish community, is to put an aged family member in a nursing home. Third- and fourth-generation Polish Americans may consider an extended-care or assisted-living facility because of work schedules and demands of care, but first-generation immigrants rarely perceive this as an option. If Polish people are to assimilate into a nursing home, the use of the Polish language and rituals may be crucial. Thus, health-care providers should assist clients in organizing these types of events for their family members or should help them select nursing homes that offer these cultural advantages.

The quality of life for elderly immigrants is an excellent area for research (Berdes & Zych, 2000). Immigrants who arrived before the age of 21 adjusted to aging much better than their elderly counterparts who arrived in America well into maturity. If the elderly Pole moved to America and was actively embraced by family and friends, adjusting to old age in America was less difficult. However, if the move to America was a forced choice, the adjustment was more difficult.

Extended family, consisting of aunts, uncles, and godparents, is very important to Poles. Long-time friends become aunts or uncles to Polish children. Numerous family rituals surround holidays, and family gatherings—such as for births, marriages, and name dates (calendar date of the patron saint for whom one is named)—are times to socialize and solidify relationships.

The goals of the family are to work, make economic contributions, and strive to enhance the position of the family in the community. The family unit comes together to help deter behaviors that might cause them shame or lower prestige in the eyes of the community. As Poles assimilate into the culture, the American value of success may prevail. Most Poles expect their children to have an education and a well-paying job and to provide for them in their old age.

ALTERNATIVE LIFESTYLES

Alternative lifestyles are seen as part of assimilation into the blended American culture. Same-sex couples are frowned upon and may even be ostracized, depending on the level of assimilation. Older second- and third-generation Poles have one of the lowest divorce rates of ethnic groups (Lopata, 1994), but patterns are changing with succeeding generations as they assimilate into the American lifestyle. Marital problems do exist, but the Polish value for family solidarity is strong and divorce is seen as truly a last resort. When divorce does result, single heads of households are accepted in the Polish American community.

Workforce Issues

CULTURE IN THE WORKPLACE

Most Polish Americans are more socially segregated than other ethnic groups. In the past, many Poles never rose above the level of foreman or supervisor. Polish American immigrants of the 1800s maintained group solidarity and could always be counted on to help their families. Because men were semiliterate and had low-level skills, they gravitated to industrial cities, such as Chicago, where they could work long hours as laborers and earn overtime pay. Because Poles were active in trade unions and maintained a sense of loyalty to the group, they were stronger supporters of unions than many other American-born workers of the 1930s and 1940s.

Polish Americans have extensive social networks, and their strong work ethic enables them to gain employment and assimilate easily into the workforce. It is still possible to spend one's entire life in the same house, be employed in the same factory, and have the majority of your social contacts inside the boundaries of Polonia. Whereas this may have helped immigrants in the past, it now acts as a deterrent to assimilation. The cultural tradition of hard work has caused employers to take advantage of this attitude. For example, Polish workers are being exploited as modern-day slave labor in Italy. Since 2000, Polish migrant workers have been recruited to the Italian countryside to harvest crops. Responding to advertisements promising well-paying contracts, the Poles paid for bus rides from Warsaw for this work opportunity. However, gangs of Polish, Italian, and Ukranian criminals held the migrant workers without pay or lodging and provided only infrequent meals of bread and water (Spolar, 2006).

ISSUES RELATED TO AUTONOMY

Some Poles entering America are underemployed and may have difficulty working with authority figures who are less educated. Poles quietly comment that they are disrespected for their educational background and that they must endure decreased status to stay in America (Lopata, 1994). Poles are usually quick learners and work hard to do a job well. The Polish characteristic of praising people for their work makes Poles strong managers, but some lack sensitivity in their quest to complete tasks.

Even though nursing in Poland is considered a profession, newer immigrants may be unprepared for the level of sophistication and autonomy of American nurses. Only since the 1980s has nursing entered the university setting in Poland. Most Polish nursing education is still completed in 1- to 2-year postsecondary education programs. As with many other professionals coming to America, if Polish nurses are willing to complete the extra courses to become registered or practical nurses, their employment as a nurse can be continued. A problem for many foreign nurses is that they may not receive credit for their work experiences in their home country. A nurse with 10 years of foreign nursing experience may have to start with the schedule, salary, and status of a new graduate. Poland's nursing students express fundamental values that are significantly influenced by a society characterized by strong religious conviction (Wronska, 2002). In the United States, nursing education's multireligious attitudes defer any discussion of religious beliefs.

Because Poles learn deference to authority at home, in the church, and in parochial schools, some may be less well suited for the rigors of a highly individualistic, competitive market. For Poles living in a country with a strong religious tradition, the American work culture may be very difficult for them to understand. Nevertheless, the strong Polish work ethic, exhibited as volunteering for overtime, being punctual, and rarely taking sick days, is valued by employers.

Native-born Polish Americans have little, if any, difficulty with the English language. Foreign-born Poles frequently have some difficulty understanding the subtle nuances of humor. Less-educated Poles tend to seek jobs as domestics or choose to perform manual labor because they are reluctant to rely on their English language and communication skills. Recent Polish immigrants, who had experience working under a Communist bureaucratic hierarchy, may have some difficulty with the structure, subtleties, and culture of the American workplace. New-wave Poles may be very naïve in acclimating to the American work culture and, therefore, may become frustrated with what is considered an acceptable work ethic.

Biocultural Ecology

SKIN COLOR AND OTHER BIOLOGICAL VARIATIONS

Most Poles are of medium height with a medium-to-large bone structure. As a result of foreign invasions over the centuries, Polish people may be dark and Mongol-looking or fair with delicate features, blue eyes, and blonde hair. Those with fair complexions are predisposed to skin cancer and other illnesses related to exposure to environmental elements. Health-care providers must be aware of these conditions when assessing Polish clients and providing health teaching.

DISEASES AND HEALTH CONDITIONS

Poles consider themselves to be a tough people with an ability to tolerate pain from injuries, illness, and disease.

Poles believe that suffering hardens individuals; therefore, they value that experience and perceive it to be good. In the Polish culture, a common belief is that enduring pain without complaining or asking for relief demonstrates virility in men and self-control in women. Young boys are taught at an early age that they can control illness, pain, or discomfort without the help of medicine and, thus, improve their inner strength. Another cultural belief is that taking medications weakens the entire system, which results in the decrease in family status. Fathers live vicariously through their children, especially their sons, and any weakness in the child is believed to reflect directly on them.

Risk factors for newer Polish immigrants are connected with their employment in industries in their homeland. Heavy industry in Poland produced prolonged, significant air pollution and environmental neglect. Living in polluted environments led to an increase in premature deliveries, low-birth-weight children, diseases of the pulmonary and circulatory systems, and various forms of cancer. The problem of occupational lead poisoning from 1970 to 1996 in Poland was documented by Szeszenia-Dabrowska and Wilczynka in 1998. Between 1972 and 1976, 8414 cases of lead poisoning, an occupational disease, were registered. A diminishing number of occupational lead poisoning cases was observed in the 1990s (Szeszenia-Dabrowska & Wilczynka, 1998). In 2005, Trzcinka-Ochocka, Jakubowski, and Razniewska published the results of their study assessing the current occupational exposure to lead and evaluating the competence of laboratories responsible for the monitoring and analysis of health risks in workers exposed to lead. The data indicate that occupational exposure to lead is still a problem and that neither the recommendations of 1996, reinforced by the Minister of Health in 2004, or the European Union directive, are universally followed. In addition, the study found that the competencies of the majority of the analytical laboratories were insufficient to evaluate the workers' exposure to lead. Another decree was issued by the Minister of Health in April 2005 that mandates accreditation of all laboratories by January 1, 2008 (Trzcinka-Ochocka et al., 2005).

In Poland, air pollution remains a serious problem because of sulfur dioxide emissions from coal-fired power plants. In addition to the air pollution problems, Poles have had a long history of excessive smoking. "At the end of the 1980s, Poland had the highest cigarette consumption in the world" (Zatorski, 2003, p. 97). In 1990, the Cancer Center and Institute, under the honorary patronage of Lech Walesa and in collaboration with the International Union Against Cancer and the American Cancer Society, hosted a conference, "A Tobacco-free New Europe." Public-health leaders from Eastern Europe were targeted; the participants heard comprehensive scientific evidence on the magnitude of health damage caused by cigarette smoking in the region. Ultimately, this conference provided the basis for health-related tobacco control legislation, which dramatically reduced the consumption of cigarettes (Zatorski, 2003).

The World Health Organization (WHO)/Europe (2004) reported that among young people, 10 percent of 13-year-olds and 21.5 percent of 15-year-olds smoke at least once a week. Unfortunately, Polish Americans have a higher rate of smoking than other European Americans. Forty percent of all Polish men and 25 percent of all women older than 15 years smoke. Thus, approximately 32 percent of the Polish adult population are smokers.

Obviously, miners and workers in heavy industry are at an increased risk for the development of pulmonary diseases. Water pollution from industrial and municipal sources and disposal from industrial waste have also become environmental problems. Once these industrial establishments comply with the current European Union codes, the pollution levels should decrease (CIA, 2006). The factors cited previously have contributed to the significant incidence of respiratory disease and lung and other cancers.

In the late 20th century, the Chernobyl incident in Russia created a concern that radiation had contaminated the land and water systems of eastern Poland. The full impact of this disaster on the incidence of cancer in Poland, as well as for Poles emigrating to other parts of the world, remains unknown.

In 2000, cardiovascular diseases (CVD) caused 56 percent of all deaths in Poland. Ischemic heart disease was the cause of 141 Polish deaths per 100,000 population, whereas cerebrovascular diseases led to 103 deaths per 100,000 population. Twenty percent of the adult population suffers from hypertension (WHO/Europe, 2004). The long-term effects of hypertension in the Polish population needs to be addressed, and awareness needs to be increased through patient education efforts (Niewada, Skowronska, Ryglewicz, Kaminski, & Czlonkowska, 2006). Zdrojewski et al. (2006) conducted individual and collective CVD risk assessments and developed individual and collective risk profiles of political and opinion leaders participating in the Polish Hygiene Society Congress. The researchers examined high blood pressure, overweight and obesity, and smoking as risk factors for those attending the conference. These results were presented to the participants, and the cumulative results were compared with the nation's current epidemiological burden caused by CVD (Zdrojewski et al., 2006). This strategy appears to be an effective way of impressing on the leaders the importance of these risk factors and improving the awareness, education, and lobbying efforts needed to establish a long-term educational program aimed at reducing the incidence of CVD risk factors.

In Poland, 10 percent of hospitalizations are attributed to cancer or other malignant neoplasms. In 2000, cancer caused 216 deaths per 100,000 Poles. In Poland, the death rate from cervical cancer is more than triple the European Union (EU)-15 average (WHO/Europe, 2004).

VARIATIONS IN DRUG METABOLISM

Documentation on the pharmacodynamics of drug metabolism in Polish individuals is limited. The health-care literature has yet to report any pharmacological studies specific to people of Polish descent.

High-Risk Behaviors

Alcohol abuse, with its subsequent physiological, psychological, and sociological effects and its related financial impact, continues to be an ongoing concern among Polish Americans. In Poland, a study by Manwell, Czabala, Ignaczak, and Mundt (2004) found high rates of depression among heavy drinkers in the primary-care population. In addition, Cherpitel, Moskalewicz, and Swiatkiewicz (2004) reported that drinking patterns and subsequent injuries among males affected the number of emergency services utilized, suggesting a high recidivism for alcohol-related injuries. These results suggest that the patient's acknowledgment of the role of alcohol in the injury may be an important factor used in developing individualized intervention strategies (Cherpitel et al., 2004).

In Poland, a high rate of alcoholic psychosis, cirrhosis of the liver, and acute alcohol poisoning exists. Other alcohol-related illnesses include cancer of the gastrointestinal tract, peptic ulcers, accidents, and suicide. An estimated 1 million Poles are dependent upon alcohol, and another 3 million are alcohol abusers. Cumulatively, 4 million of Poland's estimated 38 million people are either alcohol dependent or abusers (Manwell, Ignaczak, & Czabala, 2002). These researchers estimated that approximately 30,000 male deaths per year are considered alcohol-related, and nearly 80 percent of all cirrhosis-related deaths in men are associated with alcohol abuse (Manwell et al., 2002).

Alcohol abuse is an important part of the history of Poland. For some immigrants, alcohol was a way of relieving boredom, frustrations, and severe hardships. For other immigrants, alcohol was a way of mitigating the painful memories of WW II and reducing depression and the symptoms of post-traumatic stress syndrome. Alcohol still influences family patterns of behavior for many Polish immigrants.

Because Poles place a high value on hospitality in both Poland and America, drinking among Poles is an accepted part of the culture. Part of being a good hostess or host is to have enough alcohol for every guest. For newer immigrants and older Polish Americans, vodka is the alcohol of choice. Upper socioeconomic groups drink wine, whereas beer is consumed by all socioeconomic levels. In a study on drinking patterns of American and Polish college students, Polish students drank more than their American counterparts (Eng, Slawinska, & Hanson, 1991). Wine was the preferred drink of Polish students, and beer the preferred drink of American students.

During 2000, the average Polish adult consumed 6.6 L of pure alcohol. This amount has decreased since the 1980s, but serious concerns remain about the system of recording and the problem of underreporting (WHO/Europe, 2004). Because alcohol use and cigarette smoking are prevalent among many Poles, health-care providers must assess individual clients for abuse and provide counseling and referral for those who express an interest. Children of immigrants should especially be targeted for counseling regarding the health effects of smoking and alcohol consumption.

Illicit drug use is becoming more common among Polish urban residents. Cannabis is the most popular illicit drug. WHO/Europe (2004) reported that up to 25 percent of all Poles between 18 and 50 years of age have experimented with marijuana at least once.

HEALTH-CARE PRACTICES

As with their U.S. counterparts, the behaviors of the Polish immigrants are directly associated with their level of education, income, and lifestyle. Those with higher levels of education are very interested in weight control, preventive health behaviors, and exercise. Health-care providers need to include interventions specific to the individual's social environment (Stelmach, Kaczmarczyk-Chalas, Bielecki, & Drygas, 2005). Many Poles continue their established health-related activities after immigration.

For Poles just entering the United States, obtaining various medical benefits has often been confusing and information facilitating access to the health-care system limited. This frequently resulted in Polish people treating themselves, delivering babies at home using a lay midwife, taking folk medicines and herbal remedies, and even setting their own broken bones when necessary. The mother's or grandmother's responsibility was to know how to care for the family and their medical problems. Some additional common cultural practices included treating the symptoms of colds with herbs or poultices made from goose grease or fat. Gunpowder was ingested to promote emesis for an upset stomach. A boil was healed by soaking the heel of a loaf of white bread in milk and then placing it on the boil to draw out the core. Poor circulation or back pain was relieved by placing heated, alcohol-swabbed shot glasses, called *banki*, on the affected area. The heated banki were placed on the back or over the painful areas, causing circular, swollen areas on the skin. The Poles believed that this painless, raised area increased the circulation and reduced overall pain. Therefore, the health-care provider obviously needs to individually assess the cultural health behaviors of their Polish patients.

Health-care providers should carefully screen Polish immigrants for diseases common in their home country. Hypertension, CVDs, respiratory conditions, alcoholism, cancer (particularly leukemia), and thyroid disorders are endemic diseases of Poland that are also found in the United States. Culturally congruent health teaching strategies associated with the risk factors for these diseases must be implemented when working with this population.

Nutrition

MEANING OF FOOD

Another rather common depiction of cultural values is sometimes displayed on a wallhanging in a Polish home. The wallhanging often features a likeness of God with the inscription *Gosc W Dom, Bog W Dom*, which means "Guest in the House, God in the House."

Most Poles extend the sharing of food and drink to guests entering their homes. Eating and/or drinking with the host is perceived as social acceptance. Three important considerations influence Poles regarding food. First, Poland is primarily a land-based country with short summers and very cold winters. Thus, the major agricultural products in Poland include potatoes, vegetables, wheat, poultry, eggs, pork, and dairy products (CIA, 2006). Second, the cold weather discourages outdoor activities, while also creating a craving for hot stews, soups, and foods that produce a feeling of satiety. Unfortunately, these foods are high in carbohydrates, fat, and sodium. Meats and vegetables are cooked for a very long time, resulting in the destruction of B and other vitamins. Third, the strong Catholic influence is evidenced by attending many food-laden celebrations, festivals, and rituals, each of which has its own traditional high-calorie foods. Many Poles continue these routine dietary practices after emigrating. Health-care providers need to assess how the Polish clients' dietary habits influence their weight, blood pressure, and overall health status and then structure a diet that is culturally acceptable, promotes healthy food choices, and is sustainable.

COMMON FOODS AND FOOD RITUALS

Polish foods and cooking are similar to German, Russian, and Jewish practices. Staples of the diet are millet, barley, potatoes, onions, radishes, turnips, beets, beans, cabbage, carrots, cucumbers, tomatoes, apples, and wild mushrooms. Common meats are chicken, beef, and pork. Traditional high-fat entrees include pigs' knuckles and organ meats such as liver, tripe, and tongue. *Kapusta* (sauerkraut), *golabki* (stuffed cabbage), *babka* (coffee cake), *pierogi* (dumplings), and *chrusciki* (deep-fried bowtie pastries) are common ethnic foods. As mentioned previously, hot soups and stews are favored during the bitterly cold winters, and cold soups are preferred during the summer.

The meal plan for many Poles consists of a hearty breakfast of coffee, bread, cheese, sausage, and eggs. A midmorning snack comprises a sandwich and tea or coffee. The main meal in midafternoon includes soup, meat, potatoes, a hot vegetable, and dessert. In the evening, cold cuts, eggs, butter, sour cream, bread, and grains are common. This diet is modified depending on the availability of the food, the growing season, and the family's finances. Dill, paprika, garlic, and marjoram (used in *kielbasa*) are common herbs. Many foods may be pickled or canned for storage, which also increases their sodium content. Table 20–1 lists a variety of traditional Polish foods.

TABLE 20.1 *Polish Foods*

Common Name	Description	Ingredients
Babka	Coffee cake	Yeast bread
Barszcz	Beet soup	Served plain or with sour cream
Bigos	Hunter's stew	Stew with game, sausage, sauerkraut
Chrusciki	Polish bowties	Fried egg dough
Golabki	Cabbage rolls	Cooked cabbage stuffed with chopped meat and rice in tomato sauce
Kielbasa	Sausage	Sausage
Ogorki smietanie	Sour cream cucumbers	Sour cream, cucumbers
Pierogi	Boiled dumplings	Dumplings filled with potatoes, cheese, or sauerkraut
Sledzie	Herring	Pickled fish

DIETARY PRACTICES FOR HEALTH PROMOTION

The Polish American diet is frequently high in carbohydrates, sodium, and saturated fat. Assessing clients for increased blood sugar and cholesterol levels and high blood pressure should be routine. Interventions that require significant dietary modifications to their culturally based menus may be difficult.

Like many other economically developing countries, Poland's efforts to examine the health status of its citizens has become increasingly important. One disease with dramatic long-term consequences is insulin-dependent diabetes. Over the years, an increased incidence of this disease in Poles has been documented. Sobel-Maruniak, Grzywa, Oriowska, and Staniszewski (2006) reported the results of their study to compare the long-term trend in the incidence of insulin-dependent diabetes over 20 years (1980–1999). Their results showed a significant growth in the incidence of insulin-dependent diabetes among people aged 0 to 29 years in the Rzeszow Province. The male incidence of 6.7 significantly exceeded the 5.5 per 100,000 population rate in females. The group aged 0 to 14 years had a higher incidence (6.4/100,000) than the 15- to 29-year-old age group (5.8/100,000). Boys aged 10 to 14 had the highest incidence at 11.5 per 100,000. Obviously, there has been a increased incidence of insulin-dependent diabetes in the subjects over the 20-year observation period (Sobel-Maruniak et al., 2006). Health-care providers should be especially alert to the symptoms of diabetes in younger Polish immigrants.

VIGNETTE 20.2

John Jagojinski came to America as a young boy in the 1940s and has lived in the same Polonia and worked in a nearby steel mill his entire life. He married his neighborhood girl-friend, Sophie, and they had two children. John is proud of his family, but dislikes the idea that their adult children moved to the suburbs 15 years ago.

Until recently, John was a heavy drinker who smoked one pack of cigarettes daily for 30 years. He quit smoking 10 years ago because he felt "winded." He stopped drinking about 5 years ago because "I just couldn't hold it like I used to."

John has been feeling ill for the past month and told his wife he was drinking so much water that he was going to the bathroom all the time. John was concerned that he could barely hold his water (urine) when going to the bathroom.

A complete physical examination revealed that John's legs were swollen and that he was having trouble breathing. John was given prescriptions to treat his condition and advised to reduce his dietary sodium intake.

After 1 week, John insisted on returning to the steel mill and asked Sophie to make him his customary lunchmeat sandwiches to take to work. After 3 weeks, the swelling in his legs has worsened and his wife said she should call the doctor for an appointment. John got angry.

1. What are the most likely clinical problems that John has developed?
2. What cultural considerations must the health-care provider keep in mind when advising John and Sophie?

3. How can John's lunch be modified to reduce his sodium intake?
4. Why should Sophie or their adult children be included in managing John's condition?
5. What health promotion activities should John be encouraged to perform?

NUTRITIONAL DEFICIENCIES AND FOOD LIMITATIONS

Unfortunately, most of the land and water in Poland contains low levels of iodine. Iodine does not develop naturally in specific foods unless it is present in the soil or water. Iodine penetrates the foods that are grown in the soil, and their ingestion supplies it to the consumer. Ocean water also contains adequate amounts of iodine; thus, eating fish or other nutrients from the sea is likely to furnish sufficient amounts. Unfortunately, consuming fish on a regular basis has failed to become a part of the traditional diet in Poland.

Except for individuals living near the Baltic Sea in northern Poland who consume fish regularly, Poles are in danger of developing nutritional problems related to the lack of iodine in their diet. Iodine is an essential component for the thyroid's hormonal function, and its deficiency results in the underproduction of thyroxine and triiodothyronine. Disorders related to the inadequate production of these hormones may include (1) mental retardation, (2) neurological system defects, (3) goiters (e.g., enlarged thyroid), (4) sluggishness, (5) growth retardation, (6) reproductive failure, and (7) increased childhood mortality. Fortunately, this nutritional problem is being monitored and addressed.

Pregnancy and Childbearing Practices

FERTILITY PRACTICES AND VIEWS TOWARD PREGNANCY

Because family is very important, most Poles want children. In an agrarian society, and for early immigrants, children were considered important because they brought happiness and status to the family and were an economic necessity. In Poland, the Catholic Church strongly opposes abortion, which is the prevailing attitude of many Poles in America. However, during the years of war, poverty, and Communist rule, abortion and child spacing were considered necessities.

In 2006, the estimated birth rate was 9.85 per 1000 people, whereas the rate of death was 9.89 per 1000. The estimated fetal fertility rate for 2006 was 1.25 children born per woman (CIA, 2006), which is less than the 2.0 children required to sustain the current population. In Poland, women receive fully paid maternity leave for 90 days, and longer with partial payment, but many women are unable to take the entire leave owing to trying economic circumstances. Fertility practices are balanced between the needs of the family and the laws of the Church.

PRESCRIPTIVE, RESTRICTIVE, AND TABOO PRACTICES IN THE CHILDBEARING FAMILY

Pregnant Polish Americans are expected to seek preventive health care, eat well, and get adequate rest to ensure a healthy pregnancy and baby. Immigrant families who have experienced poverty, famine, and inadequate health care are more likely to pay attention to prenatal care. The emphasis on food and "eating for two" is a common philosophy. Health-care providers must pay special attention to ensure that pregnant Polish American women restrict their weight gain during pregnancy.

Because the process of childbirth was poorly understood by an undereducated society, folk beliefs, magicoreligious explanations, and taboos continue to surround the process. Many consider it bad luck to have a baby shower, and even now, many Polish grandmothers may be reluctant to give gifts until after the baby is born. Birthing is typically done in the hospital. Midwives may be used if there is a community feeling that they are "just as good as the doctor."

Pregnant women usually follow the physician's orders carefully. In America, Polish women seek prenatal clinics when they are unable to afford private fees. The birthing process is considered the domain of women. Newer Polish immigrants may feel uncomfortable with men in the birthing area or with family-centered care.

Women are expected to rest for the first few weeks after delivery. For many, breastfeeding is important. Health-care providers may need to provide active lactation counseling and education about appropriate care during breastfeeding (e.g., proper techniques) and to help the woman understand the balance between diet, rest, and exercise after delivery.

Death Rituals

DEATH RITUALS AND EXPECTATIONS

Most Poles have a stoic acceptance of death as part of the life process and a strong sense of loyalty and respect for their loved ones. Family and friends stay with the dying person to negate any feelings of abandonment. The Polish ethic of demonstrating caring by doing something means bringing food to share, caring for children, and assisting with household chores.

Most Polish women are quick to help with the physical needs of the dying. Home hospice care is acceptable to most Poles. Health-care providers may encounter difficulty in convincing the family that the dying member may choose to refuse food as a result of the illness rather than because of stubbornness or the caretaker's cooking. Polish women may tend to hover. Health-care providers need to help families understand that it is important for the dying person to conserve energy.

RESPONSES TO DEATH AND GRIEF

In early Poland, individuals were buried within 24 hours of their deaths. Historically, immigrant Poles continued the practice of burying the deceased from the home and having home burial ceremonies, which included a wake or vigil in which family members prayed and repeated the rosary over the dead person. Today, Polish American family members follow a funeral custom of having a wake for 1 to 3 days, followed by a Mass and religious burial. Most Poles honor their dead by attending Mass and making special offerings to the Church on All Souls' Day, November 1. Families may continue tending the gravesite for years.

Spirituality

DOMINANT RELIGION AND USE OF PRAYER

The Catholic Church, with its required attendance at Mass on Sundays and holy days, is an integral part of the lives of most Polish people. There are "holy days" in almost every month of the year, in addition to the rituals of Baptism, confirmation, marriage, sacrament of the sick, and burial. Christmas and Easter are the two biggest holidays requiring both special foods and rituals. On Christmas Eve, depending on the affluence of the family, up to 13 meatless dishes are served with the *oplatek* (similar to a large communion wafer) that everyone shares at the table. On Christmas Day, the main meal consists of *kielbasa*, goose, ham, or turkey. The Easter holiday may begin with women bringing food to the church on Easter Saturday to be blessed by the priest. On Easter Sunday, lamb or *kielbasa* and boiled eggs are served. A table ornament, usually a lamb made of salt or butter, is often displayed. Like many Americans of various ethnic backgrounds, Polish Americans have had a renewed interest in their ethnic roots. For example, their attendance at language classes, festivals, and Polish Catholic churches has become very widespread.

Religious ceremonies are a major part of maintaining Polish culture. Poles are very concerned that churches continue to act as a vehicle of Polish culture. Birthdays and name days are important religious and family events for Poles. One very popular song is *Sto Lat*, which conveys wishes that the celebrant live 100 years. Polish weddings are legendary. This is the time when family and friends get together and two families unite. One folk practice is to bring *chlebem i sola* (bread and salt) as a symbol of hospitality. Guests always receive plenty of food and drink, listen to music, and dance. In America, Polish weddings may last only 1 day, but plenty of food and alcoholic beverages are considered essential to the joyous occasion.

Primary spiritual sources are God and Jesus Christ, with many Polish immigrants praying to the Virgin Mary, saints, and angels to ward off evil and danger. Honor and special attention are paid to the Black Madonna or Our Lady of Czestachowa (Fig. 20–1). Czestachowa, a town in central Poland, displays a picture of the Virgin Mary with two scratch marks on her darkened face. Every year, many Poles join a walking pilgrimage to see the Madonna. The United States has several settings honoring the Black Madonna. During times of illness and serious family concerns, one might hear a Pole evoking *Matka Boska*, which literally translated means "Mother of God."

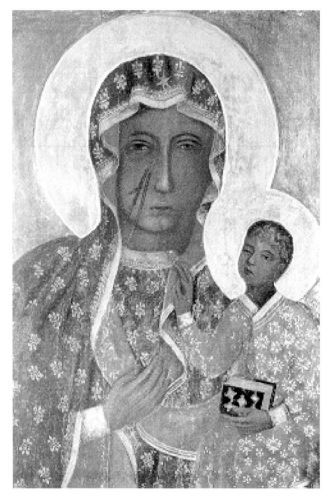

FIGURE 20–1 The Black Madonna or Our Lady of Czestachowa is an object of devotion to millions of native and immigrant Polish people. (From The Marian Library/International Marian Research Institute, Dayton, OH. http://www.udayton.edu/mary/resources/blackm/blackm03.html)

Many older Polish people believe in the special properties of prayer books, rosary beads, medals, and consecrated objects. Polish Americans commonly exhibit devotions to God, such as crucifixes and pictures of the Virgin Mary, the Black Madonna, and Pope John Paul II, in their homes.

MEANING OF LIFE AND INDIVIDUAL SOURCES OF STRENGTH

Most Polish Americans have a strong work ethic and pride themselves on being fastidious and punctual. They are loyal to friends and family, have a strong sense of Catholic ideals, are self-disciplined, and are concerned about respect and honor. Most Polish Americans enjoy music, such as the works of Chopin and other classical composers, and dancing, including the jovial Polish polka, the waltz, or polonaise. Liturgical music may be important to older and more religious Poles.

After years of living under Communist censorship, newer immigrants value freedom, independence, being respected for their work, and having status in the com-

munity. Most Polish Americans find meaning in family loyalty and show great generosity to friends and extended family. Like all cultural groups, Polish Americans want to be shown respect.

SPIRITUAL BELIEFS AND HEALTH-CARE PRACTICES

Among the early immigrants, religion had both a folk tradition and a formal Catholic element. Most believed in mythological beings, water spirits, and house ghosts. Killing or any useless slaughter of animals was condemned. All life had meaning, and if an experience was unexplainable, mysterious, or magical, folk beliefs and/or religion provided the answer.

Health-Care Practices

HEALTH-SEEKING BELIEFS AND BEHAVIORS

Most Poles put a high value on stoicism and doing what needs to be done. Many go to health-care providers only when symptoms interfere with function; then they may carefully consider the advice provided before complying. Describing anxiety and expecting nurturance are uncharacteristic of most Polish adults and children. Many Poles are reluctant to discuss their treatment options and concerns with physicians and routinely accept the proposed care plan. If Poles believe they are unable to pay the medical bill, they may refuse treatment unless the condition is life-threatening. Many have a strong fear of becoming dependent and resist relying on charity. Because many Poles consider Medicare, Medicaid, and managed care as forms of social charity, they are reluctant to apply for them. Any action that lowers their social status in their community is generally considered unacceptable. The health-care provider must describe the intent of these financial programs carefully or Poles may perceive them as charity and, therefore, unacceptable options.

Poles usually look for a physical cause of disease before considering a mental disorder. If mental health problems exist, home visits are preferred. Talk-oriented interventions and therapies without pharmaceutical or suitable psychosocial strategies are dismissed unless interventions are action oriented. In addition, Poles consult other family members and the community to assess the appropriateness of treatments. Polish Americans often seek self-help groups such as Alcoholics Anonymous before seeing a health-care provider. Assimilated Poles respect the health-care system and tend to seek specialized care when necessary.

In Poland, health care is subsidized by the state. In accordance with the National Health Fund Act of 2003, Poland has a compulsory health insurance scheme (WHO/Europe, 2004). To many immigrant Poles, the U.S. health-care system is complex, confusing, and overpriced. They perceive access to health care as difficult, and many people who can afford to pay higher fees to see a private physician are unaware of how to gain access. Some Poles return to Poland to have medical or surgical procedures performed because these are more understandable, available, and/or affordable in their homeland.

RESPONSIBILITY FOR HEALTH CARE

Given the continuation of limited access to care and the strong work ethic of this cultural group, health promotion practices are often undervalued by Polish Americans. In fact, older Polish Americans and newer immigrants commonly smoke and drink, engage in limited physical exercise outside of work, and receive poor dental care. Partial and complete dentures are common in older Poles. A number of secondary teeth are often found missing in Polish American immigrant children. This frequently surprises nurses who may be unaware of the limited number of dentists in Poland.

Attention to health promotion practices among women may be complicated by Polish American women's sense of modesty and religious background. Breast self-examination and Pap smear tests are poorly understood by many women. Health promotion practices vary greatly and are dependent on the woman's assimilation into American culture.

The Polish ethic of stoicism discourages the use of over-the-counter medications unless a symptom persists. Most Poles refuse to take time off from work to see a health-care provider until self-help measures have proved ineffective. Few Poles use vitamins unless these are suggested by a physician or a trusted family member; even then, their extrinsic value is compared with the cost.

FOLK AND TRADITIONAL PRACTICES

When a Pole is asked to undress for a physical examination, the health-care provider should pay special attention to any medals pinned to the patient's undergarments. Most of these medals have special religious significance to the wearer and should, if possible, remain on the garment. In addition, Polish Americans may use certain remedies to cure an illness, such as tea with honey and spirits to "sweat out" a cold. Herbs and rubbing compounds may also be used for problems associated with aches, pains, and inflammation from overworked joints and muscles. Because of individual differences, every client must be assessed personally and asked specifically about their use of home remedies and over-the-counter medications.

BARRIERS TO HEALTH CARE

Being unable to speak and understand English and the cost of health care and its complexity are the greatest barriers to health care for Polish immigrants. In addition to overcoming the language barrier, health-care providers need to understand Polish family values. Health-care providers also must consider that Poles often filter information through the extended family and neighborhood before accepting the recommended health-care regimen. Polish Americans who have learned English as a second language may have some difficulty with the nuances of health-care jargon and terminology.

Inadequate or miscommunication can result in tragic consequences for the client. To negate the deleterious effects of miscommunications, the Department of Health and Human Services' Office for Civil Rights issued a 1998 memorandum regarding the prohibition, under Title VI of the Civil Rights Act of 1964, against discrimination on the basis of national origin that affects people with limited English proficiency. This memorandum asserts that the denial or delay of medical care owing to language barriers constitutes discrimination. It also requires that recipients of Medicare or Medicaid funds provide adequate language assistance to patients with limited English proficiency (Flores, 2006). Unfortunately, most of the states with the greatest number of patients with limited English proficiency have not complied with the memorandum, sometimes citing cost concerns. Although, in 1993, the Office of Civil Rights issued guidelines that appear to permit health-care facilities to avoid providing language services by citing burdensome costs, Title VI provides no such exception (Flores, 2006).

Health-care providers may need to employ primary-care or case management and/or assistance to obtain a cultural bilingual health provider and interpreter from the Polish American community to help decrease the number of barriers to health care. If an interpreter is required, the Polish community can usually help provide someone. Poles are polite to authority figures and avoid offending a health-care worker by disagreeing with them. Thus, they may be reluctant to ask for clarifications on questionable issues. In addition, many Poles are primarily concerned about how a disease affects daily functioning rather than about individual survival rates.

CULTURAL RESPONSES TO HEALTH AND ILLNESS

Owing to their strong sense of stoicism and fear of being dependent upon others, many Polish Americans use inadequate pain medication and choose distraction as a means of coping with pain and discomfort. When asked, many Poles either deny or minimize their pain or level of discomfort. Poles with chronic illnesses may have similar attitudes; thus, persevering with pain is common. The health-care provider should use a visual analog scale to assess pain, assist clients with distraction techniques, and help Poles to accept pain medication when needed.

Premigration stresses (e.g., losses, catastrophic experiences, anxiety, and internment) may be combined with postmigration stressors (e.g., language difficulty, loss of relationships, cultural pride, lack of support systems) to cause mental health problems (Fenta, Hyman & Noh, 2004). Social and geographic isolation within one's own ethnic neighborhood are common, albeit somewhat restrictive, reactions to this situation. Many immigrants are able to overcome the initial shock of moving to a foreign country, but they fail to have adequate coping skills to get through the stressors of total adjustment. Lack of language skills, feelings of unfamiliarity, and fear of the unknown are some of the reasons given by those who fail to leave their Polonia. In these self-segregated cultural communities, children often become the go-betweens for their parents and the larger community. As children mature, they leave their parents and the Polonia to start their own families. Thus, the parents' avoidance of the acculturation process, even 25 years later, creates stressors leading to feelings of abandonment, loneliness, and displacement. These feelings may become significant and lead to major physical and/or mental illnesses.

Few Poles turn to psychiatrists or mental health providers for help. Those who seek help from mental health professionals do so as a last resort. Many individuals choose their priest or seek assistance from a Polish volunteer-run agency before going to a health professional for psychiatric help.

Immigration to America failed to change the Pole's concerns about the delivery of appropriate health care. Immigrants are taught from infancy to resist asking for help or assistance from others but to bear the burdens of life independently.

Successful adaptation to the new homeland requires the immigrant to voluntarily progress through the process of assimilation and acculturation. **Assimilation** requires the individual to gradually adopt and incorporate the characteristics of the prevailing culture into their own lives. **Acculturation** mandates that the immigrants willingly modify their own culture as an accomodation to their transition to accepting the general values and attitudes of their new culture and homeland. The process of acculturation may affect the association between migration and health. The bidimensional approach describes acculturation as a process of adaptation to the mainstream culture while maintaining the inherited ethnic identity (Ryder, Alden, & Paulhus, 2000).

Aroian (1992) described three types of social support needed by Polish immigrants. During the first 3 years, immigrants need help finding housing and jobs and information about getting through the system; that is, learning English, buying groceries, and learning American customs. During the next 3 to 10 years, help is required to secure credit, obtain loans, and assimilate into American life. Finally, immigrants in America for more than 10 years need support in honoring their Polish heritage through networks of other immigrants while maintaining an American support system. After immigrants are comfortable with resettlement, feelings of grief and loss begin to be acknowledged. "The psychological adaptation to migration and resettlement requires the dual task of mastering resettlement demands and grieving and removing the losses left in the homeland" (Aroian, 1990, p. 8).

VIGNETTE 20.3

Chester and Kathryn Jusczak immigrated to the United States during the 1980s. They settled in the Chicago Polonia and adjusted to a comfortable life in the neighborhood. Chester works long hours in the oil refinery, while Kathryn focused on raising their four children. After completing school, all of the children left Polonia. Chester and Kathryn remained in their neighborhood, socializing with their Polish friends.

Recently, Chester began experiencing severe right flank back pain. When the pain became unbearable, he visited his primary-care physician, Dr. Gajewski, who diagnosed a kidney stone. After it had passed, Dr. Gajewski advised the Jusczaks that Chester should go on a restricted-protein and low-sodium diet and drink more water. In addition, he gave Chester a prescription for a pain medication to take in case of another episode. After leaving the office, Chester dismissed the need for filling the prescription with the statement, "It wasn't that bad; I can handle the pain." The Jusczaks were told that the nurse would visit their home to help them structure the recommended diet.

1. How can the nurse present the dietary restrictions to Chester and Kathryn so that they are acceptable and will be implemented?
2. Why did Chester resist filling the pain medication prescription?
3. Why should the nurse request that one or more of the Jusczaks' children be present during the discussion of their diet regimen?

BLOOD TRANSFUSIONS AND ORGAN DONATION

The ethic of being useful, independent, and a good Catholic influences one to refrain from using extraordinary means to keep people alive. The individual or family determines what means are considered extraordinary. Receiving blood transfusions or undergoing organ transplantation is acceptable. However, it is important for a family to know the extent to which a patient will be able to function following organ transplantation. Cost is always an important consideration. Most Poles resist becoming a burden on their family's physical or financial resources and may attempt to convince the family that the procedure is too costly. Poles do consider it their duty to care for a sick member at home.

Health-Care Practitioners

TRADITIONAL VERSUS BIOMEDICAL PRACTITIONERS

Immigrant Poles often assess health-care providers by their demeanor, warmth, and show of respect. Health advice may be sought from chiropractors and local pharmacists as well as neighbors and extended family. Generally, professional biomedical advice is sought when a symptom persists and interferes with daily life.

Newer immigrants may fail to realize that many patients are discharged from the hospital before they have totally healed and are fully recovered. Poles may assume this practice is related to charity care, disrespect, or their financial status. Early discharges should be explained to the client and family.

STATUS OF HEALTH-CARE PROVIDERS

When caring for Polish clients, particularly the elderly, all health-care providers should make every attempt to address individuals by their surname. Although this may be difficult, many names can be phonetically pronounced. Attempting to pronounce the names demonstrates respect for the client. As a group, Poles are fiercely independent, relying on themselves or family members for almost every aspect of their social status, health, and livelihood. Nurses need to focus on the Polish client's background and upbringing and take into consideration how health care becomes accepted or rejected. Illness or being sick is considered weakness for male family members. Polish women consider it their role to care for the family members without asking for help. It is also important to consider that Polish women are modest and self-conscious and may refuse health care when asked to disrobe in front of a male health-care provider. In some cases, it may be critical to request a female provider.

When it becomes evident that only professional help will resolve a problem, the affirmative act of seeking assistance is a major decision. Communication, consideration, displaying respect, and demonstrating cultural sensitivity will help to improve the Poles' attitudes toward the health-care provider. The health-care professional will need to introduce changes in ways that are appropriate and acceptable and can be integrated into an established, culturally dominated lifestyle.

Nurses will need to understand their own cultural values, beliefs, and practices in order to avoid or prevent alienating the Polish client and family about the difficulty, complexity, and conseqences of any recommended interventions. Using an authoritarian approach to gain compliance will cause conflict. Based upon their history, Poles have a tradition of survival, sometimes through stubborness, pride, warmth, or genuineness. Therefore, being perceived as an amiable, respectful, and knowledgeable provider is integral to changing attitudes and subsequent behaviors. Communicating through the use of a bilingual family member as a liaison and finding agreements on cultural health beliefs and practices may be the best initial strategy for change when dealing with elderly immigrants or more-traditional Polish Americans.

A person's culture influences their perceptions of health and illness. How a client accepts help or allows care to be rendered depends upon their previous experiences, understanding, and trust in the provider. Respect, patience, and acceptance are important components of health care. Thus, nurses need to compassionately communicate with their clients through their professional appearance, words, actions, gestures, inflections, and postures. Clients of Polish descent interact with health-care providers, whom they perceive as authority figures, in very distinctive ways. Polite listening may determine how compliant a client may be with the recommended regimen. Nurses need to focus specifically on cultural norms when dealing with older clients if they are to meet their needs. It is often the tone or how something is said as well as the body language that accompanies it that communicates whether the nurse respects the client. Being culturally sensitive to the Polish American client will be accepted as a gift from a stranger and will be reciprocated with appreciation, genuineness, and respect.

Physicians are held in high regard in Polish communities. Poles typically follow medical orders carefully. Poles may change physicians if they believe their recovery is too slow or if a second opinion is needed. Educated Poles are more willing than those less educated to follow medical orders and continue with prescribed treatment. Poles with less education tend to change physicians if the disease fails to subside quickly enough. Poles respect physicians but need to understand the purpose of the medical treatment.

Poles expect health-care providers to appear neat and clean, provide treatments as scheduled, administer medications on time, and enjoy their work. Immigrant Poles may be unfamiliar with the advanced roles of the American nurses, who are expected to know about, plan, and be directly involved in the clients' care. Thus, many Poles may still want only the physician to explain all aspects of their care.

The World Wide Web and computer access have facilitated the production of materials that may assist the nurse and provide the client with culturally appropriate materials. McCarthy, Enslein, Kelley, Choi, and Tripp-Reimer (2002) analyzed 75 bi- and multilingual health sites available on the Internet. Such sites may be very useful for disseminating information to groups with limited English-language skills. Ethnic communities could significantly benefit from having Internet-based information about specific health conditions translated into Polish and other languages and distributed to appropriate client groups.

REFERENCES

Aroian, K. J. (1990). A model of psychological adaptation to migration and resettlement. *Nursing Research, 39*(1), 5–10.

Aroian, K. J. (1992). Sources of social support and conflict for Polish immigrants. *Qualitative Health Research, 2*(2), 178–207.

Berdes, C., & Zych, A. A. (2000). Subjective quality of life of Polish, Polish-immigrant and Polish American elderly. *International Journal of Aging and Human Development, 50*(4), 385–395.

Best, W. (2004). *Polonia.* Retrieved September 29, 2007, from http://www.encyclopedia.chicagohistory.org/pages/992.html

Bolzen, S. (2006, September 14). Polish-American pride awakens: Poland's role in Iraq finds broad support among Poles in US. *Chicago Tribune,* sect. 2, p. 3.

Brogan, P. (1990). The captive nations of Eastern Europe: 1945–1990. New York: Avon Books.

Bukowczyk, J. J. (1987). *And my children did not know me: A history of Polish Americans.* Bloomington, IN: Indiana University Press.

Centreurope.org. (2006). The domination of Poland by USSR. Retrieved September 29, 2007, from http://www.centreurope.org/pl/guide/general/ussr-poland.html.

Cherpitel, C. J., Moskalewicz, J., & Swiatkiewicz, G. (2004). Drinking patterns and problems in emergency services in Poland. *Alcohol and Alcoholism, 39*(3), 256–261.

CIA. (2006). *World FactBook: Poland.* Retrieved September 29, 2007, from https://www.cia.gov/cia/publications/factbook/print/pl.html

Eng, R., Slawinska, J. B., & Hanson, D. J. (1991). The drinking patterns of American and Polish university students: A cross national study. *Drug and Alcohol Dependence, 27,* 167–174.

Erdmans, M. P. (1998). *Opposite Poles.* University Park, PA: Pennsylvania State University Press.

Fenta, H., Hyman, I., & Noh, S. (2004). Determinants of depression among Ethiopian immigrants and refugees in Toronto. *Journal of Nervous and Mental Disease, 192*(5), 363–372.

Flores, G. (2006, July 20). Language barriers to health care in the United States. *New England Journal of Medicine, 335*(3), 229–331.

The Generations Network. (2007). *Learning: Polish names.* Retrieved September 29, 2007, from http://freepages.genealogy.rootsweb.com/~atpc/learn/tools/surname-origins.html

Grocholska, J. (1999). Polish immigration to the US. Retrieved September 29, 2007, from http://www.poloniatoday.com/immigration1.html

Jarczak, C. R. (N.D.). Polish-American contributions to our nation. Retrieved September 29, 2007, from http://www.msu.edu/user/jarczakc/polesinus.html

Library of Congress. (1992a). *Country studies: Poland: Destruction of Poland-Lithuania*. Retrieved September 29, 2007, from http://lcweb2.loc.gov/ cgi-bin/query/r?frd/cstdy:@field(DOCID+pl0032)

Library of Congress. (1992b). Country studies: Poland: Recovery of statehood. Retrieved September 29, 2007, from http://lcweb2.loc.gov/cgi-bin/query/r?frd/cstdy:@field(DOCID+pl0042)

Library of Congress. (1992c). *Country studies: Poland: Resistance at home and abroad*. Retrieved September 29, 2007, from http://lcweb2.loc.gov/cgi-bin/query2/r?frd/cstdy:@field(DOCID+pl0050)

Library of Congress. (1992d). *Country studies: Poland: World War II*. Retrieved September 29, 2007, from http://lcweb2.loc.gov/cgi-bin/query/r?frd/cstdy:@field(DOCID+pl0047)

Library of Congress. (2004). *Immigration: Polish/Russian: The Nation of Polonia*. Retrieved September 29, 2007, from http://memory.loc.gov/learn/features/immig/polish4.html

Lopata, H. Z. (1994) *Polish Americans* (2nd ed.). New Brunswick, NJ: Transaction.

Manwell, L. B., Czabala, J. C., Ignaczak, M., & Mundt, M. P. (2004). Correlates of depression among heavy drinkers in Polish primary care clinics. *International Journal of Psychiatry in Medicine, 34*(2), 165–178.

Manwell, L. B., Ignaczak, M., & Czabala, J. C. (2002). Prevalence of tobacco and alcohol use disorders in Polish primary care settings. *European Journal of Public Health, 12*(2), 139–144.

McCarthy, L. J., Enslein, J. C., Kelley, L. S., Choi, E., & Tripp-Reimer, T. (2002). Cross-cultural health education: Materials on the world wide web. *Journal of Transcultural Nursing, 13*(1), 54–60.

New Mexico Tourism Department. (2006). *2006 New Mexico Vacation guide*. Santa Fe, NM: Author.

Niewada, M., Skowronska, M., Ryglewicz, D., Kaminski, B., & Czlonkowska, A. (2006). Acute ischemic stroke care and outcome in centers participating in the Polish National Stroke Prevention and Treatment Registry. *Stroke, 37*, 1837–1843.

Organization for Economic Cooperation and Development (OECD). (2005). Poland: Country note. In *Thematic Review on Adult Learning*. Paris: OECD. Retrieved September 29, 2007, from http://www.oecd.org/dataoecd/35/49/34719950.pdf

Panna Maria, Texas: The oldest permanent Polish settlement in the USA. (2006). Retrieved September 29, 2007, from www.pannamariatexas.com

Pacyga, D. A. (2004). *Poles*. Retrieved September 29, 2007, from http://www.encyclopedia.chicagohistory.org/pages/982.html

Plawecki, H. M. (1992). Cultural considerations. *Journal of Holistic Nursing, 10*(7), 4–5.

Plawecki, H. M. (2000). The elderly immigrant: An isolated experience. *Journal of Gerontological Nursing, 26*(2), 6–7.

Polish American Center. (1997). *General Casimir Pulaski (1747–1779)*. Retrieved September 29, 2007, from http://www.polishamericancenter.org/Pulaski.html

Republic of Poland, Ministry of Foreign Affairs. (2002a). *Age structure and growth rate*. Retrieved September 29, 2007, from http://www.poland.gov.pl/Age,Structure,and,growth,rate,314.html

Republic of Poland, Ministry of Foreign Affairs. (2002b). *Borders*. Retrieved September 29, 2007, from http://www.poland.gov.pl/Borders,280.html

Republic of Poland, Ministry of Foreign Affairs.(2002c). *The collapse of a state*. Retrieved September 29, 2007, from http://www.poland.gov.pl/The,collapse,of,the,state,343.html

Republic of Poland, Ministry of Foreign Affairs. (2002d). *Education structure*. Retrieved September 29, 2007, from http://www.pologne.gov.pl/Education,Structure,315.html

Republic of Poland, Ministry of Foreign Affairs. (2002e). *Fighting on the frontlines and conducting the idoelogical battle*. Retrieved September 29, 2007, from http://www.poland.gov.pl/Fighting,on,the,frontlines,and,conducting,the,ideological,battle,360.html

Republic of Poland, Ministry of Foreign Affairs. (2002f). *Gender structure*. Retrieved September 29, 2007, from http://www.poland.gov.pl/Gender,Structure,313.html

Republic of Poland, Ministry of Foreign Affairs. (2002g). *The round table and the Polish road to democracy*. Retrieved September 29, 2007, from http://poland.gov.pl/The,Round,Table,and,the,Polish,road,to,democracy,367.html

Republic of Poland, Ministry of Foreign Affairs. (2002h). *Topographical features*. Retrieved September 29, 2007, from http://www.poland.gov.pl/Topographical,features,282.html

Republic of Poland, Ministry of Foreign Affairs. (2003). *People*. Retrieved September 29, 2007, from http://www.poland.gov.pl/Intro,312.html

Republic of Poland, Ministry of Foreign Affairs. (2004). *Foreign affairs*. Retrieved September 29, 2007, from http://www.poland.gov.pl/Foreign,policy,371.html

Ryder, A. G., Alden, L. E., & Paulhus, D. L. (2000). Is acculturation unidimensional or bidimensional? A head-to-head comparison in the prediction of personality, self-identity and and adjustment. *Journal of Personality and Social Psychology, 79*(1), 49–65.

Sobel-Maruniak, A., Grzywa, M., Oriowska-Florek, R., & Staniszewski, A. (2006). The rising incidence of type 1 diabetes in south-eastern Poland. A study of the 0–29- year-old age group, 1980–1999. *Endokrynologia Polska, 57*(2), 127–130. Retrieved September 29, 2007, from http://www.ncbi.nlm.nih.gov/entrez/query.fcgi?db=pubmed&cmd=Retrieve&dopt=AbstractPlus&list_uids=16773587&query_hl=1&itool=pubmed_docsum

Spolar, C. (2006, November 12). Poles treated as slave labor: Workers report abuses in Italy. *Chicago Tribune*, pp. 1, 14.

Statistics Canada. (2001). *Selected ethnic origins for Canada, provinces and territories*. Retrieved September 29, 2007, from http://www12.statcan.ca/english/census01/products/highlight/ETO/Table1.cfm?Lang=E&T=501&GV=1&GID=0

Stelmach, W., Kaczmarczyk-Chalas, K., Bielecki, W., & Drygas, W. (2005). How education, income, control over life and life style contribute to risk factors for cardiovascular disease among adults in a post-communist country. *Public Health, 119*, 498–508.

Szaflarski, M. (2001). Gender, self-reported health and health-related lifestyles in Poland. *Health Care for Women International, 22*, 207–227.

Szeszenia-Dabrowska, N., & Wilczynska, U. (1998). Occupational lead poisoning in Poland. *Medycyna Pracy, 49*(23), 217–222. Retrieved September 29, 2007, from http://www.ncbi.nlm.nih.gov/entrez/query.fcgi?db=pubmed&cmd=Retrieve&dopt=AbstractPlus&list_uids=9760431&query_hl=4&itool=pubmed_DocSum

Trzcinka-Ochocka, M., Jakubowski, N., & Razniewska, G. (2005). Assessment of occupational exposure to lead in Poland. *Meycyna Pracy, 56*(5), 395–404. Retrieved September 29, 2007, from http://www.ncbi.nlm.nih.gov/entrez/query.fcgi?db=pubmed&cmd=Retrieve&dopt=AbstractPlus&list_uids=16483011&query_hl=2&itool=pubmed_docsum

USA Weekend.com. (2005, May 15). *America the diverse: Chicago's Polish neighborhoods*. Retrieved September 29, 2007, from http://www.usaweekend.com/05_issues/050515travel_diversetml#to

U.S. Bureau of the Census. (2004). *Ancestry 2000: Census 2000 brief*. Retrieved March 29, 2007, from [0]http://www.census.gov/prod/2004pubs/c2kbr-35.pdf date given

von Geldern, J., & Siegelbaum, L. (2003). Solidarity and the Soviet Union. Retrieved September 29, 2007, from http://www.soviethistory.org/index.php?action= L2&SubjectID=1980solidarity &Year=1980

Wilde, R. (2001). *Tadeusz Kosciuszko (1746–1817)*. Retrieved September 29, 2007, from http://europeanhistory.about.com/library/weekly/aa060801d.htm

World Health Organization (WHO)/Europe. (2004). *10 health questions about the 10*. Copenhagen, Denmark: WHO/Europe. Retrieved September 29, 2007, from http://www.euro.who.int/document/E82865PL.pdf

Wronska, I. (2002). The fundamental values of nurses in Poland. *Nursing Ethics, 9*(1), 92–100.

Zatorski, W. (2003). Democracy and health: Tobacco control in Poland. In J. deBeyer & L. Waverley (Eds.), *Tobacco control policy: Strategies, successes & setbacks* (pp. 97–120). Washington, DC: RITC and The World Bank.

Zdrojewski, T., Babinska, Z., Katol, M., Januszko, W., Rutkowski, M., Bandosz, P., et al. (2006). How to improve cooperation with political leaders and other decision-makers to improve prevention of cardiovascular disease: Lessons from Poland. *European Jounal of Cardiovascular Prevention and Rehabilitation, 13*, 319–324.

DavisPlus | For case studies, review questions, and additional information, go to http://davisplus.fadavis.com

Chapter *21*

People of Thai Heritage

RATCHNEEWAN ROSS and JEFFREY ROSS

Overview, Inhabited Localities, and Topography

OVERVIEW

Siam, the land of the musical *The King and I*, is the former name of Thailand, a country in Southeast Asia well known for its cuisine and exotic culture. Thailand today is a unique blend of traditions that reach back to its origins as a blend of Southeast Asian peoples, a background in Buddhism, and profound influences from the cultures of both India and China. For providers of health care to Thai patients, beliefs and practices that stem from these combined traditions can present both opportunities and challenges.

Thailand began a tradition of emulating Western political, economic, and cultural ideas in the late nineteenth century. In the later decades of the twentieth century, Thailand (like several other Asian "economic tigers") began a period of explosive economic growth that continues today but that has been interrupted at times by political and economic instability. A recent example was the bloodless coup that took place in the fall of 2006. Visitors to Thailand, and especially those who learn to love and study its culture, are always impressed with the unique ways in which the people of Thailand manage an often precarious balance between contrasts of the old and the new—between the rich traditions of the past and the frenetic influences of modern economic competition and a global cultural influence.

In the context of health care, this balance very often plays out as a tension between older cultural beliefs (and sometimes superstitions) and more modern concepts of medicine grounded in research. These tensions need to be understood by providers in both their positive and their negative potentials for health care as to how they vary from individual to individual.

Thailand is located north of Malaysia, west of Laos and Cambodia, and east of Myanmar (formerly Burma). Further to the north lies the once-sleeping giant of China, now dramatically influencing Thailand's political and economic spheres. Thailand's land mass (511,770 km²) and population (over 64 million people) are similar to those of France (CIA, 2006). Over 10 million people live in the regions of greater Bangkok, the capital of Thailand. Once called the "Venice of the East" because of its historic canal system, Bangkok today is the vast and vibrantly pulsating hub of the country. More than anywhere else, it embodies the contrasts between the old and the new in the country.

Thailand has several important rivers. The main river, the Chao Praya irrigates the fertile soil of the central plains. The Mekong River in the north and northeast marks the boundary between Thailand and Laos before flowing further southeast to Vietnam. The Ping, Wang, Yom, and Nan rivers are located in the north (Hoare, 2004).

Thailand is divided into 76 provinces within four different regions: north, northeast, central, and southern. Each region is unique in its geographic and cultural characteristics. Northern Thailand is the most beautiful region geographically with high mountains, deep valleys, rivers, forests, and waterfalls. The "Golden Triangle" in the north, where drug and opium smugglers have sought asylum, lies at the junction of three countries: Thailand, Laos, and Myanmar (Hoare, 2004).

In general, Thailand has a tropical climate with three seasons. The summer, or hot season, runs from March to June. The rainy season lasts from July to November, and the cool season from December to February. Many Thais, with their good sense of humor, will tell you that the country's three seasons are called "hot, hotter, and hottest" (Hoare, 2004, p. 12). Indeed, for visitors from a temperate climate, the weather throughout most of the year in Thailand will seem very humid and hot, with some relief from the heat only during the weeks of late December and early January. Thais love the beauty of their land and are adjusted to the weather, yet many who see snow for the first time in another country usually experience overwhelming joy at such a moment.

HERITAGE AND RESIDENCE

In terms of its history, Thailand is the only Southeast Asian country that has never been colonized by Westerners. The earliest knowledge of what today is Thailand is shrouded in lost histories of the ancient peoples of Southeast Asia. New cultures arose as kingdoms shifted through the centuries. The *Dvaravati* (1st century BC to the eleventh century AD) were strongly influenced by Indian culture so that even today the Rama legends of Indian mythology form an integral part of Thailand's belief system (Hoare, 2004). The present king of Thailand is the ninth of the Rama Kings, and the Thais' perception of their king's divinity can also probably be traced to Indian origins.

The first people who are culturally considered "Thais" probably migrated from the south of China. *Sukhothai*, founded in the thirteenth century AD, is considered the first kingdom of Siam (or Thailand). Its most famous king was *Ramkhamhaeng*, who is credited with developing the first Thai alphabet. *Sukhothai* had a profound influence on the development of Buddhist theology and classical art in Thai culture (Hoare, 2004). The *Sukhothai* period was eclipsed AD 1350 by the extremely powerful kingdom of Ayutthaya on the Chao Praya River. The kings of Ayutthaya in particular further embodied the essence of divine kingship as an inheritance from Indian philosophy. Although Ayutthaya eventually met its tragic demise when the Burmese sacked the city in 1767, it still represents a magnificent blossoming of artistic and cultural expression in the history of Siam (Hoare, 2004).

After an interval known as the *Thonburi* period, the present *Rattanakosin* period of Rama kings began in 1782 with its seat in Bangkok. Rama I undertook building Bangkok from a sleepy little village into what eventually became the great city of the Grand Palace (Hoare, 2004).

Especially in the eighteenth, nineteenth, and twentieth centuries, policymakers of Thailand remained independent of European colonial powers by steering a political course as a strategic buffer zone between British Burma (today Myanmar) to the west and French Indochina (Cambodia, Laos, and Vietnam) to the east (Hoare, 2004).

Thais are very proud of their independence. In 1939, the name of the country was changed from Siam to Thailand, which literally means "The land of the free." This name change reflected a fundamental shift from supreme monarchy to constitutional monarchy as a governing system (Hoare, 2004).

In 1932, Thailand appointed its first prime minister. Thereafter, the king no longer served in any critical deci-

sion-making capacities (Hoare, 2004). Still, the lineage of Thai kingships continues, and the Thai people continue to love and deeply revere their king. This intimate relationship between royalty and the people is intertwined with Thai Buddhism and the Thai peoples' perception of their king as divinely ordained. The king is usually not directly involved in Thai politics, but if a strong moral issue arises, he generally helps in addressing the problem guided by his peace and wisdom (Hoare, 2004). In 2006, the Thais' celebrated their beloved King Rama IX's 60th anniversary. His monarchy is now the oldest in the world. Any criticism of the King and his family is not at all acceptable to Thais and is even forbidden by law. Yet, Thailand's present constitutional monarchy is a democratic form of government built around the actual governing authority of the prime minister and the parliament.

REASONS FOR MIGRATION AND ASSOCIATED ECONOMIC FACTORS

Over 150,000 Thais live in the United States (U.S. Census Bureau, 2000). In 2004, approximately 4300 Thais became U.S. citizens (U.S. Census Bureau, 2006). Approximately 66 percent of all Thais in the United States live in Los Angeles. Los Angeles is therefore often referred to as "Thailand's 77th province." Coincidental and interesting to note is that both Bangkok and Los Angeles are known as the "City of Angels." However, Thai communities are spread throughout the United States. Other cities with sizable Thai populations include Houston and Philadelphia (Wikipedia, 2006).

The first two Thai immigrants in the United States were *Eng and Chang*, the famous Siamese twins who captured the world's attention because of their conjoined chests and whose career was a public exhibition. A number of medical examinations were performed on them to learn about the true nature of their condition (Wikipedia, 2006). The first Thai student in the United States came with an American missionary in 1871. His name was Mr. He Thien and he graduated from a medical college in New York. He later became the father of former prime minister of Thailand Pote Sarasin (Wikipedia, 2006).

During the Vietnam War, many Thai women married American GIs and immigrated to the United States (Bao, 2005). Immediate family members of these American Thais often followed them and settled in the new country. From 1968 to 1976, many Thai professionals such as physicians, pharmacists, and engineers immigrated to the United States to further their studies under scholarship programs, and many of them never returned to Thailand (Wikipedia, 2006). They found professional careers and remained in the United States. In general, Thais have continued in their migration to the United States in search of better opportunities.

EDUCATIONAL STATUS AND OCCUPATIONS

In Thailand, education is compulsory for at least 9 years (grades 1–9) (Fig. 21–1). However, the Thai government provides free education to all Thais who go to government

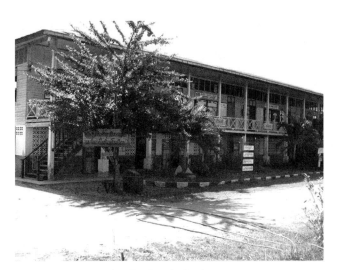

FIGURE 21–1   A grade school in Thailand.

schools up to grade 12. The literacy rate in Thailand was 92.6 percent in 2002 (CIA, 2006).

The system of higher education is well developed in Thailand, with government universities perceived as being of higher quality than private universities. Government universities are competitive, however, because of their difficult entrance examination requirements. Those students who are not accepted in government universities can still opt to enroll in the more expensive private schools. In 2002, 27.4 percent of Thais aged 17 to 24 years enrolled in college (Thailand Investor Service Center, 2004).

Many Thais with graduate degrees work in the United States in professional fields such as medicine, nursing, and engineering. Others own Thai restaurants or grocery stores and provide work for other Thais.

Communication

DOMINANT LANGUAGE AND DIALECTS

The standard Thai dialect is derived from *Pali* and *Sanskrit* (ancient South Asian languages) and is the official language in Thailand. The Thai language is a fixed tonal language having five tones. Thus, the same phonetic sound can have different meanings depending on the tone. The written alphabet is a complicated system of 44 letters with over 33 vowels or vowel combinations.

English is used in international schools, tourist places, and sometimes among Thai elite society. Although English is taught in Thai schools, the English proficiency of Thai people in general is not very high, especially when compared with certain other Southeast Asian countries such as Malaysia or Singapore. This may be due in part to Thailand's having never been colonized.

The north, northeast, and southern regions of Thailand are all areas with a unique dialect of their own. The dialect in northern Thailand is *Pasah Nua,* literally "the northern language." Thais in the Northeast speak *Pasah Isaan,* "the northeast language," which is a mixture of Laotian and other dialects. *Pasah Isaan* usually sounds very foreign to the ears of people in other regions of Thailand. The dialect of southern Thais is *Pasah Dai,* "the southern language," and is the fastest-sounding among the dialects.

CULTURAL COMMUNICATION PATTERNS

Age and status in Thailand contribute greatly to how Thais communicate with one another. According to the Thai culture, a younger person is expected to show respect for an older person through his or her gestures and language. A Thai female uses the word *"Kah"* and a Thai male uses *"Kraab"* at the end of a sentence to add politeness in a conversation. Looking in a person's eyes and conversing quietly reflect respect and politeness. A distance of 1½ to 2 feet between two speakers is preferable.

In terms of body language, kisses and hugs between a male and a female are not traditional in the Thai culture. Thais usually greet each other with the *"Wai"* motion—putting the palms of both hands together in a prayer-like gesture and bowing the head slightly. This gesture is used by both men and women of all age groups. Respect for older people, an important aspect of Thai culture, is always signaled by a younger person gesturing with the *"Wai"* to the older person first.

TEMPORAL RELATIONSHIPS

Traditional Thai families are nuclear in nature. Today, however, single families are becoming more common in Thailand. In any case, it is not uncommon for a single Thai to live with her or his sibling(s), cousin(s), aunt(s), uncle(s), grandparent(s), and/or parent(s). A friendship between two individuals who are not biologically related can often evolve into a family-like relationship. Thus, a Thai may become like a brother, a sister, an aunt, an uncle, a parent, or a grandparent to a friend.

As mentioned previously, respect for seniority is crucial among Thais. Visiting and bringing along a present or giving money to elders during the Thai New Year is an important role obligation for younger Thais. When the elders in a Thai family become too old to take care of themselves, younger members are morally required to care for them. Only in very rare circumstances do elderly Thais live alone.

FORMAT FOR NAMES

Most Thais have long first and last names. A Thai is usually referred to by her or his first name, even in an official setting like school or work. Their names usually have clear meanings. A first name is often given by a Buddhist monk or a fortune-teller based on the date, day of the week, and time of a newborn's birth. Sometimes, parents name their children themselves. When married, a woman usually uses her husband's last name. A couple's children also use their father's last name.

When Thai names are written in English, the spelling is merely a kind of phonetic translation from its real spelling in the Thai alphabet. Because Thai is a tonal language, the pronunciation of names cannot be ascertained from their spelling in English. For health-care providers in the West, the best course is to ask Thai clients how to pronounce their name and do the best one can in approximating it.

Importantly, almost all Thais have a short nickname used by their family and close friends and often by colleagues at work. A nickname normally has no relationship with the first name. They are often humorous to Thais themselves. Nicknames are usually either Thai or English words. They might be derived from names of colors, body types, fruits, or any number of other things. Health-care providers should feel free to ask their clients if they wish to be called by their nickname. The client may well prefer it.

Family Roles and Organization

HEAD OF HOUSEHOLD AND GENDER ROLES

Gender is another important aspect in Thai families. A man is the head of the household in a traditional Thai family, usually being the breadwinner and managing important tasks. This view is reflected in an elder's teaching on a wedding day: "The man is the front step of an elephant. The woman is the hind step."

In most Thai families, responsibilities involving household chores and taking care of children belong to a woman. If a woman works outside the home, a maid is sometimes hired to help with the household chores and babysitting. Many Thai men have much more leisure time than Thai women, regardless of the employment status of a woman. However, more Thai families today have begun to divide household chores between men and women.

PRESCRIPTIVE, RESTRICTIVE, AND TABOO BEHAVIORS FOR CHILDREN AND ADOLESCENTS

Thai children are taught to respect elders. Talking back to elders is discouraged. The role of children as students in school is very important. Many Thai parents choose a career deemed suited to their child's abilities and characteristics. The degree to which children assist with household chores depends upon a family's economic status; the poorer the family, the more chores children do.

Thai female adolescents have traditionally been expected to protect their virginity until marriage. Dating with a chaperone present is preferable to parents. However, more and more Thai adolescents date on their own today. Social attitudes are changing rapidly in Thailand, and those of the youth culture are strongly influenced by global trends related to music, entertainment, and social mores. These are often challenging to older traditions and can conflict with those inherited through Buddhist theology.

FAMILY GOALS AND PRIORITIES

Children are the center of the family for Thais (Fig. 21–2). Many Thai children, therefore, sleep with their parents from birth until some point in time before they reach adolescence. Thai parents do not feel comfortable leaving

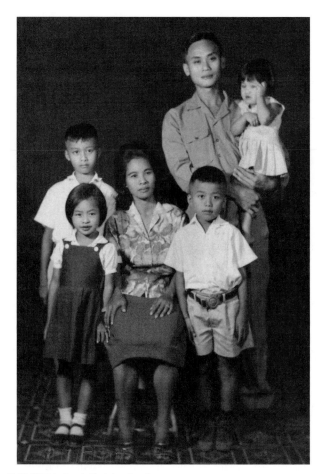

FIGURE 21–2 A Thai family photo.

their infants in a separate bedroom. Often, children are spoon-fed by adults until they are 6 to 7 years old. This can sometimes appear unusual to Westerners. Most Thai parents hope their children will go to college. They will pay whatever they can for tuition fees and support even through graduate school. Education is so vitally important for Thais that Westerners are often amazed when a Thai spouse will leave his or her partner or children behind for years to further studies aboard.

Marriages in Thailand used to be mainly arranged by the parents. Today, young Thais have more freedom to select a spouse. Nevertheless, sometimes parents may make the final decision as to whether or not a bride or groom is acceptable. However, in this context, younger Thais are clearly expected to care for older people, including older in-laws, when they are in need.

ALTERNATIVE LIFESTYLES

Gays and lesbians in Thailand are more accepted today than in the past. Before the mid 1980s, commercial lounges and bars were the main or the only places for gays and lesbians for social gatherings. Since the mid 1990s, Thai gays and lesbians have had more venues to meet and advance a positive lifestyle. These new places include launched boutiques, hotels, restaurants, karaoke clubs, pubs, and spas (Utopia, 2007).

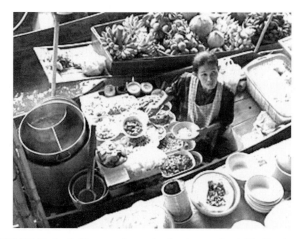

FIGURE 21–3 Selling noodles at the floating market in Thailand.

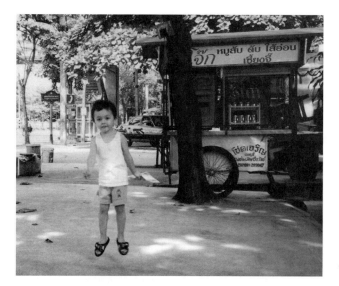

FIGURE 21–4 An interracial boy (American Thai) in front of a vendor's wagon in Thailand.

The first Thai lesbian organization was founded in Bangkok in 1986 by a popular Thai singer. Eight years later, the first Southeast Asian gay and lesbian center was established. The center is a resource for gays and lesbians to find books and presents. Both of the organizations have at least two common goals, which include a movement for lesbian and gay rights and efforts to combat HIV/AIDS (Utopia, 2007). At present, gay marriage is not supported by Thai laws.

Workforce Issues

CULTURE IN THE WORKFORCE

Most Thais usually try to avoid personal conflicts at work and are hard workers. Although the family is deemed very important for Thais, in many circumstances, especially for economic reasons, work comes before family (Fig. 21–3). For instance, a husband and his wife in Thailand often work in different provinces. A good number of the Thai couples reunite once a month. Taking a leave from work for a major surgery or a death or dying of family members besides one's spouse, child, or parent may not be supported by Thai agencies.

In general, Thai Americans tend to socialize among themselves rather than be exposed to Americans or peoples from other cultures. Therefore, Thai Americans may not deeply understand American culture. Language barriers often occur in the workplace. In order to help them adjust to an agency in the United States, an orientation program focusing on cultural differences may be helpful.

ISSUES RELATED TO AUTONOMY

Like many other American Asians, Thai Americans respect their supervisors because seniority is strongly valued in their culture. Thus, they might not be assertive at work. Therefore, supervisors may be wise to provide open discussions and expression of opportunities for their Thai American colleagues.

As mentioned previously, English proficiency among some Thais is low. Therefore, with Thai Americans who are learning English as their second language, the language used in the workplace should be clear. Slang expressions should be avoided. If used, slang expressions need to be clarified.

Biocultural Ecology

SKIN COLOR AND OTHER BIOLOGICAL VARIATIONS

An estimated 75 percent of the population in Thailand are pure "Thai"; 14 percent are Chinese; and the rest (11 percent) are Malay, Lao, Mon, Cambodian, Vietnamese, Asian Indian, Caucasian, or hill-dweller tribes—Karen, Lisu, Ahka, Lahu, Mien, and Hmong (Fig. 21–4) (CIA, 2006).

Some Thais in northeast Thailand (*Isaan*) emigrated from Laos or Cambodia. In general, *Isaan* Thais have darker skin color (dark brown) than other Thais who live in the north and central regions. The facial profile of *Isaan* Thais is akin to that of Laotians, with a relatively flat nose and broad prominent cheekbones (Fig. 21–5). Some Thais in the north immigrated to Thailand from China or Burma. They tend to have finer skin texture and lighter skin color than other Thais in the country. Their nose is a little longer and their cheekbones are narrower than those of *Isaan* Thais. Central Thais generally have medium skin color compared with that in the rest of the country. Their facial profile is a mixture of *Isaan* Thais and northern Thais. Southern Thais, some of whom migrated from Malaysia, are likely to have darker skin color. Their facial profile is similar to that of Malay.

Other Thais have combined Thai and Chinese, Vietnamese, Malaysian, Laotian, or other heritage, with skin color and facial profiles representing mixtures of such racial combinations. Overall, regardless of skin color or facial profile, the Thais' size and body structure are usually much smaller than those of Caucasians.

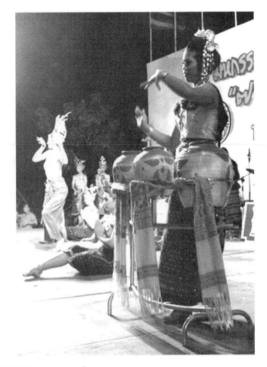

FIGURE 21–5   Isaan dance.

DISEASES AND HEALTH CONDITIONS

Thai scientists in collaboration with scientists from Riken Yokohama Institute in Japan and Yale University in the United States successfully identified a genetic pattern common to Thais by analyzing blood samples from 280 Thais from all four regions of the country (National Center for Genetic Engineering and Biotechnology [BIOTEC], 2006). This breakthrough, hopefully, will help scientists to better understand Thais' responses to a variety of antigens, drug metabolism, and genetic disorders.

Glucose-6-phosphate dehydrogenase deficiency (G6PD) is the most common genetic disorder among humans. Sixty-five percent of Thai newborns' jaundice is caused by this deficiency (Nuchprayoon, Sanpavat, & Nuchprayoon, 2002). Usually, the enzyme regulates how red blood cells function. When a person lacks the enzyme, her or his red blood cells can be hemolyzed by certain medications, foods, or infections. The condition is called "hemolytic anemia." In most cases, when the cause of the anemia is removed, symptoms disappear. In rare cases, people with G6PD deficiency have persistent anemia and need to be monitored on a regular basis (Nuchprayoon et al., 2002).

Thalassemia is another genetic disorder prevalent among Thais. Thirteen percent of Thais have inherited this disorder, and 50 percent of those who are affected by the disorder come from *Isaan,* or the northeast of Thailand (Fucharoen et al., 2006). Symptoms among Thais with Thalassemia range from asymptomatic to severe anemia (Fucharoen et al., 2006). When Thai patients show anemic symptoms, they should be tested for thalassemia and identified for care if necessary.

VARIATIONS IN DRUG METABOLISM

Different ethnic groups may have different pharmacokinetic functions (Bjornsson et al., 2003). Recent literature reporting some variations in drug metabolism between Thais and non-Thais is mostly associated with antiretroviral medications. For example, a study revealed that using indinavir/ritonavir dose (400 mg/100 mg) as a combined antiretroviral drug among Thais is more preferable than using indinavir/ritonavir dose (600 mg/100 mg) as used among Caucasians owing to the smaller body size of the Thais (Cressey et al., 2005). This lower-dose medicine results in fewer side effects and greater adherence for Thais than the higher-dose medicine. Although the lower-dose medication provided lower plasma concentrations among the Thai participants, low dose seems to be effective as evidenced by a suppression of viral replication through 48-week follow-ups (Cressey et al., 2005). Therefore, when treating Thai patients, dosing recommendations derived from Caucasian patients may not be appropriate. As a general rule, a lower dose may be more beneficial for Thais, possibly resulting in fewer severe side effects and greater adherence to the medications.

High-Risk Behaviors

HEALTH-CARE PRACTICES

The Thai Ministry of Public Health (2005) examined the most significant risk factors (during 2001–2004) negatively affecting the lives of Thai people. Results showed that unsafe sex (12.7 percent) is the leading factor, followed by smoking (6.9 percent), alcohol consumption (5.3 percent), hypertension (4.8 percent), nonuse of helmet while driving motorcycle/motorbike (4.2 percent), high body mass index (3.7 percent), illicit drug use (2.7 percent), high cholesterol (2 percent), inadequate vegetable and fruit consumption (1.5 percent), occupational injuries (1 percent), poor sanitation and malnutrition (1 percent), physical inactivity (1 percent), and pollution (0.8 percent).

As stated, unsafe sex is the number one health-behavior concern in Thailand. Because unsafe sex is related to high rates of HIV infection and AIDS in Thailand, information regarding these in connection with certain Thai sexual behaviors is presented in the next section.

HIV/AIDS

In September of 1984, the first patient with AIDS (a Thai gay man who studied in the United States and moved back to Thailand) was reported in Thailand. Since then, incidences of HIV infection have been reported throughout the country. HIV infection rates in Thailand peaked at 4 percent in 1991, with over 140,000 new cases in that year. Rates declined to 1.5 percent by 2003, partly due to the 100 percent condom use campaign promoted among high-risk groups by the Thai government (Ministry of Public Health, 2005).

In the past, high-risk groups included female commercial sex workers (CSWs) and injection drug users (IDUs). HIV-positive rates among Thai female CSWs climbed to over 33 percent in 1994 but fell to 4 to 8 percent in 2004, mainly due to the 100 percent condom use campaign (Sunthrajarn, Wongkongkateph, Onnom, & Amroncichet, 2005). The extent to which high-risk behavior among homosexual men played a part in the early spread of HIV and AIDS in Thailand is difficult to ascertain owing to a lack of reliable information. However, a recent survey revealed that 17 percent of gay men who did not frequent CSWs were HIV-positive (Cairns, 2004).

Thailand has been commended for its response to HIV/AIDS. However, Thailand has in large measure ignored the problems of HIV/AIDS among homosexual men. Adding complication, the problem is interrelated with Thailand's commercially successful male sex industry. Young male sex workers sell their services—negotiating with sex, condoms, work, and social stigma while living with the ever-present danger of an HIV infection (Mutchler, 2005). Today, the situation for gay men in Asian countries is similar to that in the West in the mid 1980s (Cairns, 2004).

Over 600,000 HIV-positive individuals live in Thailand, with over 20,000 new cases each year (Ratanasuwan, Anekthanoanom, Techasathit, Rongrungruang, Sonjai, & Suwanagool, 2005). More recently, over 80 percent of Thai HIV-positive individuals are 20 to 39 years old, and the ratio of males to females with HIV is 2:1, as opposed to 6:1 in the early 1990s (Sunthrajarn et al., 2005).

At present, the major route of HIV transmission in Thailand is through sexual activity (>85 percent in 2004). This is because many Thai males frequent female or male CSWs without using a condom (Centers for Disease Control and Prevention [CDC], 2006; Sunthrajarn et al., 2005). Even though prostitution is illegal in Thailand, the country has over 200,000 sex workers at any given point in time (Manopaiboon et al., 2003). Only 27 percent of Thai customers use a condom, whereas 52 percent of other Asian customers and 76 percent of Western customers use a condom when they visit female CSWs in Thailand (Buckingham & Meister, 2003).

Many men in Thailand have sex with women other than their wives (Sunthrajarn et al., 2005). A study revealed that 92 percent of Thai husbands had multiple sexual partners during the last 5 years of their marriage. Among the men in this study, approximate 85 percent had frequented female CSWs without using a condom. Over half of the wives were not aware of their husbands' promiscuity (Bennetts, Shaffer, Phophong, Chaiyakul, Mock, Neeyapun, et al., 1999). This pattern of sexual behavior among Thai men in Thailand may or may not be generalized to those living in the United States, Canada, or other countries in which cultural patterns are different.

Approximately 200,000 women and 1 to 2 percent of pregnant women in Thailand have contracted HIV (Joint United Nations Programme on HIV/AIDS, 2005; United Nations Children's Fund, 2005). Furthermore, one study reported that at least 80 percent of Thai pregnant women with HIV experience depression (Ross & Srisaeng, 2005). Only 76 percent of HIV-positive Thai pregnant women receive antiretroviral medications as mother-to-child transmission prophylaxis, whereas all HIV-positive pregnant women in the Unites States receive the medications if there is no contraindication (United Nations Children's Fund, 2005).

At present, newer and more prominently high-risk groups for contracting HIV include young Thai men who have sex with men, seafarers, amphetamine users, and drinkers (Sunthrajarn et al., 2005). More and more Thai youth have casual sex at a younger age. Since the mid 1980s in Thailand, the youngest age for first-time sexual intercourse has fallen from 16 to 9 years (Fongkaew, 2004). Moreover, a report shows that only 20 to 30 percent of sexually active young Thais use condoms consistently (United Nations Development Programme, 2004). Among Thai men who have sex with men, it is reported that 17.3 percent were HIV-positive in 2003 (Thanprasertsuk et al., 2005), but the rate went up to 28.3 percent in 2005 (CDC, 2006). Approximately 25 percent of these men also had sex with women without using condoms consistently (Thanprasertsuk et al., 2005).

Seafarers, highly mobile and working on boats far from land, have become a newly vulnerable group to contract HIV. Most of them are single, young Thai or immigrant (from Myanmar or Cambodia) men who stay out to sea for weeks or months at a time. When they return to land, they often drink heavily and have sex with female CSWs without condom use. Their HIV-positive rate is strikingly high at 15.5 percent (Entz, Ruffolo, Chinveschakitvanich, Soskolne, & van Griensven, 2000). After contracting sexually transmitted diseases, they tend to treat themselves by using over-the-counter medicine (Entz, Prachuabmoh, van Griensven, & Soskolne, 2001).

Amphetamine users and alcohol drinkers tend to have sex while they are high, which puts them at risk for having unsafe sex (Sunthrajarn et al., 2005). An estimated 600 million tablets of amphetamines are used annually in Thailand (Newton, Chierakul, Ruangveerayuth, Abhigantaphand, Looareesuwan, White, 2003). Thai names for amphetamines are *Yaa Bah* (literally means "crazy drug") or *Yaa Mah* (literally means "horse drug," from the horse emblem on the tablet) (Newton et al., 2003). The drug is usually taken by young people as a stimulant so that they can work for hours or days without feeling exhausted. An overuse of amphetamines can cause a person to be agitated and harm oneself or others. Withdrawal from amphetamine use generally leads to excessive sleeping and hypoglycemia (Newton et al., 2003).

Overall, incidences of HIV infection cause severe financial, physical, emotional, and social disruption for Thai patients and their families. The medical care cost for one HIV infection in Thailand is over U.S. $600 per family per year (Sunthrajarn et al., 2005). In perspective, the gross national income in Thailand is U.S. $440, as opposed to U.S. $43,740 in the United States (World Bank, 2006). The long-term burdens posed by high rates of HIV/AIDS among Thais need to be studied, especially at the community level.

For Thais, family and extended family members are all considered within the Thai culture as a *whole* unit. Thus, when any member in the greater family suffers from HIV/AIDS (or any other hardship/illness), it affects each and every member in the family. Moreover, every family member has a responsibility to support a suffering member, through either emotional, financial, or other tangible means (Ross, Sawatphanit, Suwansujarid, & Draucker, 2007). One family member's actions, whether negative or positive, belong to the whole family. The family's unique *oneness* in the Thai culture can work either positively or negatively for a Thai with HIV/AIDS. On the one hand, the concept of *oneness* can help to receive all kinds of support from one's family. For instance, the parents and siblings of sick persons are definitely expected to care for them. Also, maternal grandparents are expected to care for the sick person's child if the child's parents were to pass away owing to AIDS (Rende Taylor, 2005). On the other hand, the patient with HIV/AIDS can be abandoned owing to fears in the family of viral transmission and family disgrace (Bechtel & Apakupakul, 1999; Bennetts et al., 1999).

Studies show that when family support is not available, critical emotional support from nurses can save HIV-positive pregnant Thai women's lives and increase their self-esteem (Ross et al., 2007; Sawatphanit, Ross, & Suwansujarid, 2004). Therefore, health-care professionals should assess and offer emotional support for their Thai patients with HIV/AIDS, especially when family support for these patients does not exist.

SMOKING AND ALCOHOL CONSUMPTION

Smoking and alcohol consumption follow unsafe sex as the second and third most common risk factors found in the behavior of Thai people. Thailand has low smoking rates compared with those in other countries. From 1981 to 2004, smoking rates among Thais declined from 35.2 to 19.5 percent. Among Thai males, smoking rates fell from 63.2 to 37.2 percent, and among Thai females from 5.4 to 2.1 percent (Thailand Health Promotion Institute, 2006). These declining rates result from government campaigns that limit cigarette advertisements. Government campaigns also employ Thai celebrities as role models for nonsmoking (Ministry of Public Health, 2005).

Conversely, alcohol consumption has been an ever-increasing problem in Thailand. Alcohol consumption rates among adult Thais climbed from 26 percent in 1985 (Institute of Population and Social Research, 1985) to 32.7 percent in 2002 (Public Health Statistics, Ministry of Public Health, 2006). A report in 2003 showed that more than half of Thai drinkers consumed alcohol at least twice a week (Ministry of Public Health, 2005). The amount of alcohol consumed by Thais is found to be higher than that consumed by French, Americans, Japanese, and Filipinos.

In general, Thai men drink more alcohol than Thai women. Traditionally, Thai men have always used alcohol and smoked more than Thai women, in part due to different social expectations between men and women (Assanangkornchai, Conigrave, Saunders, 2002). Owing to factors such as globalization and the imitation of other cultures, such expectations have been changing. The number of Thai female drinkers rose from 1 percent in 1996 to over 5 percent in 2003.

The highest rates for drinking are found among young Thais, aged 15 to 24 years, one third of whom engage in drinking alcohol (Ministry of Public Health, 2005). One study found that the most common cause in the 1990s for first-time drinking among young Thais was peer pressure, followed by "wanting to try" and the socializing effects (Assanangkornchai et al., 2002). A more recent survey revealed that the number one factor causing young Thais to drink for the first time is socialization, followed by peer pressure and "wanting to try" (Ministry of Public Health, 2005).

Drinking is highly associated with road accidents around the world. In Thailand, over half of road accidents are caused by driving under the influence (DUI). In general, Thai rates for deaths from accidents are composed mostly of road accidents. The rate for deaths resulting from all accidents in 1984 was 5.74 deaths per 100,000 people. The rate had increased dramatically to 20.97 deaths per 100,000 people by 2002 (Ministry of Public Health, 2005).

The first law to specify a blood-alcohol limit for drivers in Thailand was passed several years ago, yet incidences of DUI continue to escalate (Ministry of Public Health, 2005). Clearly, there is a need for the Thai government to pass a stronger law that punishes drivers for incidences of DUI.

Nutrition

VIGNETTE 21.1

Boon, a 25 year-old Thai man, is seeing a doctor at a free mobile clinic in California. Boon came to the United States a few years ago and now works as a cook at a Thai restaurant. His English is broken, and it is hard for the doctor to understand him. The doctor calls a Thai nurse who lives in town to be an interpreter. Through the interpretations, the doctor learns that Boon has some pain in his abdomen. He comes from the northeastern region of Thailand, or Isaan; he loves to eat spicy food, especially Som-Tum, with fermented fish as one of the ingredients. Boon is worried about his liver because his father died in Thailand from liver cancer.

1. What additional information regarding his food intake should be obtained from Boon? Why?
2. How can the nurse tell whether Boon's pain is related to his stomach, his liver, or both?
3. How important is it to have a bilingual Thai-English interpreter at a clinic when a Thai American patient is not proficient in English?

MEANING OF FOOD

"We should eat to live, not live to eat" is a famous saying not only in Latin but also in Thai, reflecting the central importance and meaning of food in the Thai culture. Many Thais live their lives by following such a saying.

In general, an individual portion of a Thai dish is about one-third to one-fifth of a typical U.S. dish in terms of volume. As a result, most Thais are slim owing to these smaller portions and also the types of food they eat. Thais believe that foods containing adequate essential nutrients help to maintain life and growth and delay illness later in life (Kosulwat, 2002). A Thai balanced diet usually includes low-fat/low-meat dishes with a large percentage of vegetable and legumes. Rice and fish are main staples (Kosulwat, 2002).

COMMON FOODS AND FOOD RITUALS

In general, rice is the main source of carbohydrates in Thai dishes, but noodles are also found in many favorite recipes. Vegetables and meats are usually fried or grilled and prepared in many combined variations to supplement rice. Overall, pork or chicken is eaten more than beef. All meats are consumed more sparingly in proportion to vegetables when compared with a Western diet. Fish and other forms of seafood are also regularly enjoyed. Thailand has a long coastline, especially in the south, with an old and rich tradition of fishing as an important industry.

Communal eating is an essential part of the Thai culture. Friends and families eat seated together either on the floor or at a table. Either way, when rice is part of the meal, Thais will begin with a large amount of rice on their plates and reach to central communal plates of combined meat and vegetable recipes to add to their rice. This is done by all in a free fashion throughout the meal, with some families using a serving spoon to take from the communal dishes and others use their individual tablespoons. The tablespoons are the main instruments for eating, with the fork used only as a guide; knives are not often used because the meats in Thai recipes are usually precut. Noodle recipes are much loved by Thais and prepared with the noodles already mixed in with meats and vegetables.

For all foods, seasonings are critical to the Thai artistry of accommodating different palettes. Fish and oyster sauces are very often combined with soy sauce as a basic starting point for many recipes. Thai chili pepper is the basic ingredient added to control the degree of spiciness in foods. Many Thais love very spicy food, but not all. *Tom-Yum* is a traditional spicy Thai soup that is gaining popularity worldwide (Fig. 21–6). It has been found to have positive effects on people's health because of its ingredients, which include lemon grass, galangal roots,

kaffir lime leaves, hot chilies, red onions, and garlic (Siripongvutikorn, Thummaratwasik, & Huang, 2005). *Tom-Yum's* antioxidant effects are the result of the ingredients mentioned previously. The soup's antimicrobial effects come from its chilies, onions, and garlic (Siripongvutikorn et al., 2005). Onions and garlic can function against diabetes and hypercholesterolemia. Fresh garlic, used as an ingredient in *Som-Tum* and many other Thai dishes, has been identified as an antifungal, antiparasitic, and antiviral agent (Siripongvutikorn, Thummaratwasik, & Huang, 2005).

Som-Tum is a famous spicy Thai salad originating from the northeast of Thailand. Its ingredients include fresh shredded papaya, cut tomatoes, tamarind juice, fish sauce, salt, sugar, fresh crushed garlic, and hot chilies. Sometimes, cooked or raw fermented fish is added. *Som-Tum* is usually served with hot *sticky* (sweet) rice, which is a favorite in the Northeast. Sources of protein, such as Thai beef/pork jerky and grilled chicken are often served with *Som-Tum* and *sticky* rice. Overall, this course of *Som-Tum*, *sticky* rice, and sources of protein is considered an enjoyable delicacy by Thais in all areas of society.

In the past, many Thais became sick and died from eating raw fermented fish, which contains *Opisthorchis viverrini*, a liver fluke, found to cause cholangiocarcinoma in humans (Watanapa & Watanapa, 2002). Today, because of increased health education provided by nurses and other health professionals, Thais are more knowledgeable about the dangers of eating raw fish. Nevertheless, some Thais may persist in eating raw fermented fish because of entrenched eating habits and their attraction to its taste and smell. An assessment regarding any preference for eating raw fermented fish could be helpful.

A study conducted in Thailand revealed that many healthy Thai dishes are being replaced by foods containing a high quantity of fat and meat, related to the country's evolution from an agricultural to a newly industrialized country. Food produced in Thailand is now more important for exportation purposes and the economy than for domestic consumption (Kosulwat, 2002). Thai families have less time to cook. They tend to eat at Western-style restaurants serving foods high in fats, meat, and sugar content. As a result, obesity rates among Thai children and adults have risen dramatically since the mid 1980s (Kosulwat, 2002). A study revealed that Thai children with obesity have low self-esteem and are often ridiculed by their peers (Phakthoop & Ross, 2006).

In a study among 102 Thais in the United States, 79 percent changed their food intake habits when living in the United States (Siripongvutikorn et al., 2005). They skip more meals and consume more Western foods and snacks such as white bread, salty items, fruit juice, soft drinks, and sweets. When they dine out, they tend to go to American or Chinese restaurants. Forty percent of the participants indicated that their diet has become less healthy owing to a lack of time for food preparation and the unavailability of some Thai ingredients and/or food choices (Siripongvutikorn et al., 2005). An analysis of this study, as based on the Food Guide Pyramid, reveals that most Thai participants living in the United States consume enough fruits and vegetables; not enough bread and milk; and too much meat, fats, oils, and sweets. Health

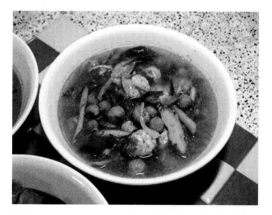

FIGURE 21–6   Tom-Yum Koong with lemon grass.

professionals in the United States should assess their Thai clients' food intake habits and encourage them to consume more fruits and vegetables. If needed, advice about an increase of bread and milk intake and limiting meat, fats, oils, and sweets should also be provided (Siripongvutikorn et al., 2005).

DIETARY PRACTICES FOR HEALTH PROMOTION

For Thais, hot or warm foods or drinks are considered healthier than cold ones. This idea is based in part on a belief in "cold and hot" or "Yin and Yang," inherited from Thailand's profound Chinese influence. Many types of herbs are considered to promote health and work against cancer development. Some herbs are considered a panacea. Therefore, Thai dishes usually contain some kind of herbs, particularly garlic and hot chilies. Positive effects of some herbs have already been described.

NUTRITIONAL DEFICIENCIES AND FOOD LIMITATIONS

Iodine deficiency (IDD) used to be a major health concern in Thailand. In 1953, IDD was first identified in the northeastern and northern regions of Thailand, where there is no sea outlet. Aware of the problem, in 1965, the Thai government initiated a pilot project of salt iodization in a northern province. Owing to its success, the project has been further expanded. The first IDD survey, conducted until 1988, was completed in 15 provinces of two regions of Thailand, showing an IDD prevalence rate of 19.3 percent. In 1993, the salt iodization project was expanded nationwide, resulting in further success with an IDD rate of 1.3 percent in 2003. At present, the Thai government examines goiter rates among school children in 15 northeast and northern provinces and uses them as the Thai IDD indicator (Ministry of Public Health, 2005).

Despite the salt iodization program success, at the 2004 Review of Progress towards Sustainable Elimination of Iodine Deficiency held in Thailand, the Thai Ministry of Public Health indicated that only 51 percent of Thai households consumed enough iodized salt (Network for Sustained Elimination of Iodine Deficiency, 2004). This is well below the international target of at least 90 percent set for the end of the year 2005. More than 34 million Thais do not ingest enough iodized salt, and 375,000 newborns may suffer from IDD. However, no evidence exists that the Thai Ministry of Industry and the U.S. Food and Drug Administration are working with salt producers in monitoring salt iodization activities (Network for Sustained Elimination of Iodine Deficiency, 2004).

In Thailand, only seven cases of anorexia nervosa have been reported (Jennings, Forbes, McDermott, Hulse, & Juniper, 2006). However, evidence exists that young Thais in particular are increasingly becoming susceptible to developing eating disorders. A study among 101 Thais in Thailand, 110 Caucasian Australians, and 130 Asian Australians found that the Thai participants reported the highest scores on eating disorder attitudes and psychopathology (Jennings et al., 2006). Recently, pressure to be thin has become more extreme in Thailand than in Australia. The evidence suggests that eating disorders may not be limited to Westerners, as we used to believe. Such disorders will become more prevalent among Thais in the near future.

Pregnancy and Childbearing Practices

FERTILITY PRACTICES AND VIEWS TOWARD PREGNANCY

Thai women view pregnancy as a special time in their lives when they need extra care physically and emotionally (Nigenda, Langer, Kuchisit, Romero, Rojas, Al-Osimy, et al., 2003). They acknowledge that this is a time when their moods can be unstable. Ideally, the age of 20 years is the optimal time for pregnancy owing to the women's physical and emotional maturity. Thai women want their husbands and their mothers to be supportive of their pregnancies. Some women state that the most common side effects of pregnancy are excessive white vaginal discharge, frequent urination, and morning sickness (Nigenda et al., 2003). Owing to modesty, especially during a vaginal examination, Thai women prefer female health-care providers over their male counterparts. They do not feel comfortable exposing their bodies to male providers (Nigenda et al., 2003).

PRESCRIPTIVE, RESTRICTIVE, AND TABOO PRACTICES IN THE CHILDBEARING FAMILY

VIGNETTE 21.2

Nin, a 35-year-old Thai, comes to the prenatal clinic. She shows a nurse a safety pin over her belly on her maternity cloth. She also states that postpartum, she will need to follow her mother's advice regarding beliefs of "hot" and "cold." When informed by her doctor about her gestational diabetes and hypertension diagnoses, Nin looks worried and states that she probably got the disorders from her "Karma."

1. What additional information should the nurse obtain from Nin regarding her "hot" and "cold" practices after delivery?
2. What should be the response of the nurse when Nin shows him or her the safety pin?
3. What should the nurse ask Nin about her belief in "Karma" and her illness?

The descriptions in this section are based on literature review and the authors' experience working with pregnant and postpartum Thai women. During the childbearing period, Thai women basically receive advice from their mothers about what to do or not do. Their mothers are the most significant persons who direct their practices during this time. Some of the practices presented herein are not stereotypical among all Thais; rather, they reflect some general practices or beliefs of some Thais in some particular areas of the country.

During pregnancy, the mothers of some pregnant Thai women may discourage their daughters from particular practices or behavior. For example, pregnant women are advised not to complain or get upset so that newborns will be happy and stay happy for the rest of their lives. They may also be advised not to sit on stairs or doorsills to avoid a difficult labor and delivery. When a pregnant mother blocks other people from going up and down stairs or in and out of a doorway, the unborn baby could be blocked inside the mother's uterus.

Astrology and animism play major roles in many Thais' lives. In general, Thai pregnant women are discouraged from visiting a hospitalized person (regardless of the kind of sickness), attending a funeral ceremony, or visiting a house where there has been a death (Kaewsarn, Moyle, & Creedy, 2003b). Such practices are believed to prevent the pregnant woman and her unborn baby from catching any illness or getting haunted by a spirit or ghost.

In northeast Thailand, some women believe that eating eggs may result in having smelly newborns (Nigenda et al., 2003). Some avoid drinking coconut juice, believing that it can cause too much vernix caseosa (fat on the newborn's skin), whereas others drink a lot of the juice, believing that it will help their newborns to have smooth and beautiful skin texture. Some believe that drinking chocolate milk, eating chocolate, or drinking coffee will cause their newborns to have a darker skin color. Most Thais view lighter skin as more favorable.

Pregnant women from the central region of Thailand are often seen with a safety pin on their outfit over their belly. The pin works against a kind of ghost who always wants to steal the unborn baby from a mother's womb. Also, pregnant Thai women, especially those with Chinese descendents and their families, may ask their obstetric physicians to perform selective cesarean sections, believing that the date and time of their babies' births can greatly affect their children's future as based on the Chinese Zodiac calendar and fortune-telling (Ross et al., 2007).

Like many other Southeast Asian women, postpartum Thai mothers practice the concept of "Yin" and "Yang" (cold and hot) (Kaewsarn, Moyle, & Creedy, 2003a). After a child is born, the mother is left cold and wet. Therefore, the mother should gain some heat to dry out her body, especially her uterus (Kaewsarn et al., 2003a). To gain heat, some Thai mothers practice *Yue Fai*, which literally means "being with fire." There are a couple of ways to perform *Yue Fai*. The new mother lies down either on a bed above a bonfire or on a wooden plank nearby. The fire is tended for as long as the mother is supposed to be near the fire, which may be from 1 to 30 days. Reasons given by Thai mothers for practicing *Yue Fai* include desiring an increase of milk, faster involution of the uterus, and illness and bone ache prevention (Kaewsarn et al., 2003a). Some drawbacks of this ritual, however, include inconvenience, discomfort, and complications, such as heat rashes, sweating, dehydration, and/or minor burns (Kaewsarn et al., 2003a). To be able to perform *Yue Fai*, space is needed and a family member must keep tending the fire. Without enough space and a 24/7 support person, *Yue Fai* is not possible.

When *Yue Fai*, the ultimate practice for gaining heat during the postpartum period, is not possible, Thai moth-

ers are advised by their mothers and/or nurses to use a combination of practices, including a perineal heat light, a hot Sitz bath, sauna heat belts, and warm showers (Kaewsarn et al., 2003a). Warm/hot drinks and foods are consumed; ice chips or ice cubes are avoided.

In general, all Thai mothers are allowed by their mothers to drink warm/hot nonalcoholic liquids. However, there is no consensus about the types of protein, vegetable, and fruit the postpartum mothers should consume. Whereas some mothers are encouraged to eat certain food items, others are not (Kaewsarn et al., 2003a). Many postpartum Thai women are not restricted to proteins, vegetables, and fruit, but some are.

Sources of protein include pork, chicken, fish, eggs, milk, catfish, internal organs, beef, water buffalo meat, and shrimp (Kaewsarn et al., 2003a). However, some mothers might be advised to not eat eggs, chicken, or buffalo meat, believing that the new mothers' perineum may not heal. On many occasions, the first author has heard the mothers of postpartum Thai mothers' give their reason as to why chicken is a taboo food for women after delivery: They stated that usually a chicken likes to scratch the ground to look for food. The chicken meat, therefore, could scratch open the perineum.

Eggs are avoided by some mothers, believing that they could cause a big scar on the perineum. Water buffalo meat is tough and cheap and, therefore, seen as unhealthy by Thais. Based on this belief, it is thought that the healing process of the new mother's perineum could be jeopardized by its consumption.

Vegetables eaten by postpartum mothers may include lettuce, banana flower, lemon grass, onion, ginger, cabbage, hairy melon, snake beans, chili, peppers, and bamboo shoots (Kaewsarn et al., 2003a). Acceptable fruits after the postpartum period may include oranges, bananas, tamarind, watermelon, jack fruit, and durian, an oval fruit with a hard spiny rind (Fig. 21–7). However, some women avoid durian because of its strong smell. For traditional Thai families, especially those from rural Thailand, the new mother might be restricted to a few items of food for the first few weeks. For example, she might be allowed to take only rice soup with salt without any protein or fruit. Some postpartum Thai women drink

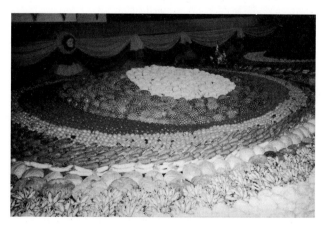

FIGURE 21–7 Beautiful Thai fruits at a commencement ceremony.

Ya Dong, a Thai nonalcoholic or alcoholic drink infused with herbs. Herbs used in *Ya Dong* may include ginseng, galangal, peppermint, cinnamon, spirulina, and plant roots. As perceived by many Thais, *Ya Dong* is famous for its medicinal qualities. When used by postpartum women, the drink helps with blood production and drying out the uterus quickly.

Death Rituals

DEATH RITUALS AND EXPECTATIONS

Because most Thais are Buddhists, only the funeral rites in connection with Buddhism are addressed here. Like other Buddhists, Thai Buddhists believe that after a person dies, the person will be reborn somewhere else based on that person's *Karma* (Dhammanada, 2002). "*Karma* means 'action' and . . . refers to the process by which a person's moral behavior or actions have consequences for the person's future, either in the present or later life" (Ross et al., 2007, p. 4).

In general, Thai Buddhists follow the custom of cremating the bodies of the deceased because, when the Buddha passed away, his body was cremated. According to the Buddha's teaching, a funeral ceremony should be simple. Unfortunately, many Thai Buddhists (and some other Buddhists) have transformed what was a traditionally simple cremation ceremony into one that is overly extravagant.

"The consciousness or mental energy of the departed person has no connection with the body left behind . . . . A dead body is simply an old rotten simple house which the departed person's life occupied. The Buddha called it 'a useless log.' Many people believe that if the deceased is not given a proper burial or if a sanctified tombstone is not placed on the grave, then the soul of the deceased will wander to the four corners of the world and weep and wail and sometimes even return to disturb the relatives. Such a belief cannot be found in Buddhism" (Dhammanada, 2002, p. 246).

In the funeral ceremony, often Buddhist monks are invited to chant verses to the dead and the family (Fig. 21–8). Food and candles are offered to the monks. Many

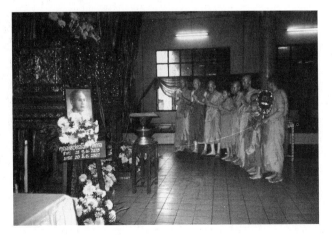

FIGURE 21–8   A Buddhist funeral.

Thai Buddhists believe that such chanting will benefit the spirit of the dead, regardless of Buddha's teaching about the unbound relationship between the body and the spirit. The ashes from the cremation are buried at a cemetery. Sometimes, a portion of the ashes is sprinkled in a river. If possible, when the family of the dead returns home after a sojourn away from Thailand, some of the ashes may be sprinkled again in a river or near the deceased's hometown.

RESPONSES TO DEATH AND GRIEF

During the funeral ceremony, the family gets together. The sons of the deceased are expected to be ordained for a short period of time, ranging from a week to 3 months. The ordination is believed to help the dead go to heaven. Female relatives normally wail quietly. The family members pray quietly to the dead before the cremation to ask for forgiveness and wish the dead to be reborn in a happy and peaceful home. Often, in their prayer, family members wish for themselves to be reborn in the same family with the same relation to the dead in their next life.

Spirituality

DOMINANT RELIGION AND USE OF PRAYER

Approximately 95 percent of the Thais are Buddhist; the rest are Muslim (4.6 percent), Christian (0.7 percent), and Hindu or other (0.1 percent) (CIA, 2006). In the United States, over three million people are Buddhist, most coming from Asian countries, including Thailand (Eck, 2001). Buddhism is an exceptionally tolerant religion with its roots in Hinduism. Although precepts grounded in Buddhism (as discussed later) are fundamental to the spiritual make-up of most Thais, animistic beliefs generally have equal meaning for them and play a parallel role in their belief system.

Although not in agreement with all other religious beliefs, Thai Buddhists are free to incorporate any other religious values and/or animism to their beliefs and practices when deemed good. Most Thais in all socioeconomic strata to some degree incorporate animism, fortune-telling, and astrology. Studies have shown that ancient spirits are prayed to by many Thai patients (or their caregivers) and fortune-telling plays a major role in how Thais deal with illnesses (Ross et al., 2007; Rungreangkulkij & Chesla, 2002).

Many families in Thailand have a *spirit house* where they believe that the ancient spirits of the land (*Pra Poom*) dwell: Two little statues of the *Pra Poom* (one male and one female) are placed inside a unique little abode that rests on a post or column. This house is usually at least as high as the eye level of an adult so as to indicate the respect of the family for the *Pra Poom.* Their abode can be either very simple or quite decorative, depending upon how much the family can afford, and faces either north or east (in the belief that these two directions are superior to the south and west). Miniature figures of a couple of horses and elephants are often placed in front of the *Pra Poom* figures to accompany them. Fresh flowers, food, and drink are placed in tiny plates, bowls, and cups as offerings. These may be placed everyday, or about once a month. The family members pray to the *Pra Poom* as often as they wish. Usually, the family prays and gives offerings to the *Pra Poom* more often when asking for blessings and faster healing of an ill family member.

MEANING OF LIFE AND INDIVIDUAL SOURCES OF STRENGTH

For most Thais, family support along with Buddhism is a crucial source of strength. In the Thai culture, parents are obliged to care for their ill children, regardless of a child's age or type of illness (Rungreangkulkij & Chesla, 2002; Sunthrajarn et al., 2005). Children or the unborn babies of HIV-positive pregnant Thai women have been identified as a major source of strength for their mothers (Jirapaet, 2001; Ross et al., 2007).

In a study among Thai mothers of schizophrenic adult children, the mothers practiced "Thum-jai" as a way to cope with a situation perceived to be unchangeable (Rungreangkulkij & Chesla, 2002). *Thum-jai* means "let it be" or "whatever will be, will be." By practicing *Thum-jai*, a person will be able to accept the reality of a challenge or problem and try to move on in his or her life with calmness and peace. The mothers in Rungreangkulkij and Chesla's study (2002) stated that when their sick children misbehaved, they smoothed their own heart with "water." For the Thai, a metaphor of "water versus fire" indicates "calmness versus anger/frustration." The "fire" should be put out by "water" in a person's heart to defeat a crisis situation. The mothers in this study offered that calmness and gentle speech usually worked better than scolding in calming down their schizophrenic children (Rungreangkulkij & Chesla, 2002).

SPIRITUAL BELIEFS AND HEALTH-CARE PRACTICES

Buddhism significantly pervades the life of many Thais (Burnard & Naiyapattana, 2004). When coping with difficulties or illnesses, many Thai lay people and health-care professionals follow Buddha's teaching (Ross et al., 2007; Sunthrajarn et al., 2005). Like most Buddhists, the ultimate goal for a Buddhist Thai is to reach *Nirvana*. This is the end of reincarnation or the cycle of rebirths. When there is no rebirth, there is no suffering. Either they are happy or suffering. "Peace" is the ultimate goal (Dhammanada, 2002). Results from a study reflect this belief by reporting that the ultimate goal of HIV-positive postpartum Thai women (alongside goals for their children) is to live with their HIV infection in peace. The women thus stated that they followed the Buddha's teachings through their beliefs in *Karma*, the *Five Precepts*, and the *Four Noble Truths* in order to live in peace with HIV (Ross et al., 2007).

As mentioned earlier, *Karma* is strongly associated with belief about rebirth. Many Thai patients (or caregivers) believe that unwholesome *Karma* from their past life has caused them to become ill in the present life. They believe that the illness can be improved by following the *Five Precepts* so that their present or next life (or the lives of

their loved ones) will be improved (Ross et al., 2007). Merit making—a way to decrease selfishness and greed and a way to be hopeful for a better present and future life—is performed by many Thais. Merit making includes activities such as freeing animals or birds, donating money to the poor or temple, offering food to monks, and tangibly helping those in need, emotionally, or financially (Ross et al., 2007; Tongprateep, 2000).

The *Five Precepts* are comparable with half of the Christian *Ten Commandments* and stress abstinence from killing, stealing, lying, sexual misconduct, and illicit drugs and alcohol consumption (Smith, 1994). A study with seven HIV-positive postpartum Buddhist Thai women revealed that the participants all decided to carry their pregnancies to term instead of ending them. They all stated that ending a pregnancy is a type of killing, which is considered a sin. Furthermore, all of the women in this study believed that such unwholesome action would follow them in their next reincarnation as bad *Karma* (Ross et al., 2007). In another study, it was found that the *Five Precepts* are observed by older Thai people to help them feel happy and peaceful (Tongprateep, 2000).

The *Four Noble Truths* reflect tenets about life, suffering, and the cessation of suffering. *The First Noble Truth* maintains that life is suffering, and that suffering as such is found in four unavoidable life moments; namely birth, illness, aging, and death. *The Second Noble Truth* maintains that the cause of all suffering is *Tanha,* or personal desire. *The Third Noble Truth* is a belief that overcoming *Tanha* is attainable. *The Fourth Noble Truth* outlines paths to end suffering (Smith, 1994).

A qualitative study reported that the *Four Noble Truths* were followed by HIV-positive pregnant Thai women to cope with their infection (Ross et al., 2007). The women stated that they began dealing with their illness by accepting the truth that everyone dies anyway at some point in life (*The First Noble Truth*) and that their suffering came from their personal desire (*The Second Noble Truth*). In other words, their desire arose by thinking of themselves as a real existence in the world rather than as an illusion. "Self" is like a mirage, or an imagined being (Flanagan, 2005). Therefore, when a person becomes selfless, the person is freed from suffering (Smith, 1994). The women in the study tried to think that their body and soul were not theirs, but instead imagined elements. To overcome desire, the participants tried to focus on universal life (*The Third Noble Truth*) by thinking about their infants instead of themselves and by meditating and praying. They also tried to follow the *Middle Way*, or a path between the two extremes of self-pleasure and self-mortification (Dhammanada, 2002), as a means to end their suffering. In accordance with the Buddha's teaching that any extremes of thoughts, behavior, or speech are not wholesome, they reported trying not to feel too badly about themselves in order to be peaceful.

Meditation and prayer are ways for many Thais to cope with an illness. Studies revealed that both Thai pregnant and nonpregnant women meditated and prayed to the Buddha and supreme beings in order to help them cope with HIV/AIDS (Dane, 2000; Jirapaet, 2001; Ross et al., 2007). Meditation is a means for Thai older people to enhance their self-awareness, peace of mind, sleep, and physical health (Tongprateep, 2000). For Thai older people in the United States, meditation and prayer also help them feel peaceful, perceive life as valuable, value tranquil relationships with family and friends, and experience meaning and confidence in death. For Thais, health and spirituality are intertwined and are important aspects of life (Pincharoen & Congdon, 2003).

In conclusion, the spiritual concepts of *Karma, Nirvana,* the *Five Precepts,* the *Middle Way,* and the *Four Noble Truths* are all important for Buddhist Thais. Ideally, when health professionals in the United States are aware of Buddhist concepts in caring for their sick or healthy Thai clients, the quality of care can be significantly enhanced.

Health-Care Practices

⊙── VIGNETTE 21.3

Wan, a 60-year-old married Buddhist Thai American, diagnosed with cervical cancer, has been coming to a hospital for chemotherapy since her diagnosis. Today, Wan is being admitted to the hospital for the therapy. While Wan's nurse is entering her room, Wan is closing her eyes with the palms of her hands put together and facing a little Buddha image she brought with her from home.

1. If you were the nurse, what would you do at that moment?
2. What additional information would you want to get from Wan in terms of her Buddha image in relation to her illness?
3. Identify a culturally related mental health problem for Wan related to her illness.
4. Identify helpful culturally congruent interventions regarding Wan's spiritual beliefs.

HEALTH-SEEKING BELIEFS AND BEHAVIORS

In Thailand, most Thais rely on government health-care facilities, especially in the northeast region, or *Isaan*. People in *Isaan* hold strong traditional beliefs and practices. They tend to be poorer and less educated than the rest of the country. In the *Isaan* area, statistical rates of gynecological problems are relatively low, yet, *Isaan* women's self-reports show high rates of gynecological complaints associated with vaginal discharge and pain "in the uterus" (Boonmongkon, Nichter, & Pylypa, 2001). This contrast is often explained by a lack of comprehension among some *Isaan* women who do not understand clearly the physiological changes of their menstrual cycle and the amount of vaginal discharge. Some of the pain "in the uterus" with which they are concerned may well be related to physiological pain during ovulation.

Boonmongkon and colleagues (2001) reported that *Isaan* women's complaints and concerns about vaginal discharge and pain in the uterus may have an extreme impact on their lives. The women believe that such problems will turn into cervical cancer. This belief causes them to visit health-care facilities often, self-treat by relying on small doses of inappropriate antibiotics, be unhappy with their sexual relationship with their husband, and suffer from worries of their "ailments" (Boonmongkon et al., 2001).

Most *Isaan* women in Boonmongkon and colleagues' study (2001) believed that their sustaining problems of vaginal discharge and pain "in the uterus" stemmed from their inappropriate practices after postpartum or significant past events. For instance, over 25 percent of the women stated that their chronic symptoms resulted from their inadequate practices of "lying by fire" and this caused their uterus to stay wet. Examples of other past experiences that the women believed caused their sustaining gynecological problems include hard work in youth, abortion, pushing too hard during delivery, and sterilization. Some women in the study indicated that they did not receive adequate information about their problems from health professionals but did not feel like asking questions for fear of being scolded. Therefore, U.S. health-care professionals should bear in mind that Thai women, especially from *Isaan,* may need more information regarding physiological changes related to their menstrual cycle and may need encouragement to ask any questions they have regarding their gynecological concerns.

RESPONSIBILITY FOR HEALTH CARE

Health promotion and disease prevention behavior among the Thais is very limited. Although all Thais are covered by some kind of health insurance, including the Universal Coverage of Health Care Scheme (75-cent health care), only 5.3 percent of the population used health promotion services, which include immunization, prenatal care, family planning, postpartum care, yearly check-ups, dental care, and some other services (Ministry of Public Health, 2005). Among those who did use such services, one-third went to urban health centers, 28.7 percent to community hospitals, and 11.3 percent to general/regional hospitals. One-third of the services used were yearly check-ups and one-third included immunization (Ministry of Public Health, 2005).

FOLK AND TRADITIONAL PRACTICES

Folk practices are common among less educated, rural Thais. Many Thais believe that bad *Karma* and/or negative supernatural power causes mental illness. Therefore, folk therapies from traditional healers are the first resource for many Thai families. When such therapies do not seem to work, they go to contemporary medical facilities as their second resource. Folk therapies may include healing ceremonies, using shamans (as a mediator) to converse with supernatural beings (such as black magic, evil beings, and/or ancient/natural spirits), negotiating with them that the sick person might be released from their illness. In such ceremonies, holy water or oil is usually used to anoint the sick (Rungreangkulkij & Chesla, 2003).

Khwan is a Thai concept about the "power inside," or the "life spirit." Thais believe that *Khwan* enters the newborn's anterior fontanel during delivery. *Khwan* is different from self-esteem; it is thought of as a "life force" that can vanish when people are in a stage of shock, mental illness, or far away from home (Burnard & Naiyapattana, 2004). In a *Khwan* ceremony, fresh flowers are offered by the sick or the person who has lost her or his *Khwan*. A monk or an older person then ties a blessed white thin string around a person's wrist, believing that the blessed string will tie the *Khawn* again to the person's body (Burnard & Naiyapattana, 2004).

BARRIERS TO HEALTH CARE

For Buddhists, when one is too extreme in one's speech, thoughts, or behavior, it is considered unwholesome, as based on their belief in the *Middle Way* (Dhammanada, 2002). In this sense, some Buddhist Thais may not seek health care until their symptoms become severe. In addition, stigmatization attached to mental illness and beliefs in animism and *Karma* tend to prevent some Thais from seeking professional help when mental health problems arise. Some may not seek assistance from health-care professionals until they realize that traditional healers, Shamans, cannot help them (Rungreangkulkij & Chesla, 2003).

CULTURAL RESPONSES TO HEALTH AND ILLNESS

Adhering to their belief in the *Middle Way*, many Thais may appear stoic in trying to withhold expressions of pain or suffering from their illness. Health-care professionals may need to rely more on nonverbal clues for pain or some psychological-emotional distress when assessing their Buddhist Thai patients.

Many Thais, and even some health professionals, equate depression with psychosis (Ross et al., 2007). Thus, when clinical depression is diagnosed, health-care professionals should make extra efforts to encourage depressed Thai patients to get help and treatment, along with assuring them that depression and psychosis are different disorders.

BLOOD TRANSFUSION AND ORGAN DONATION

No religious beliefs against blood transfusion exist for Thais. However, donating and receiving organs is another matter. Although acceptable among many Thais, belief in their rebirth might prevent some from donating their organs, believing that they might not have the organ when needed in the next life.

Health-Care Practitioners

TRADITIONAL VERSUS BIOMEDICAL PRACTITIONER

Like Hindus, Thais in the United States and elsewhere tend to consult their family and friends first when they feel ill or have medical problems. Thai women usually seek female practitioners for childbearing care and gynecological problems owing to their modesty and their culture. However, if female practitioners are not available, they are generally willing to accept male practitioners. Traditional healers, or Shamans, in relation to Thai patients are discussed earlier.

STATUS OF HEALTH-CARE PROVIDERS

Respect for seniority is a strong cultural value among Thais. Thus, less-experienced health professionals in

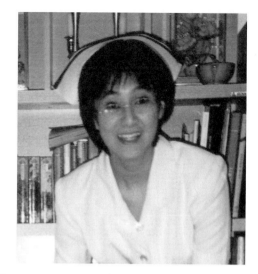

FIGURE 21–9   A nurse in a Thai nursing uniform.

Thailand are expected to respect those with more experience in the same profession. In general, when comparing physicians, head nurses, and junior nurses, Thai physicians receive the most respect, followed by the head nurses and junior nurses (Fig. 21–9). In some cases, very senior head nurses receive the same level of respect as physicians (Burnard & Naiyapatana, 2004).

Based on a concept of "Thainess" as expressed by many Thais, and especially in terms of being Buddhist, Thai nurses reported that they often incorporate Buddhist ideas and beliefs in caring for their chronically ill patients (Burnard & Naiyapattana, 2004; Sawatphanit et al., 2004).

Like many other patients in developing countries (Withell, 2000), some Thai patients, especially those with lower socioeconomic status, are typically passive in voicing their needs and requesting care and services from health-care providers (Jirapaet, 2001). Therefore, health professionals, in North America or elsewhere, are advised to evaluate the level of passivity among their Thai patients so that their needs can be addressed with an eye toward optimal quality care.

REFERENCES

Assanangkornchai, S., Conigrave, K. M., & Saunders, J. B. (2002). Religious beliefs and practice, and alcohol use in Thai men. *Alcohol and Alcoholism, 37*(2), 193–197.

Bao, J. (2005). Merit-making capitalism: Re-territorializing Thai Buddhism in Silicon Valley, California. *Journal of Asian American Studies, 8*(2), 115–142.

Bechtel, G. A., & Apakupakul, N. (1999). AIDS in southern Thailand: Stories of *krengjai* and social connections. *Journal of Advanced Nursing, 29*(2), 471–475.

Bennetts, A., Shaffer, N., Phophong, P., Chaiyakul, P., Mock, P. A., Neeyapun, K., Bhadrakom, C., & Mastro, T. D. (1999). Differences in sexual behavior between HIV-infected pregnant women and their husbands in Bangkok, Thailand. *AIDS Care, 11*, 649–661.

Bjornsson T. D., Wagner, J. A., Donahue, S. R., Harper, D., Karim, A., & Khouri, M. S. (2003). A review and assessment of potential sources of ethnic differences in drug responsiveness. *Journal of Clinical Pharmacology, 43*, 943–967.

Boonmongkon, P., Nichter, M., & Pylypa, J. (2001). *Mot Luuk* problems in northeast Thailand: Why women's health concerns matter as much as disease rates. *Social Science & Medicine, 53,* 1095–1112.

Buckingham, R., & Meister, E. (2003). Condom utilization among female sex workers in Thailand: Assessing the value of the health belief model. *California Journal of Health Promotion, 4*(4), 18–23.

Burnard, P., & Naiyapatana, W. (2004). Culture and communication in Thai nursing: a report of an ethnographic study. *International Journal of Nursing Studies, 41*(7), 755–765.

Cairns, G. (2004). *Gay HIV increases—Local or Global?* Retrieved January 25, 2007, from http://www.iasociety.org/bangkok/mainpage.aspx?pageId=288

Centers for Disease Control and Prevention. (2006). HIV prevalence among populations of men who have sex with men—Thailand, 2003 and 2005. *MMWR Morb Mortal Wkly Rep, 55*(31), 844–848.

CIA. (2006). *The World Factbook: Thailand.* Retrieved January 4, 2007, from https://www.cia.gov/cia/publications/factbook/print/th.html

Cressey, T. R., Leenasirimakul, P., Jourdain, G., Tod, M., Sukrakanchana, P., Kunkeaw, S., Puttimit, C., Tod, M., Jourdain, G., & Lallemant, M. J. (2005). Low-doses of indinavir boosted with ritonavir in HIV-infected Thai patients: Pharmacokinetics, efficacy and tolerability. *Journal of Antimicrobial Chemotherapy, 55*(6), 1041–1044.

Dane, B. (2000). Thai women: Meditation as a way to cope with AIDS. *Journal of Religion and Health, 39,* 5–21.

Dhammanada, K. S. (2002). *What Buddhists believe.* Kuala Lumpur, Malaysia: Buddhist Missionary Society Malaysia.

Eck, D. L. (2001). *A new religious America.* Retrieved December 28, 2006, from http://usinfo.state.gov/journals/itdhr/1101/ijde/eck.htm

Entz, A., Prachuabmoh, V., van Griensven, F., & Soskolne, V. (2001). STD history, self treatment, and healthcare behaviours among fishermen in the Gulf of Thailand and the Andaman Sea. *Sexually Transmitted Diseases, 77,* 436–440.

Entz, A., Ruffolo, V., Chinveschakitvanich, V, Soskolne, V., & van Griensven, G. J. P. (2000). HIV-1 prevalence, HIV-1 subtype and risk factors among fishermen in the Gulf of Thailand and the Andaman Sea. *AIDS, 14,* 1027–1034.

Flanagan, A. (2005). *Buddhism.* Retrieved November 10, 2006, from http://buddhism.about.com/cs/ethics/a/BasicsKama.htm

Fongkaew, W. (2004). *Love and sex in Thai adolescents.* Bangkok, Thailand: Beyond Enterprise.

Fucharoen, G., Trithipsombat, J., Sirithawee, S., Yamsri, S., Changtrakul, Y., Sanchaisuriya, K., & Fuchareaon, S. (2006). Molecular and hematological profiles of hemoglobin EE disease with different forms of α-thalassemia. *Annals of Hematology, 85*(7), 450–454.

Hoare, T. D. (2004). *Thailand: A global study handbook.* Santa Barbara, CA: ABC CLIO.

Institute of Population and Social Research. (1985). Retrieved September 27, 2007, from http://www.ipss.go.jp

Jennings, P. S., Forbes, D., McDermott, B., Hulse, G., & Juniper, S. (2006). Eating disorder attitudes and psychopathology in Caucasian Australian, Asian Australian and Thai university students. *Australian and New Zealand Journal of Psychiatry, 40*(2), 143–149.

Jirapaet, V. (2001). Factors affecting maternal role attainment among low-income, Thai, HIV-positive mothers. *Journal of Transcultural Nursing, 12,* 25–33.

Joint United Nations Programme on HIV/AIDS. (2005). *Uniting the world against AIDS: Thailand.* Retrieved on January 30, 2007, from http://www.unaids.org/en/Regions_Countries/Countries/thailand.asp

Kaewsarn, P., Moyle, W., & Creedy, D. (2003a). Thai nurses' beliefs about breastfeeding and postpartum practices. *Journal of Clinical Nursing, 12,* 467–475.

Kaewsarn, P., Moyle, W., & Creedy, D. (2003b). Traditional postpartum practices among Thai women. *Journal of Advanced Nursing, 41,* 358–366.

Kosulwat, V. (2002). The nutrition and health transition in Thailand. *Public Health Nutrition, 5*(1A), 183–189.

Manopaiboon, C., Bunnell, R. E., Kilmarx, P. H., Chaikummao, S., Limpakarnjanarat, K., & Supawitkul, S. (2003). Leaving sex work: Barriers, facilitating factors and consequences for female sex workers in northern Thailand. *AIDS Care, 15,* 39–52.

Ministry of Public Health. (2005). *Thailand health profile 2001–2004.* Bangkok, Thailand: Printing Press, Express Transportation Organization.

Mutchler, M. G. (2005). Money-Boys in Thailand: Sex, work, and stigma. *Journal of HIV/AIDS Prevention in Children & Youth, 6*(1), 121–128.

National Center for Genetic Engineering and Biotechnology. (2005). Gene sequence of Thais identified. Retrieved January 11, 2007, from international.biotec.or.th/documents/newsOnGAPs.pdf

Network for Sustained Elimination of Iodine Deficiency. (2004). Optimal iodine nutrition in the Americas. Retrieved January 10, 2007, from http://206.191.51.240/About_Ameet_Thai.htm

Newton, P. N., Chierakul, W., Ruangveerayuth, R., Abhigantaphand, D., Looareesuwan, S., & White, N. J. (2003). Malaria and amphetamine "horse tablets" in Thailand. *Tropical Medicine & International Health, 8*(1), 17–18.

Nigenda, G., Langer, A., Kuchisit, C, Romero, M., Rojas, G., & Al-Osimy M. (2003). Women's opinions on antenatal care in developing countries: Results of a study in Cuba, Thailand, Saudi Arabia and Argentina. *BMC Public Health, 3*(17). Retrieved January 30, 2007 from http://www.biomedcentral.com/1471-2458/3/17.

Nuchprayoon, I., Sanpavat, S., & Nuchprayoon, S. (2002). Glucose-6-phosphate dehydrogenase (G6PD) mutations in Thailand: G6PD Viangchan (871G>A) is the most common deficiency variant in the Thai population. *Human Mutation, 19*(2), 185.

Pincharoen, S., & Congdon, J. (2003). Spirituality and health in older Thai persons in the United States. *Western Journal of Nursing Research, 25*(1), 93–108.

Phakthoop, M., & Ross, R. (2006). Antecedents, consequences, and management of obesity: A descriptive qualitative study among obese children in Chonburi Province. *The Journal of the Faculty of Nursing, Burapha University, 14,* 34–48.

Public Health Statistics, Ministry of Public Health. (2006). *Thai health statistics.* Retrieved January 8, 2007, from http://web.nso.go.th/eng/ en/indicators/health_e.htm

Ratanasuwan, W., Anekthanoanom, T., Techasathit, W., Rongrungruang, Y., Sonjai, A., & Suwanagool, S. (2005). Estimated economic losses of hospitalized AIDS patients at Siriraj Hospital from January 2003 to December 2003: Time for aggressive voluntary counseling and HIV testing. *Journal of the Medical Association of Thailand, 88*(3), 335–339.

Rende Taylor, L. (2005). Patterns of child fosterage in rural northern Thailand. *Journal of Biosocial Science, 37*(3), 333–350.

Ross, R., Sawatphanit, W., Suwansujarid, T., & Draucker, C. B. (2007). Life story and depression of an HIV-positive, pregnant Thai woman who was a former sex worker: Case study. *Archives of Psychiatric Nursing, 21*(1), 32–39.

Ross, R., & Srisaeng, P. (2005, November 12). *Depression and its correlates among HIV-positive, pregnant women in Thailand.* An abstract presented at the 38th Sigma Theta Tau International Conference, Indianapolis.

Rungreangkulkij, S. & Chesla, C. (2002). Smooth a heart with water: Thai mothers care for a child with schizophrenia. *Archives of Psychiatric Nursing, 15,* 120–127.

Sawatphanit, W., Ross, R., & Suwansujarid, T. (2004). Development of self-esteem among HIV positive pregnant women in Thailand: Action research. *Journal of Science, Technology, and Humanities, 2*(2), 55–69.

Siripongvutikorn, S., Thummaratwasik, P., & Huang, Y. (2005). Antimicrobial and antioxidation effects of Thai seasoning, Tom-Yum. *Society of Food Science and Technology, 38,* 347–352.

Smith, H. (1994). *The illustrated world's religions: A guide to our wisdom traditions.* San Francisco: HarperCollins.

Sunthrajarn, T., Wongkongkateph, S., Onnom, C., & Amornwichet, P. (2005). *Health promotion: The challenge in the prevention control of HIV/AIDS.* Retrieved January 4, 2007, from http://www.anamai.moph.go.th/6thglobal/06_HPromotion.pdf.

Thailand Health Promotion Institute. (2006). *Smoking habit of the population.* Retrieved September 27, 2007, from http://www.thpinhf.org/smoking_habit_of_the_population.pdf

Thailand Investor Service Center. (2004). About Thailand: About education. Retrieved January 21, 2007, from http://www.thailandoutlook.com/thailandoutlook1/about+thailand/education/

Thanprasertsuk, S., Sirivongrangson, P., Ungchusak, K., Jommaroeng, R., Siriprapasiri, T., Phanuphak, P., et al. (2005). The invisibility of the HIV epidemic among men who have sex with men in Bangkok, Thailand. *AIDS, 19*(16), 1932–1933.

Thongprateep, T. (2000). The essential elements of spirituality among rural Thai elders. *Journal of Advanced Nursing, 31,* 197–203.

UNAIDS/WHO. (2005). *AIDS Epidemic Update-December 2005.* Geneva: Author.

United Nations Children's Fund. (2005). *The nation profile: Thailand.* Retrieved January 30, 2007 from http://lcweb2.loc.gov/frd/cs/profiles/Thailand.pdf.

United Nations Development Programme. (2004). *Report on the global AIDS epidemic.* Retrieved December 15, 2006 from http://www.unaids.org/bangkok2004/GAR2004_html/GAR2004_00_en.htm

U.S. Census Bureau—2000. Retrieved July 3, 2007, from www.census.gov/main/www/cen2000.html

U.S. Census Bureau—2006. Retrieved July 3, 2007, from quickfacts.census.gov/qfd/states/00000.html

Utopia. (2007). *Travel and resources: Thailand.* Retrieved January 25, 2007, from http://www.utopia-asia.com/tipsthai.htm

Watanapa, P., & Watanapa, W. B. (2002). Liver fluke-associated cholangiocarcinoma. *The British Journal of Surgery, 89,* 962–970.

Wikipedia. (2006). *Thai American.* Retrieved January 15, 2007, from http://en.wikipedia.org/wiki/Thai_American.

Withell, B. (2000). A study of the experiences of women living with HIV/AIDS in Uganda. *International Journal of Palliative Nursing, 6,* 234–244.

World Bank. (2006). *GNI per capita 2005.* Retrieved January 5, 2007 from http://siteresources.worldbank.org/DATASTATISTICS/Resources/GNIPC.pdf.

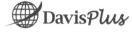 **DavisPlus**

For case studies, review questions, and additional information, go to http://davisplus.fadavis.com

Appendix

Cultural, Ethnic, and Racial Diseases and Illnesses

Causes are grouped into three categories, genetic, lifestyle, and environment.

Lifestyle causes include cultural practices and behaviors that can generally be controlled: for example, smoking, diet, and stress.

Environment causes refer to the external environment (e.g., air and water pollution) and situations over which the individual has little or no control over (e.g., presence of malarial mosquitos, exposure to chemicals and pesticides, access to care, and associated diseases).

Cultural/Racial Group	Diseases/Disorders	Causes
Black Populations	Sickle cell disease	Genetic, environment
	Hypertension	Genetic, lifestyle
	Systemic lupus erythematosus	Genetic with an environmental trigger
	Diabetes mellitus	Genetic, lifestyle
	Glaucoma	Genetic
	Cardiovascular disease	Genetic, environment, lifestyle
	Lung, colon, and rectal cancer	Environment and lifestyle
	Prostate cancer	Genetic, environment
	Lead poisoning	Environment
	Asthma	Environment and lifestyle
	HIV/AIDS	Lifestyle
	Hemoglobin C disease	Genetic
	Hereditary persistence of hemoglobin F	Genetic
	Glucose-6-phosphate dehydrogenase deficiency	Genetic
	β-Thalassemia	Genetic
	HAITIANS	
	Malaria	Environment
	Tuberculosis	Lifestyle, environment
	Diabetes mellitus	Genetic, environment, lifestyle
	Hypertension	Genetic, lifestyle
	KENYANS	
	Nasopharyngeal cancer	Lifestyle
	Esophageal cancer	Lifestyle, environment?

Cultural/Racial Group	Diseases/Disorders	Causes
	ZAIRIANS & UGANDANS	
	Stomach cancer	Lifestyle
	Duodenal ulcers	Unknown
	ZIMBABWEANS	
	Stomach cancer	Lifestyle
	SUB-SAHARAN AFRICANS	
	Liver cancer	Environment
	100 DEGREES NORTH AND SOUTH OF THE EQUATOR	
	Burkitt lymphoma	Environment
Hispanics	Lactase deficiency	Genetic
	Diabetes mellitus	Genetic, lifestyle, environment
	Cleft lip/palate	Lifestyle
	Dental caries	Lifestyle, environment
	Cardiovascular disease	Genetic, environment, lifestyle
	Tuberculosis	Environment, lifestyle
	Hypertension	Genetic, environment, lifestyle
	COSTA RICANS	
	Malignant osteoporosis	Environment? Genetic?
	PUERTO RICANS	
	Cardiovascular disease	Genetic, environment, lifestyle
	Hypertension	Genetic, environment, lifestyle
	Dengue fever	Environment
	Breast cancer	Genetic, lifestyle
	Prostate cancer	Genetic, environment, lifestyle
Arabs/Middle Easterners	Familial Mediterranean fever	Genetic
	Familial paroxysmal polyserositis	Genetic
	Tuberculosis	Environment, lifestyle
	Malaria	Genetic, environment
	Trachoma	Environment, lifestyle
	Typhoid fever	Environment
	Glucose-6-phosphate dehydrogenase deficiency	Genetic
	Sickle cell disease	Genetic, environment
	Thalassemia	Genetic
	Hepatitis A and B	Environment, lifestyle
	Schistosomiasis (bilharzia)	Environment, lifestyle
	Familial hypercholesterolemia	Genetic, lifestyle
	IRANIANS	
	Dubin-Johnson syndrome	Genetic
	Epilepsy	Genetic
	IRAQIS	
	Ichthyosis vulgaris	Genetic
	YEMENIS	
	Phenylketonuria	Genetic
	Glucose-6-phosphate dehydrogenase deficiency	Genetic
	LEBANESE	
	Dyggve-Melchior-Clausen syndrome	Genetic
	Familial hypercholesterolemia	Genetic
	EGYPTIANS	
	Schistosomiasis	Lifestyle, environment
	Trachoma	Environment, lifestyle
	Typhoid fever	Environment
	Tuberculosis	Lifestyle, environment
	β-Thalassemia	Genetic

Cultural/Racial Group	Diseases/Disorders	Causes
	SAUDI ARABIANS	
	Metachromatic leukodystrophy	Genetic
Asian/Pacific Islanders	CHINESE	
	α-Thalassemia	Genetic
	Glucose-6-phosphate dehydrogenase deficiency	Genetic
	Lactase deficiency	Genetic
	Nasopharyngeal cancer	Environment, lifestyle
	Liver cancer	Environment, lifestyle
	Stomach cancer	Unknown, lifestyle and/or environment
	Cardiovascular disease	Genetic, lifestyle, environment
	Hepatitis B	Genetic, lifestyle, environment
	Tuberculosis	Environment, lifestyle
	Diabetes mellitus	Genetic, lifestyle, environment
	JAPANESE	
	Vogt-Koyanagi-Harada syndrome	Genetic
	Cardiovascular disease	Genetic, lifestyle, environment
	Asthma	Lifestyle, environment
	Takayasu disease	Genetic
	Acatalasemia	Genetic
	Cleft lip/palate	Lifestyle, genetic
	Oguchi disease	Genetic
	Lactase deficiency	Environment, lifestyle
	Stomach cancer	Genetic, lifestyle, environment
	Hypertension	Genetic, lifestyle, environment
	ASIAN INDIANS	
	Cancer of the cheek	Lifestyle
	Ichthyosis vulgaris	Genetic
	Tuberculosis	Lifestyle, environment
	Malaria	Environment
	Rheumatic heart disease	Environment
	Cardiovascular disease	Genetic, lifestyle, environment
	Sickle cell disease	Genetic
	FILIPINOS	
	Diabetes mellitus	Genetic, environment, lifestyle
	Hyperuricemia	Lifestyle
	Cardiovascular disease	Genetic, lifestyle, environment
	Hypertension	Genetic, lifestyle, environment
	Thalassemia	Genetic
	Glucose-6-phosphate dehydrogenase deficiency	Genetic
	THAILANDERS	
	Glucose-6-phosphate dehydrogenase deficiency	Genetic
	Thalassemia	Genetic
	Lactase deficiency	Genetic
	VIETNAMESE	
	Nasopharyngeal cancer	Lifestyle, environment
	Lactase deficiency	Genetic
	Post-traumatic stress disorder	Environment
	Tuberculosis	Lifestyle, environment
	Malaria	Environment
	Hepatitis B	Environment, lifestyle
	Melioidosis	Environment, lifestyle
	Paragonimiasis	Environment, lifestyle
	Leprosy	Genetic

Cultural/Racial Group	Diseases/Disorders	Causes
	HMONGS & LAOTIANS	
	Nasopharyngeal cancer	Lifestyle, environment
	Lactase deficiency	Genetic
	Tuberculosis	Environment, lifestyle
	Hepatitis B	Genetic, environment, lifestyle
	KOREANS	
	Stomach cancer	Lifestyle
	Liver cancer	Genetic, environment
	Hypertension	Genetic, lifestyle, environment
	Schistosomiasis	Environment, lifestyle
	Hepatitis A and B	Environment, lifestyle
	Lactase deficiency	Genetic
	Osteoporosis	Genetic, lifestyle
	Peptic ulcer disease	Lifestyle, environment
	Lactose intolerance	Genetic
	Tuberculosis	Environment and lifestyle
	Astestosis	Environment
	Insulin autoimmune deficiency disease	Genetic
	Renal failure	Lifestyle
European American Ethnic White Populations	Skin cancer	Environment, lifestyle
	Appendicitis	Unknown
	Diverticular disease	Lifestyle, genetic?
	Colon cancer	Lifestyle, genetic?
	Hemorrhoids	Lifestyle, unknown
	Cardiovascular disease	Genetic, lifestyle, environment
	Varicose veins	Genetic
	Diabetes mellitus	Genetic, lifestyle
	Multiple sclerosis	Environment
	Obesity	Lifestyle
	ENGLISH	
	Cystic fibrosis	Genetic
	Hereditary amyloidosis, type III	Genetic
	Rosacea	Genetic
	FRENCH CANADIANS	
	Sickle cell disease	Genetic, environment
	Osteoporosis	Lifestyle, genetic
	Osteoarthritis	Genetic
	Cardiovascular disease	Genetic, lifestyle, environment
	Lung cancer	Environment, lifestyle
	Breast cancer	Genetic, lifestyle
	Cystic fibrosis	Genetic
	Phenylketonuria	Genetic
	Tyrosinemia	Genetic
	Morquio syndrome	Genetic
	Familial hypercholesterolemia	Genetic, lifestyle
	Breast and ovarian cancer	Genetic, environment
	Spastic ataxia Charlevoix-Saguenay type	Genetic
	Cytochrome lipase deficiency	Genetic
	Phenylketonuria	Genetic
	GERMANS	
	Myotonic muscular dystrophy	Genetic
	Hereditary hemochromatosis	Genetic
	Sarcoidosis	Genetic, environment
	Dupuytren's disease	Genetic

Cultural/Racial Group	Diseases/Disorders	Causes
	Peyronie's disease	Genetic
	Cholelithiasis	Genetic, lifestyle
	Stomach cancer	Genetic, lifestyle, environment
	Cystic fibrosis	Genetic
	Hemophilia	Genetic
GREEKS		
	Tay-Sachs disease	Genetic
	Cardiovascular disease	Genetic, environment, lifestyle
	Malaria	Environment
	Tuberculosis	Environment, lifestyle
	Glucose-6-phosphate dehydrogenase deficiency	Genetic
	Hepatitis A and B	Environment, lifestyle
FINLANDERS		
	Stomach cancer	Lifestyle, environment
	Congenital nephrosis	Genetic
	Generalized amyloidosis, type V	Genetic
	Polycystic liver disease	Genetic
	Retinoschisis	Genetic
	Aspartylglycosaminuria	Genetic
	Diastrophic dwarfism	Genetic
	Choroideremia	Genetic
ITALIANS		
	Vogt-Koyanagi-Harada syndrome	Genetic
	β-Thalassemia	Genetic
	Recurrent polyserositis	Genetic
	Hypertension	Lifestyle, genetic
	Nasopharyngeal cancer	Lifestyle
	Stomach cancer	Lifestyle
	Liver cancer	Lifestyle
	Familial Mediterranean fever	Genetic
	Glucose-6-phosphate dehydrogenase deficiency	Genetic
JEWS		
	Lactase deficiency	Genetic
	Werdnig-Hoffmann disease	Genetic
	Mucolipidosis IV	Genetic
	Phenylketonuria	Genetic
	Kaposi sarcoma	Genetic
	Gaucher disease	Genetic
	Niemann-Pick disease	Genetic
	Tay-Sachs disease	Genetic
	Riley-Day syndrome	Genetic
	Torsion dystonia	Genetic
	Factor XI plasma thromboplastin antecedent (PTA) deficiency	Genetic
	Cystinuria	Genetic
	Ataxia-telangiectasia	Genetic
	Familial Mediterranean fever	Genetic
	Metachromatic leukodystrophy	Genetic, unknown
	Bloom syndrome	Genetic, lifestyle
	Myopia	Genetic, lifestyle
	Polycythemia vera	Genetic
	Hypercholesterolemia	Genetic
	Breast cancer	Environment, lifestyle
	Diabetes mellitus	Genetic, lifestyle, environment

Cultural/Racial Group	Diseases/Disorders	Causes
	POLES	
	Phenylketonuria	Environment
	Respiratory diseases	Environment, lifestyle
	Cardiovascular diseases	Lifestyle
	APPALACHIANS	
	Black lung	Environment, lifestyle
	Emphysema	Unknown, environment, lifestyle
	Tuberculosis	Genetic, lifestyle, environment
	Hypochromic anemia	Environment, lifestyle
	Cardiovascular disease	Genetic, lifestyle
	Sudden infant death syndrome	Genetic
	Diabetes mellitus	Genetic
	Otitis media	Lifestyle
	SCANDINAVIANS	
	Cholelithiasis	Genetic, lifestyle
	Sjögren-Larsson syndrome	Genetic
	Krabbe disease	Genetic, environment, lifestyle
	Phenylketonuria	Genetic
	IRISH	
	Phenylketonuria	Genetic
	Neural tube defects	Genetic
	Cardiovascular disease	Genetic
	Alcoholism	Genetic, environment, lifestyle
	Skin cancer	Genetic
	AMISH	
	Limb-girdle muscular dystrophy	Genetic
	Ellis–van Creveld syndrome	Genetic
	Dwarfism	Genetic, unknown
	Polydactylism	Genetic
	Cartilage hair hypoplasia	Genetic
	Phenylketonuria	Genetic
	Glutaric aciduria	Genetic
	Manic-depressive disorder	Genetic
	Pyruvate kinase deficiency	Genetic
	Hemophilia B	Genetic
	RUSSIANS	
	Alcoholism	Lifestyle, genetic, environment
	Hypertension	Lifestyle, environment
	Pulmonary disorders	Lifestyle, environment
	Hyperlipidemia	Lifestyle, genetic
	Diabetes mellitus	Lifestyle, genetic
	Depression	Lifestyle, environment
	Gastrointestinal disorders	Lifestyle
Native Americans/ Alaskan Natives	Diabetes mellitus	Genetic, lifestyle, environment
	Cholelithiasis	Lifestyle
	Lactase deficiency	Genetic
	Liver disease	Environment, lifestyle
	Hepatitis B	Environment, lifestyle
	Nasopharyngeal cancer	Environment, lifestyle
	Tuberculosis	Environment, lifestyle
	Alcoholism	Lifestyle, genetic

Cultural/Racial Group	Diseases/Disorders	Causes
	NAVAJOS	
	Ear anomalies	Genetic
	Arthritis	Genetic
	Severe combined immunodeficiency syndrome	Genetic
	Navajo neuropathy	Genetic
	Albinism	Genetic
	Tuberculosis	Environment, lifestyle
	HOPIS	
	Tyrosinase-positive albinism	Genetic
	Trachoma	Environment, lifestyle
	PUEBLOS	
	Albinism	Genetic
	ZUNIS	
	Tyrosinase-positive albinism	Genetic
	ESKIMOS	
	Hereditary amyloidosis	Genetic
	Congenital adrenal hyperplasia	Genetic
	Methemoglobinemia	Genetic
	Lactase deficiency	Genetic
	Pseudocholinesterase deficiency	Genetic
	Haemophilus influenza type B	Genetic?
TURKS	Sickle cell	Genetic, environment
	Goiter	Genetic, environment
	Helminthiasis	Environment, lifestyle
	Behçet's disease	Genetic
	Thalassemias	Genetic
	Lactase deficiency	Genetic
	Tuberculosis	Environment, lifestyle
	Cardiovascular disease	Genetic, lifestyle
	Diabetes mellitus	Genetic, lifestyle

Abstracts

People of Baltic Heritage: Estonians, Latvians, and Lithuanians

RAUDA GELAZIS

The Baltic countries today are democratic, growing economically, and successful when compared with many other former Soviet Union countries where poverty and dictatorships have been predominant. All three Baltic countries have established strong ties to Western democratic countries and have been accepted into the North Atlantic Treaty Organization (NATO) and the European Union. Since the mid-1990s, the Baltic countries have experienced a "brain drain" to some extent, because many of their highly educated people have emigrated to the United States and Europe.

People of Baltic descent share thoughts and feelings readily. The stereotype of quiet, stoic individuals is not borne out by observation or research. Older individuals from these cultural groups are generally first-generation Americans or immigrants who came to the United States after World War II. Many individuals are not as acculturated as younger people and often prefer to speak their own languages. Health-care professionals need to be sure that any instructions given to these patients are well understood. The father or father figure is the head of the household in the typical family of Baltic heritage, although both men and women in the family may have jobs and discuss major decisions. Health-care and other major decisions are often made jointly by both spouses. Because both spouses tend to work, child care may be shared by grandparents and should be included in health teaching.

People of Baltic descent adapt readily to American values of timeliness in the workplace. Most have no difficulty maintaining their sense of autonomy and readily assume work roles and responsibility for decision-making. They usually do not like to directly confront those in authority and find ways to deal with difficult situations or people through the use of humor or deference. Recent immigrants who have lived under the Soviet regime may not be accustomed to making decisions for themselves or acting autonomously, and this must be considered when they are hired.

Recent immigrants from Estonia, Latvia, and Lithuania may be at risk for cancer because of the current industrial pollution, including radiation exposure resulting from the Chernobyl nuclear disaster in 1988. Some immigrants are survivors of political torture, having spent years in prison labor camps in Siberia. When performing health assessments, health-care providers need to be alert to ill health resulting from the conditions that immigrants endured because of the political situations in their countries of origin.

Americans of Baltic descent are health conscious and believe that a well-balanced lifestyle maintains health and well-being. For example, well-being among Lithuanian Americans is typically described as a holistic concept—that is, a state of being in which the person's physical, spiritual, psychological, and social health are in balance. Moderation is perceived as desirable for living a healthy life. Natural foods are preferred, and whenever possible, vegetables and fruits are homegrown.

Americans of Baltic descent use modern Western medicine practices, are likely to obtain early prenatal medical care, and are likely to be receptive to health teaching for prenatal and postnatal care. Because they prefer natural processes, some women and families prefer natural childbirth and breastfeeding.

Grief is expressed by sadness, crying, and talking about the deceased with fondness and respect. Emotions are readily expressed but not in highly dramatic ways. Decorum is maintained in public and with strangers.

Estonian Americans and Latvian Americans are predominantly Lutherans but include some Catholics. Lithuanian Americans are predominantly Roman Catholic. Most Americans of Baltic descent consider prayer an individual expression of their faith. The nurse or health-care professional should allow the client and family to take the lead with regard to prayer. Because prayer is individualized, some patients welcome time for individual or shared prayer, whereas others do not wish to pray. Many have been sustained through hardships by their strong religious faith and continue to have strong religious needs. Clients find considerable comfort in speaking with the clergy in times of crises and serious illness.

Some stigma is attached to mental illness, but medical care is sought. The family encourages compliance with prescription medications and treatments. Most people of Baltic descent accept physical handicaps, mental illness, and mental retardation. The family usually cares for the individual at home. The community is also supportive. Americans of Baltic descent do not enjoy the sick role and avoid it when possible. People of Baltic descent are used to both men and women giving direct physical care. Physicians in the Baltic countries may be female. Health-care practitioners need to provide for privacy and consider the modesty needs of female and male clients of these cultures as they would for any client.

People of Brazilian Heritage

MARGA SIMON COLER

Brazilians are a mixture of Portuguese, French, Dutch, German, Italian, Japanese, Chinese, African, Arab, and native Brazilian Indians. Information about Brazilian culture is unidentifiable in the professional health-care literature, which tends to incorporate Brazilians into aggregate data on Hispanics. Most Brazilians in the United States are concentrated in communities around Boston; New York; Newark, New Jersey; and Miami.

Portuguese is the official language of Brazil and continues to dominate the Brazilian communities in the United States. Brazilians, in general, are not punctual, arriving late—from minutes to hours—especially for social occasions. However, those in professional circles are punctual. Health-care providers may need to carefully explain the necessity of showing up on time for health appointments.

Gender roles vary according to socioeconomic class and education. Brazilian society is one of *machismo*, with the middle and upper classes being patriarchal in structure. As women assert their equality, more-egalitarian relationships are becoming evident. However, lower-socioeconomic households tend to be more matriarchal in nature. Godparents are a very important family extension to Brazilians. Poor families frequently ask their *patron* or *patrona* (employer and his wife) to be godparents to their child. Godparent responsibilities include clothing, schooling, and caring for the child in case of the parents' death. Health-care providers need to be nonjudgmental regarding Brazilian family decision-making patterns.

Brazilians value diplomacy over honesty, as shown in their tendency to promise to attend to something the next day, knowing that it will be impossible. This is due in part to their fatalistic beliefs and in part to the need to save face. Most Brazilians in the workforce show up for work on time and generally respect authority. They are more comfortable in employment situations in which rules and job specifications are well-defined. Brazilians often have a lesser sense of responsibility than is seen in the dominant American culture. When educated people believe that they can do something more efficiently, they are apt not to ask permission from their supervisor to do what they believe is required to complete the job.

Specific diseases related to the regional topography and climate of Brazil include dengue fever, meningitis, rabies, and yellow fever. In addition, Chagas' disease, schistosomiasis, typhoid fever, Hansen's disease, hepatitis, and tuberculosis are present in various parts of Brazil. Because intestinal worms are common in Brazilian immigrants, parasitic diseases should be considered during health assessments.

The undocumented status of Brazilian immigrants places them at a high risk for nonassimilation into the culture of the community in which they live. Brazilians in America have become vitamin- and health food–conscious. The preference, especially among young Brazilian women, is to rely on vitamins instead of a heavy diet to help them remain thin. Undocumented Brazilians who are here to earn fast money may experience malnutrition.

Brazilian immigrants generally practice birth control so that pregnancy will not interfere with their reason for leaving Brazil. At times, single women become pregnant to facilitate their chance of remaining permanently in their new country. This opportunity is greatly enhanced if the child is born in the United States and has been able to attend school. Many restrictions are related to pregnancy. Women are encouraged not to do heavy work or swim. Taboos also warn against having sexual relations during pregnancy. During pregnancy, some foods are to be avoided and other specific foods are recommended.

The meaning of life is found in religion, economy, fatalism, and reality. The greatest source of strength for Brazilians is their immediate and extended families. Tradition and folk religion are other sources of strength.

Most Brazilians do not talk about their illnesses unless these are very serious. Generally, illness is discussed only within the family. Many Brazilians feel that talking about an illness such as cancer negatively influences their condition. Because many Brazilians tend to shun hospitals, when they are hospitalized, their families accompany them and stay around the clock. Brazilian families are eager to participate in patient care and, thus, can be taught various procedures and care activities.

Responses to death and grief depend on the family. To a poor family, a continuously suffering person is rescued. The fatalistic expression, "It was God's will," helps the grieving among the rich and the poor. Older people wear black for various lengths of time depending on the relationship of the family member. Frequently, the final portrait is hung in the family *chaper* or near the family altar, and prayers are recited. An eternal light burns.

The Brazilian culture is rich in folk practices that depend on geographic region, ethnic background, socioeconomic factors, and generation. Traditional and homeopathic pharmacies are supplemented by *remedios populares* (folk medicines) and *remedios caseiros* (home medicines). Health-care providers need to specifically ask about their use. Brazilians generally do not like to talk about pain. However, once the emotional barrier is removed, they feel relieved to be able to discuss their discomfort. Many pain-relieving medicines are available without a prescription in Brazil. Frequently, a person requiring these on a regular basis will request that friends or friends of friends bring a supply from Brazil.

The folk-health field has many types of health-care practitioners for Brazilians. *Curandeiros* are divinely gifted; *rezadeiras* (praying women) help exorcise an illness; *card readers* can predict fortunes; *espiritualistas* are able to summon souls and spirits; *conselheiros* are counselors or advisors; and *catimbozeiros* are sorcerers. All have the power to heal their believers. Health-care providers need to specifically ask Brazilian clients about their use of folk healers and the treatments prescribed.

People of Greek Ancestry

IRENA PAPADOPOULOS and LARRY D. PURNELL

The Greek and Greek Cypriot diaspora is of considerable size and is spread to all continents and numerous countries. The largest Greek community outside Greece is in America, whereas the largest Greek Cypriot community outside Greece is in Britain. The characteristics of Greek and Greek Cypriot communities vary considerably according to the time of immigration; rural, island, or urban residence; and other primary and secondary characteristics of culture.

Despite considerable temporal and geographic variation, several core themes are common to people who retain affiliation with a Greek community: emphasis on family, honor, religion, education, and Greek heritage. The core values of honor, respect, and shame are key when considering the experience of Greeks and Greek Cypriots. Because Greeks and Greek Cypriots value warmth, expressiveness, and spontaneity, northern Europeans are often viewed as "cold" and lacking compassion. Eye contact is generally direct, and speaking and sitting distances are closer than those of other European Americans. Whereas innermost feelings such as anxiety or depression are often shielded from outsiders, anger is expressed freely, sometimes to the discomfort of those from less-expressive groups. Thus, health-care providers must not take personal offense with verbal and nonverbal communication practices that are different from theirs.

Greek children are included in most family social activities and tend not to be left with babysitters. The child may be disciplined through teasing, which is thought to "toughen" children and make them highly conscious of public opinion. Providers must interpret these child-rearing practices within their cultural context.

Treatment of older people reflects the themes of closeness and respect within the family. Grandparents tend to participate fully in family activities. Families feel responsible to care for their parents in old age, and children are expected to take in widowed parents. Failure to do so results in a sense of dishonor for the son and guilt for the daughter. Health-care providers need to thoroughly assess the family beliefs when considering long-term care.

In regard to the workforce, probably no single characteristic applies so completely to members of the Greek and Greek Cypriot communities as the emphasis on self-reliance within a family context. Greeks and Greek Cypriots in North America, Britain, Australia, and Sweden stress this trait, seen as reluctance to be told what to do and given as a major reason for their pattern of establishing their own businesses as soon as possible.

Two important genetic conditions, thalassemia and glucose-6-phosphate dehydrogenase (G-6-PD), are seen in relatively high proportions among Greek populations. Drugs such as aspirin, primaquine, quinidine, thiazolsulfone, dapsone, furzolidone, nitrofural, naphthalene, toluidine blue, phenylhydrazine, and chloramphenicol can induce a hemolytic crisis. This threat is sufficiently severe that the World Health Organization recommends that all hospital populations in areas with high proportions of Greeks and Greek Cypriots be screened for G-6-PD deficiency before drug therapy is offered.

Fasting is an integral part of the Greek Orthodox religion. General fast days are Wednesdays and Fridays; nowadays, these are observed only by some older people. Greek Orthodox wishing to take Holy Communion observe at least 3 days of fasting. However, people with health conditions and small children are exempt from fasting. The prevalence of lactose maldigestion among Greek adults is about 75 percent; however, milk intolerance is rarely seen in children. Health-care providers should use this knowledge when counseling clients with these conditions.

If a pregnant woman remarks that a food smells good, or if she has a craving for a particular food, it should be offered to her; otherwise the child may be "marked." This is the usual explanation for birthmarks.

After a death in the Greek community, pictures and mirrors may be turned over. During a wake, women may sing dirges or chant. In some regions, people practice "screaming the dead," in which they cry a lament, the *miroloyi*. This ritual may involve screaming, lamenting, and sobbing by female kin. After death, family and close relatives, who stay at home, mourn for 40 days. Close male relatives do not shave, as a mark of respect.

The Greek Orthodox religion emphasizes faith rather than specific tenets. Easter is considered the most important of holy days, and nearly all Greeks and Greek Cypriots in America and Britain attempt to honor the day. Women often consider faith an important factor in regaining health. Family members may make "bargains" with saints, such as promises to fast, be faithful, or make church donations if the saint acts on behalf of an ill family member.

Three traditional folk-healing practices are particularly notable: those related to *matiasma* (bad eye or evil eye), *practika* (herbal remedies), and *vendouses* (cupping). *Matiasma* results from the envy or admiration of others. Whereas the eye is able to harm a wide variety of things including inanimate objects, children are particularly susceptible to attack. Common symptoms of *matiasma* include headache, chills, irritability, restlessness, and lethargy; in extreme cases, *matiasma* has resulted in death.

Ponos (pain) is the cardinal symptom of ill health and an evil that needs eradication. The person in pain is not expected to suffer quietly or stoically in the presence of family. The family is relied on to find resources to relieve the pain or, failing that, to share in the experience of suffering. However, in the presence of outsiders, the lack of restraint in pain expression suggests lack of self-control. Although the experience of physical pain is acknowledged publicly, emotional pain is hidden within the privacy of the family.

Many Greeks and Greek Cypriots display a general distrust of all professionals and may "shop around" for physicians and other professionals to obtain additional opinions. The use of several physicians simultaneously may result in untoward drug interactions from conflicting multiple drug use.

People of Cuban Heritage

DIVINA GROSSMAN and LARRY D. PURNELL

Over 1.2 million Cuban Americans live in the United States, representing the third largest Hispanic group, after Mexican Americans and Puerto Ricans. The experience of Cubans in their homeland and in the United States is distinct from that of other Hispanic groups. Under the Cuban Adjustment Act of 1966, Cubans were welcomed by the U.S. Government and were provided with support. Cubans have managed to adjust to mainstream American culture while remaining close to their Cuban roots. However, young adults and adolescents who were educated in Cuba with strict Communist ideation and who emigrated with their parents may find the clash in values between Cuba and their new country confusing and negative.

Some Cuban Americans consider English to be their dominant language, others consider Spanish to be their dominant language, whereas still others are completely bilingual. Because many Cubans live and transact business in Spanish-speaking ethnic enclaves, they have little need or motivation to learn English and are less likely to acculturate.

Cubans value **simpatia** and **personalismo** in their interactions with others. *Simpatia*, the need for smooth interpersonal relationships, is characterized by courtesy, respect, and the absence of harsh criticism or confrontation. *Personalismo* emphasizes intimate interpersonal relationships over impersonal bureaucratic relationships.

Conversations among Cubans are characterized by animated facial expressions, direct eye contact, hand gestures, and gesticulations. Voices tend to be loud, with a fast rate of speech. Great emphasis is paid to current issues and problems rather than projections into the future.

Family is the most important social unit and source of emotional and physical support among Cubans. The traditional family structure is patriarchal, although the more-acculturated families have become more egalitarian. *La casa*, the house, is considered the province of the woman, and *la calle*, the street, the domain of the man. Extended, multigenerational households are common, with grandparents often part of the nuclear family.

Most Cuban Americans are white. Because of their predominantly European ancestry, Cuban Americans have skin, hair, and eye colors that vary from light to dark. A minority who are of African Cuban extraction are dark-skinned.

The Cuban cultural perspective of the "healthy body" is an obstacle to good nutritional practices. A healthy and beautiful Cuban infant is fat by U.S. standards. Even among adults, a little heaviness is considered attractive. *Que gordo estas*! (How fat you are!) is considered a compliment. The traditional Cuban diet, high in calories, starches, and saturated fats, predisposes individuals to the development of obesity and cardiovascular diseases.

Many Cuban folk beliefs and practices surround pregnancy. Some Cuban women believe that they have to eat for two during the pregnancy and end up gaining excessive weight. Some believe that morning sickness is cured by eating coffee grounds; that eating a lot of fruit ensures that the baby will be born with a smooth complexion; and that wearing necklaces during pregnancy causes the umbilical cord to be wrapped around the baby's neck.

Although, traditionally, it was not acceptable for Cuban men to attend the birth of their children, the younger and more-acculturated Cuban fathers tend to be present to support their wives during labor and delivery. In the postpartum period, ambulation, exposure to cold, and going barefoot place the mother at risk for infection.

Thus, family members and relatives often care for the mother and baby for about 4 weeks postpartum.

Bereavement is expressed openly among Cuban Americans, with loud crying and other physical manifestations of grief considered socially acceptable. Death is an occasion for relatives living far away to visit and commiserate with the bereaved family. Women from the immediate family usually dress in black during the period of mourning. Approximately 85 percent of Cuban Americans are Roman Catholics, with the remaining 15 percent being Protestants, Jews, and believers in the African Cuban practice of *Santeria*. Roman Catholicism as practiced by Cubans is personalistic, rather than institutional, in nature. The religious practice of Cuban Catholics is characterized by devotion and intimate, confiding relationships with the Virgin Mary, Jesus, and the saints.

Santeria is a 300-year-old African Cuban religious system that combines elements of Roman Catholicism with ancient Yoruba tribal beliefs and practices. Followers of Santeria believe in the magical and medicinal properties of flowers, herbs, weeds, twigs, and leaves. Sweet herbs are used for attracting good luck, love, money, and prosperity. Bitter herbs are used to banish evil and negative energies.

When someone is sick, that person's physical complaints may be diagnosed and treated by a physician, but the *santero* may be summoned to assist in balancing and neutralizing the various aspects of the illness. Compared with their peers from previous migration waves, recent Cuban immigrants may be less likely to be Catholic. Further, large numbers of Cubans consider themselves adherents of Catholicism and Santeria simultaneously.

When Cuban clients consult health-care providers, in all likelihood, they have already tried some folk remedies recommended by older women in their family or obtained from a botanica. Most folk remedies are harmless and do not interfere with biomedical treatment. Health-care providers should be alert to the frequent practice of sharing prescription medications in families and among relatives. Cubans may use traditional medicinal plants in the form of teas, potions, salves, or poultices.

Barriers to accessing health care among Cubans include language, poverty, time lag, and transportation, especially if they do not live in an urban environment. Others indicate that the red tape and paper work required by health-care facilities are deterrents to accessing care, especially preventive care and health wellness checkups. For some, overdependence on family and folk practices may also be a barrier to accessing care.

Among Cuban Americans, dependency is a culturally acceptable sick role. Sick family members are showered with attention and support. Cuban Americans tend to express their pain and discomfort. Verbal complaints, moaning, crying, and groaning are culturally appropriate ways of dealing with pain. The expression of pain itself may serve a pain-relieving function and may not necessarily signify a need for administration of pain medication.

People of Hindu Heritage

LARRY D. PURNELL

Hindus represent a segment of Asian Indians that includes Sikhs, Punjabis, Moslems, and Christians. Different religious sectors share many common cultural beliefs and practices, and they differ according to the primary and secondary characteristics of culture. Asian Indians leave their country for a variety of reasons, the most important of which is to attain a higher standard of living. The prospect of greater material prosperity, combined with better working conditions, enhances the appeal of a wider range of job opportunities in the United States.

Women are expected to strictly follow deference customs—that is, direct eye contact is avoided with men, although men can have direct eye contact with one another. Direct eye contact with older people and authority figures may be considered a sign of disrespect. Touching and embracing are not acceptable for displaying affection. Even between spouses, a public display of affection such as hugging or kissing is frowned upon.

Most Hindus have become part of the skilled workforce in America. Hard work, interest in saving and investment, and business acumen enable many to become financially successful. Because of their educational and professional backgrounds, it is not difficult for most to find suitable employment and improve their economic status.

Adolescents face tremendous pressure to keep up the image of "whiz kids" and to meet the expectations of their parents, which may override individual aptitudes and choices. This may create anxiety and frustration, thereby leading to failure and anger toward parents, which may dispose adolescents to use drugs as a coping strategy.

Vegetarianism is firmly rooted in the culture and the term *nonvegetarian* is used to describe anyone who eats meat, eggs, poultry, fish, and cheese. Foremost among the perceptions of Hindus is the belief that certain foods are "hot" and others "cold" and, therefore, should be eaten only during certain seasons and not in combination. The geographic differences in the hot and cold perceptions are dramatic; many foods considered hot in the north are considered cold in the south. Such perceptions and distinctions are based on how specific foods are thought to affect body functions. Dietary habits within the Indian subcontinent are complex, regionally varied, and strongly influenced by religion.

Physical examinations and procedures, particularly pelvic examinations, are especially traumatic to Hindu American women who may not have experienced or heard about these examinations in the past. It is important to explain the procedures, provide privacy, and assign a female health-care provider to decrease the stress and discomfort associated with a pelvic examination.

Childbirth is a social and religious event in the Hindu culture. Pregnancy rituals are performed during specific months of pregnancy to protect the pregnant mother and the unborn child from evil spirits. The birth of a son is considered a blessing, not only because the son carries the family name but also because he is expected to care for his parents in their old age. Furthermore, a son is also required for the performance of many sacred rituals. In contrast, the birth of a daughter is cause for worry and concern because of traditions associated with *dowry*, a ritual that can impoverish the lives of those who are less affluent.

Hindus prefer to die at home. The eldest son is responsible for the funeral rites and completes prayers for ancestral souls. Death is considered rebirth. Women may respond to the death of a loved one with loud wailing, moaning, and beating their chests in front of the corpse,

389

attesting their inability to bear the thought of being left behind to handle situations by themselves. This is significant for women because widowhood is considered inauspicious. Health-care providers need to offer support and understanding of the Hindu culture with respect for death and grief beliefs.

Hinduism is both a religious and a social system. The philosophical explanation of *caste* as the gradual progress of the individual soul to a state of union with the divine principle was made to concur with the social explanation of caste as the division of humankind into complementary functional groups. Health-care providers must understand the Hindu religious beliefs and practices to provide culturally congruent care for Hindu clients.

Within the traditional system of medicine in India, the primary emphasis is on the prevention of illnesses. Individuals are responsible for meeting their own health needs. One of the principles of **Ayurveda** includes the art of living and proper health care, advocating that one's health is a personal responsibility.

Because of religious beliefs related to karma, Hindus attempt to be stoic and may not exhibit symptoms of pain. Furthermore, pain is attributed to God's will, the wrath of God, or a punishment from God and is to be borne with courage. As a result, health-care providers may need to rely more on the nonverbal aspects of pain when assessing the comfort needs of Hindu clients.

Because of the stigma attached to seeking professional psychiatric help, many Hindus do not access the health-care system for mental-health problems. Instead, family and friends seem to be the best help, and there is a general belief that time is the best healer. Physical and mental illnesses are considered God's will and are associated with a fatalistic attitude. The sick role is assumed without any feelings of guilt or ineptness in doing one's tasks.

Women generally seek female health-care providers for gynecological examinations. Health-care providers need to respect their clients' modesty by providing adequate privacy and assigning same-gender caregivers whenever possible. In the area of mental health, traditional healers, such as *Vaids*, practice an empirical system of indigenous medicine; *mantarwadis* cure through astrology and charms; and *patris* act as mediums for spirits and demons. Health-care providers must specifically ask whether their Hindu clients are using these folk practitioners and what treatments have been prescribed.

People of Irish Heritage

SARAH A. WILSON

The history of the Irish in America has not been harmonious. Early immigrants were subjected to religious persecution and economic discrimination. Irish Americans are a diverse group, and health-care providers must be careful to avoid generalizations or assumptions, such as the Irish being superstitious, heavy drinkers, and practical jokers, because these do not apply to all Irish. Religious persecution and deplorable economic conditions were primary reasons for early immigration to America. Ireland had a population of 8.5 million until the Great Potato Famine of 1846 to 1848, when the population decreased to 3.4 million. During the famine, thousands of Irish died from malnutrition, typhus epidemics, dysentery, and scurvy, and millions immigrated to America.

The Irish use low-context English, in which many words are used to express a thought. This low-contextual use of the language has its roots in the Celtic folk tradition of storytelling. Humility and emotional reserve are considered virtues. Displays of emotion and affection in public are avoided and often difficult in private. The people often rely on humor and teasing as expressions of affection and may use this form of humor with health-care providers.

Kinship and sibling loyalty are important to the Irish. Irish families emphasize independence and self-reliance in children. Boys are allowed and expected to be more aggressive than girls. Girls are raised to be respectable, responsible, and resilient. Children are expected to have self-restraint, self-discipline, and respect and obedience for their parents and older people. Over time, the Irish have made a place for themselves in the workforce in the United States or wherever they have migrated and are represented in all occupations and professional roles.

Most Irish are either dark haired and fair skinned or have red hair, ruby cheeks, and fair skin. However, as with other ethnic groups, variations in hair and skin color exist. The fair complexion of the Irish places them at risk for skin cancer. The major cause of infant mortality in Ireland is congenital abnormalities. Other conditions with a high incidence among the Irish are phenylketonuria (PKU), neural tube defects, and alcoholism. Most states require screening all newborns for PKU; health-care providers may need to encourage women who give birth at home to seek PKU screening for their infants.

Alcohol problems in Ireland are among the highest internationally. Purnell and Foster in their multinational review of the literature on alcohol use, report that the percentage of people in the United States, Ireland, and England who drink is the same; however, behavior problems are greater among the Irish. Because drinking may be a way of coping with problems, the health professional needs to assist Irish American clients to explore more-effective coping strategies and caution them against the dangers of mixing alcohol with medications.

The Irish believe that not eating a well-balanced diet or not eating the right kinds of food may cause the newborn to be deformed. In addition, the Irish share the belief common to many other ethnic groups that the mother should not reach over her head during pregnancy because the baby's cord may wrap around its neck. A taboo behavior in the past, which some women still respect, is that if the pregnant woman sees or experiences a tragedy during pregnancy, a congenital anomaly may occur.

The Irish reaction to death is a combination of their pagan past and current Christian beliefs. The Celts denied death and ridiculed it with humor. The Irish are fatalists and acknowledge the inevitability of death. The American emphasis on technology and dying in the hospital may be incongruent with the Irish American belief that family members should stay with the dying person. The Irish wake continues as an important phenomenon in contemporary Irish families and is a time of melancholy, rejoicing, pain, and hopefulness.

The predominant religion of most Irish is Catholicism, and the church is a source of strength and solace for many Irish Americans. In times of illness, Irish Catholics receive the Sacrament of the Sick, which includes Anointing, Communion, and a blessing by the priest. Prayer is an individual and private matter. In the health-care setting, clients should be given privacy for prayer, whether or not a clergy member is present. Some Irish Americans wear religious medals to maintain health. These emblems provide them with solace and should not be removed by the health-care provider.

The Irish's fatalistic outlook and external locus of control influences health-seeking behaviors. Irish Americans use denial as a way of coping with physical and psychological problems. Many Irish limit and understate symptoms when ill. For some Irish Americans, illness behavior does little to relieve suffering and perpetuates a self-fulfilling prophecy. Illness or injury may be linked to guilt and the result of having done something morally wrong. The behavioral response of the Irish to pain is stoic, usually ignoring or minimizing it. Irish deny pain and delay seeking medical treatment longer than Italians.

In most Irish families, nuclear family members are consulted first about health problems. Mothers and older women are usually the family members who possess the knowledge of folk practices to alleviate common problems such as colds. When home remedies are not effective, the Irish seek the care of biomedical practitioners.

People of Italian Heritage

SANDRA M. HILLMAN

This chapter describes the beliefs and practices of Italian Americans from the mainland of Italy, although some of these characteristics may be shared by Italian Americans with a heritage from Sicily and Sardinia.

The willingness to share thoughts and feelings among family members is a major distinguishing characteristic of the Italian American family. Many times, a fluctuating emotional climate exists within the family, with expressions of affection erupting briefly into what appears to an outsider as anger or hostility. Italians are sentimental and not afraid to express their feelings, and this extends into the health-care environment. Even though traditional roles remain strong in Italian American families, a trend toward more-egalitarian relationships is evolving. Families maintain close relationships: Daughters have close ties with both parents, particularly as they approach old age.

Italians believe strongly in the work ethic, are punctual, and rarely miss work commitments owing to a cold, headache, or minor illnesses. If completing their work requires staying later, they do so. Although the family is of utmost importance to Italians, work takes priority over family unless serious family situations arise. This cultural predisposition parallels the North American work ethic.

People of Italian ancestry have some notable genetic diseases, such as familial Mediterranean fever, Mediterranean-type glucose-6-phosphate dehydrogenase (G-6-PD) deficiency, and β-thalassemia. Thus, administration of sulfonamides, antimalarial agents, salicylates, and naphthaquinolones should be avoided. A recommendation is to screen all people of Italian heritage for these conditions before administering medications.

A close association between food and mothering results in some predictable problems. Many Italians believe that bigger babies are healthier. The size of the baby is perceived as an index of the successful maintenance of maternal and wifely responsibilities. The belief that a mother does not conceive while nursing continues to be held by many Italian women. Among traditional Italians, a postpartum woman is not allowed to wash her hair, take a shower, or resume her domestic chores for at least 2 or 3 weeks after birth so she can rest. New mothers are expected to breastfeed, restoring the health of the reproductive organs and keeping the mother and baby free of infections.

In the Italian American family, death is a great social loss and brings an immediate response from the community. Sending food and flowers (chrysanthemums), giving money, and congregating at the home of the deceased are expected. The funeral procession to the cemetery is a symbol of family status. There is great pride in the size of the event, which is determined by the number of cars in the procession. Although there is a tendency today to decrease the elaborateness of the funeral, it remains very much a family and community event.

Emotional outpourings can be profuse. Women may mourn dramatically, even histrionically, for the whole family. They do not merely weep; they may rage against death for the harm it has done to the family. Family members may moan and scream for the deceased throughout the church. Screaming is an effort to ensure that Jesus, Mary, and the saints hear what the bereaved are thinking and feeling.

Their predominant religion, Roman Catholicism, includes folk religious practices. Most Italians pray to the Virgin Mary, the Madonna, and a number of saints. Many traditional first-generation and newer Italian American families display shrines to the Blessed Virgin in their backyards. God is an all-understanding, compassionate, and forgiving being. Prayer and having faith in God and saints help Italian Americans through illnesses. The health-care provider may need to help the client obtain the basic rites of the Sacrament of the Sick, which includes Anointing, Communion, and if possible, a blessing by the priest.

The concept of family, the most dominant influence on the individual, is the most credible source of health-care practices. Italians believe that the most-significant moments of life should take place under their own roofs. The extended family is the front-line resource for intensive advice on emotional problems. Mental-health specialists are frequently perceived as inappropriate agents for meeting problems that are beyond the expertise of the family and local community.

Individuals can protect themselves from the evil eye by using magical symbols and by learning the rituals of the *maghi*, "witch." Amulets are worn on necklaces or bracelets, held in a pocket, or sewn into clothing. *Cornicelli*, "little red horns," can still be purchased in Little Italies as good luck charms. These should not be removed from patients' bedsides or from their clothing because they provide significant solace for some.

Both age and gender mediate ethnic differences in the expression of pain for Italian Americans. Older Italian Americans, especially women, are more likely to report pain experiences, express symptoms to the fullest extent, and expect immediate treatment. Italians tend to be more verbally expressive with chronic pain. The sick role for many Italian Americans is one not entered into without personal feelings of guilt; thus, they may keep sickness a secret from family and friends and are not inclined to describe the details because they blame themselves for the health problem.

People of Puerto Rican Heritage

LARRY D. PURNELL

Puerto Ricans are the third largest Hispanic cultural subgroup, with a population of approximately 3 million living in the continental United States. Most Puerto Ricans on the mainland live in metropolitan areas in the northeastern United States. Puerto Ricans have a unique pride in their country, culture, and music. They self-identify as *Puertorriqueños* or *Boricuans* (Taíno Indian word for Puerto Rican), or *Niuyoricans* for those born in New York.

Puerto Ricans are known for their hospitality and the value placed on interpersonal interaction such as *simpatia*, a cultural script in which an individual is perceived as likable, attractive, and fun-loving. They often expect the health-care provider to exchange personal information when beginning a professional relationship. The health-care provider may wish to set boundaries with discretion and *personalismo*, emphasizing personal rather than impersonal and bureaucratic relationships.

From childhood through adolescence, children are socialized to have respect for adults, especially older people. Great significance is given to the concept of familism, and any behavior that shifts from this ideal is discouraged and may be perceived as a disgrace to the family. Puerto Ricans value the unity of the family. Because grandparents assume an active role in rearing grandchildren, supporting the family, babysitting, teaching traditions, disciplining, and enforcing educational activities, they should be included in health teaching.

Whereas most migrant Puerto Ricans are task oriented and meticulous about the presentation of their work, some have a relativistic view of time and may not value regular attendance and punctuality in the workforce. Most Puerto Ricans are cheerful, have a positive attitude, and value personal relationships at work. Work is perceived as a place for social and cultural interactions.

Puerto Ricans on the mainland face a high incidence of chronic conditions such as mental illness among younger adults and cardiopulmonary and osteomuscular diseases among older people. Acute conditions among Puerto Ricans include a disproportionate number of acute respiratory illnesses, injuries, infectious and parasitic diseases, and diseases of the digestive system. Dengue fever, a mosquito-transmitted disease caused by any of the four viral serotypes of the *Aedes aegypti* mosquito, is an endemic disease that migrants may bring to the mainland. Health-care providers need to advise Puerto Rican clients and families traveling to Puerto Rico to avoid exposure to endemic areas and to use mosquito repellent and protective clothing at all times.

Puerto Ricans celebrate, mourn, and socialize around food. Food is used (1) to honor and recognize visitors, friends, family members, and health-care providers; (2) as an escape from everyday pressures, problems, and challenges; and (3) to prevent and treat illnesses. Puerto Rican clients may bring homemade goods to health-care providers as an expression of appreciation, respect, and gratitude for services rendered. Refusing these offerings may be interpreted as a personal rejection.

Many Puerto Ricans ascribe to the hot-and-cold classifications of foods for nutritional balance and dietary practices during menstruation, pregnancy, the postpartum period, infant feeding, lactation, and aging. Health-care providers should become familiar with these food practices when planning culturally congruent dietary alternatives.

Death is perceived as a time of crisis in Puerto Rican families. The body is considered sacred and guarded with great respect. News about the deceased should be given first to the head of the family, usually the oldest daughter or son. Because of cultural, physical, and emotional responses to grief, health-care providers should use a private room to communicate such news and have clergy or a minister present when the news is disclosed.

The family of the deceased freely express themselves through loud crying and verbal expressions of grief. Some may talk in a thunderous way to God. Others may express their grief through a sensitive but continuous crying or sobbing. Some believe that not expressing their feelings could mean a lack of love and respect for the deceased.

Most Puerto Ricans have a curative view of health. They tend to underuse health promotion and preventive services such as regular dental or physical examinations and Pap smears. Many use emergency health-care services for acute problems, rather than preventive health-care services. Most Puerto Ricans believe in "family care," rather than self-care. Women are seen as the main caregivers and promoters of family health and the source of spiritual and physical strength. Health-care providers should incorporate the participation of the family in the care of the ill.

Natural herbs, teas, and over-the-counter medications are often used as initial interventions for symptoms of illness. Many consult family and friends before consulting a health-care provider. Over-the-counter medications and folk remedies are often used by Puerto Ricans to treat mental-health symptoms, acute illnesses, and chronic diseases. Health-care providers should inquire about those practices and encourage clients to bring their medications to every visit. Engaging in friendly conversation encourages clients to reveal their use of folk treatments, over-the-counter medications, and concurrent use of folk healers. Because mental illness carries a stigma for many Puerto Ricans, obtaining information or talking about mental illness with Puerto Rican families may be difficult. Some might not disclose the presence or history of mental illnesses, even in a trusting environment.

Many Puerto Ricans use traditional and folk healers such as *espiritistas* and *santeros* along with Western health-care providers. Some *espiritismo* practices are used to deal with the power of good and evil spirits in the physical and emotional development of the individual. *Santeros*, individuals prepared to practice *santería*, are consulted in matters related to the belief of object intrusion, diseases caused by evil spirits, the loss of the soul, the insertion of a spirit, or the anger of God.

Navajo Indians

OLIVIA HODGINS and DAVID HODGINS

The Bureau of Indian Affairs (BIA) recognizes over 500 different American Indian tribes that extend throughout the United States and Canada. Navajo Indians claim the distinction of being the largest tribe, consisting of approximately 352,862 people. The Navajo tribe has one of the largest reservations in the United States, covering portions of Arizona, Utah, and New Mexico. Because of severe economic conditions and high unemployment rates, significant migration occurs into and out of the reservations. Many who leave the reservation experience culture shock resulting from a rapid and drastic change in their environment. Many Indians return to their reservation on a regular basis to refresh and renew themselves through *Blessingway* ceremonies.

American Indians have consistently been identified as the most underrepresented of all minority groups in colleges and universities. Traditional educational values for most American Indians are reflected in learning the tribal culture and clarifying their roles in the clan and the community.

The Navajo language was not written until the 1970s; consequently, many older Navajos speak only their native language and few are literate in English. The few older Navajos who are bilingual speak limited Spanish or English. The younger populations are usually bilingual, with their native tongue spoken primarily in the home. Minor variations in pronunciation may change the entire meaning of a word or phrase. Thus, it is safer to use a trained interpreter.

Among Navajo Indians, talking loudly is considered rude; voice tones are quiet, but not monotone. Navajos generally do not share inner thoughts and feelings with anyone outside their clan. Navajo Indians are comfortable with long periods of silence. Failing to allow adequate

time for information processing may result in an inaccurate response or no response.

Touch among Navajos is unacceptable unless one knows the person very well. If contact is made, it is in the form of a handshake. Rather than pointing a finger, which is considered rude, to indicate a direction, individuals shift their lips toward the desired direction. Direct eye contact is considered rude and, possibly, confrontational for the Navajos. Even close friends do not maintain eye contact; this rule does not change with socioeconomic status.

Navajo society is matrilineal. The land is not owned, but grazing rights are passed from mothers to daughters. Although men are seen as important, grandmothers and mothers are at the center of Navajo society. When family care is to be provided, no decision is made until the appropriate older woman is present.

A primary social premise is that no person has the right to speak for another. Thus, Navajo children are frequently allowed to make decisions that other cultures might consider irresponsible. Older children are taught to be stoic and uncomplaining. Social status is determined by age and life experiences. Status is not derived from standing out in the clan or tribe. Group activities are an important norm in the Navajo culture.

Skin color among the Navajos varies from light brown to very dark brown. Navajos have epithelial eye folds and are generally taller and thinner than other American Indian tribes. The Navajos have traditionally been good runners and excel in relay races and long-distance running.

Health conditions with high frequency are upper respiratory illnesses, acute otitis media, heart disease, malignant neoplasm, motor vehicle accidents, unintentional injuries, diabetes mellitus, alcoholism, and suicide. Other health problems include the plague, tick fever, and recently, the

Muerto Canyon Hantavirus, severe combined immunodeficiency syndrome (SCIDS), and Navajo neuropathy.

Among the Navajos, food is not generally associated with promoting health or illness. American Indian diets may be deficient in vitamin D because many individuals suffer from lactose intolerance or do not drink milk.

Large families are looked on favorably because, in times past, many children died at an early age. In the past, many traditional Navajo women did not seek prenatal care because pregnancy was not considered a physical state requiring health care. Many Navajo women are reluctant to deliver their babies in hospital settings because pregnant women should not be around the dead or in a place where people have died. Purchasing clothes for an infant before birth is a taboo practice among the Navajos. Outsiders may interpret this practice as the mother not wanting the baby. In reality, preparing for the baby before birth is forbidden by Indian tradition.

Many Navajos start the day with prayer, meditation, corn pollen, and running in the direction of the rising sun. Navajos believe wellness is a state of harmony with one's surroundings. When people are ill or out of harmony, the medicine man or, in some cases, a diagnostician tells them what they have done to disrupt their harmony.

They are returned to harmony through the use of a healing ceremony.

Navajos view pain as something to be endured, and thus, they do not ask for analgesics and may not understand that pain medication is available. Other times, herbal medicines are preferred and used without the knowledge of the health-care provider. Those with physical or mental handicaps are not seen as different; rather, the limitation is accepted and a role is found for them within the society.

For the American Indian, cultural perceptions of the sick role are based on the ideal of maintaining harmony with nature and with others. Ill people have obviously done something to place themselves out of harmony or have had a curse placed on them.

Native healers are divided into three categories: those working with the power of good, the power of evil, or both. Generally, they are divinely chosen and promote activities that encourage self-discipline and self-control and that involve acute body awareness. Navajo tribal practitioners divide their knowledge into preventive measures, treatment regimens, and health maintenance. Acceptance of Western medicine is variable with a blending of traditional health-care beliefs.

People of Turkish Heritage

GULBU TORTUMLUOGLU

The 202,000 people of Turkish descent in the United States live in 42 states, with over half living in New York, California, New Jersey, and Florida. Just over half of the individuals in this group were born outside the United States, and most arrived since 1980. Most Turks practice Islam and come from a collectivist culture in which an individual's behavior is expected to conform to the norms or traditions of the group, which has important implications for health-care providers advocating health promotion and wellness; illness, disease, and injury prevention; and health-maintenance restoration.

Modern Turkish women tend to be more Westernized than some of their Middle Eastern or Muslim counterparts, resulting in more-egalitarian decision-making. Older people in Turkish culture are attributed authority and respect until they become weak or retired, at which time, their authoritative roles diminish. However, respect always remains a factor. Individuals are socialized to take care of older parents, regarding it as normal rather than an added burden. Grandparents play a significant role in raising their grandchildren, especially if they live in the same home.

Turkey is known for its high-power distance (the psychological and emotional distance between superiors and subordinates), respect for authority, centralized administration, and authoritarian leadership style. In Turkish culture, a manager's authoritative control is often more important than the achievement of organizational goals; thus, the U.S. workforce culture must be explained to ensure satisfactory working relationships.

Helminthiasis (intestinal worm), hepatitis, tuberculosis, and malaria have not been fully eradicated in Turkey. Endemic goiter associated with iodine deficiency is a major health problem among Turks. Turkey also has some of the highest rates of occupational diseases and work accidents in Europe. Thus, health-care providers may need to provide education regarding safety issues in occupational health and assess newer Turkish immigrants for intestinal parasites, tuberculosis, malaria, and other health conditions found in Turkey.

Turkish cuisine is influenced by the many civilizations encountered by nomadic Turks over the centuries as well as by a mixture of delicacies from different regions of the vast Ottoman Empire. Therefore, food choices are varied and tend to provide a healthy, balanced diet. Food is a highly valued symbol of hospitality and communicates love and respect to those for whom it is prepared. The Islamic tradition of *Ramazan* is a month of fasting observed by practicing Muslims throughout the world. During Ramazan, one is not allowed to eat or drink anything from sunrise to sunset, necessitating adjustments in medication administration. Generally, pregnant and postpartum women, travelers, and those who are ill are excused from fasting.

Motherhood, and therefore pregnancy, is accorded great respect, and pregnant women are usually made comfortable in any way possible, including satisfying their cravings. Pregnant women may continue their daily activities or work as long as they are comfortable. In traditional Turkish culture, one of the most important desires of a married woman is to have a child. A woman who has not had a child is faced with social pressure and accusations and, thus, may try to use some traditional practices to increase fertility. Newborns are treated as cherished gifts. A small blue bead, *nazar boncuk*, protects the child from the "evil eye" and is usually placed on the child's left shoulder. This practice protects the child from the evil angel whispering in the left ear, often portrayed in Christian religious art.

399

Traditional rituals after death are closing the eyes of the deceased, tying the chin, turning the head toward Mecca, putting the feet next to each other, putting the hands together on the abdomen, and removing clothing. After the burial, the deceased is honored with a meal that signifies moving the deceased into the afterlife, emphasizing the need to eat and drink, and filling the void that will occur in the community. If these rituals are not completed, the spirit of the deceased will be left behind.

Turks who emigrate to the West tend to be very moderate Muslims. Traditional prayer is practiced five times each day and can take place anywhere, as long as one is facing the holy city of Mecca. A special small rug is used for praying. Health-care providers may need to assist clients to prepare for prayers.

Most Turks rely on Western medicine and highly trained professionals for health and curative care. However, remnants of traditional beliefs have an impact on health-care practices. A common explanation for the cause of illness is an imbalance of hot and cold. For example, diarrhea is thought to come from too much cold or heat; pneumonia results from extreme cold.

Terminally ill clients are generally not told the severity of their conditions. Informing a client of a terminal illness may take away the hope, motivation, and energy that should be directed toward healing, or it may cause the client additional anxiety related to the fear of dying and concern about those being left behind. Thus, the health-care provider should discuss a terminal illness with the family spokesperson before informing the patient.

Depression is a major public health problem in Turkey; high-risk groups include women, individuals in middle adulthood, and those in nuclear rather than extended families. Such groups may well describe a large portion of Turkish immigrants in the United States, requiring careful assessments. Physicians, and to a lesser extent nurses and midwives, have historically been held in very high esteem. Moreover, practitioners should ask about a same-gender health-care provider for those who practice Islam.

People of Vietnamese Heritage

LARRY D. PURNELL

Approximately 1.2 million Vietnamese live in the United States. Vietnamese immigrants confront a unique set of problems, including dissimilarity of culture, lack of family or relatives to offer initial support, and a negative identification with the unpopular Vietnam War. Many Vietnamese are involuntary immigrants. Their expatriation was unexpected and unplanned, and their departures were often precipitous and tragic. Escape attempts were long, harrowing, and for many, fatal. Survivors were often placed in squalid refugee camps for years.

Whenever confronted with a direct but delicate question, many Vietnamese cannot easily give a blunt "no" as an answer, because such an answer may create disharmony. Self-control, another traditional value, encourages keeping to oneself, whereas expressions of disagreement that may irritate or offend another person are avoided. Expressing emotions is considered a weakness and interferes with self-control. At times of distress or loss, they often complain of physical discomforts, such as headaches, backaches, or insomnia.

A person's age is calculated roughly from the time of conception; most children are considered to already be a year old at birth and gain a year each *Tet*, the Asian Lunar New Year. A child born just before Tet could be regarded as 2 years old when only a few days old by American standards. Because the practice of determining age is so different in Vietnam, many immigrants may have difficulty determining their exact birth date and are often given January 1 as a date of birth for official records.

The traditional Vietnamese family is strictly patriarchal and is almost always an extended family structure, with the man having the duty of carrying on the family name through his progeny. Young people are expected to respect their elders and to avoid behavior that might dishonor the family. As a result of the effects of their exposure to Western cultures, a disproportionate share of young people have difficulty adapting to this expectation. A conflict often develops between the traditional notion of filial piety, with its requisite subordination of self and unquestioning obedience to parental authority, and the pressures and needs associated with adaptation to American life.

Most Vietnamese respect authority figures with impressive titles, achievement, education, and a harmonious work environment. They may be less concerned about such factors as punctuality, adherence to deadlines, and competition. Other traditions include a willingness to work hard, sacrificing current comforts and saving for the future to ensure that they assimilate well into the workforce. Because many fear losing their jobs if they speak out about inequities, they are likely to be taken advantage of by some more-unscrupulous employers.

The Vietnamese family may try various home remedies, allowing the condition to become serious before seeking professional assistance. Once a physician or nurse has been consulted, the Vietnamese are usually quite cooperative and respect the wisdom and experience of health-care professionals. Hospitalization is viewed as a last resort and is acceptable only in case of emergency, when everything else has failed. With respect to mental health, Vietnamese do not easily trust authority figures, including treatment staff, because of their refugee experiences.

A predominant aspect of the traditional Asian system of health maintenance is the principle of balance between two opposing natural forces, known as *am* and *duong* in Vietnamese. These forces are represented by foods that are considered hot (*duong*) or cold (*am*). Illness or trauma may require therapeutic adjustment of hot-and-cold balance to restore equilibrium. The *am*-and-*duong* balance of forces continues during pregnancy and postpartum. Because body heat is lost during delivery, Vietnamese women avoid cold foods and beverages and increase consumption of hot foods to replace and strengthen their blood. Ice water and other cold drinks are usually not welcome, and most raw vegetables, fruits, and sour items are taken in lesser amounts.

Most Vietnamese have an aversion to hospitals and prefer to die at home. Some believe that a person who dies outside the home becomes a wandering soul with no place to rest. Family members think that they can provide more comfort to the dying person at home. Vietnamese families may wish to gather around the body of a recently deceased relative and express great emotion. Traditional mourning practices include the wearing of white clothes for 14 days, the subsequent wearing of black armbands by men and white headbands by women, and the yearly celebration of the anniversary of a person's death.

Vietnamese religious practices are influenced by the Eastern philosophies of Buddhism, Confucianism, and Taoism. Confucianism stresses harmony through maintenance of the proper order of social hierarchies, ethics, worship of ancestors, and the virtues of chastity and faithfulness. Taoism teaches harmony, allowing events to follow a natural course that one should not attempt to change. These beliefs have contributed to an attitude characterized by maintenance of self-control, acceptance of one's destiny, and fatalism toward illness and death that may be perceived as passive by Westerners.

Good health is achieved by having harmony and balance with the two basic opposing forces, *am* (cold, dark, female) and *duong* (hot, light, male). An excess of either force may lead to discomfort or illness. The belief that life is predetermined is a deterrent to seeking health care. For many Vietnamese, diagnostic tests are baffling, inconvenient, and often, unnecessary. Common treatments practiced in Vietnam and continued, to some degree, in the United States are *cao gio*, *giac*, *be bao*, *xong*, *moxibustion*, and *acupuncture*. Fatalistic attitudes and the belief that problems are punishment may reduce the degree of complaining and expression of pain among the Vietnamese, who view endurance as an indicator of strong character. One accepts pain as part of life and attempts to maintain self-control as a means of relief.

Traditional Asian male practitioners do not usually touch the bodies of females and sometimes use a doll to point out the nature of a problem. Young and unmarried women are more comfortable with female health-care providers.

Glossary

A

aagwachse Amish folk illness, referred to in English as *livergrown*, with symptoms of abdominal distress believed to be caused by too much jostling, especially occurring in infants during buggy rides.

abnemme Amish folk illness characterized by "wasting away"; usually affects infants or young children who seem to be too lean and not active.

abwaarde Amish term for ministering to someone by being present and serving when someone is sick in bed.

Acadia Part of the Canadian Maritime Provinces.

Acadian Early French settler of Acadia; a French dialect spoken by people in Acadia.

acculturate To modify or give up traits from the culture of origin as a result of contact with another culture.

achegewe Amish term for warm hands.

adab Egyptian term for politeness.

Ainu Indigenous people of uncertain origin in northern Japan.

Allah Greatest and most inclusive of the names of God. Arabic word used to describe the God worshipped by Muslims, Christians, and Jews.

am Pervasive force in Vietnamese traditional medicine, associated with cold conditions and things that are dark, negative, feminine, and empty.

Americanos Hispanic term for people from the European American culture.

amor propio Filipino term for saving face.

Anabaptist Adherent of the radical wing of the Protestant Reformation who espouses baptism of adult believers.

antyesti Hindu equivalent of last rites.

Appalachian Regional Commission Federal Commission established in the 1960s to improve economic conditions in Appalachia. This includes appropriations for improving and building roads, establishing loans for small businesses, and attracting industry to the area.

Arabic Semitic language of the Arabs.

arwah Egyptian term for the spirits.

asafetida bag Odorous combination of roots and herbs, usually made into a poultice, enclosed in a bag, and worn around the neck or some other part of the body for the purpose of warding off contagious illnesses.

Ashkenazi Descended from Eastern Europe and Russia.

assimilate To gradually adopt and incorporate the characteristics of the prevailing culture.

attitude State of mind or feeling with regard to some matter of a culture.

augmented families Term used in African American culture to refer to children who are raised in households in which they are not related to the head of that household.

ay bendito! Frequently used Puerto Rican phrase, expressing astonishment, surprise, lament, or pain.

Ayurveda Traditional Asian Indian medicine.

B

bahala na Filipino term for it is up to God.

barrenillos Spanish term for obsessions.

baten Iranian term for inner self.

be bao or bat gio Vietnamese folk practice in which the skin is pinched in order to produce ecchymosis and petechiae; practiced to relieve sore throats and headaches.

Bedouins Desert inhabitants of Egypt.

Behçet's disease Endemic disease in Turkey; characterized by chronic inflammatory disorders of the blood vessels with recurrent ulcerations of the oral and pharyngeal mucous membranes and the genitalia, skin lesions, severe uveitis, retinal vasculitis, and optic atrophy.

being Essence of existence in an unqualified state; conceived as an essential of nature in which one does not need to be actively engaged in an activity.

belief Something accepted as true, especially a tenet or a body of tenets accepted by people in an ethnocultural group.

Black English Dialect used by African Americans.

boat people Haitian or Cuban immigrants who arrive in small boats; usually of undocumented status.

bonzuk   Russian term for the cup used in performing cupping.

Boricua   Puerto Rican term used with great pride; name given to Puerto Rico by the Taino Indians.

botanica   Traditional Cuban or other Spanish store selling a variety of herbs, ointments, oils, powders, incenses, and religious figurines used in Santería.

brauche   Folk healing art common among Pennsylvania Germans.

braucher   Amish practitioner of *brauche*, a folk healer.

bris or **brit milah**   Ritual circumcision of a male Jewish child.

Burakumin   Japanese term for Korean descendants or descendants of the *burakumin*, the "untouchable" caste who cared for the dead and tanned leather in feudal times.

Bureau of Indian Affairs (BIA)   Federal agency responsible for ensuring services to Native Americans, Alaskan Indians, and Eskimo tribes.

C

caida de la mollera   Condition of fallen fontanelle, believed to occur because the infant was withdrawn too harshly from the nipple; common among some Spanish-speaking populations.

cao gio   Vietnamese practice of placing ointments or hot balm oil across the chest, back, or shoulders and rubbing with a coin; used to treat colds, sore throats, flu, and sinusitis.

cariñoso(a)   Hispanic term for caring, in both verbal and nonverbal communications.

catimbozeiros   Portuguese word for sorcerer; can be a folk practitioner.

Celtic   Belonging to a group of Indo-European languages: Irish, Welsh, or Breton.

cheshm-i-bad   Iranian term for evil eye.

Chiac or **ciac**   French dialect used in New Brunswick.

Chicano(a)   Mexican American.

Chondo Kyo   Korean naturalistic religion that combines Confucianism, Buddhism, and Daoism.

choteo   Cuban term for a lighthearted attitude, involving teasing, bantering, and exaggeration.

clan   Division of a tribe tracing descent from a common ancestor.

collectivist culture   Group of people who place a higher value on the family than on the individual.

comadre   Portuguese term for godmother.

community   Group of people having a common interest or identity; goes beyond the physical environment to include the physical, social, and symbolic characteristics that cause people to connect.

compadrazgo   Spanish term for a system of personal relationships in which friends or relatives are considered part of the family whether or not there is a blood relationship.

compadre   Portuguese term for godfather.

confianza   Hispanic term for trust developed between individuals; essential for effective communication and interpersonal interactions in health-care settings.

Conservative   Jewish term for the religious group between Reform and Orthodox in terms of religious practice.

contadini   Italian term for peasants.

Copts   Christian Egyptians.

cornicelli   Italian red horns; a symbol of good luck.

cosmology   Branch of philosophy that deals with the origin, processes, and structure of the universe.

Creole   Rich and expressive language derived from two other languages, such as French and Fon, an African tongue.

crystal gazer   Navajo folk healer who interprets dreams.

cultural awareness   Appreciation of the external signs of diversity such as the arts, music, dress, and physical characteristics.

cultural competence   Having the knowledge, abilities, and skills to deliver care congruent with the client's cultural beliefs and practices. (*See* Chapter 1 for a more extensive definition.)

cultural imperialism   Practice of extending the policies and practices of one organization (usually the dominant one) to disenfranchised and minority groups.

cultural imposition   Intrusive application of the majority cultural view onto individuals and families.

cultural relativism   Belief that the behaviors and practices of people should be judged only from the context of their cultural system.

cultural sensitivity   Having to do with personal attitudes and not saying things that may be offensive to someone from a cultural or ethnic background different from the health-care provider's background.

culturally conscious   Having an awareness of one's own existence, sensations, thoughts, and environment and not letting them have an undue influence over the cultural characteristics of another individual, family, group, or community.

culture   Totality of socially transmitted behavior patterns, arts, beliefs, values, customs, lifeways, and all other products of human work and thought characteristics of a population of people that guides their worldview and decision-making. Patterns may be explicit or implicit, are primarily learned and transmitted within the family, and are shared by the majority of the culture.

curandeiro   Portuguese folk practitioner whose healing powers are divinely given.

curandero   Traditional folk practitioner common in Spanish-speaking communities; treats traditional illness not caused by witchcraft.

D

daadihaus   Amish grandparents' cottage adjacent to farmhouse.

dan wei   Functional unit of Chinese society; work unit or neighborhood unit responsible to and for the Chinese people's way of life.

dao   Balance between *yin* and *yang*.

dayah   Arab midwife.

decensos   Spanish term for fainting spells.

demut   German term for humility, a priority value for the Amish, the effects of which may be seen in details such as the height of the crown of an Amish man's hat, as well as in very general features such as the modest and unassuming bearing and demeanor usually shown by Amish in public. This behavior is reinforced by frequent verbal warnings against its opposite, *hochmut*, pride or arrogance, which is to be avoided.

Deitsch/Duetsch Pennsylvania German (sometimes incorrectly anglicized as Pennsylvania Dutch); American dialect derived from several uplands and Alemanic German dialects, with an admixture of American English vocabulary.

Diet Japanese parliament.

dulse Iodine-rich edible seaweed used in clarifying beer and wine and as a suspension medium in some medicines; also known as *Irish moss*.

duong Vietnamese force used in traditional health practice, associated with things positive, masculine, light, and full.

E

ebo Sacrificial offering made to establish communication between the spirits and human beings in the Santería religion.

Eid Iranian term for celebration of a feast; for example, *Eid Gorgan* (day/feast ending pilgrimage to Mecca); *Eid Fetr* (last day of the month of Ramadan).

Eire Gaelic name for Ireland.

el ataque/ataque de nervios Hyperkinetic spasmodic activity common in Spanish-speaking groups. The purpose is to release strong feelings or emotions. The person requires no treatment, and the condition subsides spontaneously. It is an expression of deep anger or depression.

empacho Condition common among some Spanish-speaking populations; believed to be caused by a bolus of food stuck in the gastrointestinal tract. Massage of the abdomen is believed to relieve the condition.

endropi Greek term for shame.

escondido Portuguese term for hidden; refers to undocumented aliens who remain hidden.

espiritualista (espirituista) Spanish or Portuguese folk practitioners who receive their talent from "God"; treat conditions believed to be caused by witchcraft.

ethic of neutrality Avoiding aggression and assertiveness, not interfering with others' lives unless asked to do so, avoiding dominance over others, and avoiding arguments and seeking agreement.

ethnic group Group of people who have had experiences different from those of the dominant culture in status, background, residence, religion, education, or other factors that functionally unify the group and act collectively on one another. Pertains to a religious, racial, national, or cultural group.

ethnic identity Subjective sense of social boundary (social emphasis) or a self-definition that answers the question, "Who am I?"

ethnocentrism Universal tendency for human beings to think that our own ways of thinking, acting, and believing are the only right, proper, and natural ones and to believe that those who differ greatly are strange, bizarre, or unenlightened.

ethnocultural Group of people who have had experiences different from those of the dominant culture in status, ethnic background, residence, religion, education, or other factors that functionally unify the group and act collectively on one another.

F

falling out Sudden collapse, paralysis, and inability to see or speak; noted among African Americans during a funeral or other tragic experiences.

familism Social pattern in which family solidarity and tradition assume a superior position over individual rights and interests.

family Two or more people who are emotionally involved with each other. They may, but not necessarily, live in close proximity to each other.

fatalism Acceptance that occurrences in life are predetermined by fate and cannot be changed by human beings.

fatback Salt pork.

Filipino Preferred term for someone from the Philippines; same as Pilipino.

Francophone People living in Canada using French as their first language.

Frau German title for a married woman; equivalent to "Mrs." in English.

Fraulein German title for an unmarried woman; equivalent to "Miss" in English.

freindschaft Amish three-generational extended family network of relationships.

G

galang Filipino term for respect.

garm Iranian term for hot.

garmie Iranian digestive problem caused from eating too much hot food.

gelassenheit Amish term for submission, yielding, surrender of self and ego to the higher will of the group or deity.

generalization Reducing numerous characteristics of an individual or group of people to a general form that renders them indistinguishable.

geophagia Eating of nonfood substances such as clay, cornstarch, or charcoal during pregnancy.

giac Vietnamese dermabrasive procedure performed with cup suctioning.

giagia Greek term for grandma.

giri Japanese term for the sense of obligation that exists between people who are socially interconnected.

gohan Japanese term for rice, particularly the sticky rice preferred by Japanese.

Great Eid Islamic feast of 4 days.

Great Potato Famine Time in Ireland (1848–1850s) when the main crop, potatoes, failed; millions of Irish emigrated to escape starvation.

guanxi Chinese term defining how relatives are expected to help each other through connections, used by Chinese society in a manner similar to the use of money in other cultures.

Gullah Creole language spoken by African Americans who reside on or near the sea islands off Georgia and the Carolinas.

H

hadith Oral tradition of the Prophet Muhammad; collection of words and deeds that form the basis of Muslim law.

Halakha   Jewish laws or commandments.

halal   The lawful—that which is permitted by Allah; also, the term used to describe ritual slaughter of meat.

Han   Largest ethnic group of Chinese

hand trembler   Navajo traditional healer.

hanyak   Korean traditional herbal medicine used to create harmony between oneself and the larger cosmology; a healing method for body and soul.

haram   The unlawful—that which is prohibited by Allah; anyone who engages in what is prohibited is liable to incur punishment in the hereafter (as well as legal punishment in countries that incorporate Islamic law into legal codes).

Hasidic   Jewish ultra-Orthodox sect.

health   State of wellness defined by the people within their ethnocultural group; generally includes physical, mental, and spiritual states as they interact with the family, community, and global society.

Hebrew   Language of Israel and of Jewish prayer.

hejab   Iranian term for any behavior that expresses modesty in public; e.g., in women, modest attire (loose dress or head scarf) or shy, self-limiting behavior in relating to the other gender.

Herr   German title for a man; equivalent to "Mr." in English.

high blood   Too much blood in circulation in the body or pressure that is too high. Term commonly used by African Americans and Appalachians.

hijab   Modest covering of a Muslim woman; conceals the head and the body, except for the hands and face, with loosely fitting, nontransparent clothing.

hilot   Filipino folk healer and massage therapist.

hindi ibang tao   Filipino term for insider.

Hispanic   American of Spanish or Latin American origin.

hiya   Filipino term for shame.

hoca   Turkish traditional healer.

hochmut   Amish term for pride and arrogance.

hogan   Earth-covered Navajo dwelling.

home   In the Appalachian context, a connectedness to the land more than to a physical dwelling.

honor   Spanish term for goodness or virtue; can be diminished or lost by an immoral or unworthy act.

hot-and-cold theory   Hispanic concept that illness is caused when the body is exposed to an imbalance of hot and cold; foods are also classified as hot or cold.

hwa-byung   Korean traditional illness that occurs from repressing anger or other strong emotions.

hwangap   Significant celebration in Korean society—at the age of 60, a person starts the calendar cycle over again.

I

ideology   Thoughts and beliefs that reflect the social needs and aspirations of an individual or an ethnocultural group.

igang tao   Filipino term for outsider.

il mal occhio   Italian term for evil eye.

imam   Muslim leader of the prayer; usually the most learned member of the local Islamic community.

Indian Health Service   Federal agency that has the responsibility for providing health services to Native Americans.

Indochinese   Individuals originating from Vietnam, Cambodia, or Laos.

insallah   Arabic term for if God wills.

insider   Someone known to and accepted by the group; usually has special knowledge regarding the values and beliefs of the group.

Islam   Monotheistic religion in which the supreme deity is Allah; according to Muslim belief, God imparted his final revelations—the Holy Qur'an—through his last prophet, Mohammed, thereby completing Judaism and Christianity.

issei   First-generation Japanese immigrant.

itami   Japanese term for pain.

itheram   Egyptian term for respect.

J

jenn   Egyptian term for the devil.

jerbero   Spanish folk practitioner who specializes in treating health conditions through the use of herbal therapy.

jing   Chinese term for passages throughout the body that are interrelated and connected; includes the 14 meridians called the *jing luo*.

jinn   In Iran, spirits created by God from smokeless fire; they inhabit a world parallel to that of humans; some are righteous and others are evil.

Joual   French dialect incorporating English words into a syntax and grammar that is essentially French.

K

kaddish   Jewish prayer said for the dead.

kampo   Japanese term for East Asian or Chinese medical practices and botanical therapies.

karma   Hindu term for actions performed in the present life and the accumulated effects from past lives.

kashrut or kashrus   Jewish laws that dictate which foods are permissible under religious law.

khwan   Thai term for power inside or life spirit.

ki   Japanese or Korean term for the energy that flows through living creatures.

Koran   *See* Qur'an.

kosher   Kashrut laws in the Jewish religion.

koumbari   Greek term for coparents.

L

la gente de la raza   Phrase denoting a genetic determination to which all Spanish-speaking people belong, regardless of class differences or place of birth.

lace curtain Irish   Name given to Irish in America who left inner-city enclaves and moved to the suburbs.

Ladino(a)   Originally, a person with Jewish and Spanish background.

Latino(a)   Person from Latin America.

laying on of hands   Spiritual practice of placing one's hands on an individual for the purpose of healing.

lien   Vietnamese concept that represents control over and responsibility for moral character.

limerick   Irish humorous poem of 5 lines receiving its name from the County of Limerick in Ireland.

low blood   Too little blood, too low blood count, or too thin blood; commonly used by African Americans and Appalachians.

M

maalesh Arabic term meaning never mind, it doesn't matter; substantial efforts are directed at maintaining pleasant relationships and preserving dignity and honor; hostility in response to perceived wrongdoing is warded off by an attitude of *maalesh*.

machismo Sense of masculinity that stresses virility, courage, and domination of women; includes the need to display physical strength, bravery, and virility.

magissa Greek folk healer.

mal ojo Spanish term for the evil eye, a hex condition with unspecific signs and symptoms believed to be caused by an older person admiring a younger person; condition can be reversed if the person doing the admiring touches the person being admired.

marielitos Cuban immigrants who arrived in 1980 on a massive boatlift from Muriel Harbor, Cuba, to Key West, Florida.

masallah Turkish term for God bless and protect.

matiasma Greek term for the evil eye.

Matka Boska Poland's patroness to help in time of need; literally mother of God.

Métis People of mixed Native American and European, especially French Canadian, heritage.

mestizo(a) Person of mixed Spanish and Native American heritage.

mezuzah Container with biblical writings; placed on the doorpost of homes or hung around the neck on a necklace.

mien Vietnamese concept based on wealth and power.

mikveh Jewish term for a ritual bath, after a woman's menstrual period is over.

minyan Ten adults needed for prayer in the Jewish faith.

Mohammed Prophet of God and founder of Islam.

Mohel Ritual circumciser in the Jewish faith.

moreno Portuguese Brazilian individual who has black or brown hair and dark eyes.

morita therapy Indigenous Japanese school of psychotherapy.

Moslem *See* Muslim.

mosque Muslim place of worship.

moxibustion Vietnamese health-care practice in which pulverized wormwood is heated and placed directly on the skin at specified meridians to counter conditions associated with excess cold.

mukrah Arabic term for undesirable but not forbidden.

Mulatto Person of mixed European and African heritage.

mundang Korean folk healer who has special abilities for communicating with the spirits and in treating illnesses after all other means of treatment are exhausted.

muska Turkish tradition of writing a prayer on a piece of paper, wrapping it in fabric, and hiding it in the home or worn by a person seeking help for emotional problems.

Muslim Person who follows the Islamic faith, the world's second largest religion.

N

naharati Iranian term for generalized distress.

Navajo neuropathy Neurological condition confined to Navajo Indians; characterized by a complete absence of myelinated fibers resulting in short stature, sexual infantilism, systemic infection, hypotonia, areflexia, loss of sensation in the extremities, corneal ulcerations, acral mutilation, and painless fractures.

nazar Turkish term for envy.

nazar boncuk Small blue bead used among Turkish people to protect a child from the evil eye.

nervioso(a) Hispanic term used to describe signs and symptoms of nervousness, anxiety, sadness, and grief.

nevra Greek folk illness.

Nihon/Nippon Japanese name for Japan.

Nihonjin Japanese term for a native of Japan.

nisei Japanese term for the second generation of an immigrant family.

Niuyorican Term used to identify the cultural pride of Puerto Rican generations born and reared in New York.

O

obi Sash for a Japanese kimono, or an abdominal binder.

o-cha Japanese term for green tea.

office lady Young woman who works in a Japanese office providing hospitality to visitors and performing limited clerical functions.

o-furo Japanese bath.

Old Order Amish Most conservative and traditionalist group among the followers of Jacob Ammann; today simply called *Amish*, but technically known as *Old Order Amish Mennonite*, to distinguish them from other related Amish and Mennonite groups.

onore della famiglia Italian term for family honor.

oplatek Polish wafer that everyone shares; served at Christmas time.

oppression Haitian ailment related to asthma; describes a state of anxiety and hyperventilation.

ordnung Codified rules and regulations that govern the behavior of a local Amish church district, or congregation; local consensus of faith and practice; also the German term for order.

orishas Gods or spirits in Santería.

Orthodox Traditional Judaism.

o-shogatsu Japanese New Year; celebrated for several days around January 1.

outsider Someone who is not known to members of the group; it is assumed that they do not have the special knowledge regarding the values and beliefs that an insider has.

P

padrone Italian word for master, head of the family.

pakikisama Filipino term for yielding to the leader or the majority.

pakiramdam Filipino term for shared inner feeling with another person.

panikhida Russian Orthodox special prayer vigil over the deceased.

pappous Greek word for grandfather.

Pasah Dai Dialect in southern Thailand.

Pasah Isaan Dialect in northeastern Thailand.

Pasah Nua Dialect in northern Thailand.

pazienza Italian word for patience/long suffering.

person Human being who is constantly adapting to their environment biologically, psychologically, and socially.

personalismo Spanish word for emphasis on intimate, personal relationships as more important than impersonal, bureaucratic relationships.

philptimo Greek term for respect.

phylacto Greek amulet worn to ward off envy.

pidgin Simplified language used for communicating between speakers of different languages.

Pilipino Filipino term for Filipino.

pogrom Organized persecution or massacre of a minority group.

Polonia Communities heavily occupied by Polish immigrants and descendants of Polish Nationals.

postmodernism Holds the stance that everything is social construction, which leads to contention that context is all important.

practika Greek herbal remedies.

primary characteristics of culture Nationality, race, color, gender, age, and religious affiliation.

pseudofamilies Vietnamese households made up of close and distant relatives and friends that share accommodations, finances, and fellowship.

Pu tong hua Recognized language of China.

Q

qi One of five substances or elements of traditional Chinese medicine; encompasses the foundation of the energy of the body, environment, and universe; includes all sources and expenditures of energy.

Quebecer Descendant of early French settlers, now living in Quebec Province, Canada.

Qur'an or Koran Muslim holy book; believed by Muslims to contain God's final revelations to humankind.

R

rabbi Jewish religious leader.

race Having to do with genetic differences such as blood type, skin color, and other physical characteristics.

Ramadan or Ramazan The 9th month of the Islamic year during which Muslims are required to fast during daylight hours for 30 days.

reconstructionism Mosaic of the three main branches of Judaism; is an evolving religion of the Jewish people; seeks to adapt Jewish beliefs and practices to the needs of the contemporary world.

refakatci Turkish term for someone who stays overnight in the hospital with a sick person.

Reform Liberal or Progressive Judaism.

refugee Someone who flees from their home country owing to political, religious, or other type of oppression; host country assigns refugee status.

remedios caserios Portuguese (Brazilian) home medicine or remedy.

remedios populares Portuguese (Brazilian) folk medicine practitioner.

respeto Hispanic term denoting respect; refers to the qualities developed toward others such as parents, the elderly, and educated people who are expected to be honored, admired, and respected.

S

sake Japanese rice wine; used ritually as well as socially.

sand painting Navajo art work originally designed on the hogan floor and then destroyed and returned to the earth; currently, sand paintings are created and sold commercially.

sansei Japanese term for the third generation of an immigrant family.

Santería 300-year-old Afro-Cuban religion that syncretizes Roman Catholic elements with ancient Yoruba tribal beliefs and practices.

santero Practitioner of Santería.

sard Iranian term for cold.

sardie Iranian digestive problem; occurs from eating too much cold food.

secondary characteristics of culture Includes educational status, socioeconomic status, occupation, military experience, political beliefs, urban or rural residence, enclave identity, marital status, parental status, physical characteristics, sexual orientation, gender issues, and reason for migration (sojourner, immigrant, or undocumented status).

Sensei Japanese term for master; used to address teachers, physicians, or those in seniority in a corporate setting.

sephardic Jewish term for being descended from Spain, Portugal, the Mediterranean, Africa, or Central or South America.

severe combined immune deficiency syndrome Immune deficiency syndrome (unrelated to AIDS), characterized by a failure of antibody response and cell-mediated immunity.

shanty Irish Term for Irish who lived in urban Irish ethnic enclaves.

shiatsu Japanese term for acupressure therapy.

Shinto Indigenous religion of Japan.

sikkeenah Egyptian term for knife.

simpatia Spanish term for smooth interpersonal relationships; characterized by courtesy, respect, and the absence of harsh criticism or confrontation.

sit a spell Process of engaging in nonhierarchical relaxed conversation in order to get to know the beliefs and feelings of others.

Small Eid Islamic holy feast of 3 days.

sobador Spanish folk practitioner, similar to a chiropractor, who treats illnesses and conditions affecting the joints and musculoskeletal system.

sojourner Someone who relocates with the intention of remaining only a short time and then returning home.

Solidarity Union of interests, purposes, and sympathies promoting fellowship with Polish nationals.

Som-tum Spicy Thai salad.

soul food Traditional diet of African Americans.

Spanglish Sentence structure that includes both English and Spanish words.

speaking in tongues Praying in a language that is not understood by anyone except the person reciting the prayer.

stereotyping Oversimplified conception, opinion, or belief about some aspect of an individual or group of people.

sto lat Polish phrase meaning that the celebrant should live a hundred years.

subculture Group of people who have had experiences different from those of the dominant culture in status, ethnic background, residence, religion, education, or other factors that functionally unify the group and act collectively on one another.

susto "Magical fright," a condition believed to be caused by witchcraft; symptoms can be quite varied and include both mental and physical concerns.

synagogue Jewish house of worship.

T

ta'arof Iranian ritual expressing courtesy.

tae kyo Korean term, literally fetus education, with the objective being health and well-being of fetus and mother through art, beautiful objects, and a serene environment.

tae mong Korean term signifying the beginning of pregnancy; the pregnant woman dreams of conception of the fetus.

Tagalog Filipino national language.

Taglish Dialect mixing English and Tagalog.

tatami Traditional Japanese floor coverings made of straw.

Tet Asian Lunar New Year; celebrated in January or February.

Torah Five books of Moses; referred to in the Jewish faith.

treyf Jewish term for forbidden or unclean.

tribe Native American social organization comprising several local villages, bands, districts, lineages, or other groups who share a common ancestry, language, and culture.

Tridosha Theory that the body is made up of five elements: fire, air, space, water, and earth.

Turkiye Turkish word for the country Turkey.

U

universal ethics Belief that each culture decides what is right or wrong and what is good or bad.

utang na loob Filipino term for gratitude.

V

values Principles and standards that are important and have meaning and worth to an individual, family, group, or community.

velorio Spanish term for a wake; a festive occasion following the burial of a person.

vendouses Greek practice of cupping.

verguenza Spanish term for a consciousness of public opinion and the judgment of the entire community.

via nuova Italian word for new way.

via vecchia Italian word for old way.

viandas Spanish term for root vegetables.

visiting High-frequency custom of family-to-family home visits that help to maintain kinship and church ties and the flow of information within the Amish community.

voudou or voodoo Vibrant religion born from slavery and revolt; the term means sacred in the African language of Fon.

W

waham Egyptian term for cravings during pregnancy.

wake Watch over a deceased person before burial; usually accompanied by a celebration, which may include feasting.

warm hands Healing art related to therapeutic touch; regarded by Amish as a gift to be applied for the good of others in need of healing; a form of *brauche*.

Western ethics Beliefs that are held by individualistic societies can be applied to all cultural groups.

wetback Derogatory term applied to undocumented aliens of Mexican or Latin American descent.

wind Classification for Vietnamese foods that is closely related to cold foods.

worldview Way an individual or group of people look upon their universe to form values about their life and the world around them.

Y

yang In Chinese belief system, one of two opposing principles of the balance of life; can be either a single phenomenon or a state of being of a phenomenon. *See yin.*

yangban Korean term for upper class.

yarmulke Jewish head covering.

yerbero *See jerbero.*

Yiddish Language often spoken by elderly Jews.

yin In Chinese belief system, one of two opposing principles of the balance of life; can be either a single phenomenon or a state of being of a phenomenon. *See yang.*

Z

zaher Iranian term for public persona.

zar Egyptian transmeditative ceremony.

zong Vietnamese herbal preparation; relieves motion sickness or cold-related problems.

Index

Note: Page numbers followed by f refer to figures; those followed by t refer to tables.